Cognition and Acquired Language Disorders

An Information Processing Approach

Richard K. Peach, PhD
Professor
Department of Communication Disorders and Sciences
College of Health Sciences
Rush University
Chicago, Illinois

Lewis P. Shapiro, PhD
Professor
School of Speech, Language, and Hearing Sciences
College of Health and Human Services
San Diego State University
San Diego, California

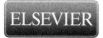

ELSEVIER
MOSBY

3251 Riverport Lane
St. Louis, Missouri 63043

Vice President and Publisher: Linda Duncan
Executive Editor: Kathy Falk
Managing Editor: Jolynn Gower
Publishing Services Manager: Julie Eddy
Project Manager: Jan Waters
Design Direction: Karen Pauls

Working together to grow
libraries in developing countries

www.elsevier.com | www.bookaid.org | www.sabre.org

ELSEVIER | BOOK AID International | Sabre Foundation

Printed in the United States of America

Last digit is the print number: 9 8 7 6 5 4 3 2 1

Dedication

To Patti and Kevin
For reminding me every day what's important
Richard

To Mitzi, Joelle, and Dillon
My candles in the dark
Lew

CONTRIBUTORS

Alfredo Ardila, PhD, ABPN
Professor
Department of Communication Sciences
   and Disorders
Florida International University
Miami, Florida

Kathleen Brumm, PhD pending
SDSU/UCSD Joint Doctoral Program
School of Speech, Language, and Hearing
   Sciences
San Diego State University
San Diego, California

Michael Cannizzaro, PhD, CCC-SLP
Assistant Professor
Graduate Program Coordinator
Department of Communication Sciences
   and Disorders
The University of Vermont
Burlington, Vermont

Thomas H. Carr, PhD, MS
Professor
Department of Psychology
Michigan State University
East Lansing, Michigan

Carl Coelho, PhD
Professor and Department Head
Communication Sciences Department
University of Connecticut
Storrs, Connecticut

Matthew L. Cohen, MS
Department of Clinical & Health
   Psychology
College of Public Health and Health
   Professions
University of Florida
Gainesville, Florida

Bruce Crosson, PhD
Department of Veterans Affairs
   Brain Rehabilitation Research Center of
   Excellence
Malcolm Randall VA Medical Center
Department of Clinical & Health Psychology
College of Public Health and Health Professions
University of Florida
Gainesville, Florida

G. Albyn Davis, PhD
Communicative Sciences and Disorders
New York University
New York, New York

Argye E. Hillis, MD, MA
Executive Vice Chair and Professor
Co-director, Cerebrovascular Division
Department of Neurology
School of Medicine
Johns Hopkins University
Baltimore, Maryland

Jacqueline J. Hinckley, PhD, CCC-SLP
Associate Professor Emeritus
Department of Communication Sciences
   and Disorders
University of South Florida
Tampa, Florida

Susan Kemper, PhD
Roberts Distinguished Professor
Department of Psychology
University of Kansas
Lawrence, Kansas

Swathi Kiran, PhD, CCC-SLP
Associate Professor
Speech Language and Hearing Sciences
Sargent College of Health & Rehabilitation
   Sciences
Boston University
Assistant in Neurology
Massachusetts General Hospital
Boston, Massachusetts

Tracy Love, PhD
Professor
School of Speech, Language, and Hearing
   Sciences
San Diego State University
Center for Research in Language
University of California, San Diego
San Diego, California

Nadine Martin, PhD, CCC-SLP
Professor
Department of Communication Sciences
   and Disorders
College of Health Professions and Social Work
Temple University
Philadelphia, Pennsylvania

Randi Martin, PhD, MS
Elma Schneider Professor
Department of Psychology
Rice University
Houston, Texas

Richard K. Peach, PhD
Professor
Department of Communication Disorders
   and Sciences
College of Health Sciences
Rush University
Chicago, Illinois

Josée Poirier, PhD
Research Scientist
Language Processes Laboratory
School of Speech, Language, and Hearing
   Sciences
San Diego State University
San Diego, California

Liana S. Rosenthal, MD
Department of Neurology
School of Medicine
Johns Hopkins University
Baltimore, Maryland

Chaleece Sandberg, PhD Student
Speech Language and Hearing Sciences
Sargent College of Health & Rehabilitation
   Sciences
Boston University
Boston, Massachusetts

Lewis P. Shapiro, PhD
Professor
School of Speech, Language, and Hearing
   Sciences
College of Health and Human Services
San Diego State University
San Diego, California

L. Robert Slevc, PhD
Assistant Professor
Department of Psychology
Program in Neuroscience and Cognitive Science
University of Maryland
College Park, Maryland

Leanne Togher, B App Sc (Speech Path), PhD
NHMRC Senior Research Fellow
Associate Professor
Discipline of Speech Pathology
The University of Sydney
Sydney, Australia

Julie A. Van Dyke, MSc, PhD
Senior Research Scientist
Haskins Laboratories
New Haven, Connecticut

Clinical practice associated with acquired language disorders has evolved in important ways in the past 30 years as a result of advances in our understanding of the cognition of language. In 1982, the Committee on Language of the American Speech-Language-Hearing Association (ASHA) defined language as a rule-governed behavior that can be described by at least five parameters—phonological, morphological, syntactic, semantic, and pragmatic—for which "learning and use are determined by the interaction of biological, cognitive, psychosocial, and environmental factors" (ASHA, 1983). The separation of language and cognition in this definition was reinforced in a subsequent report by a subgroup of the same committee (the Subcommittee on Language and Cognition) to address the roles of the speech-language pathologist in the habilitation and rehabilitation of cognitively impaired individuals (ASHA, 1987). In that report, cognition was described, using Neisser's (1967) definition, as "the processes by which sensory input is transformed, reduced, elaborated, stored, recovered, and used" and was considered separately from language. In portraying "cognitive-language relationships," the report went on to list the "specific cognitive impairments that may affect language" by contributing "to deficits in the semantic, syntactic, phonologic, and/or pragmatic aspects of language." The independence of the communication problems arising from these "cognitive" deficits from other types of language disorders was emphasized and thus gave rise to the category of so-called *cognitive-communication impairments*. Cognitive-communication impairments were defined as "communicative disorders that result from deficits in linguistic and nonlinguistic cognitive processes" (p. 54). The distinction between cognitive-communication and language disorders was further highlighted in the scope of practice for speech-language pathology (ASHA, 1990) with statements partitioning the practice for language versus cognitive-communication disorders. These distinctions continue to be upheld in more recent updates of these clinical practice documents (ASHA, 2003, 2005, 2007). The descriptor *cognitive-communication impairments* has evolved in some quarters into the even more problematic term *cognitive-linguistic deficits*.

These approaches suggest, as Davis (this volume) explains, "that cognition *plays a role* in language and communication, or that it is *related to* language and communication, as if 'language' and 'cognition' are different things." They are not. Language is part of cognition, part of our higher mental processes. The study of human language provides a unique way to understand human nature, to do cognitive science, to dig deep into the science of mental life (Boeckx, 2010). This is the goal of psycholinguistics, the study of the mental processes and types of knowledge involved in understanding and producing language in both its oral and written forms. Psycholinguistics examines "listening, speaking, reading, and writing, trying to discover the cognitive machinery and knowledge structures that underlie these skills and what role they play in linguistic behavior" (De Groot, 2011, p. 2).

In the case of language, impairments to such intrinsic cognitive processes, whether they are attentional, memorial, linguistic, or executive, can produce language disorders. Breakdowns are not ones of processes that "interact" with language abilities. Rather, such breakdowns occur in processes that are fundamental to language itself. For this reason, we use the term *acquired language disorders* in this text in lieu of the less desirable but well-entrenched term *cognitive-communication impairments* to emphasize the unity of cognition and language. From a cognitive neuropsychological perspective, acquired language disorders are but one example of the larger class of cognitive disorders (Lezak, Howieson, & Loring, 2004; Rapp, 2002). Identification of the processing impairments that contribute to different types of acquired language disorders provides a basis for informed approaches to language intervention and rehabilitation.

Cognition and Acquired Language Disorders is designed to be used as a primary textbook in graduate courses addressing the cognitive aspects of communication. Information is assembled in a consistent framework composed of (1) normal cognitive processing for language in adults, (2) the cognitive impairments underlying language disorders arising from a variety of neurological conditions, and (3) current assessment and treatment strategies for the management of these disorders. The text is organized using an information processing approach to acquired language disorders and thus can be set apart from more traditional syndrome-based approaches (e.g., stroke, dementia, and traumatic brain injury). In syndrome-based approaches, numerous neurological conditions that produce acquired language disorders (e.g., tumor, infection, degenerative diseases, and multiple strokes) are often ignored. In the current processing approach, the language disorders that result from a variety of neurological conditions are treated as being more similar than the specific etiologies themselves. As just one example, working memory and attention are considered "domain-general" operations that are disrupted in several types of disordered populations. Similarly, the processing approach allows for the descriptions and treatments to be applied across multiple neurological groups who share specific cognitive deficits.

The chapters of this text describe how attentional, memorial, linguistic, and executive processes coalesce in language functioning. The language characteristics of individuals presenting with a variety of neurological conditions that impair these processes are also addressed, as well as the assessment and treatment of the resulting language disorders with reference to the specific types of underlying impairments. The intent is to provide an advanced discussion of this material for both graduate coursework in speech-language pathology and clinical neuropsychology and to offer a reference for practicing clinicians in these disciplines.

The text is divided into four sections. The first section provides an overview of cognition and language, as well as tutorials describing the effects of aging on normal language processing and the neurological conditions that are associated with acquired language disorders. The second section provides an in-depth discussion of normal processing for attention, memory, language, and executive functioning and serves as a foundation for the subsequent discussion of language disorders. The third section examines the cognition of acquired language disorders, and the fourth section provides guidance for the clinical management of these disorders. Assessment and treatment protocols that are provided are based on a review of current evidence so that students and clinicians will have a ready clinical resource for managing language disorders due to deficits in attention, memory, linguistic operations, and executive functions.

Following the introductory material, the text provides three chapters—one on normal processing, one on disorder characteristics, and one on clinical approaches—for each of the cognitive domains associated with language functioning and acquired language disorders. Although each of the chapters of this text can be studied independently of the others, the structure of the text is designed to encourage instructors to complete the readings for normal processing across all cognitive domains before proceeding to discussions of their applied counterparts (i.e., disorders and interventions). This approach allows readers to fully appreciate the relations among cognitive domains (e.g., attention and working memory, working memory, and the central executive) before proceeding to discussions of deficits within these domains in acquired language disorders due to neurological impairments.

We want to express our thanks to the authors, all experts in their chosen areas, for agreeing to contribute their work to this text. We are confident that the breadth, depth, and overall excellence of their work will make this the most authoritative source available regarding cognition and acquired language disorders. Finally, we would like to thank Jolynn Gower, our managing editor at Elsevier, for providing outstanding support and guidance for the development of this text. We hope that you will find it to be a helpful resource for the clinical management of acquired language disorders.

RKP

LPS

REFERENCES

American Speech-Language-Hearing Association. (1983). Committee on Language: Definition of language. *Asha, 24,* 44.

American Speech-Language-Hearing Association. (1987). The role of speech-language pathologists in the habilitation and rehabilitation of cognitively impaired individuals: A report of the subcommittee on language and cognition. *Asha, 29,* 53–55.

American Speech-Language-Hearing Association. (1990). Scope of practice, speech-language pathology and audiology. *Asha, 32* (Suppl. 2), 1–2.

American Speech-Language-Hearing Association. (2003). *Evaluating and treating communication and cognitive disorders: Approaches to referral and collaboration for speech-language pathology and clinical neuropsychology* [Technical Report]. Available from www.asha.org/policy.

American Speech-Language-Hearing Association. (2005). *Roles of speech-language pathologists in the identification, diagnosis, and treatment of individuals with cognitive-communication disorders: Position Statement* [Position Statement]. Available from www.asha.org/policy.

American Speech-Language-Hearing Association. (2007). *Scope of practice in speech-language pathology* [Scope of Practice]. Available from www.asha.org/policy.

Boeckx, C. (2010). *Language in cognition: Uncovering mental structures and the rules behind them.* Chichester, West Sussex, UK: Wiley-Blackwell.

Davis, G. A. (2012). The cognition of language and communication. In R. K. Peach & L. P. Shapiro (Eds.), *Cognition and acquired language disorders* (p. 1). St. Louis: Elsevier Mosby.

De Groot, M. B. A. (2011). *Language and cognition in bilinguals and multilinguals: An introduction.* New York: Psychology Press.

Lezak, M. D., Howieson, D. B., & Loring, D. W. (2004). *Neuropsychological assessment* (4th ed.). New York: Oxford University Press.

Neisser, U. (1967). *Cognitive psychology.* New York: Appleton, Century, Cross.

Rapp, B. (2002). *The handbook of cognitive neuropsychology: What deficits reveal about the human mind.* Philadelphia: Psychology Press.

CONTENTS

CHAPTER 1

The Cognition of Language and Communication

CHAPTER OUTLINE

G. Albyn Davis

For a long time, *language* has had a curious relationship to *cognition* in the vocabularies of rehabilitation practitioners, as well as laypersons. Diagnosticians have neatly divided and packaged disorders into separate categories. "Language" has been viewed descriptively with assistance from linguistics (e.g., phonology, morphology, syntax), whereas "cognition" has been identified broadly with "intelligence" and specifically with mental functions such as attention, perception, and memory. In some quarters, morphology and memory have been considered to be two separate entities, despite the reality that we store morphology in our memory. To assess memory, we use tests of cognition; to assess morphology, we use tests for aphasia.

It has been suggested that cognition *plays a role* in language and communication or that it is *related to* language and communication, as if "language" and "cognition" are different things. However, if cognition is identified with information processing and we think of language use as information processing, then it is consistent to think of language functions as embedded in cognition. Language comprehension and formulation are part of the cognitive system. When linguists characterize what we know about language, they are speaking of something in memory.

This first chapter introduces cognition and how it is studied, mainly in cognitive psychology. For the study of language processes, psycholinguists and many speech-language pathologists use the methods to be discussed. Then, the chapter provides an orientation to later topics of attention, memory, executive function, and language. Subsequent chapters will be more specific and expansive as to how cognition fuels language comprehension, formulation, and communication. Mainly, the present chapter sets up the thinking behind the investigation of cognition.

ASSUMPTIONS IN THE STUDY OF COGNITION

Cognition is "an umbrella term for all higher mental processes . . . the collection of mental processes and activities used in perceiving, remembering, thinking, and understanding" (Ashcraft & Radvansky, 2010, p. 9). In contemplating their history, "cognitive psychologists generally agree that the birth of cognitive psychology should be listed as 1956" (Matlin, 2009, p. 7). Around this time, key publications and conferences steered psychology away from behaviorism. This change was driven by the Skinner-Chomsky debate over nurture versus nature, George Miller's measure of short-term memory as being around seven units, and interest at Carnegie-Mellon University in the computer as an analogy for human information processing. The shift was complete when the *Journal of Verbal Learning and Verbal Behavior* became the *Journal of Memory and Language* in the early 1980s. Essentially, psychologists admitted that mental processes exist.

This section introduces three of four assumptions underlying the study of mental processes. They are presented as a hierarchy of dichotomies in Figure 1-1. First, *there is a working distinction between behavior (as evidence) and what happens in our heads (as theory).* Similarly for clinical diagnosis, we consider the relationship of what we can observe (symptoms) to what we cannot observe (diagnosed impairment). Scientists avoid writing statements like "comprehension is a behavior" so that they do not think carelessly and confuse one for the other.

Now that we are thinking inside the box, *the second assumption differentiates the brain as a material thing from cognition as a mental thing.* Because cognition is what the brain does and, therefore, is not truly independent of the brain, this dualism is largely a contrivance that is reflective of a research strategy. Cognitive psychologists approached their work *as if* "the mind can be studied independently from the brain" (Johnson-Laird, 1983). Through the 1980s, cognitive psychology texts barely mentioned the brain. At that time, Flanagan (1984) stated that cognitive psychologists "by and large, simply seem not to worry about the mind-brain problem."

This dualistic approach was necessary, because technology for observing the brain (e.g., fuzzy structural imaging) was not matching the constructs for measurement of mental operations. Now, with the emerging fine-tuned technologies of functional neuroscience (Cabeza & Kingstone, 2006; Gazzaniga, Ivry, & Mangun, 2008), current editions of texts on cognition include chapters on the brain and sometimes are regaled with colorful pictures from brain imaging (e.g., Ashcraft & Radvansky, 2010). Nevertheless, one can conduct experimental cognitive psychology without considering the brain and, as a result, can restrict theory to functional matters (e.g., how memory works, as opposed to how the brain works).

In our everyday vocabularies, "brain" and "mind" often refer to the same thing. Yet, saying that someone has "lost his mind" does not mean that he has misplaced his brain (Box 1-1).

In his text for speech-language pathologists, Davis (2007a) encouraged clear thinking by recommending that we keep what happens to the brain (e.g., stroke, trauma) logically distinct from what happens to cognition (e.g., aphasia, amnesia). We can say that stroke causes aphasia (not that aphasia causes stroke). Neurosurgeons treat the brain, speech-language pathologists treat cognition, and so on. Whether cognitive-language therapy re-wires the brain is a current question. At least, to understand the nature of aphasia, we should have some idea of what happens to cognition.

Putting aside the brain, the third assumption focuses on cognition. *Cognition consists of a fairly stable knowledge base and fleeting processes.* This distinction was helpful when clinical pioneer Hildred Schuell proclaimed that what we do about aphasia depends on what we think aphasia is (Sies, 1974). A frequent question has been whether aphasia is an erasure of language knowledge or a disruption of language processing (while knowledge remains intact). The answer informs the broad approach to therapy, namely, whether it involves teaching words anew (because of a "loss" of

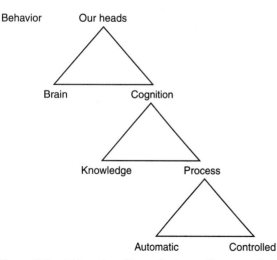

Figure 1-1   A hierarchy of increasingly specific assumptions underlying the study of cognition.

Box 1-1

Dialogue from a 1988 Episode of *Miami Vice*

Interrogator: What about the fact that he can't remember any of his actions? Isn't that a convenient lapse of memory?

Physician: The answer to your question is that I'm a neurosurgeon. You're questioning Detective Crockett's mental capacities. That determination should be made by a psychiatrist.

knowledge) or exercising an impaired mental process that accesses a healthy store of vocabulary. Despite a layperson's inclination to define *aphasia* as a "loss" of language, Schuell's (1969) clinical experience led her to believe that "the language storage system is at least relatively intact" (p. 336). This belief, now supported by research, led her to advocate a "stimulation" approach to therapy.

APPROACHES TO THE STUDY OF COGNITION

Just as archaeologists build models of Troy based on analysis of unearthed floors and walls, cognitive scientists construct the most likely "functional architecture" of the mind from hundreds of carefully crafted experiments. Theoretical models are helpful in characterizing phenomena that are too big, too small, too old, or too obscure to be observed in everyday experience or "with the naked eye" (Davis, 1994). A layperson's idea of "theory" can be heard in putdowns such as "it's only a theory," as if to say that such an explanation is *only a guess*. A scientific theory, however, is a collection of coordinated hypotheses built from appropriate evidence (Stanovich, 2007). Appropriate evidence of global climate change, for example, would be long-term worldwide temperature trends, as opposed to looking out the window (Box 1-2).

Clinical research sometimes entails collecting data and then exploring theoretical possibilities regarding the cause of observed behavior, called *post hoc* analysis. Theory-motivated clinical research, on the other hand, tends to lean on an established theory before an experiment is conducted. A useful theory, *a priori*, leads to a valid method and some predictions (i.e., "appropriate evidence"). The theory should be so clearly related to the experimental task that predictions of performance would logically and transparently follow from the theory. An investigator may think through what a person must do mentally to perform the task. Another approach, unfortunately, is to choose an established task created for other reasons (e.g., from a clinical test) without considering what a participant must do cognitively to carry out the task. A journal peer review may challenge an investigator to explain how a task demonstrates operation of the process purported to be studied. This disciplined and collaborative strategy maximizes the likelihood that a theoretical explanation is the correct one.

Any experiment consists of at least one comparison, either between groups of participants or between conditions. In clinical research, a study often contains both types of comparison. Differences between conditions are often labeled as special "effects," such as the word frequency effect, the semantic priming effect, or the garden path effect. For example, a task with common words usually has fewer errors than a task with rare words. A theory of accessing the lexicon may predict this word frequency effect and then provide an explanation for why it does or does not occur.

A fundamental tenet is that a theory should be *falsifiable*, meaning that "in telling us what *should* happen, the theory must also imply that certain things will *not* happen. If these latter things *do* happen, then we have a clear signal that something is wrong with the theory" (Stanovich, 2007, p. 20). A common type of nonfalsifiable theory is one that is so general that it can explain anything (see Shuster, 2004). Explanations that are hard to test, such as appealing to motivations, are also difficult to falsify. Several comparisons should produce a pattern of results consistent with a theory, and the comparisons should also allow for the possibility of other patterns that could be suggestive of another theory. What follows are some of the basic approaches to making these comparisons in cognitive science.

A classic approach to experimentation is called *mental chronometry* or *additive/subtractive methodology*. Inspired by research to determine the speed of neural impulses, Franciscus Donders, a Dutch physician in the 1800s, used a subtraction method to measure the speed of mental operations in simple responses to lights. The experiment was a comparison between similar tasks. The general idea was that when one task takes longer, the difference in time is a measure of the operation that made the task take longer. In the 1960s, Sternberg (1975) worried that two tasks could differ in more than one way, spoiling theoretical interpretation. His solution, in order to study short-term memory scanning, included the comparison of several conditions differing in one respect (i.e., additive method).

Box 1-2

What Is Appropriate Evidence?

Appropriate evidence is that which can be logically identified with or related to the mystery being studied. A National Geographic Network series about the science of migrations noted that we have not known what elephant seals do in the ocean for 10 months of the year. Our only data were based on watching them dive in. Speculation turned into scientific theory when data arrived in the form of tracking sensors attached to the seals as they swim, like electrodes on the skull to track neural activity hidden in the brain.

While mental chronometry was paving the way for disciplined study of human participants, the computer metaphor for the human mind encouraged studies of *computational modeling or simulation* (based on "connectionist models"). Implying a comparison to human beings, research consists of "programming computers to model or mimic some aspects of human cognitive functioning" (Eysenck, 2006). Applying simulation to clinical populations, some investigators would artificially lesion a program to mimic a disorder (Dell & Kittredge, 2011). Wilshire (2008) made note of one strength in the simulation approach that is favored by cognitive theorists in general, namely, theoretical parsimony, or explaining the widest range of observations with the fewest assumptions.

A third approach is *cognitive neuropsychology*, in which brain-injured subjects are studied to test theories of cognition. Viewed broadly, this discipline can be any study of cognition involving brain-damaged people that has the goal of understanding normal function as well as dysfunction. In one branch of this field, "CN" focuses on single cases as examples of a lesion that hypothetically knocks out one component of a processing model underlying a simple task (Rapp, 2001; Whitworth, Webster, & Howard, 2005). A typical model of reading aloud given in Figure 1-2 provides a menu of possible impaired components. Although proponents of CN speak of testing theories of language in general, their research is restricted to single words. This narrow window on language and the absence of an automatic-controlled processing distinction were a concern for Wilshire (2008; also, Davis, 1989). She noted that computer simulation has an additional advantage of explaining how and the extent to which a cognitive component may be malfunctioning.

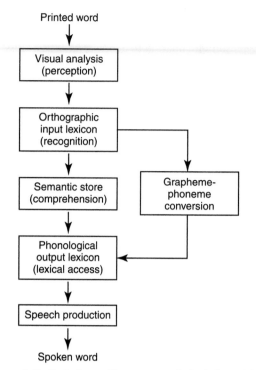

Figure 1-2 Typical cognitive neuropsychological model of stages in reading words aloud. Functional equivalents are noted in parentheses. [From Davis, G. A. (2007). *Aphasiology: Disorders and clinical practice* (2nd ed.). Boston: Allyn & Bacon/Longman.]

ATTENTION

We must be aroused or alert (i.e., conscious) for intentional communication to occur and, once aroused, we establish awareness of our surroundings so that simple communication makes sense. This is the base level of attention. Then, when faced with multiple simultaneous stimuli in a conversation, we focus on something for in-depth processing. Inability to ignore irrelevant inputs can be an impediment to successful communication (i.e., the "cocktail party problem").

"We use the term *attention* to describe a huge range of phenomena" (Ashcraft & Radvansky, 2010, p. 112). It is commonly considered to be a cognitive process that concentrates mental effort on an external stimulus or an internal representation or thought. Attending to external stimuli may be called "input attention," which

is the basic mechanism for selecting sensory information for cognitive processing. Input-directed attention includes an *orienting reflex* that directs us toward an unexpected stimulus and *attention capture*, which is driven by physical characteristics, namely, significance, novelty, and social cues.

Higher-level attention consists of different mechanisms. *Selective attention* (i.e., focusing) goes along with resisting distraction so that cognition becomes manageable. Another term, "spotlight attention," is used for a focusing mechanism that prepares the processor to deal with information based on expectations. Selective attention is studied by presenting two stimuli and requiring response to one of them. *Divided attention* confronts multiple stimuli or processes at the same time. A dual task is used whereby a participant responds to two stimuli or performs two tasks simultaneously. A researcher is interested in the effect of dealing with one stimulus or task on the other. Discussions of attention mechanisms overlap with other aspects of cognition in that they contribute to resource allocation in working memory and the management of multiple tasks associated with executive function.

MEMORY

Ashcraft (1989) wrote that cognition is "the coordinated operation of active mental processes within a multicomponent memory system" (p. 39). A simple definition of *memory* is any retention of information in the mind beyond the life of an external stimulus (i.e., minimal memory). The ability to hold information in our head is fundamental to the mind's (or brain's) ability to perform even the simplest functions such as perception and recognition. Following the knowledge-process distinction mentioned earlier, the major components of the memory system consist of long-term memory (LTM) for passive storage of information and working memory (WM) for constraining the activity of processing.

Before these components are introduced, let us consider two questions that apply to both components of memory. How does information become represented in our heads, and what form does it take? This inner form is called a **mental representation,** which occurs either in permanent storage or in a transient state. A theory of *neural* representation can appeal to tissues and chemicals. Characterizing a memory in *mental* terms is more problematic. Resorting to analogy, we may think that a mental representation for a visual input might replicate the stimulus, like a photograph. An auditory stimulus may be replicated like a tape (or digital) recording. Testable hypotheses about mental representation are included in the collection of hypotheses comprising a theory of a language function.

Long-Term Memory

A library is a common analogy for characterizing our LTM system. A library acquires books, stores them, and has procedures for access and retrieval (i.e., input-storage-output). Like a library, LTM contains different types of information. Knowledge may have a verbal representation like novels and a photographic representation like picture books. Tulving (1972) proposed the following types of knowledge:

- **Episodic memory** for individually experienced events *(autobiographical memory)*
- **Semantic memory** for general conceptual knowledge of the world
- **Lexical memory** for word forms and information about words
- **Procedural memory** for skills like swinging a golf club

Aphasiologists take particular note of the separate stores for words and world knowledge. The concept of trees may be a universal element of semantic memory, but the word for it varies from language to language and is stored in lexical memory. An aphasic person knows what he or she wants to convey but just cannot access the words. In general, the validity of these LTM stores is supported by many case studies showing that neuropathologies can impair access to one type of memory but not others (Schacter, 1996).

Because we are most interested in language, let us focus on semantic memory. Its core is universal in the sense that most people have the same basic knowledge of objects and actions, living and nonliving things. Fringes of world knowledge vary according to locale, culture, or expertise. Semantic memory is central to comprehension and the meaningful use of words. In fact, it can be said that semantic memory contains word meanings. The simplest unit of semantic memory is a *concept,* which may be defined as the representation of a class of objects or actions. Although concepts are stored separately from words, the two stores are intimately connected (Box 1-3).

Organization is important for storage and access in a library so that we do not wander around all day looking for a particular book. In this way, static structure influences dynamic action. There have been different theories of semantic memory structure (i.e., feature lists, hierarchies). The prevailing view is that it takes the form of a *semantic network*. In the spatial metaphor used to characterize the network, a concept is represented as a *node* connected to other nodes (Figure 1-3). Related concepts are close together like "neighbors," and less-related concepts are more distant denizens of other neighborhoods. As a mental reaction to a stimulus, a node activates and then, like in a web of neurons, this activation spreads to nearby nodes. Relative "distances" between concepts are among the collection of hypotheses leading to predictions of processing times (Collins & Loftus, 1975). We may imagine that the semantic

Box 1-3

Separate but Connected

There are various anecdotal supports for the connected but separate relationship between semantic memory and lexical memory. The word *web* has been stored in the lexicon for a long time, linked to conceptual areas of spiders and intrigue. Then, not too long ago, the new concept of the Internet was connected to the old word *web*. Conversely, the concept of headgear is shared universally but linked to different lexical forms (i.e., chapeau, sombrero, hat). Expanding our vocabularies involves linking a new word form to an old idea or linking a new idea to an old word form. Sometimes both are new like *prebituary, slackonomics,* or maybe *refudiate.*

network characterizes the contents of the semantic store in the reading model of Figure 1-3.

Vague proposals for the impairment of LTM have recently been supplemented with more specific or refined proposals. Investigators have contemplated different kinds of damage by referring to a total or partial disappearance of information or a degradation of information. A suggestion of "graceful degradation" in Alzheimer's dementia stands for "gradual loss of connections between features and the concepts which they represent, mirroring the likely neurodegenerative effect of AD" (Almor, Aronoff, MacDonald, et al., 2009, p. 9).

Working Memory

The encroaching dementia of old age seems to bypass memory for the past (i.e., LTM) and assault memory for the present. A memory for the present holds onto representations of current input or what just happened

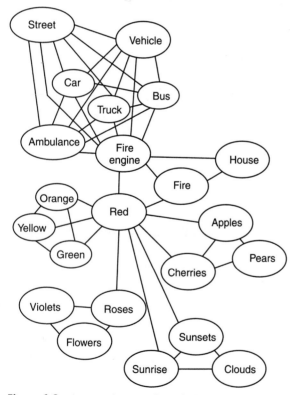

Figure 1-3 A semantic network in which concepts are identified by words. Distances are indicative of relatedness between concepts. [From Collins, A. M., & Loftus, E. F. (1975). A spreading-activation theory of semantic processing. *Psychological Review*, 82, 412. American Psychology Association, publisher.]

(i.e., the preceding phrase or sentence in what you are reading). Initially called short-term memory (STM), it has a limited capacity for transient representations. Information in STM either decays or, more likely, is pushed out by the relentless tide of incoming stimulation (i.e., interference). Digit span tests became a staple for cognitive research and clinical assessment. "In the field of intelligence testing, it is almost unthinkable to devise a test *without* a memory-span component" (Ashcraft & Radvansky, 2010, p. 148).

Baddeley (2004) tells a story of his early memory research in the 1970s. "One lunchtime, over coffee, we began to discuss some of our misgivings about the general field of short-term memory at the time" (p. 41). Transient memory constraints have as much to do with the capacity for doing work as they do for storing content. Baddeley and colleagues considered that the notion of "STM" should be expanded to become a *working memory* (WM) or "work space" for any cognitive activity (Baddeley, Eysenck, & Anderson, 2009). STM, now called a buffer, is one component of WM. The memory span test merely tells us the amount of a stimulus that can be represented in the buffer. It does not tell us about the capacity for simultaneous processes such as scanning buffered input and activating stored concepts.

Considering that WM capacity is limited, a fundamental challenge for cognition is its management of inputs from the environment and from LTM. Here is where theories of divided attention and WM resources overlap. Both domains are pertinent for the public concern with *multitasking* (e.g., texting while driving). In his chapter on multitasking, Eysenck (2006) noted that "we believe ourselves capable of performing two tasks at once . . . because we think it will save us precious time compared to the traditional approach of doing one thing at a time" (p. 127). At Stanford University recently, researchers compared frequent multitaskers to infrequent multitaskers with several experimental tasks and surprisingly found that the frequent multitaskers did worse in several respects, especially in failing to filter out irrelevant information (Box 1-4) (Gorlick, 2009).

Information Processing in Working Memory

A cognitive process, like activation of the semantic network mentioned previously, can be a quick mental response to a stimulus. It is the "light bulb turning on." In fact, the metaphors of activating lights and churning gears are presented on the cover of Ashcraft and Radvansky's (2010) text on cognition. Processes are temporal, and measuring their duration is the basis for the chronometric approach introduced earlier. The lights act quickly, and the gears can churn slowly. As indicated in Figure 1-1, *processing may be automatic, or it may be controlled.*

Box 1-4

Divided Attention

In the novel *Deaf Sentence* by the humorist David Lodge, the narrator is a retired linguistics professor who is hard-of-hearing. Watching television is a multitasking problem: " . . . when I watch using headphones and subtitles together I hear spoken words and phrases which are missing from the subtitles, which I'm sure I would not have heard using the headphones alone. Presumably my brain is continuously checking the two channels of communication against each other. . . . It might be worth writing up for a psycholinguistics journal if I could be bothered. But I can't" (Lodge, 2008, pp. 36–37).

Presented with a stimulus, the brain reacts without our conscious control. What cognitive functions are served by this reaction? The blink of activation, "without thinking," is commonly referred to as **automatic processing.** It has the following characteristics:

- It is subconscious (unconscious) or beneath our awareness
- It is obligatory (i.e., mandatory)
- It takes up little or no room in WM

In a book about visual processing called *The First Half Second* (Ögmen & Breitmeyer, 2006), the authors noted that "a considerable level of behaviorally relevant information processing occurs at unconscious levels" (p. ix) . . . "rich representations must be modified or newly constructed by the visual system in a period of time lasting from 250 to 500 ms" (p. 1). Scientists program computers to present so-called *fast tasks,* putting a few milliseconds between stimuli and measuring the duration of quick responses. Intuitions or self-reports can be misleading for discovering what happens automatically, and a fast task sometimes yields a "counterintuitive" result.

Rehabilitation specialists are more experienced with assessment involving **controlled processing,** which has the following features:

- It can be conscious or in our awareness
- It can be intentional and, therefore, optional
- It is effortful and takes up room in WM

Also known as *strategic processing,* controlled processing is studied with *slow tasks* that allow enough time for conscious decision-making or planning to occur. Unlike automatic processes, strategic processes clog WM. When a patient scans picture-choices in a clinical comprehension task, there is time for all sorts of conscious processing to occur. Language processes become particularly effortful in "metalinguistic" tasks, such as editing a manuscript or contemplating the coherence of a meandering lecture. One cannot "tag" (like the elephant seals) automatic processes with slow tasks.

WM receives input from two "directions": from outside and inside the cognitive system. Processes, such as orienting reflexes and attention capture, are **bottom-up** (or *stimulus driven; data-driven*) to the extent that they are influenced by characteristics of environmental input. Length and complexity of a sentence can influence comprehension processes. Processing, such as spotlight attention, is **top-down** (or *concept-driven*) to the extent that it is directed by what we already know. Experiments may emphasize one or the other, but cognitive activity usually depends on both.

An implication of the two processing directions for research is that variables in any cognitive activity consist of internal factors, as well as commonly manipulated external ones in stimuli. Our knowledge of language provides top-down directed expectations that enable us to "fill in the blanks" as in studies of reading despite missing letters (i.e., phonological restoration effect). We "read between the lines" to provide context and interpret motives. Comprehension in conversation is determined by knowledge of a topic or familiarity with the partner.

Finally, a hypothesis crisscrossing most arenas of cognitive research has to do with the **modularity** of processes. An assumption of modularity has been essential to the localization of variously defined functions in the brain. The question has been whether cognitive systems (i.e., language in general) or processes (i.e., lexical access) are independent of other systems or processes. A modular process is said to be self-contained or "encapsulated." Because a cognitive function is likely to depend on more than one process, a further question is whether the operation of such multiple processes is *serial* (i.e., sequential) or *parallel* (i.e., simultaneous). Many models in cognitive neuropsychology are serial, because components or processes are believed to operate one at a time without overlap. Serial processing has also been assumed in chronometric (additive/subtractive) approaches. However, current findings favor more parallel or overlapping processing for most functions (Ashcraft & Radvansky, 2010).

EXECUTIVE FUNCTION

An executive supervisory system, or "a little person in the head to direct behavior" (Andrewes, 2001, p. 135), can be hard to find in some texts for cognitive psychology (e.g., Ashcraft & Radvansky, 2010). A "central executive" for managing dual-task attention was part of Baddeley's WM. However, he worried that his initial definition was "so vague as to serve as little more than a ragbag into which could be stuffed all the complex strategy selection, planning, and retrieval checking that clearly goes on . . . " (Baddeley, 1996, p. 6). As this "ragbag," it has presented a challenge for conjuring appropriate methods for obtaining evidence of its nature and role.

The idea of an executive function may have originated in an information processing conference at Carnegie-Mellon University in 1958. The conference inspired Miller, Galanter, and Pribram (1960) to write an influential book on the importance of an overseer that guides complex human behavior toward meeting a goal. Later, Norman and Shallice (1986) cited several elements of an executive system, and some of them follow:

- Initiation, or activation of a cognitive system
- Goal maintenance or task persistence
- Organization of action-sequences
- Awareness, or self-monitoring and modification (flexibility)

Since then, lists of the components of this system have varied somewhat, but most include initiation, planning, and organization.

Currently, elaboration of executive function appears to be mainly a neuropsychological development and is invoked for characterizing problems caused by traumatic brain injury. It is commonly associated with the frontal lobes (e.g., Collette & Van der Linden, 2002). Andrewes (2001) wondered "whether we should be using such a term" for such a complex and fluid construct that has been related to multiple tests with questionable intercorrelations. Assessment generally consists of a task with multiple steps having a logical arrangement.

LANGUAGE AND COMMUNICATION

A collection of case studies and a large treatment study in the Netherlands reflect a broad agreement that there are two complementary approaches to aphasia treatment (De Jong-Hagelstein, van de Standt-Koenderman, Prins, et al., 2010; Martin, Thompson, & Worrall, 2008). One approach is impairment-oriented, focusing on repairing language or cognitive deficits. The other approach is labeled as communication-oriented or consequence-oriented. The current book is aimed primarily at areas of impairment, namely, the cognitive systems related to and responsible for language functions and, thus, appears to be most compatible with the impairment approach.

Language-related issues are studied in a branch of experimental cognitive psychology known as *psycholinguistics* (Traxler & Gernsbacher, 2006). Some of the early work in this field started with an assumption of serial processing and with a chronometric strategy for studying sentence verification. This approach to sentence verification was applied briefly to the study of aphasia by predicting response times for conditions that were assumed to differ by a single mental process (Just, Davis, & Carpenter, 1977). This section highlights the functions of word and sentence comprehension, discourse comprehension, and pragmatic communication.

Earlier in this chapter, it was said that a researcher thinks through what a listener or reader must do mentally, let us say, to comprehend a word. The problem is that we comprehend a familiar word instantaneously, and cognitive theory is suggestive of events than can occur in the blink of an eye. *Our brain activates a meaning automatically. The meaning is represented as a concept in a semantic network. Activation of the concept spreads automatically to its nearest neighbors. This spreading activation should influence the processing of a subsequent word.* This is the thinking that goes into designing a semantic priming task in which one word precedes another (McNamara, 2005). Referring to Figure 1-3, let us say that the first word is RED, activating nearby nodes so that a second word FIRE is recognized faster than if the first word were GREEN. Subconscious activation after the first word is detected by its influence on simple response to the second word. This priming effect occurs even with merely a tenth of a second between words and is evidence of instantaneous events.

Sentence comprehension is explored with the assumption that the cognitive system, like the brain, activates automatically as soon as a sentence is initiated and continues as the sentence is heard or read. *On-line* methods seem to be the appropriate source of evidence for processing as it occurs in real time or "as it happens." Participants in a study usually respond to a point within a sentence, before its presentation is completed. Response time is indicative of relative processing load at that point. Many on-line techniques are used to study comprehending a word in a sentence or to study assigning a syntactic structure to a sentence (Carreiras & Clifton, 2004).

Syntax is a puzzlement, because we cannot literally hear or see a structure like we can hear and see words, which may be why some language researchers steer clear of syntax. Linguists provide us with "tree-structures" to help us visualize syntactic relations. The following *USA Today* headline, aided by its spacing, may convince us of the psychological reality of the top-down assignment of structure:

**Cruise ship dumping poisons
seas, frustrates U.S. enforcers**

If we stop at the end of the first line, it reads *the ship is dumping poisons*. When we continue to the next line, we have to correct the original structural assignment, because the headline was meant to be understood as *the dumping poisons the seas*. The difference in meaning is slight, but this structural ambiguity (called a *garden-path sentence*) shows that structural relations exist and determine interpretation. The minimal comparison in an on-line study consists of measuring processing load at the point an error would be recognized to the same point in a similar sentence without the ambiguity.

Syntactic parsing (or structural assignment) has been a topic of enthusiastic theoretical debate. The basic issue has been whether the syntactic processor is modular from the start, acting automatically on its own, or whether syntactic assignment necessarily interacts with all sorts of contextual information from the beginning of a sentence. A modular theory suggests that the parser, in its haste, subconsciously assigns the simplest possible structure (i.e., *ship is dumping poisons*) and then corrects itself when an error is discovered. This correction predicts a "garden-path effect" of extra processing time at the crucial point in the sentence. The processing load at critical points is often detected by the on-line measurement of eye-fixations while reading (eye-tracking). Many studies demonstrate a context-effect that eliminates the garden path and supports an interactive theory of processing (see reviews in Traxler & Gernsbacher, 2006).

While basic word and sentence comprehension occurs comfortably within processing capacity, discourse (or text) comprehension can be demanding of WM with its stream of input and thirst for interpretive information from LTM (Baddeley et al., 2009; Zwaan & Rapp, 2006). In the study of discourse, this constraint on processing is known as the "bottleneck problem." One of the demands of language input is the requirement of linking or integrating two or more elements across the discourse, within long sentences or among different sentences. A theorist, striving for parsimony, need appeal only to a few cognitive mechanisms to account for comprehending a range of phenomena. One example is the problems of pronoun comprehension and gap-filling, both likely to involve integrating a semantically "empty" space with a referent occurring earlier in a long sentence or in another sentence (Box 1-5).

Finally, let us turn briefly to the area of cognitive studies that approaches communication-oriented or consequence-oriented rehabilitation. An important feature of this domain is the assumption of or presence of another participant in the exchange of messages (i.e., a speaker when studying comprehension; a listener when studying production). In cognitive psychology,

Box 1-5

A Psycholinguistic Operation

Examples of the similarity between pronoun and trace comprehension are found in a study of aphasia (Zurif, Swinney, Prather, et al., 1993). Elements requiring a link to a referent (the baby) are *who* in the first sentence and a trace [t] for an object to fed in the second sentence.

- The passenger smiled at the baby in the blue pajamas who drank milk at the train station.
- The passenger smiled at the baby that the woman in the pink jacket fed [t] at the train station.

Comprehending each involves linking a semantic gap back to a referent earlier in the sentence.

the domain of social cognition is relevant (Fiske & Taylor, 1991: Moskowitz, 2005). The mind described to this point is the mind that participates in conversation, and the young field of **cognitive pragmatics** is being developed to study the mind's automaticity, as well as its strategies, when presented with real communicative problems. "The challenge," according to Davis (2007b), "is to construct experiments in a way that reflects the more authentic problems of natural communication and that is consistent with fundamental paradigms for the study of cognition" (p. 114).

In interpersonal communication, people convey and comprehend more than the literal interpretation of an utterance. A problem for cognitive pragmatics is to figure out how someone utilizes communicative contexts to infer or convey meaning beyond the literal. Theorists tap into general psycholinguistic processes such as activating multiple meanings, selecting contextually appropriate meaning, and suppressing inappropriate meanings (Long, Johns, & Morris, 2006). Moreover, these processes are considered in attempts to understand comprehension deficits in right hemisphere–damaged individuals (e.g., Tompkins, Fassbinder, Blake, et al., 2004).

A CLOSING EDITORIAL

This chapter opened with a comment on the way that language and cognition have been related to each other, especially when thinking about the nature of aphasia. This has been problematic when language and cognition are thought to be different things. On the one hand, people with aphasia insist on public awareness of their competence, in accordance with an understanding of aphasia as a language disorder largely sparing other cognitive functions. The following slogan is common among support groups: "APHASIA, loss of language, not intellect." On the other hand, some researchers are collecting evidence of deficits in cognition beyond language processing. For example, Murray and Clark (2006) observed that "aphasia is commonly accompanied by problems of attention, memory, and executive functioning" (p. 30). Is this a conflict? Do people with aphasia have cognitive deficits, or do they not?

Proposing a theory to explain certain features of aphasia, McNeil, Hula, and Sung (2011) have had a fairly unique way of articulating the relationship between certain cognitive functions and language functions. They recently argued that "the most parsimonious account for the disparate phenomena of aphasia is an impairment of a language dedicated (executive) attentional system, with secondary, rather than primary impairments of the linguistic computational or STM component of the WM system" (p. 569). A language-dedicated executive and a linguistic computational/STM component may be original configurations (see this chapter's discussion of STM), but this account appears to be generally consistent with thinking of language functions as embedded in cognition. Another articulation may be that computational (or psycholinguistic) mechanisms (e.g., spreading activation in LTM, structural assignment, gap-filling, and so on) occur in WM, dependent on temporary storage of buffered input. Clinical practitioners have reason to be puzzled by the various configurations of cognitive elements that go into explanations of aphasia.

In addition, McNeil and his colleagues pitted their particular cognitive explanation against a "loss of language" viewpoint, also calling it a "centers and pathways" view. Mixed into this ingenious brew was the linguistic theory of trace deletion for one type of aphasia (Grodzinsky, 1989). They claimed that "the overwhelming majority of researchers" hold a "nearly blind adherence" to the loss/centers view and that "a relatively small minority" hold a cognitive processing view. Quite to the contrary, a majority actually recognize that the "loss of language" theory has not been taken literally since Schuell, as discussed earlier in this chapter regarding the knowledge-process dichotomy (see Brookshire, 2007; Davis, 2007a). Currently, the term "loss" shows up mainly in slogans and book titles for the general public, with no intention of contributing to theory.

In examining the positions on aphasic language processing, we can find variation in the way that researchers portray the cognitive processing that is considered to be impaired. Some investigators, such as McNeil and others (their "minority"), have dealt with cognition at the general level of attention and memory.

Others have tackled specific processes such as spreading activation in a semantic memory store and syntactic gap-filling (e.g., Copland, Chenery, & Murdoch, 2002; Shapiro & Levine, 1990; Tompkins et al., 2004; Zurif et al., 1993). On a few occasions, we may discover that one of these types of explorers ignores the territory of the other type or considers another view to be hostile territory incompatible with life at home. In these situations, there actually may be no conflict when another view incorporates different but complementary features of cognition underlying a different experimental problem.

So, what are we to make of McNeil's assertions, especially regarding the nature of aphasia? Shuster and Thompson (2004) argued that "one cannot falsify resource theory . . . because resource theory is so vague and ill-defined that it can be used to explain any finding" (p. 852). In this debate, McNeil and others (2004) essentially agreed but considered this limitation to be an insufficient basis for rejecting the possibility that WM constraints have something to do with aphasia. Murray and Kean (2004) advised that we pay attention to general cognitive processes, but we should note the wording cited earlier, namely, the phrase "accompanied by." Just as aphasia the language disorder can be accompanied by hemiplegia, dysarthria, and apraxia of speech depending on location and size of the lesion, it can be accompanied by diminished awareness, delayed thought, and some disorganization. McNeil took a unique position that general cognitive processes explain the essence of aphasia. Murray seems to have suggested that general cognition may be deficient in some cases in addition to a language-specific impairment.

Clarity about the role of cognition in aphasic language impairment may be valuable in the courtroom, such as the case of Ruby McDonough, a resident of a nursing home in Massachusetts. She was the victim of a horrible assault by a nurse's aide (Miller, 2010). Although her basic cognitive competence was recognized despite her expressive aphasia, she was denied the right to accommodations in giving testimony in a district court. Later, the Massachusetts Supreme Judicial Court ruled that she should be allowed accommodations. Despite her possible deficits of attention and resource management, the court learned that Ms. McDonough could testify under conditions that recognize her strengths of situational recognition, episodic memory, and reasoning. Her testimony was to be simplified by answering yes-no questions, and she was to be given more than the usual time to respond. These commonly used compensations are consistent with a person who has intact linguistic knowledge but a deficit of some type in the processing of language.

CONCLUSIONS

In this chapter, some of the thinking that goes into the study of cognition was introduced. It also provided an orientation to general cognitive systems of attention, memory, and executive function; and it pointed out that language is processed within these systems. Comprehension and production draw from knowledge stored in LTM and are constrained by the capacity of WM. Both functions are accomplished with bottom-up and top-down informational flow and both operate at automatic and controlled levels. In addition, language comprehension relies on basic mechanisms of representation, scanning, activation, integrative matching (e.g., gap-filling), and so on. Psycholinguistic processes are considered to be function-specific cognitive mechanisms; and, therefore, we should repress an inclination to think of "cognition" as something that is qualitatively different.

Argument about the nature of aphasia is battered by various ways in which investigators frame the issues. This chapter singled out resource theory because it is an example of applying cognition to aphasia and its advocates have cast a wide net. A productive strategy for future research will be to compare different theories of the same thing by using appropriate experiments (not just with logic). Hiking these trails with their shadows, twists and turns, and dead-ends can be guided by a thorough understanding of how language is processed with general and specific cognitive mechanisms that are automatic or controlled. Understanding comes from a good education in cognitive psychology in general and psycholinguistics in particular provided by primary investigators in these fields. Subsequent chapters will be more specific as to how cognition fuels language comprehension, formulation, and communication.

REFERENCES

Almor, A., Aronoff, J. M., MacDonald, M. C., Gonnerman, L. M., Kempler, D., Hintiryan, H., Hayes, U. L., & Andersen, E. S. (2009). A common mechanism in verb and noun naming deficits in Alzheimer's patients. *Brain and Language, 111*, 8–19.

Andrewes, D., (2001). *Neuropsychology: From theory to practice.* Hove, UK: Psychology Press.

Ashcraft, M. H. (1989). *Human memory and cognition.* Glenview, IL: Scott, Foresman.

Ashcraft, M. H., & Radvansky, G. A. (2010). *Cognition* (5th ed.). Boston: Prentice Hall.

Baddeley, A. D. (2004). *Your memory: A user's guide.* Buffalo, NY: Firefly Books.

Baddeley, A. D. (1996). Exploring the central executive. *Quarterly Journal of Experimental Psychology, 49A,* 5–28.

Baddeley, A. D., Eysenck, M. W., & Anderson, M. C. (2009). *Memory.* New York: Psychology Press.

Brookshire, R. H. (2007). *Introduction to neurogenic communication disorders* (7th ed.). St. Louis, MO: Mosby Elsevier.

Cabeza, R., & Kingstone, A. (Eds.). (2006). *Handbook of functional neuroimaging of cognition* (2nd ed.). Cambridge, MA: MIT Press.

Carreiras, M., & Clifton, C., Jr. (Eds.). (2004). *The on-line study of sentence comprehension: Eye-tracking, ERPs and beyond.* Brighton, UK: Psychology Press.

Collette, F., & Van der Linden, M. (2002). Brain imaging of the central executive component of working memory. *Neuroscience & Neurobehavioral Reviews, 26,* 105–125.

Collins, A. M., & Loftus, E. F. (1975). A spreading activation theory of semantic processing. *Psychological Review, 82,* 407–428.

Copland, D. A., Chenery, H. J., & Murdoch, B. E. (2002). Hemispheric contributions to lexical ambiguity resolution: Evidence from individuals with complex language impairment following left-hemisphere lesions. *Brain and Language, 81,* 131–143.

Davis, G. A. (1989). The cognitive cloud and language disorders. *Aphasiology, 3,* 723–734.

Davis, G. A. (1994). Theory as the base on which to build treatment of aphasia. *American Journal of Speech-Language Pathology, 3,* 8–10.

Davis, G. A. (2007a). *Aphasiology: Disorders and clinical practice* (2nd ed.). Boston: Allyn & Bacon/Longman.

Davis, G. A. (2007b). Cognitive pragmatics of language disorders in adults. *Seminars in Speech and Language, 28,* 111–121.

De Jong-Hagelstein, M., van de Sandt-Koenderman, W. M. E., Prins, N. D., Dippel, D. W. J., Koudstaal, P. J., & Visch-Brink, E. G. (2010). Efficacy of early cognitive-linguistic treatment and communicative treatment in aphasia after stroke: A randomised controlled trial (RATS-2). *Journal of Neurology, Neurosurgery and Psychiatry,* DOWNLOADED October 13, 2010.

Dell, G., & Kittredge, A. (2011). Connectionist models of aphasia and other language impairments. In J. Guendouzi, F. Lonke, & Williams, M. J. (Eds.), *The handbook of psycholinguistic and cognitive processes: Perspectives on communication disorders* (pp. 169–188). New York: Psychology Press.

Eysenck, M. W. (2006). *Fundamentals of cognition.* New York: Psychology Press.

Fiske, S. T., & Taylor, S. E. (1991). *Social cognition* (2nd ed.). New York: McGraw-Hill.

Flanagan, O. J. (1984). *The science of the mind.* Cambridge, MA: MIT Press.

Gazzaniga, M. S., Ivry, R. B., & Mangun, G. R. (2008). *Cognitive neuroscience: The biology of the mind* (3rd ed.). Norton.

Gorlick, A. (2009, August). Media multitaskers pay mental price, Stanford study shows. *Stanford Report.* Retrieved November, 9, 2009, from http://news.stanford.edu/news/2009/august24/multi-task-research-study-082409.html.

Grodzinsky, Y. (1989). Agrammatic comprehension of relative clauses. *Brain and Language, 37,* 480–499.

Johnson-Laird, P. N. (1983). *Mental models.* Cambridge, UK: Cambridge University Press.

Just, M. A., Davis, G. A., & Carpenter, P. A. (1977). A comparison of aphasic and normal adults in a sentence-verification task. *Cortex, 13,* 402–423.

Lodge, D. (2008). *Deaf sentence.* London: Penguin Books.

Long, D. L., Johns, C. L., & Morris, P. E. (2006). Comprehension ability in mature readers. In M. J. Traxler & M. A. Gernsbacher (Eds.), *Handbook of psycholinguistics* (2nd ed.) (pp. 801–834). London: Elsevier.

Martin, N., Thompson, C. K., and Worrall, L. (Eds.). (2008). *Aphasia rehabilitation: The impairment and its consequences.* San Diego, CA: Plural Publishing.

Matlin, M. W. (2009). *Cognition* (7th ed.). Wiley: Hoboken, NJ.

McNamara, T. P. (2005). *Semantic priming: Perspectives from memory and word recognition.* New York: Psychology Press.

McNeil, M. R., Hula, W. D., Matthews, C. T., & Doyle, P. J. (2004). Resource theory and aphasia: A fugacious theoretical dismissal. *Aphasiology, 18,* 836–839.

McNeil, M. R., Hula, W. D., & Sung, J. E. (2011). The role of memory and attention in aphasic language performance. In J. Guendouzi, F. Lonke, & M. J. Williams (Eds.), *The handbook of psycholinguistic and cognitive processes: Perspectives on communication disorders* (pp. 551–578). New York: Psychology Press.

Miller, G. A., Galanter, E., & Pribram, K. H. (1960). *Plans and the structure of behavior.* New York: Henry Holt.

Miller, N. (2010). Ruby McDonough allowed to testify in Sudbury sexual assault case. *MetroWest Daily News.* Retrieved November, 29, 2010, from http://www.metrowestdailynews.com/features/x298229494/Ruby-McDonough-allowed-to-testify-in-Sudbury-sexual-assault-case

Moskowitz, G. B. (2005). *Social cognition: Understanding self and others.* New York: Guilford Press.

Murray, L. L., & Clark, H. M. (2006). *Neurogenic disorders of language: Theory driven clinical practice.* Clifton Park, NY: Thomson Delmar.

Murray, L. L., & Kean, J. (2004). Resource theory and aphasia: Time to abandon or time to revise? *Aphasiology, 18,* 830–835.

Norman, D. A., & Shallice, T. (1986). Attention to action: Willed and automatic control of behaviour. In R. J. Davidson, G. E. Schwartz, & D. Shapiro (Eds.), *Consciousness and self-regulation: Advances in research and therapy* (pp. 1–18). New York: Plenum.

Ögmen, H., & Breitmeyer, B.G. (2006). *The first half second.* Cambridge, MA: MIT Press.

Rapp, B. (Ed.). (2001). *The handbook of cognitive neuropsychology.* Philadelphia: Psychology Press.

Schacter, D. L. (1996). *Searching for memory: The brain, the mind, and the past.* New York: Basic Books.

Schuell, H. M. (1969). Aphasia in adults. In *Human communication and its disorders—An overview.* Bethesda, MD: U.S. Department of Health, Education, and Welfare.

Shapiro, L. P., & Levine, B. A. (1990). Verb processing during sentence comprehension in aphasia. *Brain and Language, 38,* 21–47.

Shuster, L. I. (2004). Resource theory and aphasia reconsidered: Why alternative theories can better guide our research. *Aphasiology, 18,* 811–830.

Shuster, L. I., & Thompson, J. C. (2004). Resource theory: Here, there, and everywhere. *Aphasiology, 18,* 850–854.

Sies, L. F. (Ed.). (1974). *Aphasia theory and therapy: Selected lectures and papers of Hildred Schuell.* Baltimore: University Park Press.

Stanovich, K. E. (2007). *How to think straight about psychology* (8th ed.). Boston: Allyn & Bacon.

Sternberg, S. (1975). Memory scanning: New findings and current controversies. In D. Deutsch & J. A. Deutsch (Eds.), *Short-term memory* (pp. 195–231). New York: Academic Press.

Tompkins, C. A., Fassbinder, W., Blake, M. L., Baumgartner, A., & Jayaram, N. (2004). Inference generation during text comprehension by adults with right hemisphere brain damage: Activation failure versus multiple activation. *Journal of Speech, Language, and Hearing Research, 47,* 1380–1395.

Traxler, M. J., & Gernsbacher, M. A. (Eds.). (2006). *Handbook of psycholinguistics* (2nd ed.). London: Elsevier.

Tulving, E. (1972). Episodic and semantic memory. In E. Tulving & W. Donaldson (Eds.), *Organization of memory* (pp. 382–403). New York: Academic Press.

Whitworth, A., Webster, J., & Howard, D. (2005). *A cognitive neuropsychological approach to assessment and intervention in aphasia: A clinician's guide.* Hove, UK: Psychology Press.

Wilshire, C. E. (2008). Cognitive neuropsychological approaches to word production in aphasia: Beyond boxes and arrows. *Aphasiology, 22,* 1019–1053.

Zurif, E. B., Swinney, D., Prather, P., Soloman, J., & Bushell, C. (1993). An on-line analysis of syntactic processing in Broca's and Wernicke's aphasia. *Brain and Language, 45,* 448–464.

Zwaan, R. A., & Rapp, D. N. (2006). Discourse comprehension. In M. J. Traxler & M. A. Gernsbacher (Eds.), *Handbook of psycholinguistics* (2nd ed., pp. 725–764). London: Elsevier.

CHAPTER 2

The Effects of Aging on Language and Communication

CHAPTER OUTLINE

Susan Kemper

Consider the two language samples presented in Box 2-1. Both were produced by 75-year-old men who had completed 4 years of college education. Neither of the men had a history of neurological disease, diabetes, ischemic heart disease, significant hearing loss, or other major medical conditions. Speaker A is fluent and articulate. He expresses himself clearly with little repetition or redundancy; he uses a range of different grammatical structures and lexical items and few fillers. Speaker B is struggling to express himself; his speech is fragmented and marked by many repetitions and fillers. When he does manage to produce a complete sentence, it is short and grammatically simple. This chapter will consider a variety of explanations for the marked differences in the fluency, grammatical complexity, and linguistic content of Speakers A and B.

WORKING MEMORY, AGING, AND LANGUAGE PROCESSING

One difference between Speaker A and Speaker B is their working memory capacity. On conventional tests of working memory span, Speaker A scores very well, with span scores typically in the same range as those observed in young adults. His Forward Digit Span score was 7.6; his Backward Digit Span was 6.3; and he attained a score of 4.5 on a Reading Span test. In contrast, Speaker B has a more limited working memory capacity, with a Forward Digit Span score of 5.4; a Backward Digit Span of 3.0; and a Reading

Span of 2.0. (These tests are more fully described in Appendix 2-1.)

Working memory limitations are generally assumed to contribute to age-related declines in language and communication. This section begins with an overview of working memory, focusing on tests used to assess two types of working memory limitations: limitations of working memory capacity and limitations of executive function including a breakdown of inhibition. Following a brief review of how aging affects the neurological basis of working memory, the section concludes by assessing how working memory affects older adults' language processing and communication.

Concept of Working Memory

Working memory is essential to many everyday tasks that involve the retention of information; working memory has two functions: the short-term retention of information and the manipulation of information. The prevailing model of working memory, as proposed by Baddeley (1986) and Baddeley and Hitch (1974), involves three components: two temporary storage mechanisms that buffer visual information (e.g., the visual scratchpad) and auditory information (e.g., the phonological loop) and a central executive processor. A fourth component, an episodic buffer linked to long-term memory, was added by Baddeley (2000). Cowan (1995, 2001), McElree (2001), and Oberauer and Kliegl (2006), among others, have proposed mixture models linking attention and working memory. A chief characteristic of

Box 2-1

Language Samples from Speakers with Distinct Working Memory Capacities

Speaker A

Question: What are some good things and bad things about living in Lawrence?

I find [MAIN] that there are [THAT] mostly good things about Lawrence.

And [FILL] >

The bad ones are [MAIN] so routine that you don't notice [THAT] them.

You'll see [MAIN] them anywhere you are [REL].

But Lawrence has [MAIN] a lot of uniqueness to it.

And the students make [MAIN] the town in a lot of ways and there's [MAIN] a good relationship between town and gown.

I ran [MAIN] into a lady who was [REL] my neighbor down in Shawnee Kansas.

She graduated [MAIN] from KU and then she went [MAIN] back and got married.

And she had [MAIN] a family and everything like that.

And her daughters are living [MAIN] in Lawrence.

And they said [MAIN] "why don't you just come [MAIN] back here, now that dad's [SUB] gone."

You know [FILL] >

So >

She moved [MAIN] back to Lawrence.

And she just is [MAIN] so excited about it.

You know [FILL] >

It's [MAIN] just really a turn-on for her.

And she's [MAIN] older than I am [REL].

She is [MAIN] really neat.

But anyway, except for some stupidity that goes [REL] on in the city commission I think [MAIN] basically it's [THAT] pretty good here.

Speaker B

Question: What are some good things and bad things about living in Lawrence?

The good things about Lawrence >

Is [MAIN] >

Honestly uhh, >

I spent [MAIN] some time in Wichita.

And [FILL] umm >

That (that) to me is [MAIN] cultural shock.

Lawrence is [MAIN] now >

Lawrence is [MAIN] >

Ahh, ahh >

A very good place >

I mean [MAIN] ahh >

There's [MAIN] pretty much >

Everybody >

As a matter fact the neighborhood I'm [MAIN] in >

Halfway between >

Between umm >

The high school and KU >

So [FILL] >

The neighborhood I'm [MAIN] in >

Most, ahh >

A lot of people work [MAIN] for KU.

But [FILL] >

And [FILL] umm >

Across the street >

A couple of students did [MAIN] move in.

But they're [MAIN] graduates.

They are [MAIN] graduate students.

What's [MAIN] bad about Lawrence?

You can't ahh >

On a Saturday >

You can't ahh >

There's [MAIN] no place to park [INF].

I have [MAIN] trouble there.

But I bet [MAIN] a lot of people have umm >

Yeah.

Note: All main clause verbs [MAIN], infinitives [INF], gerunds [GER], relative clauses [REL], that-clause complements [THAT], and subordinate clauses [SUB] are marked as well as all lexical fillers [FILL]. Sentence fragments are marked with angles >.

these multicomponent systems is that the system has limited capacity – to temporarily store information or to divide attention among processing tasks. Each component is also assumed to have unique characteristics: the auditory buffer is speech-based, while the visual buffer is spatially defined.

Executive function itself has been typically defined very broadly, as "those capacities that enable a person to engage successfully in independent, purposive, self-serving behavior" (Lezak, Howieson, Loring, et al., 2004, p. 35), or as "a multidimensional construct referring to a variety of loosely related higher-order cognitive processes including initiation, planning, hypothesis generation, cognitive flexibility, decision-making, regulation, judgment, feedback utilization, and self perception" (Spreen & Strauss, 1998, p. 171), and as a bundle of "general purpose control mechanisms that modulate the operation of various cognitive subprocesses" (Miyake, Friedman, Emerson, et al., 2000, p. 50). Executive component itself includes different functions such as attentional allocation and selection, inhibition, and information updating.

Evidence for functional separation of these components of working memory comes from studies of healthy and impaired individuals responding to different task manipulations: (1) On tests of immediate serial recall, performance is worst for phonologically similar word lists, suggesting that verbal information is held in a phonologically-based short-term store. (2) Serial recall also varies with word length and with reading time, suggesting this phonologically-based buffer has a limited capacity. (3) The continuous articulation of irrelevant speech (e.g., repeating "the, the, the . . . ") impairs recall, eliminates the phonological-similarity effect, and the word length effect, again suggesting that this buffer is speech-based. (4) Concurrent engagement in a spatial tracking task such as pointing to the source of a moving sound while blindfolded impairs performance on spatial memory tests, suggesting that the sketchpad is spatial in nature.

Measuring Working Memory

One challenge to understanding the role of working memory in language and communication is the multiplicity of tests and assessments used to measure individual differences in working memory. Working memory is typically defined by tests of working memory span and by tests of executive function (Box 2-2). Executive function itself is measured by neuropsychological tests such as the Wisconsin Card Sorting Test, or specific tests of inhibition, time-sharing, updating, and switching. These tests are briefly described in Appendix 2-1. Many variants of each test have been developed. In addition, the speed of information processing in working memory also affects language and communication and a variety of approaches have been used to assess processing speed.

There is considerable debate as to whether these tests assess separate but correlated executive functions or a unitary construct, and their relationship to general intelligence. For example, Engle, Tuholski, Laughlin, and Conway (1999) suggest that span tasks may be differentiated into simple span tests assessing short-term memory and complex span tests involving executive processes. A further issue is working memory can be subdivided into verbal and nonverbal (or visual/spatial)

Box 2-2

Tests of Working Memory and Executive Function

WORKING MEMORY TESTS
Verbal Span
  Forward and Backward Digit Span
  Counting Span
  Reading and Listening Span
  Operational Span
Visual-Spatial Span
  Corsi Blocks
  Visual Patterns

EXECUTIVE FUNCTION
Neuropsychological Tests
  Wisconsin Card Sorting
  Trail-Making
  FAS Verbal Fluency
  Tower of Hanoi
Inhibition
  Stroop task
  Stop Signal Task
Time-sharing
  Counting Backwards plus Connections
  Tracking plus Paired Associations
Updating
  Digit monitoring
  N-Back
Switching
  Plus/Minus Switching
  Letter-Letter Switching
  Local-Global Switching

---

domains. See also the "users guide" developed by Conway, Kane, Bunting, et al. (2005) for a discussion of many methodological and procedural problems in measuring working memory capacity using counting, operational span, and reading span tests.

There is no single measure that serves as the "gold standard" for the assessment of executive function. Salthouse, Atkinson, and Berish (2003), noting the complexity and breadth of notions of executive function, undertook an examination of the construct validity of executive function in a sample of 261 adults ranging in age from 18 to 84 years. Their approach was to examine convergent and discriminate validity among a set of neuropsychological and cognitive tasks typically associated with executive function, and also a set of psychometric tasks including measures of verbal ability, fluid intelligence, episodic memory, and perceptual speed.

A series of structural equation analyses were then conducted to look at the relations among these sets of variables. Their results indicated that the various neuropsychological measures were not very highly related to one another and were fairly highly related to other variables, particularly fluid intelligence. They concluded that individual differences in measures of working memory may in fact reflect differences in much broader abilities, such as fluid intelligence.

Miyake and colleagues (Friedman & Miyake, 2004; Miyake et al., 2000) have addressed similar questions but took a somewhat different approach and reached different conclusions. Miyake et al. (2000) reported a study addressing "the unity and diversity of executive functions" (p. 49) using confirmatory factor analysis and structural equation modeling. They found that a three-factor solution fit the data better than any of the one- or two-factor solutions, indicating that there are three separable dimensions of executive function. The authors conclude from this study that the three executive functions they measured (updating, shifting, inhibition) are "clearly distinguishable" and that each plays a different role in more complex executive function measures such as the Wisconsin Card Sorting Test and the Tower of Hanoi.

Aging and Working Memory

The questions of how aging affects working memory have not been clearly answered by either the Salthouse study or the Miyake studies. As measured by simple and complex span tests, working memory increases in childhood (Dempster, 1980; Gathercole, 1999; Park, Smith, Lautenschlager, et al., 1996; Pickering, 2001) and declines in late adulthood. What drives this U-shaped increase, then decrease in working memory is the subject of considerable debate. Salthouse (1994, 1996) has argued for processing speed as the fundamental mechanism; Lindenberger and Baltes (1994; Baltes & Lindenberger, 1997) have argued for neural integrity as measured by sensory acuity and postural balance and gait as the critical factor; and Hasher and Zacks (1988) have argued for a breakdown in inhibitory functions. Inhibition is critical for blocking irrelevant information from entering working memory, deleting irrelevant information from working memory, and restraining prepotent responses. Under this hypothesis, older adults with poor inhibitory mechanisms may not only be more susceptible to distraction, but they may also be less able to switch rapidly from one task to another and they may rely on well-learned "stereotypes, heuristics, and schemas" (p. 123) (Yoon, May, & Hasher, 1998). Lustig, May, and Hasher (2001) have demonstrated that working memory span in older adults can vary dramatically

as a function of test format, comparing the traditional format for testing memory span uses a sequence of trials in which set size increased from 2 to 3 to 4 to 5 items with a format designed to minimize interference in which set size decreased from 5 to 4 to 3 to 2 items. Whereas this manipulation did not affect span estimates for young adults, it did for older adults, implying that the traditional test measures not only working memory capacity but also inhibition.

Another issue is whether cognitive abilities dedifferentiate with age, becoming more highly correlated (Cornelius, Willis, Nesselroade, & Baltes, 1983; Li, Lindenberger, Homnel, et al., 2004). Dedifferentiation is assumed to arise from the decline of a basic, fundamental mechanism, such as processing speed, whereas differentiation is assumed to arise from the development or breakdown of process-specific mechanisms. Rabbitt and Lowe (2000; Rabbitt, 1993) have suggested that aging leads to increasing individual differences, reflecting different rates and trajectories of change of underlying processes and/or neural structures.

To investigate these questions, Hull, Martin, Beier, et al. (2008) used an approach similar to that used by Miyake et al. (2000) and administered a battery of tests of shifting, updating, and inhibition to a panel of middle-aged and older adults along with two criterion tests of executive function, the Wisconsin Card Sorting Test and the Tower of Hanoi test and tests of verbal and nonverbal knowledge. Their analysis suggested two underlying factors: shifting and updating with minimal overlap between these two factors. Performance on the two criterion tests was best predicted by updating, the ability to maintain information and track rule changes in working memory. Shifting, the ability to activate alternative rules, did not contribute to performance on the Card Sorting and Tower of Hanoi tests. Somewhat surprisingly, Hull et al. found no evidence for a third inhibition factor, perhaps due to a lack of measurement sensitivity for the Stroop and antisaccade tests used to assess inhibition. They also note that aging appears to affect the relative contributions of underlying factors; in the Miyake et al. (2000) study, shifting was the primary predictor of performance on the Card Sorting test whereas Hull et al. found that updating was the best predictor. Thus, as aging affects different components of working memory, the relative balance among preserved components may be altered. A decline in working memory capacity may lead increased reliance on efficiency; hence executive function in younger adults may be more dependent on the capacity to store multiple representations in working memory whereas executive function in older adults may be more dependent on the efficiency at which information can added to or deleted from a (reduced) working memory.

A similar conclusion was reached by McDowd et al. (2011) in a recent study that compared how young and older adults' performance on a variety of verbal fluency tests covaried with other measures of cognition including measures of processing speed, inhibition, working memory capacity, and verbal ability. Letter fluency (e.g., words beginning with "M"), semantic fluency (e.g., "colors" or "fluids"), and action fluency (e.g., "ways you can talk") were tested; processing speed was assessed by performance on the digit symbol and letter comparison tests (see later); working memory capacity was measured by forward and backward digit span and by reading span; inhibition was determined by performance on the Wisconsin Card Sorting Test and on the Stroop and Trail-Making Tests; and verbal ability was measured by performance on the Boston Naming (Kaplan, Goodglass, & Weintraub, 1983) vocabulary test. The group differences were very similar across fluency measures and types: in general, young adults produced more correct responses, fewest perseverations, and fewest intrusions and the older adults produced fewer correct responses, more perseverations, and more intrusions. To examine how individual differences in processing speed, verbal ability, working memory, and inhibition affected performance on the verbal fluency tests, a series of regression models was evaluated separately for the young and older adults. For young adults, these models were nonsignificant, perhaps reflecting the restricted range of young adults' performance on these tests but also supporting the differentiation of cognitive abilities into separable components. For older adults, processing speed and inhibition were the best predictors of performance on the fluency tests, suggesting that the speed of information retrieval from semantic memory as well as the ability to select and focus retrieval operations are key determinates of verbal fluency. Vocabulary size and working memory capacity do not appear to affect older adults' ability to retrieve letter, category, and action exemplars whereas processing speed and inhibition do, perhaps because speed and efficiency become a more critical determinates of verbal fluency performance as aging leads to declines in working memory capacity as well as increases in vocabulary.

Aging and the Neurological Basis of Working Memory

Working memory and executive function are believed to be subserved by the prefrontal cortex (Raz, 2005) and the nigrostriatal dopamine neurotransmitter system (Arnsten, Cai, Steere, & Goldman-Rakic, 1995; Volkow,

Wang, Fowler, et al., 1998). Both are affected by aging and, in turn, affect performance on working memory and executive function tasks. Although there is an overall reduction in brain volume with advancing age, this loss is accelerated in the prefrontal cortex (Dennis & Cabeza, 2008; Raz, 2005; Raz, Gunning, Head, et al., 1997; Raz, Lindenberger, Rodrigue, et al., 2005; Salat, Kaye, & Janowsky, 1999), arising from neuronal shrinkage and declines in synaptic density (Huttenlocher & Debholkar, 1997; Peters, Morrison, Rosene, & Hyman, 1998). This loss of brain volume results in reduced prefrontal activation (Grady, McIntosh, & Craik, 2005; Grady, McIntosh, Rajah, et al., 1999). Figure 2-1 compares regional brain volume changes in healthy adults.

Although many neurotransmitter systems are affected by aging, the most dramatic changes appear in the dopamine system (Bäckman & Farde, 2005; de Keyser, Herregodts, Ebinger, et al., 1990; Suhara, Fukuda, & Inoue, 1991; Volkow et al., 1998). Age-related declines in the dopamine system, in turn, result in reduced input to the frontal cortex, reflecting the functional interconnectedness of a frontalstriate circuit (Volkow et al., 2000). These dopaminergic pathways are illustrated in Figure 2-2.

Cabeza (2002) has proposed that frontal activity is less strongly lateralized in older adults than in young adults, implying that older adults compensate for neurocognitive deficits by recruiting both hemispheres to perform tasks that require only a single hemisphere in young adults. This pattern of age-related asymmetry reductions appears during tests of paired associate learning (Cabeza, McIntosh, Tulving, et al., 1997), word stem recall (Bäckman, Almkvist, Andersson, et al., 1997), and word recognition (Madden, Langley, Denny, et al., 2002), as well as on verbal working memory tests (Reuter-Lorenz, Jonides, Smith, et al., 2000).

In addition to changing the brain's structure and organization, aging may affect the neurochemical basis of cognition by altering or modulating signal transmission between and among neurons (Li, 2005; Li & Silkström, 2002). As a result, stimulus-response relations may be altered, reducing sensitivity to stimuli, increasing the temporal variability of responses, and increasing "noise" or random activations (Li, Lindenberger, & Fransch, 2000). One further consequence may be that events and stimuli are encoded less distinctively, resulting in a blurring of episodic memories, an increasing in the variability of performance, and the dedifferentiation of cognitive abilities as they become more correlated (Li et al., 2005).

As a result of these changes to the prefrontal cortex, the dopamine system, the lateralization of function, and neuromodulation, working memory appears to be

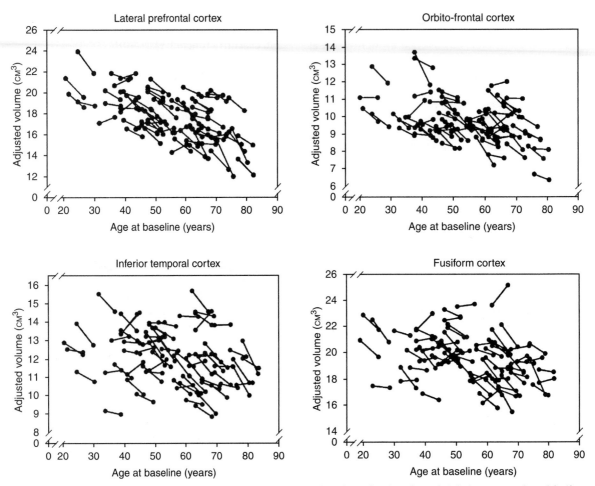

Figure 2-1 Longitudinal changes in adjusted volumes of the lateral prefrontal, orbito-frontal, inferior temporal, and fusiform cortices as a function of baseline age. [Adapted from "Regional brain changes in aging healthy adults: General trends, individual differences, and modifiers" by N. Raz, U. Lindenberger, K. M. Rodrigue, D. Head, A. Williamson, C. Dahle, D. Gerstorf, and J. D. Acker, 2005, *Cerebral Cortex, 15*, 1676–1689. Copyright 2005 by Oxford University Press. Reprinted with permission.]

Figure 2-2 Major dopaminergic pathways in the human brain: (*1*) the nigrostriatal system projecting to the basal ganglia; (*2*) the mesolimbic system projecting to the accumbens (Acc) and the limbic cortex; (*3*) the mesocortical system projecting to the neocortex. [Adapted from L. Bäckman & L. Farde. (2005). The role of dopamine systems in cognitive aging. In R. Cabeza, L. Nyberg, & D. Park (Eds.), *Cognitive neuroscience of aging*, pp. 59–84. Copyright 2005 by Oxford University Press. Reprinted with permission.]

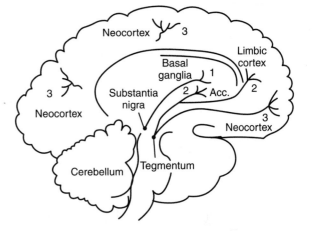

progressively compromised in older adults. The consequences for language processing are pervasive.

Working Memory Constraints on Language Processing

There is widespread agreement that working memory is critical to a wide range of cognitive abilities that affect older adults' language and communication. Support for the hypothesis that working memory limitations constrain older adults' production and comprehension of language are largely correlational. A variety of observations support this hypothesis; for example, performance on the reading and listening span tests of Daneman and Carpenter (1980) has been shown to be related to performance on reading and listening comprehension, learning to read, reading ability, arithmetic ability, and reasoning ability (Daneman & Blennerhassett, 1984; Daneman & Green, 1986; Daneman & Tardif, 1987; Hitch et al, 2001; Leather & Henry, 1994). Daneman and Merikle (1996) reviewed 77 studies involving 6,179 participants, confirming the link between reading/ listening span measures and language comprehension, reporting correlations of .41 and .52 with global and specific tests of comprehension.

Older adults have typically been found to have smaller working memory spans than young adults and such span measures have been found to correlate with measures of language processing (Borella, Carretti, & De Beni, 2008; Norman, Kemper, Kynette, et al., 1991; Stine, Wingfield, & Myers, 1990; Tun, Wingfield, & Stine, 1991). One approach has been to examine the relationship between measures of language production, obtained from elicited language samples, and measures of working memory, obtained from span or other tests. Language sample analysis relies on a variety of metrics to evaluate language including measures of fluency, grammatical complexity, and content. Typical metrics are summarized in Box 2-3 and further described in Appendix 2-2; the application of the DLevel and PDensity metrics is illustrated in Appendix 2-3. A variety of specialized software is available to assist with language sample analysis including the Systematic Analysis of Language Transcripts (SALT) software developed by Chapman and Miller (1984) and the Computerized Propositional Idea Density Rater (CPIDR) (Brown, Snodgrass, Kemper, et al., 2008). In addition, the on-line calculator Coh-metrix (Graesser, McNamara, Louwerse, & Cai, 2004) may be used to obtain additional measures; although originally developed to assess the coherence of written documents, it may be used to conduct analyses of elicited language samples. Table 2-1 illustrates the application of these metrics by comparing the two language samples from Box 2-1, one

Box 2-3
Metrics for Language Sample Analysis

Mean Length of Utterance (MLU): length in words
Mean Clauses per Utterance (MCU): length in clauses
Developmental Level (DLevel): sentence complexity
Propositional Density (PDensity): propositional content
Type-Token Ratio (TTR): lexical diversity
Fillers: retrieval failures, false starts, hedges
Fragments: retrieval failures, false starts, distractions
Speech Rate: speed of processing words per minute

Table 2-1 Application of Language Sample Metrics to 3 Examples

	Speaker A	Speaker B	Speaker C
MLU	10.00	4.70	4.86
MCU	1.35	0.48	0.83
DLevel	2.50	1.13	0.21
PDensity	5.82	2.02	5.13
Speech rate, wpm	124 wpm	96 wpm	84 wpm
TTR	.62	.87	.59
Fragments, %	20	71	66

Note. MLU, Mean length of utterance in words; *MCU,* mean clauses per utterance; *DLevel,* developmental level; *PDensity,* propositional density; *TTR,* type/token ratio; *wpm,* words per minute.

elicited from an older adult with excellent working memory and one elicited from an older adult with poor working memory, as well as a third language sample discussed later.

Cheung and Kemper (1992) used structural modeling to investigate interrelationships among many language sample metrics as well as measures of working memory capacity and verbal ability using language samples elicited from young and older adults. Cheung and Kemper showed that age-related declines in working memory were highly correlated with age-related declines in grammatical complexity assessed by metrics that are sensitive to the length of grammatical constituents, how many clauses are embedded within a sentence, and how those clauses are embedded. Kemper and Sumner (2001) extended this approach to investigate the relationship between language sample measures and traditional measures of verbal ability, working memory, and verbal fluency. They reported that grammatical complexity was correlated with span measures of working memory. In contrast, propositional content was correlated with measures of verbal fluency and reading rate, suggesting that processing speed and efficiency limit how information can be conveyed linguistically. Verbal ability, assessed by performance on vocabulary tests, constituted a third factor unrelated to the language sample measures of grammatical complexity or propositional content. These correlational analyses suggest that working memory imposes a ceiling on how many sentence relations can be formulated at one time. Each embedded or subordinate clause increases the burden on working memory by imposing additional requirements for subject-verb agreement, pronominal choice, the linear ordering of adjectives, and the application of other grammatical rules.

A Ceiling on Language Production
If older adults' language production is functionally limited, it should be evident in how young and older adults respond in controlled production experiments in which participants are given words or sentence fragments and asked to compose a sentence. In a series of studies, Kemper, Herman, and Lian (2003a) and Kemper, Herman, and Liu (2004) varied the number of nouns and the types of verbs given to the participants and scored the length, grammatical complexity, and propositional or informational content of each sentence produced and the time taken to respond. Older adults' responses were similar to those of younger adults when given 2 or 3 words. When given 4 words, the older adults were slower to respond, made more errors, and their responses were shorter, less complex and less informative than the younger adults' responses. When different types of verbs were provided, young and older adults responded similarly with simple intransitive (*smiled*) and transitive (*replaced*) verbs but older adults encountered problems using verbs like *expected* that preferentially are used with embedded clauses, e.g., . . . *expected the package to be delivered*. Older adults responded very slowly yet produced shorter, grammatically simpler, and propositionally less informative sentences.

Other researchers have shown that working memory limitations affect older adults' language processing using tests of text comprehension and recall. Kwong See and Ryan (1996) examined whether individual differences in text processing are attributable to working memory capacity, processing speed, or the breakdown of inhibitory processes. Working memory capacity was estimated by backward digit span, processing speed by color naming speed, and inhibition by performance on the Stroop task. Their analysis suggested that older adults' text processing difficulties can be attributed to slower processing and less efficient inhibition, rather than to working memory limitations.

Van der Linden et al. (1999) also sought to distinguish the effects of working memory limitations from those due to reductions of processing speed or a breakdown of inhibitory processes by examining performance on a wide range of language tasks using structural equation modeling. Young and older adults were tested on their ability to understand texts and recall sentences and words. They were also given a large battery of tests designed to measure processing speed, working memory capacity, and the ability to inhibit distracting thoughts. The analysis indicated that these three general factors (speed, working memory, inhibition) did account for age-differences in performance on the language processing tasks. Further, the analysis indicated that "age-related differences in language, memory and comprehension were explained by a reduction of the capacity of working memory, which was itself influenced by reduction of speed, [and] increasing sensitivity to interference . . . " (p. 48).

Syntactic Processing Limitations
A limitation of these studies is age-related changes to language processing are inferred from performance on recall measures, answers to comprehension questions, or global measures of reading speed. A more specific set of hypothesis about the nature of age-related changes to language processing have been examined in a series of studies using more "direct" methods to examine the role of working memory in syntactic processing. Just and his colleagues (Just & Carpenter, 1992; Just & Varma, 2002; King & Just, 1991; MacDonald, Just, & Carpenter, 1992) have claimed that working memory capacity constrains the interpretation of temporary syntactic ambiguities, limiting the ability of older or low span readers to make and sustain multiple interpretations of ambiguous phrases. According to the Just and Carpenter (1992) capacity-constrained (CC) theory (see also the 3CAPS model of Just & Varma, 2002), older or low span readers should have difficulty processing temporary syntactic ambiguities and should exhibit garden-path effects, initially misinterpreting reduced relative clause constructions as main verbs only to reinterpret the constructions once disambiguating information is encountered. Young or high span readers should be able to avoid garden-path effects, by constructing multiple syntactic interpretations of the ambiguous phrases and retaining these interpretations until disambiguating information is encountered.

This hypothesis has been carefully examined by Caplan and Waters (1999) who have considered a number of lines of evidence from studies of young and older adults as well as individuals with aphasia and dementia. They distinguish between immediate, interpretive syntactic processing and post-interpretative semantic and pragmatic processing. Caplan and Waters argue that there is little evidence to support the hypothesis that working memory limitations affect immediate syntactic processes; rather, they conclude that working memory limitations affect postinterpretative processes involved in retaining information in memory in order to recall it or use it (e.g., to answer questions or match sentences against pictures). In a variety of studies comparing adults stratified into groups based on measures of working memory, Caplan and Waters (1999) note that effects of syntactic complexity do not differentially affect high versus low span readers or listeners. And they report that secondary tasks that impose additional processing demands on working memory do not differentially affect the processing of complex sentences. Caplan and Waters consider aphasic patients such as B. O. who had a digit span of only 2 or 3 digits but who was able to perform as well as normal healthy older adults on a wide range of tasks with complex sentences. They also note that patients with Alzheimer's dementia, who also show severely limited working memory capacity, are able to make speeded acceptability judgments of complex sentences as accurately as nondemented controls.

Waters and Caplan (1996a, 1996b, 1997, 2001) have directly examined the hypothesis that working memory limitations affect older adults' ability to process complex sentences. These studies have used the auditory moving windows paradigm. This technique allows the listener to start and stop the presentation of sentence and permits the analysis of phrase-by-phrase listening times, analogous to visual moving windows paradigms, which permit the analysis of word-by-word or phrase-by-phrase reading times. The studies by Caplan and Waters typically examine the processing of subject and object relative clause constructions, such as those that follow:

OBJECT SUBJECT RELATIVE CLAUSE: The dancer
found the music$_{i, j}$ that (t_j) delighted the director.
SUBJECT OBJECT RELATIVE CLAUSE: The music$_{i, j}$
that the dancer found (t_i) (t_j) delighted the
director.

The object subject relative clause construction imposes few processing demands on the reader or the listener, the object of the main clause, (t_i), is also the subject of the embedded relative clause, (t_j). The subject object relative clause construction challenges the reader

or listener to assign the correct syntactic relations, the subject of the main clause, (t_j), must also be interpreted as the object of the embedded clause, (t_i).

Waters and Caplan (2001) compared how young and older readers allocate listening times to critical phrases of relative clause sentences. Despite differences in working memory, listening times were distributed similarity by young and older listeners. All paused longer when they heard the embedded verb in the complex object relative clause sentences than when they heard the corresponding verb in the simple subject relative clause version; this additional time is attributable to the extra processing required to recover its direct object. They found no evidence that differences in age or working memory lead to different processing strategies, supporting their theory.

A recent study by Kemper, Crow, and Kemtes (2004) using eye-tracking methodology re-examined these issues. Eye-tracking is a more naturalistic task that imposes few restrictions on readers; they are free to skip words or phrases, read ahead and glance backwards, and re-read entire segments. Using this technology, Kemper et al. examined three aspects of reading: first fixations to key phrases, regressions to earlier phrases, and the total time key phrases were fixated. They examined reduced relative clause sentences such as those below:

REDUCED RELATIVE CLAUSE SENTENCE: Several
angry workers warned about the low wages
decided to file complaints.
MAIN CLAUSE SENTENCE: Several angry workers
warned about the low wages during the holiday
season.
FOCUSED REDUCED RELATIVE CLAUSE SENTENCE:
Only angry workers warned about the low wages
decided to file complaints.

Kemper, Crow, and Kemtes (2004) found partial support for Waters and Caplan's theory: young and older adults' first pass fixations were alike and both groups showed a clear "garden-path" effect: a peak in fixation time at the second verb in reduced relative clause sentences but not at the verb in main clause sentences. This garden-path effect suggests that all readers initially interpret the first verb as the main verb and must reanalyze it when they encounter the second verb in the reduced relative clause sentence. However, Kemper et al. also observed an increase in regressions and in regression path fixations for older readers for the reduced relative clause sentences, suggesting that older adults were unable to correctly parse these sentences. Further, low span readers, identified by their scores on a battery of working memory tests, also produced more regressions and an increase in regression path fixations for reduced relative clause sentences, suggesting that they were unable to correctly parse the sentences. The results from the eye-tracking analysis of the focused reduced relative clauses sentences also posed problems for Caplan and Water's theory: high span readers initially allocated additional processing time the first noun phrase and then were able to avoid the "garden path" because the focus operator "only" led them to correctly interpret the first verb phrase as a reduced relative clause.

Kemper and Liu (2007) also used eye-tracking to compare young and older adults' processing of unambiguous object-relative sentences and subject-relative sentences, such as those given next, which differed in the locus of embedding and the form of the embedded sentences. Young and older adults showed similar patterns of the first pass fixation times, regression path fixations, and leftward regressions to critical regions for both types of cleft sentences and for object-subject relative clause sentences. However, older adults generally needed more time to process subject-object relative clause sentences than young adults; they made more regressions back to both the main clause subject and the embedded clause subject than did young adults and, consequently, their regression path fixations for these critical regions were longer. These findings directly contradict Waters and Caplan's hypothesis (2001) that working memory and sentence processing are unrelated. They also indicate that age group differences, reflecting differences in working memory, arise for some, but not all types of sentences. Whereas fixation patterns of young and older adults were similar for both cleft subject and cleft object sentences and object subject sentences, subject object sentences gave rise to marked age group differences in regressions and regression path fixations. Cleft subject and object subject sentences can be parsed as two sequential clauses: the main clause is followed by an embedded clause signaled by a "that" complementizer that is indexed to the preceding noun phrase. Cleft object sentences are somewhat more challenging to parse since the cleft object also serves as the object of the embedded clause and must be temporarily buffered while the embedded clause is processed. Subject object sentences impose yet greater demands for parsing since the subject of the main clause must also be assigned as the object the embedded clause; further, the embedded clause interrupts the main clause, so that the main clause subject must be temporarily buffered if it is to be correctly linked with its verb. It may be that there is a threshold for parsing complexity such that differences due to age

group, and by inference, working memory span, are not apparent until this threshold is surpassed. What is apparent is that there are differences in the size of the temporary buffer required for syntactic analysis of subject object sentences, mirroring age differences in working memory as measured by traditional span measures. Compared to young adults, older adults, with smaller syntactic processing buffers, must make more regressions and allocate additional processing time to establish the main clause subject and relative clause subject of subject object sentences.

CLEFT SUBJECT:	It was the tailor that altered the suit coat.
CLEFT OBJECT:	It was the suit coat that the tailor altered.
OBJECT SUBJECT:	The dancer found the music that delighted the director.
SUBJECT OBJECT:	The music that the dancer found delighted the director.

DISTRACTION, AGING, AND LANGUAGE PROCESSING

Now consider the third language sample from Speaker C in Box 2-1. Speaker C is in fact the same individual as Speaker A, the well-educated man with excellent working memory. Now, however, he is talking while attempting to track a very rapidly moving visual target. The demands of talking while simultaneously engaged in this demanding visual-motor task not only affect his speech rate but also his grammatical complexity: he produces many sentence fragments, uses many fillers, and the few complete sentences he produces are generally simple constructions. What has happened to Speaker A? In addition to the effects of working memory on language processing, a variety of other age-associated factors can affect language, including inhibitory deficits, distractions, and the demands of dual- or multi-tasking.

Inhibitory Deficits

Distraction appears to exacerbate the effects of age-related changes to language processing. Hasher and Zacks (1988) proposed that older adults are more vulnerable to distractions as a result of a weakening of inhibitory mechanisms with age. Irrelevant thoughts, personal preoccupations, and idiosyncratic associations disrupt and impair older adults' comprehension and recall. Hasher, Zacks, and May (1999) postulate three functions of inhibition: preventing irrelevant information from entering working memory, deleting irrelevant information from working memory, and restraining probable responses until their appropriateness can be assessed. They argue that older adults suffer from a variety of processing impairments that can be attributed to decreased inhibitory mechanisms. Hence, older adults' language processing may mirror that of young adults whenever the task requires the active application of processing strategies since excitatory mechanisms are spared, whereas older adults' language processing may be impaired, relative to young adults', whenever inhibitory mechanisms are required to block out distractions, clear way irrelevancies, or switch between activities. Individuals with poor inhibitory mechanisms may not only be more susceptible to distraction, but they may also be less able to switch rapidly from one task to another and they may rely on well-learned "stereotypes, heuristics, and schemas" (p. 123) (Yoon, May, & Hasher, 1998).

Off-Target Verbosity

Hasher & Zacks (1988; Zacks & Hasher, 1997) have suggested that off-target verbosity (Arbuckle & Gold, 1993; Pushkar Gold & Arbuckle, 1995) is a characteristic of older adults resulting from the breakdown of inhibitions. Pushkar Gold, Andres, Arbuckle, and Schwartzman (1988) observed that a minority of older adults not only talk a lot but drift from topic to topic, weaving into their conversations many unrelated and irrelevant topics. They refer to this style as "off-target verbosity."

Pushkar Gold, Basevitz, Arbuckle, et al. (2000) and Arbuckle, Nohara-LeClair, and Pushkar Gold, (2000) have carefully examined the speech, social skills, conversational style, and referential communication skill of older adults identified as demonstrating high levels of off-target verbosity. From a panel of 455 older adults, they scored off-target verbosity defined as copious speech and a high degree of content unrelated to the questions during a structured interview. The 35 highest scoring participants were designated as the high off-target verbose participants. This group did more poorly on inhibition tasks including the Stroop test; however, they were not distinguishable from the other participants in terms of their scores on a variety of measures of social support and social skills. During "get acquainted" conversations with other participants, they also talked more, revealed more personal information and tended to ask fewer questions of their partners and to recall less about their partners (Pushkar Gold et al., 2000). On a referential communication task, they were less efficient in giving directions in that they produced more hedged or qualified directions and gave more redundant directions (Arbuckle et al., 2000). Pushkar Gold et al. conclude that these older adults are self-absorbed and self-preoccupied.

They also emphasize that off-target verbosity characterizes a minority of older adults, and is not a general characteristic of older adults. They conclude, "It is possible that older people who are experiencing losses generated by declining cognitive skills are more motivated by self-affirmation as a communicative goal, leading them to more egocentric behavior in conversational settings."

Communication Goals

Whereas off-target verbosity has been cited as providing support for inhibitory deficit theory, Burke (1997) argues that this speech style is limited to social settings in which older adults' construe their task differently than do young adults—as monologue, responsive to an internal chain of associations. James, Burke, Austin, and Hulme (1998) examined speech samples collected from young and older adults. Those from the older adults were, indeed, more verbose but only when they were describing personal, autobiographical topics. However, these autobiographical narratives were rated as more informative and interesting than the more focused, less verbose narratives produced by young adults. Trunk and Abrams (2009) also suggest that age differences in communicative goals may contribute to the perception that older adults are off-target and verbose; older adults may indeed be "more talkative" than young adults because young adults value succinctness, conciseness, and efficiency over expressiveness and elaboration. Burke (1997) has argued that research on semantic priming, the activation of word meanings, and the detection of ambiguity provides "no support" for claims that "older adults are deficient in suppressing contextually irrelevant meaning or that they activate more irrelevant semantic information than young adults or that they retrieve more high frequency, dominant, or typical information than young adults" (p. 257).

Distractions

A variety of language processing difficulties have been reported for older adults in distracting situations such as when older adults are attempting to ignore noise or other distractions. Disfluencies during spontaneous speech have often been noted as increasing when background noise is presented (Hassol, Margaret, & Cameron, 1952; Heller & Dobbs, 1993; Jou & Harris, 1992; Southwood & Dagenais, 2001). Disfluencies include hesitations, false starts, filled and unfilled pauses, and vague, disorganized "scattered" speech. One interpretation is that language processing is disrupted by the attentional demands of blocking out or ignoring distractions as implied by the inhibitory deficit theory. An alternative hypothesis is that older adults are more susceptible to distraction than younger adults because sensory and perceptual processes require more effort, detracting from how well they can attend to and process semantic and syntactic information.

Reading with Distraction

These alternative explanations have been explored using a variety of different research paradigms examining how auditory and visual distractions affect older adults. The reading with distraction paradigm presents a text contains distracting words printed in a different typeface and participants are monitored as they read the text. Young adults are able to ignore the distracting material, even when it is related to the text, whereas older adults are not able to ignore the distracting material, which slows their reading, impairs their comprehension, and renders them subject to memory distortions (Connelly, Hasher, & Zacks, 1991; Zacks & Hasher, 1997). Although originally used to support the inhibitory deficit theory, this interpretation has been challenged by Dywan and Murphy (1996), who modified the procedure to include a surprise word recognition test for the interposed material. They found that the young adults had superior recognition memory for the distracter words, a result that is difficult to explain if the young adults are assumed to have been successful at inhibiting processing of the distracters. Further, Kemper and McDowd (2006) have suggested that perceptual deficits may affect the ability of older adults to detect the change in font. If older adults cannot discriminate between targets and distracters, they may be forced to rely on slower, more effortful semantic and syntactic processes to determine the mis-fit between the text and distracters, affecting both their reading speed and comprehension.

Hearing Loss and Effortfulness

Age-related sensory changes may not only result in declines in visual and auditory acuity but also result in impairments of higher-level cognitive and linguistic processes that may be revealed by the presence of distractions. In a simple demonstration of this, Murphy, Craik, Li, and Schneider (2000) compared serial recall curves for young adults when the auditory stimuli were presented in quiet or in noise. Noise had no effect on recall of the final 2 words in the sequence but suppressed recall of the first 3 items. Thus, they conclude that the words were correctly heard but not encoded into memory. When they tested young and older adults, they found a similar pattern: equivalent recall of the final 2 words but greatly suppressed recall of the first 3 words by the older adults. They suggested that both normal aging and background noise result in an

impoverished signal that is susceptible to rapid memory decay (see also Schneider & Pichora-Fuller, 2000).

Wingfield, Tun, and McCoy (2005) also suggested that hearing loss not only affects the ability of older adults to detect and discriminate speech sounds with regard to frequency discrimination and temporal resolution, but also affect their ability to engage in more effortful semantic and syntactic processing. They argue that the effort older adults must expend to overcome even mild hearing loss may come at great cost to processing resources that could otherwise be used to higher-level processing. For example, McCoy, Tun, Cox, et al. (2005) presented a sequence of words for recall, interrupting the presentation unexpectedly to probe for recall of the last 3 words presented. Although young and older adults had excellent recall of the final word, recall of the preceding two words was greatly reduced for older adults with hearing loss. This pattern suggests that the older adults with hearing loss expended additional effort to identify each new target word, which affected their ability to encode the words in memory.

This "effortfulness" hypothesis (Rabbitt, 1966) is consistent with findings from studies using the "irrelevant speech" paradigm in which distracters are presented auditorally while the participant is engaged in a visual or auditory memory task. The typical pattern is that recall declines when irrelevant speech is presented, not when white noise is presented. Some studies report equivalent patterns of disruption (Bell & Buchner, 2007; van Gerven, Meijer, Vermeeren, et al., 2007), whereas others find older adults' recall is more disrupted than young adults' (Bell, Buchner, & Mund, 2008). Tun, O'Kane, and Wingfield (2002) asked young and older adults to listen to lists of words while ignoring irrelevant speech. They varied whether the irrelevant speech was meaningful (read in English) or meaningless (read in Dutch by the same speaker). Whereas young adults were capable of ignoring the irrelevant speech, the older adults' recall of the target words was severely impaired by the irrelevant speech. This irrelevant speech effect was greater for older adults when the competing speech was in English than when it was in Dutch (a language that closely resembles English phonology and prosody), suggesting that the effect is due to both sensory and attentional factors (see also Tun & Wingfield, 1999). Tun et al. conclude that the older adults' recall of the target words is impaired by the demands of filtering out the irrelevant speech. Under this account, as processing the target information becomes more difficult as a result of increasing speech rate or syntactic complexity, the effects of aging and hearing loss should become more pronounced (Murphy, Daneman, & Schneider, 2006; Schneider, Daneman, & Murphy, 2005; Tun, McCoy, &

Wingfield, 2009; Wingfield, McCoy, Peelle, et al., 2006; Wingfield, Peelle, & Grossman, 2003).

The "effortfulness hypothesis" has broad implications for older adults' ability to dual- or multi-task. For example, Stine, Wingfield, and Myers (1990) examined younger and older adults' recall of information from a television newscast that was presented in auditory format, auditory supplemented with a written transcript, or the original auditory and visual recording. Although the written transcript and visual presentation aided younger adults' recall of the information, older adults did not benefit from a written transcript, suggesting they were unable to divide their attention between the two sources of information.

Dual-Tasking and Multitasking

Dual-task procedures can be used to study how individuals trade-off competing task demands, such as responding as rapidly as possible versus responding as accurately as possible. Dual-task costs may reflect the operation of a central bottleneck (Pashler, 1994) in selecting between the tasks or strategic differences how the tasks are coordinated (Meyer & Kieras, 1997a, 1997b). Recent investigations (see the meta-reviews by Riby, Perfect, & Stollery, 2004, and Verhaeghen, Steitz, Sliwinski, & Cerella, 2003) suggest that older adults' experience greater dual-task costs than young adults, especially with tasks that involve controlled processing as well as executive functions such as task switching, time-sharing, and updating. Göthe, Oberauer, and Kliegl (2007) suggest that there are persistent differences in how young and older adults combine two tasks, even well-practiced tasks. Göthe et al. have suggested that older adults adopt a "conservative" approach to dual-task demands that trades reduced speed for improved accuracy whereas young adults use a more risky approach that emphases speed over accuracy.

The dual-task approach can be used to examine how aging and task demands affect language production by requiring young and older adults to respond to probe questions while concurrently carrying out secondary tasks. When cognitive and motor tasks are performed simultaneously, older adults typically show greater dual-task costs than young adults (Li, Lindenberger, Freund, & Baltes, 2001; Lindenberger, Marsiske, & Baltes, 2000), although young and older adults may differ in how they trade-off costs to one task versus the other (Doumas, Rapp, & Krampe, 2009; Li et al., 2001; Verrel, Lövdén, Schellenbach, Schaefer, & Lindenberger, 2009).

In a series of studies using dual-task comparisons, Kemper and her colleagues (Kemper, Herman, & Lian, 2003; Kemper, Herman, & Nartowicz, 2005; Kemper, Schmalzried, Herman, Leedahl, & Mohankumar, 2009) found that young and older adults responded differentially to dual-task demands when they are asked to talk while performing simple motor tasks, such as walking or tapping a finger, or when they are listening to noise. In baseline, single-task conditions, young adults use a complex speech style, whereas older adults use a more restricted speech style composed of shorter, simpler sentences (Kemper, Kynette, Rash, et al., 1989). In dual-task conditions, both young and older adults spoke more slowly and young adults' also used shorter, simpler sentences although the length and complexity of older adults' speech did not vary. Thus, the restricted speech style of older adults arises as an accommodation to age-related declines in working memory and processing speed (Kemper & Sumner, 2001); these restrictions imposed by working memory also reduces older adults' vulnerability to dual-task demands because they are able to maintain this speech style while engaged in a concurrent activity.

To further probe the limits on older adults' ability to maintain their speech style under dual-task conditions, Kemper, Schmalzried, Herman, et al. (2009) combined pursuit rotor tracking (McNemar & Biel, 1939) with a language production task. In this task, participants track a moving target displayed on a computer screen while responding to questions. This task provides a continuous record of performance that can be synchronized with language production. The costs of concurrent speech on pursuit tracking were similar for young and older adults: tracking performance, as measured by average time on target and average distance from the target, declined when the participants were talking while tracking compared to baseline condition. However, tracking had different costs for language production in the two groups. Although both groups spoke more slowly in the dual-task condition than in the baseline condition, young adults experienced greater dual-task costs to speech than did older adults, consistent with prior research (Kemper et al., 2003b, 2005). In particular, concurrent tracking impaired young adults' verbal fluency and grammatical complexity, such that young adults used shorter, simpler sentences under dual-task conditions than they did in the baseline condition. Older adults were less vulnerable to dual-task demands than young adults, in that concurrent tracking slowed older adults' speech but did not otherwise affect their fluency, grammatical complexity, or linguistic content, compared to the baseline condition.

However, there are limits on older adults' ability to maintain this speech style as Speaker C demonstrates in Box 2-4.

Kemper, Schmalzried, Hoffman, and Herman (2010) examined the consequences of varying the speed of the

Box 2-4

Language Sample from a Speaker Tracking a Visual Target

SPEAKER C

Question: Which President do you most admire and why?

I've [MAIN] always admired President Truman.
You know [FILL] >
I can [MAIN] remember umm >
The first election I ever remember [REL] was [MAIN] >
President Roosevelt, uh, umm>
1932 >
I was [MAIN] four years old.
I think [MAIN] I remember [THAT].
I remember [MAIN] very well the 1936 umm, umm >
Well [FILL] >
And then well [FILL] he was [MAIN] president right up until I was [SUB] >
You know [FILL] ahh >
seventeen >
I was [MAIN] in high school.
Amazing >
And then Truman came [MAIN] along.
I mean [MAIN] umm, Roosevelt.
Well [FILL] ahh >

I won't [MAIN] go into that.
But uh, uh >
Truman came [MAIN] along.
And as I say [SUB] >
I am [MAIN] fond of saying [GER] umm >
I say [MAIN] he was [THAT] the last uh >
He was [MAIN] a civilian president.
And he was [MAIN] umm >
The fact that >
I admired [MAIN] uh, ahh >
Well [FILL] >
I admired [MAIN] him because of his intelligence.
He was [MAIN] an intelligent man.
He was [MAIN] honest.
I think [MAIN] he was [THAT] an honest man.
And for a president that is [MAIN] >
Well [FILL] >
He was [MAIN] a man of great decisions.
He was [MAIN] known for >
And [FILL] >
In his umm >
Running [GER] this country >
Well [FILL] ahh, umm >

Note: All main clause verbs [MAIN], infinitives [INF], gerunds [GER], relative clauses [REL], that-clause complements [THAT], and subordinate clauses [SUB] are marked as well as all lexical fillers [FILL]. Sentence fragments are marked with angles >.

---

pursuit rotor for young and older adults. Speaker C is talking while tracking a very rapidly moving visual target and his speech is now highly fragmented with reduced grammatical complexity and propositional content. Kemper et al. conclude that older adults have developed a simplified speech register that is resistant but not immune to dual-task demands. By slowing down, older adults are able to maintain their (reduced) level of grammatical complexity. However, as dual-task demands exceed some threshold, older adults are unable to maintain their simplified speech and their speech becomes highly fragmented, marked by many fillers and disfluencies, and composed of short, simple sentences. Their speech comes to resemble the speech of older adults with dementia (Kemper, LaBarge, Ferraro, et al., 1993; Lyons, Kemper, LaBarge, Ferraro, et al., 1994): it is composed of many sentence fragments, as well as short, grammatically simple sentences, and lacks semantic cohesion, informativeness, and lexical diversity. Speech that is highly fragmented, ungrammatical, incoherent, disrupted by many word finding problems, and repetitive, and redundant is highly

stigmatized and associated with negative stereotypes of older adults (Hummert, Garstka, Ryan, & Bonnesen, 2004). Such speech is dysfunctional in that it results in delays, requests for clarifications, confusions, and other forms of communication breakdown.

CONCLUSIONS

The comparison of the three language samples in Box 2-1 and Box 2-4 illustrates how aging, working memory limitations, and distractions affect speech. This chapter has reviewed a number of explanations for these changes, including constraints on language production imposed by working memory limitations and distractions. These age-associated changes to language are evident in the speech of healthy older adults as a result of nonpathological changes to the brain's structure and organization affecting the function of the prefrontal cortex, the lateralization of functions, and neuromodulation. As a result, working memory limitations constrain older adults' ability to produce and understand complex grammatical constructions, and make them more susceptible to the effects of distractions, sensory loss, and dual-task or multitask demands.

ACKNOWLEDGMENTS

Preparation of this chapter was supported in part by grants from the National Institutes of Health (NIH) to the University of Kansas through the Mental Retardation and Developmental Disabilities Research Center, Grant P30 HD-002528, and the Center for Biobehavioral Neurosciences in Communication Disorders, Grant P30 DC-005803, and by Grants RO1 AG06319, RO1 AG09952, and RO1 AG025906 from the National Institute on Aging to Susan Kemper. The contents are solely the responsibility of the author and do not necessarily represent the official views of the NIH.

REFERENCES

Arnsten, A. F. T., Cai, J. X., Steere, J. C., & Goldman-Rakic, P. S. (1995). Dopamine D2 receptor mechanisms contribute to age-related cognitive decline: The effects of quinpirole on memory and motor performance in monkeys. *The Journal of Neuroscience, 15,* 3429–3439.

Arbuckle, T., & Gold, D. P. (1993). Aging, inhibition, and verbosity. *Journal of Gerontology: Psychological Sciences, 48,* P225–P232.

Arbuckle, T., Nohara-LeClair, M., & Pushkar, D. (2000). Effects of off-target verbosity on communication efficiency in a referential communication task. *Psychology and Aging, 15,* 65–77.

Bäckman, L., Almkvist, O., Andersson, J., Nordberg, A., et al. (1997). Brain activation in young and older adults during implicit and explicit retrieval. *Journal of Cognitive Neuroscience, 9,* 378–391.

Bäckman, L., & Farde, L. (2005). The role of dopamine systems in cognitive aging. In R. Cabeza, L. Nyberg, & D. Park (Eds.), *Cognitive neuroscience of aging* (pp. 59–84). Oxford: Oxford University Press.

Baddeley, A. D. (1986). *Working memory.* Oxford, UK: Clarendon Press.

Baddeley, A. D. (2000). The episodic buffer: A new component of working memory? *Trends in Cognitive Science, 4,* 417–423.

Baddeley, A. D., & Hitch, G. (1974). Working memory. In G. H. Bower (Ed.), *The psychology of learning and motivaton: Advances in research and theory* (Vol. 8, pp. 48–89). New York: Academic Press.

Baltes, P. B. (1994). Theoretical propositions of life-span developmental psychology on the dynamics between growth and decline (trans I. Ariyevich). *Psikhologicheskiy Zhurnal, 15,* 60–80.

Baltes, P. B., & Lindenberger, U. (1997). Emergence of a powerful connection between sensory and cognitive functions across the adult lifespan: A new window to the study of cognitive aging? *Psychology and Aging, 12,* 12–21.

Bell, R., & Buchner, A. (2007). Equivalent irrelevant-sound effects for old and young adults. *Memory & Cognition, 35,* 352–364.

Bell, R., Buchner, A., & Mund, I. (2008). Age-related differences in irrelevant-speech effects. *Psychology and Aging, 23,* 377–391.

Benton, A. L., & Hamsher, K. D. (1989). *Multilingual Aphasia Examination.* Iowa City: AJA Associated.

Borella, E., Carretti, B., & De Beni, R. (2008). Working memory and inhibition across the adult life-span. *Acta Psychologica, 128,* 33–44.

Brown, C., Snodgrass, T., Covington, M. A., Herman, R., & Kemper, S. (2008). Measuring propositional idea density through part-of-speech tagging. *Behavioral Research Methods, 40,* 540–545.

Burke, D. (1997). Language, aging, and inhibitory deficits: Evaluation of a theory. *Journal of Gerontology: Psychological Sciences, 52B,* P254–P264.

Cabeza, R. (2002). Hemispheric asymmetry reduction in older adults: The HAROLD model. *Psychology and Aging, 17,* 85–100.

Cabeza, R., Grady, C. L., Nyberg, L., McIntosh, A. R., et al. (1997). Age-related differences in neural activity during memory encoding and retrieval: A positron emission tomography study. *The Journal of Neuroscience, 17,* 391–400.

Cabeza, R., McIntosh, A. R., Tulving, E., Nyberg, L., & Grady, C. L. (1997). Age-related differences in effective neural connectivity during encoding and recall. *Neuroreport: An International Journal for the Rapid Communication of Research in Neuroscience, 8,* 3479–3483.

Caplan, D., & Waters, G. (1999). Verbal working memory and sentence comprehension. *Behavioral and Brain Sciences, 22,* 114–126.

Case, R., Kurland, D. M., & Goldberg, J. (1982). Operational efficiency and the growth of short term memory span. *Journal of Experimental Child Psychology, 33,* 386–404.

Catts, H. W., & Kamhi, A. G. (Eds.). (2005). *The connections between language and reading disabilities.* Mahwah, NJ: Erlbaum.

Chapman, R., & Miller, J. (1984). *SALT: Systematic analysis of language transcripts.* Madison, WI: University of Wisconsin.

Cheung, H., & Kemper, S. (1992). Competing complexity metrics and adults' production of complex sentences. *Applied Psycholinguistics, 13,* 53–76.

Connelly, S. L., Hasher, L., & Zacks, R. T. (1991). Age and reading: The impact of distraction. *Psychology and Aging, 6,* 533–541.

Conway, A. R. A., Kane, M. J., Bunting, M. F., Hambrick, D. Z., Wilhelm, O., & Engle, R. W. (2005). Working memory span tasks: A methodological review and user's guide. *Psychological Bulletin and Review, 12,* 769–786.

Cornelius, S. W., Willis, S. L., Nesselroade, J. R., & Baltes, P. B. (1983). Convergence between attention variables and factors of psychometric intelligence in older adults. *Intelligence, 7,* 253–269.

Cowan, N. (1995). *Attention and memory: An integrated framework.* Oxford, UK: Oxford University Press.

Cowan, N. (2001). The magical number 4 in short-term memory: A reconsideration of mental storage capacity. *Behavioral and Brain Sciences, 24,* 87–185.

Daneman, M., & Blennerhassett, A. (1984). How to assess the listening comprehension skills of prereaders. *Journal of Educational Psychology, 76*, 1372–1381.

Daneman, M., & Carpenter, P. A. (1980). Individual differences in working memory and reading. *Journal of Verbal Learning and Verbal Ability, 19*, 450–466.

Daneman, M., & Green, I. (1986). Individual differences in comprehending and producing words in context. *Journal of Memory and Language, 25*, 1–18.

Daneman, M., & Merikle, P. M. (1996). Working memory and language comprehension: A meta-analysis. *Psychonomic Bulletin and Review, 3*, 422–433.

Daneman, M., & Tardiff, T. (1987). Working memory and reading skill re-examined. In M. Coltheart (Ed.), *Attention and performance XII: The psychology of reading* (pp. 491–508). Hillsdale, NJ: Erlbaum.

de Keyser, J., Herregodts, P., & Ebinger, G. (1990). The mesoneocortical dopamine neuron system. *Neurology, 40*, 1660–1662.

Dempster, F. N. (1980). Memory span: Sources of individual and developmental differences. *Psychological Bulletin, 19*, 450–466.

Dennis, N. A., & Cabeza, R. (2008). Neuroimaging of healthy cognitive aging. In F. I. M. Craik & T. A. Salthouse (Eds.), *The handbook of aging and cognition* (3rd ed., pp. 2001–2054). New York: Psychology Press.

Doumas, M., Rapp, M. A., & Krampe, R. T. (2009). Working memory and postural control: Adult age differences in potential for improvement, task priority, and dual tasking. *The Journals of Gerontology: Series B: Psychological Sciences and Social Sciences, 64B*, 193–201.

Dywan, J., & Murphy, W. E. (1996). Aging and inhibitory control in text comprehension. *Psychology and Aging, 11*, 199–206.

Engle, R. W., Tuholski, S. W., Laughlin, J. E., & Conway, A. R. A. (1999). Working memory, short-term memory, and general fluid intelligence: A latent-variable approach. *Journal of Experimental Psychology: General, 128*, 309–331.

Friedman, N. P., & Miyake, A. (2004). The reading span test and its predictive power for reading comprehension ability. *Journal of Memory and Language, 51*, 136–158.

Göthe, K., Oberauer, K., & Kliegl, R. (2007). Age differences in dual-task performance after practice. *Psychology and Aging, 22*, 596–606.

Grady, C. L., McIntosh, A. R., & Craik, F. I. M. (2005). Task-related activity in prefrontal cortex and its relation to recognition memory performance in young and old adults. *Neuropsychologia, 43*, 1466–1481.

Grady, C. L., McIntosh, A. R., Rajah, M. N., Beig, S., & Craik, F. I. M. (1999). The effects of age on the neural correlates of episodic encoding. *Cerebral Cortex, 9*, 805–814.

Graesser, A. C., McNamara, D. S., Louwerse, M. M., & Chai, Z. (2004). Coh-Metrix: Analysis of text cohesion and language. *Behavior Research Methods, Instruments, and Computers, 36*, 193–202.

Hasher, L., & Zacks, R. T. (1988). Working memory, comprehension, and aging: A review and a new view. In G. H. Bower (Ed.), *The psychology of learning and motivation* (Vol. 22, pp. 193–226). New York: Academic.

Hasher, L., Zacks, R. T., & May, C. P. (1999). Inhibitory control, circadian arousal, and age. In D. Gopher & A. Koriat (Eds.), *Attention and performance XVII: Cognitive regulation of performance: Interaction of theory and application* (pp. 653–675). Cambridge, MA: MIT Press.

Hassol, L., Magaret, A., & Cameron, N. (1952). The production of language disorganization through personalized distraction. *Journal of Psychology, 33*, 289–299.

Heller, R. B., & Dobbs, A. R. (1993). Age differences in word finding in discourse and nondiscourse situations. *Psychology and Aging, 8*, 443–450.

Hitch, G. J., Towse, J. N., & Hutton, U. (2001). What limits children's working memory span? Theoretical accounts and applications for scholastic development. *Journal of Experimental Psychology: General, 130*, 184–198.

Hull, R., Martin, R. C., Beier, M. E., Lane, D., & Hamilton, A. C. (2008). Executive function in older adults: A structural equation modeling approach. *Neuropsychology, 22*, 508–522.

Hume, G. E., Welsch, M. C., Retzlaff, P., & Cookson, N. (1997). Towers of Hanoi and London: reliability and validity of two executive function tests. *Assessment, 4*, 249–257.

Hummert, M. L., Garstka, T. A., Ryan, E. B., Bonnesen, J. L. (2004). The role of age stereotypes in interpersonal communication. In J. F. Nussbaum, & J. Coupland (Eds.), *Handbook of communication and aging research* (2nd ed., pp. 91–114). Mahwah, NJ, US: Lawrence Erlbaum Associates Publishers.

Huttenlocher, P., & Dabholkar, A. (1997). Developmental anatomy of prefrontal cortex. In N. Krasnegor, G. Reid Lyon, & P. Goldman-Rakic (Eds.), *Development of the prefrontal cortex: evolution, neurobiology, and behavior* (pp. 69–84). Baltimore: Brooks.

James, L. E., Burke, D. M., Austin, A., & Hulme, E. (1998). Production and perception of "verbosity" in younger and older adults. *Psychology and Aging, 13*, 355–368.

Jou, J., & Harris, R. J. (1992). The effect of divided attention on speech production. *Bulletin of the Psychonomic Society, 30*, 301–304.

Just, M. A., & Carpenter, P. A. (1992). A capacity theory of comprehension: Individual differences in working memory. *Psychological Review, 99*, 122–149.

Just, M., & Varma, S. (2002). A hybrid architecture for working memory: A reply to MacDonald & Christiansen (2002). *Psychology Review, 109*, 55–65.

Kaplan, E., Goodglass, H., & Weintraub, S. (1983). *Boston Naming Test*. Philadelphia: Lea & Febiger.

Kemper , S., Crow, A., & Kemtes, K. (2004). Eye fixation patterns of high and low span young and older adults: Down the garden path and back again. *Psychology and Aging, 19*, 157–170.

Kemper, S., Herman, R. E., & Lian, C. (2003a). Age differences in sentence production. *Journals of Gerontology: Series B: Psychological Sciences and Social Sciences, 58*, 260–269.

Kemper, S., Herman, R. E., & Lian, C. H. T. (2003b). The costs of doing two things at once for young and older adults: Talking while walking, finger tapping, and ignoring speech or noise. *Psychology and Aging, 18*, 181–192.

Kemper, S., Herman, R., & Liu, C. J. (2004). Sentence production by young and older adults in controlled contexts. *Journals of Gerontology: Psychological Sciences, 59B*, P220–224.

Kemper, S., Herman, R. E., & Nartowicz, J. (2005). Different effects of dual task demands on the speech of young and older adults. *Aging, Neuropsychology, and Cognition, 12,* 340–358.

Kemper, S., Kynette, D., Rash, S., & O'Brien, K. (1989). Life-span changes to adults' language: Effects of memory and genre. *Applied Psycholinguistics, 10,* 49–66.

Kemper, S., LaBarge, E., Ferraro, R., Cheung, H. T., Cheung, H., & Storandt, M. (1993). On the preservation of syntax in Alzheimer's disease: Evidence from written sentences. *Archives of Neurology, 50,* 81–86.

Kemper, S., & Liu, C. J. (2007). Eye movements of young and older adults during reading. *Psychology and Aging, 22,* 84–94.

Kemper, S., & McDowd, J. (2006). Eye movements of young and older adults while reading with distraction. *Psychology and Aging, 21,* 32–39.

Kemper, S., & McDowd, J. (2008). Dimensions of cognitive aging: Executive function and verbal fluency. In S. M. Hofer & D. F. Alwin (Eds.), *Handbook of cognitive aging: Interdisciplinary perspectives* (pp. 181–192). Thousand Oaks, CA: Sage.

Kemper, S., Schmalzried, R., Herman, R., Leedahl, S., & Mohankumar, D. (2009). The effects of aging and dual task demands on language production. *16,* 241–259.

Kemper, S., Schmalzried, R., Hoffman, L., & Herman, R. (2010). Aging and the vulnerability of speech to dual task demands. *Psychology and Aging, 25,* 949–963.

Kemper, S., & Sumner, A. (2001). The structure of verbal abilities in young and older adults. *Psychology and Aging, 16,* 312–322.

Kimberg, D. Y., D'Esposito, M., & Farah, M. J. (2000). Frontal lobes II: Cognitive issues. In M. J. Farah & T. E. Feinberg (Eds.), *Patient-based approaches to cognitive neuroscience* (pp. 317–326). Cambridge, MA: MIT Press.

King, J., & Just, M. A. (1991). Individual differences in syntactic processing: The role of working memory. *Journal of Memory and Language, 30,* 580–602.

Kwong See, S. T., & Ryan, E. B. (1996). Cognitive mediation of discourse processing in later life. *Journal of Speech Language Pathology and Audiology, 20,* 109–117.

Leather, C. V., & Henry, L. A. (1994). Working memory span and phonological awareness tasks as predictors of early reading ability. *Journal of Experimental Child Psychology, 58,* 88–111.

Lezak, M. D., Howieson, D. B., Loring, D. W., Hannay, H. J., & Fischer, J. S. (2004). *Neuropsychological assessment* (4th ed.). New York: Oxford University Press.

Li, K. Z. H., Lindenberger, U., Freund, A. M., & Baltes, P. B. (2001). Walking while memorizing: Age-related differences in compensatory behavior. *Psychological Science, 12,* 230–237.

Li, S. C. (2005). Neurocomputational perspectives linking neuromodulation, processing noise, representational distinctiveness, and cognitive aging. In R. Cabeza, L. Nyberg, & D. Park, (Eds.), *Cognitive neuroscience of aging: Linking cognitive and cerebral aging* (pp. 354–379). New York: Oxford University Press.

Li, S. C., Lindenberger, U., & Frensch, P. A. (2000). Unifying cognitive aging: From neuromodulation to representation to cognition. *Neurocomputing: An International Journal, 32–33,* 879–890.

Li, S. C., & Silkström, S. (2002). Integrative neurocomputational perspectives on cognitive aging, neuromodulation, and representation. *Neuroscience & Biobehavioral Reviews, 26,* 795–808.

Li, S. C., Lindenberger, U., Hommel, B., Aschersleben, G., Prinz, W., & Baltes, P. B. (2004). Transformations in the couplings among intellectual abilities and constituent cognitive processes across the life span. *Psychological Science, 15,* 155–163.

Lindenberger, U., & Baltes, P. B. (1994). Sensory functioning and intelligence in old age: A strong connection. *Psychology and Aging, 9,* 339–355.

Lindenberger, U., Marsiske, M., & Baltes, P. B. (2000). Memorizing while walking: Increase in dual-task costs from young adulthood to old age. *Psychology and Aging, 15,* 417–436.

Logan, G. D. (1994). Spatial attention and the apprehension of spatial relations. *Journal of Experimental Psychology: Human Perception and Performance, 20,* 1015–1036.

Logie, R., Zucco, G. M., & Baddeley, A. (1990). Interference with visual short term memory. *Acta Psychologia, 75,* 54–74.

Lustig, C., May, C. P., & Hasher, L. (2001). Working memory span and the role of proactive interference. *Journal of Experimental Psychology: General, 130,* 199–207.

Lyons, K., Kemper, S., LaBarge, E., Ferraro, F. R., Balota, D., & Storandt, M. (1994). Language and Alzheimer's disease: A reduction in syntactic complexity. *Aging and Cognition, 50,* 81–86.

MacDonald, M., Just, M. A., & Carpenter, P. A. (1992). Working memory constraints on the processing of syntactic ambiguity. *Cognitive Psychology, 24,* 56–98.

Mackworth, J. F. (1959). Paced memorizing in a continuous task. *Journal of Experimental Psychology, 58,* 206–211.

Madden, D. J., Langley, L. K., Denny, L. L., Turkington, T. G., Provenzale, J. M., Hawk, T. C., et al. (2002). Adult age differences in visual word identification: Functional neuroanatomy by positron emission tomography. *Brain and Cognition, 49,* 297–321.

McCoy, S. L., Tun, P. A., Cox, L. C., Colangelo, M., Stewart, R. A., & Wingfield, A. (2005). Hearing loss and perceptual effort: Downstream effects on older adults' memory for speech. *The Quarterly Journal of Experimental Psychology A: Human Experimental Psychology. Special Issue: Cognitive Gerontology: Cognitive Change in Old Age, 58A,* 22–33.

McDowd, J., Hoffman, L., Rozek, E., Lyons, K., Pahwa, R., Burns, J., & Kemper, S. (2011). Understanding verbal fluency in healthy aging Alzheimer's disease and Parkinson's disease. *Neuropsychology, 25,* 210–225.

McElree, B. (2001). Working memory and focal attention. *Journal of Experimental Psychology: Learning, Memory, and Cognition, 27,* 817–835.

McNemar, Q., & Biel, W. C. (1939). A square path pursuit rotor and a modification of the Miles pursuit pendulum. *Journal of General Psychology, 21,* 463–465.

Meyer, D. E., & Kieras, D. E. (1997a). A computational theory of executive cognitive processes and multiple-task performance: I. Basic mechanisms. *Psychological review, 104,* 3–65.

Meyer, D. E., & Kieras, D. E. (1997b). A computational theory of executive cognitive processes and multiple-task performance: Part 2. Accounts of psychological refractory-period phenomena. *Psychological review, 104,* 749–791.

Milner, B. (1971). Interhemispheric differences in the localization of psychological processes in man. *British Medical Bulletin, 27*, 272–277.

Miyake, A., Friedman, N. P., Emerson, M. J., Witzki, A. H., & Howerter, A. (2000). The unity and diversity of executive functions and their contributions to complex "frontal lobe" tasks: A latent variable analysis. *Cognitive-Psychology, 41*, 49–100.

Murphy, D. R., Schneider, B. A., Speranza, F., & Moraglia, G. (2006). A comparison of higher order auditory processes in younger and older adults. *Psychology and Aging, 21*, 763–773.

Murphy, D. R., Craik, F. I. M., Li, K. Z. H., & Schneider, B. A. (2000). Comparing the effects of aging and background noise of short-term memory performance. *Psychology and Aging, 15*(2), 323–334.

Murphy, D. R., Daneman, M., & Schneider, B. A. (2006). Why do older adults have difficulty following conversations? *Psychology and Aging, 21*, 49–61.

Navon, D. (1977). Forest before trees: The precedence of global features in visual perception. *Cognitive Psychology, 9*, 353–383.

Norman, S., Kemper, S., Kynette, D., Cheung, H., & Anagnopoulos, C. (1991). Syntactic complexity and adults' running memory span. *Journal of Gerontology, 46*, P346–351.

Oberauer, K., & Kliegl, R. (2006). A formal model of capacity limits in working memory. *Journal of Memory and Language, 55*, 601–626.

Park, D. C., Smith, A. D., Lautenschlager, G., Earles, J. L., & et al. (1996). Mediators of long-term memory performance across the life span. *Psychology and Aging, 11*, 621–637.

Pashler, H. (1994). Dual-task interference in simple tasks: Data and theory. *Psychological Bulletin, 116*, 220–244.

Peters, A., Morrison, J. H., Rosene, D. L., & Hyman, B. T. (1998). Are neurons lost from the primate cerebral cortex during normal aging? *Cerebral Cortex, 8*, 295–300.

Pickering, S. J. (2001). The development of visuo-spatial working memory. *Memory, 9*, 423–432.

Pushkar Gold, D., Basevitz, P., Arbuckle, T., Nohara-LeClair, M., Lapidus, S., & Peled, M. (2000). Social behavior and off-target verbosity in elderly people. *Psychology and Aging, 15*, 361–374.

Pushkar Gold, D., Andres, D., Arbuckle, T., & Schwartzman, A. (1988). Measurement and correlates of verbosity in elderly people. *Journal of Gerontology: Psychological Sciences, 43*, 27–33.

Pushkar Gold, D., & Arbuckle, T. Y. (1995). A longitudinal study of off-target verbosity. *Journal of Gerontology: Psychological Sciences, 50B*, P307–325.

Rabbitt, P. (1966). Recognition: Memory for words correctly heard in noise. *Psychonomic Science, 6*, 383–384.

Rabbitt, P. (1993). Does it all go together when it goes? The Nineteenth Bartlett Memorial Lecture. *The Quarterly Journal of Experimental Psychology A: Human Experimental Psychology, 46A*, 385–434.

Rabbitt, P., & Lowe, C. (2000). Patterns of cognitive ageing. *Psychological Research/Psychologische Forschung. 63*, 308–316.

Raz, N. (2005). The aging brain observed in vivo: Differential changes and their modifiers. In R. Cabeza, L. Nyberg, & D. Park (Eds.), *Cognitive neuroscience of aging: Linking cognitive and cerebral aging* (pp. 19–57). New York: Oxford University Press.

Raz, N., Lindenberger, U., Rodrigue, K. M., Kennedy, K. M., Head, D., Williamson, A., et al. (2005). Regional brain changes in aging healthy adults: General trends, individual differences and modifiers. *Cerebral Cortex, 15*, 1679–1689.

Reuter-Lorenz, P. A., Jonides, J., Smith, E. E., Hartley, A., Miller, A., Marshuetz, C., et al. (2000). Age differences in the frontal lateralization of verbal and spatial working memory revealed by PET. *Journal of Cognitive Neuroscience, 12*, 174–187.

Riby, L. M., Perfect, T. J., & Stollery, B. T. (2004). The effects of age and task domain on dual task performance: A meta-analysis. *European Journal of Cognitive Psychology, 16*, 868–891.

Rosenberg, S., & Abbeduto, L. (1987). Indicators of linguistic competence in the peer group conversational behavior of mildly retarded adults. *Applied Psycholinguistics, 8*, 19–32.

Salat, D. H., Kaye, J. A., & Janowsky, J. S. (2002). Greater orbital prefrontal volume selectively predicts worse working memory performance in older adults. *Cerebral Cortex, 12*(5), 494–505.

Salthouse, T. A. (1988). The role of processing resources in cognitive aging. In M. L. Howe & C. J. Brainerd (Eds.), *Cognitive development in adulthood: Progress in cognitive development research* (pp. 185–239). New York: Springer-Verlag.

Salthouse, T. A. (1994). How many causes are there of aging-related decrements in cognitive functioning? *Developmental Review, 14*, 413–437.

Salthouse, T. A. (1996). The processing-speed theory of adult age differences in cognition. *Psychological Review, 3*, 403–428.

Salthouse, T. A., Atkinson, T. M., & Berish, D. E. (2003). Executive functioning as a potential mediator of age-related cognitive decline in normal adults. *Journal of Experimental Psychology: General, 132*, 566–594.

Salthouse, T. A., & Miles, J. D. (2002). Aging and time-sharing aspects of executive control. *Memory and Cognition, 30*, 572–582.

Schneider, B. A., Daneman, M., & Murphy, D. R. (2005). Speech comprehension difficulties in older adults: Cognitive slowing or age-related changes in hearing? *Psychology and Aging, 20*, 261–271.

Schneider, B. A., & Pichora Fuller, M. K. (2000). Implications of perceptual deterioration for cognitive aging research. In F. I. M. Craik, T. A. Salthouse, & A. Timothy (Eds.), *The handbook of aging and cognition* (2nd ed., pp. 155–219). Mahwah, NJ: Lawrence Erlbaum Associates.

Spreen, O., & Strauss, E. (1991). *A compendium of neuropsychological tests: Administration, norms, and commentary*. New York: Oxford University Press.

Spreen, O., & Strauss, E. (1998). *A compendium of neuropsychological tests* (2nd ed.). New York: Oxford.

Southwood, M. H., & Dagenais, P. (2001). The role of attention in apraxic errors. *Clinical Linguistics and Phonetics, 15*, 113–116.

Stine, E. L., Wingfield, A., & Myers, S. D. (1990). Age differences in processing information from television news: The effects of bisensory augmentation. *Journals of Gerontology, 45*, P1–P8.

Suhara, T., Fukuda, H., Inoue, O., Itoh, T., Suzuki, K, Yamasaki, T., et al. (1991). Age-related changes in human D1 dopamine receptors measured by positron emission tomography. *Psychopharmacology, 103*, 41–45.

Trunk, D. L., & Abrams, L. (2009). Do younger and older adults' communicative goals influence off-topic speech in autobiographical narratives? *Psychology and Aging, 24*, 324–337.

Tun, P. A., McCoy, S., & Wingfield, A. (2009). Aging, hearing acuity, and the attentional costs of effortful listening. *Psychology and Aging, 24*, 761–766.

Tun, P. A., O'Kane, G., & Wingfield, A. (2002). Distraction by competing speech in young and older adult listeners. *Psychology and Aging, 17*, 453–467.

Tun, P. A., & Wingfield, A. (1999). One voice too many: Adult age differences in language processing with different types of distracting sounds. *Journals of Gerontology: Series B: Psychological Sciences and Social Sciences, 54b*, P317–P327.

Tun, P. A., Wingfield, A., & Stine, E. A. (1991). Speech-processing capacity in young and older adults: A dual-task study. *Psychology and Aging, 6*, 3–9.

Turner, A., & Greene, E. (1977). *The construction and use of a propositional text base*. Boulder, CO: University of Colorado Psychology Department.

Turner, M. L., & Engle, R. W. (1989). Is working memory capacity task dependent? *Journal of Memory and Language, 28*, 127–154.

Van der Linden, M., Hupet, M., Feyereisen, P., Schelstraete, M.-A., Bestgen, Y., Bruyer, R., . . . et al. (1999). Cognitive mediators of age-related differences in language comprehension and verbal memory performance. *Aging, Neuropsychology, and Cognition, 6*, 32–55.

Van Gerven, P. W. M., Meijer, W. A., Vermeeren, A., Vuurman, E. F., & Jolles, J. (2007). The irrelevant speech effect and the level of interference in aging. *Experimental Aging Research, 33*, 323–339.

Verhaeghen, P., Steitz, D. W., Sliwinski, M. J., & Cerella, J. (2003). Aging and dual-task performance: A meta-analysis. *Psychology and Aging, 18*, 443–460.

Verrel, J., Lövdén, M., Schellenbach, M., Schaefer, S., & Lindenberger, U. (2009). Interacting effects of cognitive load and adult age on the regularity of whole-body motion during treadmill walking. *Psychology and Aging, 24*, 75–81.

Volkow, N. D., Chang, L., Wag, G. J., Fowler, J. S., Lenoido-Yee, M., Franseschi, D., . . . et al. (2000). Association between age-related decline in brain dopamine activity and impairment in frontal and cingulated metabolism. *American Journal of Psychiatry, 157*, 75–80.

Volkow, N. D., Wang, G. J., Fowler, J. S., Ding, Y. S., Gur, R. C., Gatley, J., . . . et al. (1998). Parallel loss of presynaptic and postsynaptic dopamine markers in normal aging. *Annals of Neurology, 44*, 143–147.

Waters, G., & Caplan, D. (1996a). Processing resource capacity and the comprehension of garden path sentences. *Memory and Cognition, 24*, 342–355.

Waters, G. S., & Caplan, D. (1996b). The capacity theory of sentence comprehension: Critique of Just and Carpenter (1992). *Psychological Review, 103*, 761–772.

Waters, G. S., & Caplan, D. (1997). Working memory and on-line sentence comprehension in patients with Alzheimer's disease. *Journal of Psycholinguistic Research, 26*, 337–400.

Waters, G., & Caplan, D. (2001). Age, working memory, and on-line syntactic processing in sentence comprehension. *Psychology and Aging, 16*, 128–144.

Wechsler, D. (1958). *The measurement and appraisal of adult intelligence*. Baltimore: Williams & Wilkins.

Wingfield, A., Peelle, J. E., & Grossman, M. (2003). Speech rate and syntactic complexity as multiplicative factors in speech comprehension by young and older adults. *Aging, Neuropsychology, and Cognition, 10*, 310–322.

Wingfield, A., Tun, P. A., & McCoy, S. L. (2005). Hearing loss in older adulthood: What it is and how it interacts with cognitive performance. *Current Directions in Psychological Science, 14*, 144–148.

Yoon, C., May, C. P., & Hasher, L. (1998). *Aging, circadian arousal patterns, and cognition*. Philadelphia, PA: Psychology Press.

Zacks, R., & Hasher, L. (1997). Cognitive gerontology and attentional inhibition: A reply to Burke and McDowd. *Journal of Gerontology: Psychological Sciences, 52B*, P274–P283.

Tests of Working Memory and Executive Function

Working Memory tests include tests of verbal and visual-spatial span. Tests of Executive Function include neuropsychological tests as well as tests of specific executive functions such as Inhibition, Time-Sharing, Updating, and Switching

WORKING MEMORY TESTS

Verbal Span

Forward and Backward Digit Span tests (Wechsler, 1958): requires participants to recall a series of sets of digits in the correct serial order, either a forward order or backward order. The sets progressive increase in size, from 2 to 9 digits per set. The measure of working memory capacity is the highest number of digits that can be correctly recalled in 2 of 3 sets at that length. Many variants of letter and word span tests have also been developed.

Counting Span tests (Case, Kurland, & Goldberg, 1982): widely used with children and clinical populations due to its simplicity. Participants count shapes, such as green dots, presented in a random visual array interspersed among other shapes, such as yellow dots, and remember the count total. A series of sets, increasing from 1 to 5 arrays per set, is presented. The dependent variable is the highest level at which the participant is able to get two of three sets correct.

Reading Span and Listening Span tests (Daneman & Carpenter, 1980): requires participants to read (or listen to) sentences and remember the final word of each sentence. Progressively larger sets of sentences (13 to 16 words in length) are presented, increasing from two to six sentences in a set with 3 sets being tested at each level. Reading span is defined as the level at which the participant is able to recall all of the items in 2 of the 3 sets tested at that level. Reading span has been shown to be highly predictive of reading skill (Daneman & Merikle, 1996; Daneman & Tardiff, 1987).

Operational span (Ospan) test (Turner & Engle; 1989): involves a presenting a sequence of trials, each consisting of a set of 2, 3, 4, or 5 pairs of mathematical operations and to-be-remembered words. The mathematical operations, e.g., $9/3 - 2 = 1$, are read aloud and then verified as correct or incorrect and the target word is read aloud and remembered. Operational span is defined as the level at which the participant is able to recall of the words in two of three sets.

Visual-Spatial Span

Corsi blocks test (Milner, 1971): requires participants to remember a sequence of spatial locations, pointing to the correct sequence in either a forward or a backward order. Wooden blocks are unevenly distributed over a flat board and the experimenter taps a sequence of blocks and the subject is asked to tap out the same sequence or the reverse sequence. The sequences are random and the difficulty level is progressively raised by increasing the number of blocks tapped. There are three trials at each difficulty level. The subject's spatial span is conventionally taken to be the longest sequence in which at least two out of the three sequences are correctly reproduced.

Visual Pattern Test (Logie, Zucco, & Baddeley, 1990): is designed to assess non-verbal visual short-term memory. The participant is presented with checkerboard patterns, which have been designed to be difficult to code verbally. A visual pattern was created by filling in half the squares in a grid. The grids progress in size from the smallest, a 2×2 matrix (with two filled cells), to the largest, a 5×6 matrix (with 15 filled cells), complexity being steadily increased by adding two more cells to the previous grid. The patterns are displayed in a series of stimulus cards and the participant is asked to reproduce the pattern by marking squares in an empty grid of the same size as the one bearing the pattern just presented. The dependent measure is the number of filled cells in the most complex pattern recalled in the range from 2–15 cells.

EXECUTIVE FUNCTION NEUROPSYCHOLOGICAL TESTS

Wisconsin Card Sorting Test; a computerized version has been developed by Kimberg, D'Esposito, & Farah (2000); asks participants to sort cards based on color, number, or shape. Participants are not told the sorting criterion but receive feedback concerning their sorts and continue sorting 1 card at time until 8 correct sorts have been performed at which point the sorting criterion changes and participants must again sort cards until 8 correct sorts have been made. The test continues until 15 sorting categories or 288 sorts have been made. The dependent measure is the number of perseverative errors when the sorting criterion is changed but the participant failed to change sorting pattern.

Trail Making test (Spreen & Strauss, 1991): another commonly used neuropsychological test of executive function. It involves two tasks. Task A is a simple connect-the-dots task requiring the participant to connect sequentially numbered dots; Task B requires the participant to connect dots using an alternating sequence of letters and numbers. A difference score (B-A) or proportional difference score (B-A/A) is usually computed.

FAS verbal fluency test (Benton & Hamsher, 1989): widely used by neuropsychologists. Participants generate as many words as possible that meet some criterion, such as beginning with a target letter, e.g., F, A, or S, in a limited amount of time. The dependent measure is the total number of correct responses although perseverations (i.e., repeating a response), and intrusions (i.e., incorrect responses) are often scored. There are many variants of the basic fluency test including semantic category and action fluency tests and there is a current debate over how best to assess performance on these tests (see Kemper & McDowd, 2008).

Tower of Hanoi test; a computerized version was developed by Hume, Welsch, Retzlaff, & Cookson (1997); Participants re-arrange a set of disks varying in size placed on 3 pegs in order to match a target configuration. Moves are constrained such that only 1 disk can be moved at a time and a larger disk cannot be placed on a smaller disk. The dependent measure is the total number of moves required to complete the 2 problems.

Executive Function: Inhibition

Stroop task: involves 2 blocks of trials. On the first block of trials, strings of XXXXs are presented printed in different color inks and the participant must name the color of the ink for as many strings as possible during 1 minute; on the second block of trials, the words "red", "green", "blue", and "yellow" are printed in ink of a contrasting color and participant again must name the color of the ink for as many words as possible in 1 min. A difference score (Color words – XXXs) or proportional difference score (Color words – XXXs/color words) is computed.

Stop signal task (Logan, 1994): involves 2 blocks of trials. In the first block of 24 trials, participants categorize a sequence of words as animal/non-animal as rapidly as possible. In the second block of 192 trials, participants are instructed NOT to respond when they hear a tone (presented on 48 randomly selected trials – stop trials). The dependent measure is the proportion of stop trials on which the participant produces categorical responses.

Executive Function: Time-Sharing

Counting backwards plus connections task (Salthouse et al., 2003): participants try to connect a series of numbered dots in order (the dots are scattered about the page) while counting backwards by 3. The dependent measure is the average time per subtraction.

Tracking plus paired associates task (Salthouse & Miles, 2002): participants to use a track ball to keep a cursor on a randomly moving white circle while at the same time performing a paired-associate learning task. The difficulty of tracking task is individually adjusted to match a pre-specified level of accuracy. The learning task involves listening to a series of word pairs followed by the presentation of the first member of each pair and recall of the matching word. The dependent variable is number of correct responses.

Executive Function: Updating

Digit monitoring task (Salthouse et al., 2003): participants listen to a series of digits and to respond to every 3rd odd digit by pressing the letter Z and all other items by pressing the letter M. The primary dependent variable is the percentage of correct responses. In the letter memory (Morris & Jones, 1990) lists of letters are presented. The task is to recall the last 4 letters presented in the list. The number of letters (5, 7, 9, or 11) varies randomly across trials. The dependent measure is the proportion of letters recalled correctly.

N-back task (Mackworth, 1959): requires the participant to listen to a sequence of digits and to repeat the digit that occurred n items back; 1-back, 2-back, etc. tests can be used. The dependent variable is the number of errors.

Executive Function: Switching

Plus-minus switching task (Miyake et al., 2000): consists of 3 lists of 2-digit numbers. On the first list, participants add 3 to each, on the second, they subtract 3, and on the third, they alternate adding and subtracting 3 from each number. A difference score is computed between the time to complete the alternating list and the average time to complete the addition and subtraction lists; a proportional difference score can also be computed.

Letter-letter switching task (Miyake et al., 2000): presents a number and letter pair in 1 of 4 quadrants of a computer screen. Participants are instructed to indicate whether the number was odd or even if the pair was presented in either of the 2 upper quadrants or whether the letter was a vowel or consonant when the pair was presented in either of the 2 lower quadrants. The number-letter pair is presented only in the 2 upper quadrants for a block of 32 trials, then only in the 2 lower quadrants for a block of 32 trials, and then alternating among all 4 quadrants for a block of 32 trials. The dependent measure is the difference in reaction time for 3rd block of trials minus the average reaction time for the first two blocks of trials; a proportional difference score can also be computed.

Local-global switching task (Navon, 1977): requires a participant to focus on either a global figure (e.g., a triangle) or its component "local" figures (e.g., small squares) that compose the global figure. Participants are cued to say aloud the number of lines of the global figure (1 for circle, 2 for X, 3 for triangle, 4 for square) or the number of lines in the local figures. The focus may shift across trials or not. A difference reaction time is computed for the response latencies between shift and no-shift trials; a proportional difference score can also be computed.

2-2

Metrics Used in Language Sample Analysis

Mean Length of Utterance (MLU) reflects the average sentence length in words for a language sample.

Mean Clauses per Utterance (MCU) obtained by identifying each main and embedded or subordinate clause and determining the average number of clauses per utterance for the entire language sample.

Developmental Level (DLevel) based on a scale originally developed by Rosenberg and Abbeduto (1987). The scale ranges from simple one-clause sentences worth 1 point to complex sentences with multiple forms of embedding and subordination worth 7 points. The DLevel for a sample is the average points per sentence based on this scale.

Propositional Density (PDensity) calculated according to the procedures described by Turner and Greene (1977) for decomposing each utterance into its constituent propositions, which represent propositional elements and relations between them. The PDensity for each language sample is defined as the average number of propositions per 100 words.

The lexical diversity of a language sample measured by Type Token Ratio (TTR). The number of different lexical items (types) is compared to the total number of words (tokens). The repetition of pronouns, auxiliary verbs, and other "closed-class" items will reduce type-token ratios.

The incidence of fillers. Both lexical and non-lexical fillers commonly occur in spontaneous speech. Lexical fillers include expressions such as "well" and "you know." Non-lexical fillers include "uh," "umm," and "duh." Fillers markers may serve as placeholders as the speaker attempts to "buy" time for lexical retrieval or syntactic formulation, may mark conceptual or linguistic errors, or serve other pragmatic functions such as hedging or weakening assertions.

The incidence of sentence fragments or the percentage of grammatical sentences in a language sample: Sentence fragments are incomplete sentences lacking either a subject or predicate, other obligatory grammatical constituent. They may result from word finding problems, syntactic planning problems, or other distractions or interruptions. Sentence fragments can also arise from "run-on" sentences as the speaker or writer adds additional information to an already completed sentence.

The rate of speech determined by counting the number of words (or syllables) in a language sample of known duration. Speech rates will be reduced by pauses, non-lexical fillers, and other hesitation phenomena.

Application of the DLevel and PDensity Metrics

Developmental Level (DLevel)

Points are assigned to each sentence and then averaged. Points are determined by grammatical complexity, reflecting the order of emergence of these structures in the speech of children. Points: 0: sentence with a single main clause; 1: sentence with a main clause plus an embedded infinitive; 2: sentence with a main clause plus a wh-clause used in the predicate or a conjoined or compound sentence; 3: sentence with main clause plus a relative clause or a that-clause used in the predicate; 4: sentence main clause plus a gerund used in the predicate or a comparative construction; 5: sentence with a main clause plus a relative clause, wh-clause, that-clause, infinitive clause, or gerund used in subject; 6: sentence with a main clause plus a subordinate clause; 7: sentence with a main clause plus two or more of the above constructions.

Propositional Density (PDensity)

All propositions are identified in a language sample and the average number of propositions per 100 words is computed. Propositions include predicates and relations plus their arguments; propositions may be embedded within other propositions, or link two or more propositions. Predicates typically refer to actions, events, or states and correspond to verbs; arguments refer to persons, objects, times, places, etc. and correspond to nouns. Relations include logical, causal, and temporal connections between propositions such as negation, conjunction or disjunction, and qualities, quantities, or other attributes of arguments.

Example

The English essayist William Hazlitt wrote "Good style is neither more nor less than the way a man who is intelligent, well-educated, urbane, witty and well-traveled, would normally speak."

DLevel = 7

    1 main clause: style is . . .
    2 comparatives: [way is] more than . . .
    [way is] less than . . .
    1 relative clause: man speaks
    5 coordinate relative clauses:
    man is intelligent
    man is well-educated
    man is urbane
    man is witty
    man is well-traveled

PDensity = 6.52 (15 propositions, 23 words)

1. is, style, good
2. speaks, man, way
3. neither, p4
4. more than, p1, p2
5. nor, p6
6. less than, p1, p2
7. speaks, man, normally
8. is, man, intelligent
9. is, man, educated
10. educated, well
11. is, man, urbane
12. is, man, witty
13. is, man, traveled
14. traveled, well
15. and p8, p9, p10, p11, p12, p13, p14

CHAPTER 3

Neuropathologies Underlying Acquired Language Disorders

CHAPTER OUTLINE

Liana S. Rosenthal and Argye E. Hillis

Although it has long been recognized that distinct impairments of language are associated with damage to different locations of the brain, predominantly in the left cortex (Broca, 1865; Dax, 1865; Wernicke, 1881), there has been much less interest in the etiology (underlying disease or other cause) of the brain damage. For example, there has been quite a bit of controversy over the cause of aphasia in Broca's originally described patient, or "Tan," who had a progressive illness that has never been clearly identified (Broca, 1865; Selnes & Hillis, 2000). Often studies of aphasia recovery and rehabilitation combine various etiologies of aphasia as though the cause is unimportant, but this assumption may be unwarranted.

The neurological and systemic diseases that can cause language disorders encompass the entire spectrum of etiologies in medicine (vascular, infectious/postinfectious, traumatic, autoimmune, metabolic/toxic, idiopathic, neoplastic, congenital/hereditary, degenerative). Medical and surgical treatment for these diseases has been met with varying degrees of success, with patients returning to baseline after some disorders, others remaining stable with effective management, while still others deteriorating despite interventions. However, regardless of the probability of clear improvement, even individuals with the most rapidly progressive illness can often benefit from consultation with a speech-language pathologist, as well as other rehabilitation specialists, as indicated. A basic understanding of the disease processes and the likely course of the disease with or without medical intervention will help inform both the limits and expectations of therapy, as well as contribute to the counseling of patients and their families.

For the purpose of gaining a broader understanding of what to expect in patients with specific illnesses, we have divided the causes of language disorders based on the expected disease course (Box 3-1). This classification includes diseases that are acute at onset then slowly improve, those that wax and wane, those that are episodic, and those in which function slowly deteriorates over time. The classic example of diseases that have acute onset and usually slowly improve with medical treatment and therapies is

Box 3-1

Neurological Diseases that Can Result in Language Impairments

ACUTE-ONSET DISEASES THAT REMAIN STABLE OR IMPROVE
Stroke
Acute ischemic stroke
Intracerebral hemorrhage
Subarachnoid hemorrhage
Subdural hemorrhage
Traumatic brain injury
Abscesses
Encephalitis
Acute disseminated encephalomyelitis (ADEM)

IMMUNOCOMPROMISED PATIENTS
Progressive multifocal leukoencephalopathy
Immune reconstitution inflammatory syndrome (IRIS)
HIV infection/AIDS

DISEASES THAT RELAPSE AND REMIT, THEN GENERALLY TREND DOWNWARD
Multiple sclerosis (MS)
Systemic lupus erythematosus (SLE)

DISEASES THAT MAY WORSEN OVER TIME
Alzheimer disease (AD)
Parkinson disease (PD)
Primary progressive aphasia (PPA)
Behavioral variant frontotemporal dementia (bvFTD)
Progressive supranuclear palsy (PSP)
Corticobasal degeneration syndrome (CBD)
Multisystem atrophy (MSA)
Creutzfeldt-Jakob disease (CJD)
Brain tumors

DISEASES THAT ARE EPISODIC
Transient ischemic attacks (TIAs)
Seizures
Migraines

our best efforts. Finally, there are three neurological diseases that are episodic, in which the patient should always return to baseline: seizures, migraines, and transient ischemic attacks (TIAs).

ACUTE-ONSET DISEASES THAT REMAIN STABLE OR IMPROVE

The most well known example of a disease that presents with language impairment is stroke. While most strokes in the United States are acute ischemic strokes (AISs), a sizeable minority of patients present with primary intracerebral hemorrhage (Brazis, Masdeu, & Biller, 2007). Subarachnoid hemorrhage accounts for an even smaller percentage of strokes. AIS and intracerebral hemorrhage (ICH) share some common risk factors, including hypertension, smoking, diabetes, and obesity. If the AIS or ICH affects the language networks in the brain, patients and observers will describe a sudden onset in difficulty speaking or understanding as well as additional neurological symptoms. Subarachnoid hemorrhage usually presents very differently but can result in delayed AIS from vasospasm. Direct sequelae of the subarachnoid hemorrhage, including diffuse cognitive deficits, as well as possible interventions will be discussed in detail later.

Acute Ischemic Stroke

For patients with AIS, the first few days after the stroke are the critical period during which some brain tissue may be saved. If the patient is admitted within several hours of onset of symptoms, the initial focus will be on saving brain tissue and restoring immediate brain function, by restoring blood flow to ischemic tissue via thrombolytic agents, clot retrieval, surgical intervention, or other methods. The medical team caring for the stroke patient will then likely institute blood pressure, glucose, and temperature management to reduce the risk of brain swelling or worsening of the patient's neurological deficits and will take measures to reduce complications of stroke, such as deep venous thrombosis, aspiration pneumonia, and contractures. They will also search for the etiology of the AIS to prevent recurrence. Of patients with AIS, the 30-day case fatality is about 25% (although this rate is lower in dedicated stroke units), with the greatest predictor of mortality being stroke severity (Hankey, 2003). Death is usually secondary to the stroke itself and its resulting sequelae. Especially in the first 3 to 5 days post stroke, significant brain swelling may occur that can result in herniation and subsequent death. Overall, however, patients with small to moderate-size AIS generally do well, with a rapid improvement in

stroke. In diseases whose symptoms wax and wane over time, patients may at first return to baseline between exacerbations of the disease, but eventually many patients slowly accumulate deficits and ultimately demonstrate a slow, downhill progression. Multiple sclerosis is the most well known of this disease type. There are also numerous neurodegenerative diseases, including primary progressive aphasia, for which there is currently no disease-modifying therapy. Patients with these illnesses therefore slowly worsen over time, usually developing more symptoms despite deficits within the first week to months after the ischemic event and then a slowing in the rate of improvement over the next year. Although it is often taught that patients show minimal improvement after 1 year from the precipitating event, there is no basis for this teaching. Many patients continue to show functional recovery for the remaining years of their life, if they continue to work toward learning new ways to function better. The mechanisms of recovery are likely to change over time. In the first few days, restoration of tissue function likely accounts for early recovery of language. Reorganization of structure-function relationships, in which undamaged parts of the brain assume functions of the damaged parts, is likely an important part of subacute recovery days to weeks after AIS onset, a process that can be facilitated by intense speech-language therapy (and perhaps augmented by certain medications that affect neurotransmitter release and reuptake) (Hillis, 2005). Finally, reorganization of cognitive processes underlying language and compensation can take place for months or years after stroke and can be facilitated by intense practice at home, guided by a speech-language pathologist, family member, or other coach.

The language function in AIS can fluctuate in the first few days and weeks after stroke, and these fluctuations can reflect changes in cerebral blood flow (Croquelois, Wintermark, Reichhart, et al., 2003; Hillis, 2007; Ochfeld, Newhart, Molitoris, et al., 2009) and/or changes in neurotransmitter release and reuptake reflected in, or caused by, fluctuation in motivation, mood, response to rehabilitation, positive and negative responses to medications, and so on. The etiology of AIS is important in understanding the course, the probability if recurrence, and possibility of recovery. For example, AIS due to coagulopathy caused by cancer is likely to recur unless the cancer can be cured. AIS caused by carotid stenosis might never recur if the patient is a candidate for endarterectomy to reverse the carotid stenosis. AIS due to atrial fibrillation will be much less likely to recur if atrial fibrillation can be reversed with cardioversion to a normal cardiac rhythm, and somewhat less likely to recur if the patient is anticoagulated with blood thinner chronically. The course of lacunar strokes (strokes smaller than 1 cm or 1.5 cm) is nearly always stable; the course of strokes caused by narrowing of the middle cerebral artery may be stuttering or progressive over several days (Figure 3-1).

Deficits observed in AIS can be explained by the affected vascular territories. The classic aphasia classifications are vascular syndromes, or collections of language symptoms that commonly co-occur because the functions

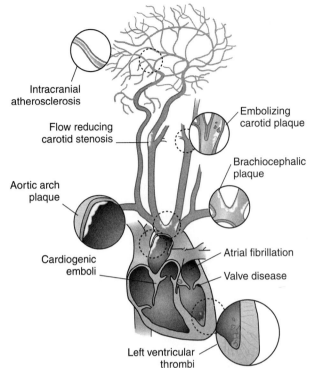

Figure 3-1 Cardiogenic and arterial atherosclerotic sources for stroke. [From Townsend. (2007). *Sabiston textbook of surgery* (18th ed.). Philadelphia: Saunders Elsevier.]

affected are localized to a particular vascular territory. Therefore, the relationship between dysfunction in a particular area (low blood flow or infarct in a vascular territory) and a particular aphasia syndrome is much stronger in the acute stage of stroke than in chronic stroke, after some patients have shown significant recovery but still have the lesion (Croquelois et al., 2003; Ochfeld et al., 2009). For example, blockage in the superior division of the left middle cerebral artery (MCA) typically results in ischemia to the left posterior inferior frontal cortex and a Broca's aphasia. These patients typically have nonfluent, apractic, agrammatic speech output, poor repetition, and relatively spared comprehension at least of simple syntactic structures at onset. As the motor strip is often also involved, these patients typically also have right face and arm weakness greater than right leg weakness. The *left* face, arm, and leg as well as visual fields will be spared. If the lesion is relatively restricted to this area, many recover relatively quickly and may have no deficits 6 months later (Ochfeld et al., 2009). In contrast, ischemia in the posterior superior temporal cortex secondary to a blockage in the inferior division of the left MCA generally leads to fluent but meaningless speech output, poor repetition, and poor comprehension, classified as Wernicke's aphasia (Croquelois et al., 2003; Ochfeld et al., 2009). These patients may also have a subtle, usually clinically under-appreciated, right-sided hemispatial neglect as well as superior quadrantanopia but no arm or leg weakness. Because emboli from the heart tend to travel down the inferior division, rather than up the superior division of the MCA, cardioembolic strokes are more likely to cause Wernicke's aphasia than Broca's aphasia (Urbinelli, Bolard, Lemesle, et al., 2001), again underscoring that these are vascular syndromes (Figure 3-2).

"Watershed" strokes are a special case of AIS with a somewhat different mechanism from simple occlusion of an artery leading to loss of blood flow to the territory of one artery. They often occur when there is severe narrowing of one or more cerebral vessels, combined with sudden drop in blood pressure. Imagine having two sprinklers that provide water to your yard. You have positioned them such that they just cover the yard but do not overlap. If suddenly the water pressure drops, there will be a strip of yard between the two sprinklers where the water from neither sprinkler will reach. Likewise, if there is a sudden drop in blood pressure, especially if there is narrowing of the carotid artery that supplies the MCA and anterior cerebral artery (ACA), there will be a strip of brain that will not receive adequate blood from either the MCA or the ACA. Ischemia in the watershed areas between the left MCA and left ACA territories generally results in transcortical motor aphasia with relatively preserved comprehension and repetition but nonfluent speech with difficulty initiating and organizing responses (Hillis, 2007). In addition, patients with a transcortical motor aphasia

may also have right leg greater than arm weakness and a relative sparing of facial musculature, because the leg area of the motor strip, medial to the arm and face is in this "watershed" area. Ischemia in the watershed area between the left MCA and left posterior cerebral artery (PCA) often results in a transcortical sensory aphasia in which the patient has poor comprehension and mean-ingless speech but relatively preserved repetition. These patients may also have a hemianopsia and a hemihyp-esthesia, where patients have difficulty on the affected side with two-point discrimination and stereoagnosia because parts of the sensory strip lie in this territory. There are, of course, numerous other aphasia syn-dromes and aphasic deficits that do not fit within vascular syndromes, which are beyond the scope of the chapter (Figure 3-3).

While not strictly resulting in aphasia, right hemi-sphere strokes will also lead to communication disor-ders. These deficits include reduced understanding of the humor, intent, connotation, and affective prosody of speech, in part because of difficulty integrating lan-guage and its context. Patients with right hemisphere lesions have difficulty understanding the nonliteral meaning of words and sentences. For example, when observing someone carrying a load of books, a patient with a right hemisphere lesion might reply "yes" when asked "could you open the door for me?" Most others would understand that the book-carrier actually wants the door opened for them (Mitchell & Crow, 2005). Patients with right hemisphere lesions can also have great difficulty understanding the emotion conveyed by a person's tone of voice or can have trouble convey-ing emotion through prosody (Ross & Monnot, 2008).

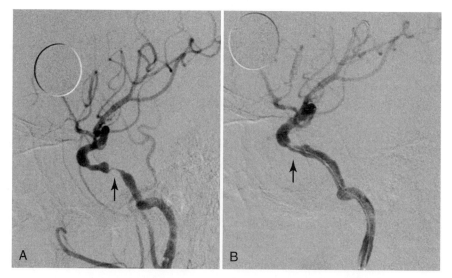

Figure 3-2   A, Intracranial high-grade symptomatic stenosis. **B,** This patient failed aggressive medical therapy and responded only to angioplasty and stenting. [From Ferri, F. F. (2010). *Clinical advisor 2011.* Philadelphia: Elsevier Saunders.]

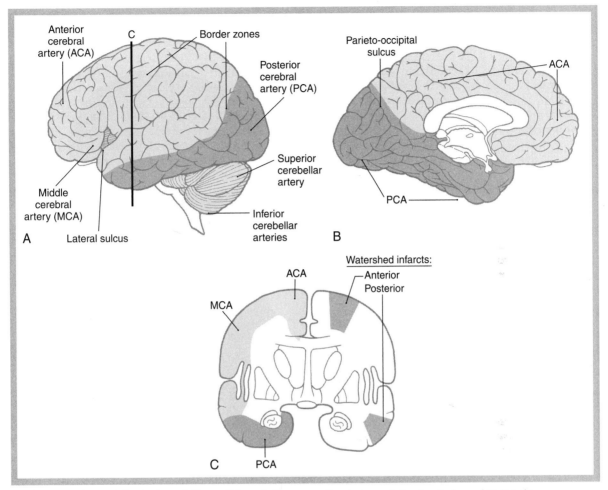

Figure 3-3 A, Lateral, **B,** medial, and **C,** cross-sectional views of the hemisphere showing the regions served by the anterior cerebral *(light grey)*, middle cerebral *(medium grey)*, and posterior cerebral *(dark grey)*, arteries. The distal territories of these vessels overlap at their peripheries and create border zones. These zones are susceptible to infarcts **(C)** in cases of hypoperfusion of the vascular bed. Small border zones also exist **(A)** between superior *(no shading)* and inferior *(light grey)* cerebellar arteries. [From Haines, D. E. (2006). *Fundamental neuroscience for basic and clinical applications* (3rd ed.). St Louis: Elsevier.]

For example, the phrase "She stole my money" has slightly different meanings if the emphasis is placed on the *she* versus an emphasis on the *my* or the *money*. Patient with right cortical lesions also sometimes have difficulty with metaphors. Subjects with right cortical lesions asked to select which of two drawings conveyed the meaning of the phrase "he had a heavy heart" more often chose the photograph with the literal meaning of a person stumbling with a large heart tied to his back as opposed to the photograph of a person crying (Winner & Gardner, 1977). Some of these patients also perform poorly on tasks of discourse comprehension, such as understanding the main theme of a paragraph or a conversation (Hough, 1990). The relationships between site of lesion and type of communication deficit have not been clearly identified after right hemisphere ischemic stroke but are under investigation.

Intracerebral Hemorrhage

ICH accounts for approximately 10% to 15% of all strokes in the United States (Brazis et al., 2007) and has a significantly higher mortality compared to AIS, with only 38% of affected patients surviving the first year (Qureshi, Tuhrim, Broderick, et al., 2001). A low score on the Glasgow Coma Scale (GCS), a large volume of the hematoma, and the presence of intraventricular blood on the initial CT scan are three factors that have consistently been associated with a high mortality rate (Qureshi et al., 2001). The increased mortality associated with intraventricular blood may be secondary to a direct mass effect of the blood on periventricular structures or may relate to the development of obstructive hydrocephalus.

In an effort to decrease the morbidity and mortality associated with intraventricular blood, these patients often have catheters placed in their ventricles to facilitate external drainage of cerebrospinal fluid. The goal is to relieve the pressure buildup and hydrocephalus that develop because of the blood clotting in the ventricles. These catheters are not ideal because they have a high infection risk and they often clot with the very blood they are supposed to be draining. There is, therefore, continued interest in administering thrombolytic agents into the ventricles of patients with intraventricular hemorrhages, and small studies have shown an improvement in mortality with this approach (Qureshi et al., 2001).

Management of ICH may also involve surgical evacuation of the clot. This surgery serves to relieve the pressure of the blood on the brain, prevents the release of neuropathic products from the hematoma, and prevents prolonged interaction between blood and normal brain tissue. In practice, hemorrhages that are deep within the brain in the basal ganglia and thalamus are not evacuated as the damage to more superficial brain structures would be too great. Cerebellar bleeds and cortical bleeds, however, could benefit from surgical evacuation based on their locations but large randomized control trials have yet to show benefit.

Similar to AIS, the deficits related to ICH are directly related to the localization of the damaged tissue. ICHs, however, do not respect the vascular territories so patients do not present with the classic aphasia syndromes described earlier. Instead, ICHs have five typical locations where they occur: the cerebral lobes ("lobar hemorrhage"), basal ganglia, thalamus, brainstem, and cerebellum (Figure 3-4). Patients with hemorrhage in the deep brain structures of the left hemisphere including the basal ganglia, internal capsule, and the adjacent white matter lesions have been noted to suffer from articulatory impairment in addition to comprehension and naming impairments. Left hemisphere thalamic lesions led to impairments in naming and repetition. Right hemisphere thalamic lesions led to a deficit in the elaboration of narratives and integrating elements within a context. For example, these patients had difficulty describing the

activity of the subjects in a picture (Radanovic & Scaff, 2003). Patients with large ICHs typically present with a decreased level of consciousness. In addition, patients often have headaches, nausea, and emesis due to increased intracranial pressure and may have meningismus secondary to blood in the ventricles.

The most common risk factor for ICH is idiopathic hypertension, especially ICH in the basal ganglia, thalamus, or brainstem. However, ICH may also be secondary to amyloid angiopathy, arteriovenous malformations, intracranial aneurysms, and other vascular malformations. Arteriovenous malformations are abnormal communications between arteries and veins that tend to bleed; their treatment with radiosurgery, surgery, or embolization is controversial, as rebleeding is common with and without treatment (Stapf, Mohr,

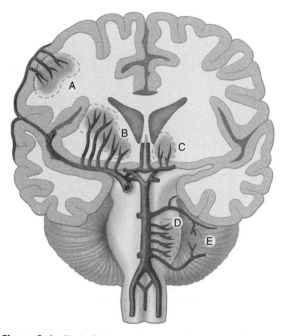

Figure 3-4 Typical sites and sources of intracerebral hemorrhage. Intracerebral hemorrhages most commonly involve the cerebral lobes and originate from penetrating cortical branches of the anterior, middle, or posterior cerebral arteries (*A*); the basal ganglia and originate from ascending lenticulostriate branches of the middle cerebral artery (*B*); the thalamus and originate from ascending thalamogeniculate branches of the posterior cerebral artery (*C*); the pons and originate from paramedian branches of the basilar artery (*D*); and the cerebellum and originate from penetrating branches of the posterior inferior, anterior inferior, or superior cerebellar arteries *E*. [From Qureshi, A. I., Tuhrim, S., Broderick, J. P., et al. (2001). Spontaneous intracerebral hemorrhage. *New England Journal of Medicine, 344*, 1450–1460.]

Choi, et al., 2006). In addition, dural venous sinus thrombosis can lead to an ICH as can an intracranial primary neoplasm or metastasis of a systemic neoplasm. Melanoma, renal cell carcinoma, and choreocarcinoma are cancers that commonly bleed. Other common cancers that metastasize to the brain and sometime hemorrhage are breast and lung cancer. Cocaine and alcohol use have also been associated with an increased ICH risk. Finally, the ICH may be secondary in part to a coagulopathy, most often caused by anticoagulant use (Qureshi et al., 2001). Venous hemorrhage can be caused by thrombosis of the cerebral veins (also called cerebral sinuses). It is common for large AISs to show hemorrhagic conversion, but this does not change the prognosis for the AIS unless it is large and causes acute

increased intracranial pressure (e.g., in some cases after thrombolysis); hemorrhagic conversion of ischemic stroke is not considered ICH.

Although patients with ICH initially seem much more ill and have a lower level of consciousness than do patients with AIS, if they survive the acute period, they generally do well. Once the blood is reabsorbed, there may be little permanent damage. An exception to this brighter prognosis is the increasingly recognized etiology of cerebral amyloid angiopathy, the most common cause of lobar hemorrhage, particularly in people over 60. It is typically diagnosed by the presence of multiple microhemorrhages in the cortex (see Figure 3-5) and is associated with high risk of recurrent lobar hemorrhage and progressive dementia and, to a lesser extent, with infarct and SAH.

Cerebral Amyloid Angiopathy Case

A previously healthy 53-year-old woman developed progressive confusion, memory lapses, hallucinations, and difficulties completing activities of daily living. She was started on antipsychotics and antidepressants and moved in with her daughter, who could assist her. She also had a brief admission to psychiatry due to her hallucinations. Her condition continued to worsen, and 7 months after the onset of symptoms the patient was taken to the emergency department for further evaluation. Neurological examination revealed that she was oriented only to person. She could name simple objects and follow simple commands. Mini-Mental Status Examination score was 19 of 30. Head CT scan in the emergency department showed an intraventricular hemorrhage, possibly originating from the left choroid plexus, as well as diffuse periventricular patchy hypoattenuation. MR images demonstrated innumerable small bleeds (see Figure 3-5). Workup for lymphoma, a metastatic process, and sarcoidosis was negative. Given the patient's young age, a brain biopsy was performed to confirm the diagnosis. Pathology revealed cortical and leptomeningeal vessels containing beta amyloid, confirming the diagnosis of cerebral amyloid angiopathy (CAA). This case may represent an index case of familial CAA, in view of her young age.

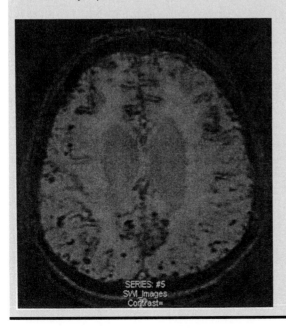

Figure 3-5 Cerebral amyloid angiopathy case: The susceptibility weighted MRI of the patient showing numerous areas of hypointensity is consistent with small bleeds.

Subarachnoid Hemorrhage

SAH accounts for most of the remaining 2% to 5% of all strokes. The average case-fatality rate is about 51%. While SAH accounts for 5% of deaths from stroke, it accounts for 27% of all stroke-related years of potential life lost before the age of 65 (Suarez, Tarr, & Selman, 2006). This high morbidity rate reflects the fact that SAH often occurs at a younger age than other strokes. About 85% of all nontraumatic SAHs are the result or a ruptured intracranial aneurysm (Van Gijn & Rinkel, 2001). Head trauma is the most common cause of SAH, but SAH is rarely the isolated injury in these cases (Figure 3-6).

Headache and decreased level of consciousness are the most common presentations of aneurysmal SAH. Localizable deficits are related to the location of the ruptured aneurysm and subsequent bleed. Common initial signs include a third nerve palsy, a sixth nerve palsy, bilateral lower extremity weakness, abulia, visuospatial neglect, or the combination of hemiparesis and aphasia. Subsequent localizable deficits are often secondary to vasospasm, which is symptomatic in 46% of patients after SAH (Suarez et al., 2006). Delayed cerebral vasospasm, causing infarcts and increased intracranial

pressure, is now the leading cause of death and disability among patients with aneurysmal SAH (Brazis et al., 2007). Other common sequelae include hydrocephalus in 20% of patients and rebleeding in 7% of patients (Suarez et al., 2006).

Initial management of SAH generally includes a conventional angiogram for evaluation of a possible aneurysm. If an aneurysm is found, early management of the aneurysm with either microvascular surgical clipping or endovascular coiling improves mortality and allows for better management of neurological complications (Whitfield & Kirkpatrick, 2001). Both methods of securing a ruptured aneurysm have been shown to be effective, and the decision regarding which method to use is based on characteristics of both the patient and the aneurysm.

Further management of the patient often involves starting an antiepileptic medication prophylactically and monitoring for complications. Possible vasospasm is monitored through transcranial Doppler ultrasound and, if it develops, treated with hypertension, hypervolemia, and hemodilution. Should hydrocephalus develop, an intraventricular catheter may be placed. These patients are also at risk for medical complications

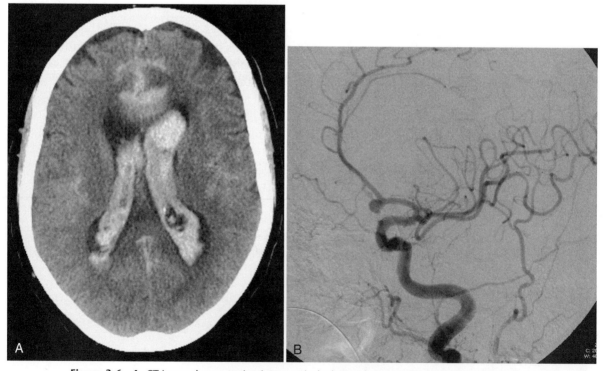

Figure 3-6   A, CT image demonstrating intraventricular hemorrhage as well as subarachnoid hemorrhage in a patient with a ruptured left anterior communicating aneurysm. **B,** The aneurysm is demonstrated on the oblique anteroposterior view of the catheter left carotid cerebral angiogram. [From Haaga, J. R. (2009). *CT and MRI of the whole body* (5th ed.). Philadelphia: Elsevier Mosby.]

including pulmonary edema and electrolyte abnormalities, so patients are also monitored in a critical care setting and treated appropriately.

Most survivors of SAH are able to live with their families and gain independence in activities of daily living. In one study, two-thirds of the patients who had been working prior to the SAH had returned to that position 1 year later; on average, they were away from work for 20 weeks (Hackett & Anderson, 2000). Despite these positive outcomes, many survivors report difficulties with neuropsychological functioning. One year after SAH, there was a significant reduction in patient-reported health-related quality of life and difficulties with memory, mood, speech, and self-care. Overall, one-third to one-half of the patients report reductions in their ability to perform their social role (Hackett & Anderson, 2000). The grade, or severity, of SAH is the best predictor of impairment of cognition and memory (Ogden, Mee, & Henning, 1993). Many benefit from cognitive rehabilitation to return to work.

Subdural Hematoma

Similar to strokes, subdural hematomas (SDHs) (Figure 3-7) may also present with aphasia or other focal neurological deficits (Dell, Batson, Kasdon, & Peterson, 1983; Kaminski, Hlavin, Likavec, & Schmidley, 1992; Mori & Maeda, 2001; Moster, Johnston, & Reinmuth, 1983). The focal presentations are often secondary to the blood pushing on the brain and therefore inhibiting cortical function. Alternative presentations include headache, seizure, and psychiatric abnormalities (Ernestus, Beldzinski, Lanfermann, & Klug, 1997). SDHs may be acute or chronic and are most often a result of trauma. Other etiologies include neurosurgical treatment for other reasons, anticoagulant therapy, coagulopathy, and alcoholism (Mori & Maeda, 2001; Ernestus et al., 1997). Management usually involves correcting any coagulopathy, considering prophylactic antiepileptic medication, and also considering surgical evacuation. For acute SDHs, surgical evacuation is recommended for all SDHs with a thickness greater than 10 mm or those that result in midline shift greater than 5 mm. For

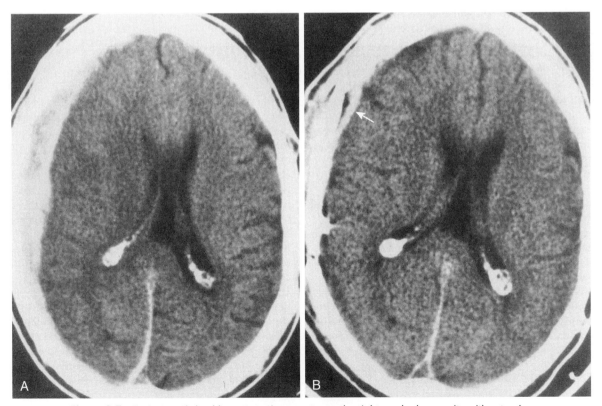

Figure 3-7　A, Acute subdural hematoma is present over the right cerebral convexity with extension into the interhemispheric fissure posteriorly. **B,** Postoperative scan reveals small residual hematoma *(arrow).* [From Haaga, J. R. (2009). *CT and MRI of the whole body* (5th ed.). Philadelphia: Elsevier Mosby.]

smaller SDHs or those with less of a midline shift, surgical evacuation should be performed in patients with a rapidly decreasing GCS score, an enlarged pupil, and/or an intracranial pressure greater than 20 mm Hg (Bullock, Chesnut, Ghajar, et al., 2006). Surgical evacuation in chronic subdural hematomas often follows similar guidelines. For smaller, chronic SDHs, that do not appear to be leading to devastating neurological sequalae, or in patients with too high of a surgical risk, it is reasonable to manage the SDH expectantly. Patients often undergo numerous computed tomography (CT) scans and monitoring of their neurological symptoms and, overtime, the SDH may spontaneously resolve (Parlato, Guarracino, & Moraci, 2000).

Mortality is generally high in patients with acute SDH, but there is a wide range of rates noted, with death occurring in 12% of patients in one study and in 60% of patients in another (Bershad, Farhadi, Suri, et al., 2008; Koc, Akdemir, Oktem, et al., 1997). The difference in prognosis seems to rest primarily on whether surgical intervention is warranted, with higher mortality seen in patients who require surgical evacuation of the blood (Senft, Schuster, Forster, et al., 2009). Poor prognosis is also associated with advanced age, low GCS score on admission, signs of elevated intracranial pressure clinically, and CT findings of a large hematoma volume and midline shift. Coagulopathy prior to acute SDH, most often secondary to anticoagulation treatment, has also been associated with worse prognosis in some studies (Bershad et al., 2008) but other studies report no mortality difference (Senft et al., 2009). Most of the studies in the literature discuss mortality as the primary outcome and data on neurological morbidity are therefore difficult to determine.

In contrast to acute SDH, most patients with chronic SDH have a good outcome, although most of the literature reviews only patients who underwent surgical evacuation. One case series reported about 89% of patients having a good recovery, while 8% of patients showed no change in their deficits and about 2% worsened (Mori & Maeda, 2001). If the patient responds well to treatment and the SDH resolves, the neurological deficits also improve. One case series of 104 patients reported that about 70% were discharged from the hospital without any neurological deficit or with only mild deficits (Ernestus et al., 1997).

Traumatic Brain Injury

Traumatic brain injury (TBI) can result in numerous neuropsychiatric and neurological manifestations beyond the scope of this chapter. Mild TBI, consisting of only a brief loss or alteration of consciousness, is associated with delayed memory and fluency in the acute period (Belanger, Curtiss, Demery, et al., 2005). While most patients with mild TBI recovered within 3 to 12 months after the event, pending litigation was associated with stabilization or worsening of neurological deficits over time (Carroll, Cassidy, Peloso, et al., 2004). Patients with severe TBI, usually associated with a more prolonged loss of consciousness including coma for longer than 1 week, are afflicted with long-term difficulties, often in the realm of psychiatric symptomatology, decreased cognitive function, and difficulties with social functioning. These difficulties often result in trouble with employment as well as difficulties with independent functioning (Hoofien, Gilboa, Vakil, & Donovick, 2001). Patients with severe TBI do have the capacity to improve, specifically in areas of cognitive speed, visuoconstruction, and verbal memory (Millis, Rosenthal, Novack, et al., 2001). In children, TBI has been associated with language difficulties in both the acute and chronic stage, with children demonstrating difficulties with propositions and cognitive organization of speech as late as 3 years after the TBI (Ewing-Cobbs, Brookshire, Scott, & Fletcher, 1998).

Infections and Postinfectious Inflammatory Conditions

Language disorders may also be secondary to inflammation of the brain parenchymal tissue. This brain inflammation may be the result of an infection, including abscess or encephalitis, or an inflammatory disease such as acute disseminated encephalomyelitis. Brain infections may occur in both immunocompetent and immunocompromised patients, although the latter are at risk for additional infections and inflammatory reactions. Meningitis is one of the better known brain infections; it is inflammation of the meninges surrounding the brain and therefore should not result in a language disorder and will not be further discussed here, although it can be devastating to the afflicted patient.

Brain Abscesses

Brain abscesses are a rare type of infection in the United States, with about 1500 to 2500 cases reported yearly (Mamelak, Mampalam, Obana, & Rosenblum, 1995). With improvement in surgical techniques and antibiotic therapy, the mortality from abscesses has declined significantly since the 1970s and has remained steady at less than 10% since the 1990s (Mathisen & Johnson, 1997; Yang & Zhao, 1993). Brain abscess (Figure 3-8) is a focal, intracerebral infection that begins as a localized area of cerebritis and develops into a collection of pus

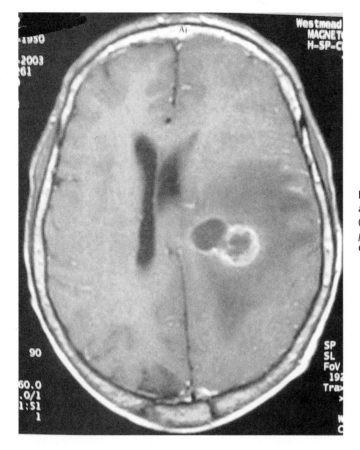

Figure 3-8 Brain abscess. MRI showing *Nocardia* brain abscess. [From Mandell, G. L., Bennett, J. E., & Dolin, R. (2010). *Mandell, Douglas, and Bennett's principles and practice of infectious diseases* (7th ed.). Philadelphia: Churchill Livingstone.]

surrounded by a well-vascularized capsule (Mathisen & Johnson, 1997). Abscesses are classified based on the most likely entry point of the infection, which is usually direct or indirect spread from infection in the paranasal sinuses, middle ear, or teeth. Metastastic seeding of the brain from distant extracranial sources such as the heart valves is another important source of infection.

The most common presenting complaint of brain abscess is a nonspecific, dull headache. Mental status changes, focal neurological deficits, and fever are also common, with these symptoms occurring in about 30% to 60% of cases. Similar to stroke, the focal deficits are related to the brain function in the area of the abscess. A patient with a large abscess may present with signs of increased intracranial pressure including increased somnolence, generalized confusion, and even papilledema (Tunkel, 2005). Imaging is the primary method of diagnosing the abscess, with both CT scanning and magnetic resonance (MRI) imaging having characteristic findings. Treatment usually consists of antimicrobial therapy and drainage of the abscess (Mathisen & Johnson, 1997). Outcome is most closely related to neurological status on admission, and one case series determined that about 62% of patients have a favorable outcome, defined in this case as not being in a vegetative state and not being completely dependent for all activities of daily living (Xiao, Tseng, Teng, & Tseng, 2005).

Development of a brain abscess is associated with specific risk factors. For example, patients with poorly controlled diabetes are at particular risk for fungal abscesses. Furthermore, numerous case reports indicate that the breakdown of the blood-brain barrier associated with ischemic (Chen, Tang, & Ro, 1995; Miyazaki, Ito, Nitta, et al., 2004) and hemorrhagic strokes (Nakai, Yamamoto, Yasuda, & Matsumura, 2006) is an increased risk factor for abscesses in those locations. Neoplasms may also serve as a nidus of infection, although not secondary to surgical manipulation at the tumor site. Instead, bacteremia and sinusitis were the primary etiology, indicating a spread of the organism through the blood (Kalita, Kala, Svebisova, et al., 2008).

Encephalitis

While an abscess is an actual collection of pus in the brain, encephalitis is an inflammation of the brain parenchyma or tissue itself. Patients with encephalitis often present with somnolence, even appearing to fall asleep during the examination. Focal findings are comparatively rare in patients with encephalitis, being observed in only about 10% to 20% of all patients (but much more common in herpes encephalitis, as described later). Encephalitis may occur secondary to a virus or bacterium that directly invades the brain or may manifest as the result of a postinfectious, autoimmune inflammatory condition.

Regardless of the etiology, the result is an acute inflammatory reaction with neuronal necrosis or damage. As a result, the brain tissue becomes edematous and possibly demyelinated and subsequently develops white matter lesions as well as hemorrhages, hypoperfusion, and diminished cerebrovascular reserves (Goozee & Murdoch, 2009). Morbidity and mortality are related to the etiology of the encephalitis and availability of medical care, with outcomes ranging from no neurological sequelae to death. Among patients who survive, there is a broad range of cognitive and language problems reported. Most of the literature focuses on viral encephalitis cases, and lasting communication problems ranging from dysarthria through mutism have been reported (Goozee & Murdoch, 2009).

While a discussion of every type of viral and bacterial encephalitis (Figure 3-9) is beyond the scope of this chapter, special attention is warranted to herpes simplex encephalitis (HSE). HSE is the most common, fatal, sporadic encephalitis in humans, with about 2000 cases annually in the United States. Untreated, HSE has a mortality rate of about 70% with fewer than 3% of survivors returning to normal function. Even with treatment, mortality remains about 20% to 30% (Whitley, Alford, & Hirsch, 1986). Patients with HSE often present with confusion, fever, personality changes, and focal neurological findings including aphasia. Fascinating cases of category-specific semantic deficits caused by HSE have been described (Warrington & Shallice, 1984). Studies investigating the neurological sequelae of HSE mostly predate our current treatment paradigms, so morbidity rates may overestimate the sequelae of the disease. These studies indicated that approximately 38% of patients return to normal function after HSE (Whitley, 2006). Thus, at least until recently, most patients have had significant neurological impairment. The neurological sequelae of the virus is reflected in its predilection for the mesial temporal lobes, with patients often showing significant dysnomia, decreased verbal intelligence, and moderate-to-severe impairments of new learning and memory.

Herpes Simplex Encephalitis Case

A 32-year-old man with a history of mood disorder was admitted to the neurology service following a generalized tonic-clonic seizure. He had been on the psychiatric service 3 days prior to admission. While on the psychiatric service he was noted to be febrile and no source was found. Once discharged home from psychiatry, he had headaches, fever, and chills and was confused and forgetful. On admission, neurologic examination was notable only for a Wernicke's aphasia, with fluent, grammatical speech, but limited content, frequent semantic paraphasias, and poor word comprehension. His naming was especially poor for living things (animals, fruits, and vegetables). The patient was started on intravenous acyclovir for suspected herpes encephalitis. Lumbar puncture revealed a lymphocytic pleocytosis, and the herpes simplex virus polymerase chain reaction returned with a positive result a few days later. MRI revealed a left temporal lobe hyperintensity. During the hospitalization, the patient became agitated and confused, and a subsequent CT scan showed a large left temporal hemorrhage and uncal herniation. The patient did well with aggressive treatment of increased intracranial pressure, and he was ultimately discharged home with an examination notable for decreased ability to name low-frequency items with semantic paraphasias, difficulty repeating complicated phrases, and verbal memory deficits. His most recent evaluation was 9 years after his herpes simplex encephalitis diagnosis. While he was able to return to work full-time in a high-level position, he reported continued difficulty with word retrieval and recall of verbal information. Neuropsychological testing was broadly within normal limits, however.

West Nile virus can cause an almost identical encephalitis with aphasia and verbal memory deficits.

Acute Disseminated Encephalomyelitis

An encephalitis can also develop from a postinfectious, immune-mediated inflammatory disorder, the most common of which is termed *acute disseminated encephalomyelitis* (ADEM). ADEM predominantly affects the white matter of the brain and spinal cord and is more common in pediatric patients than in adults. It is classically a monophasic disorder, although there are numerous reports of relapses. Patients present with a rapid-onset encephalopathy and multifocal neurological deficits including aphasia, determined by the location

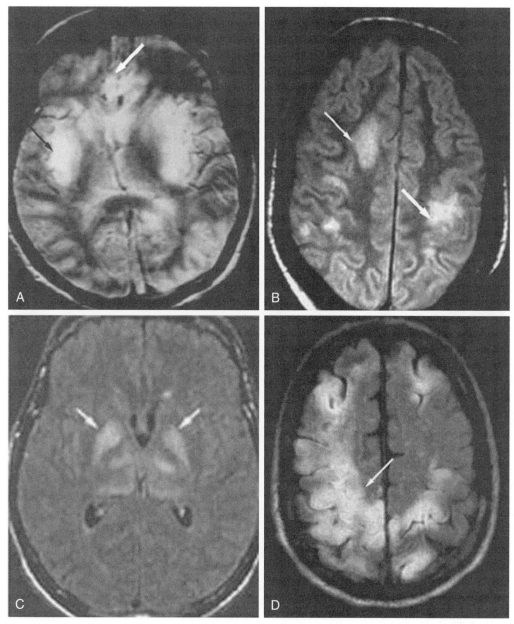

Figure 3-9   Typical MRI changes associated with viral encephalitis. **A,** Herpes simplex virus type 1 encephalitis with increased T2-weighted signal in bilateral temporal lobes. Increased signal does not extend beyond the insular cortex *(thin arrow)* but does involve the cingulated gyrus *(thick arrow).* **B,** Varicella-zoster virus vasculopathy on proton-density MRI scan with multiple areas of infarction in both hemispheres *(arrows).* **C,** West Nile virus encephalitis with increased signal on FLAIR MRI of the basal ganglia *(arrows).* **D,** Enterovirus encephalitis with increased signal intensity on FLAIR MRI in both hemispheres, greater on the right, in the posterior cerebral hemisphere *(arrow).* [**A, B, D** from Gilden, D. H., Mahalingam, R., Cohrs, R. J., & Tyler, K. L. (2007). Herpesvirus infections of the nervous system. *Nature Clinical Practice Neurology, 3,* 83. **C** from Debiasi, R. L., & Tyler, K. L. (2006). West Nile virus meningoencephalitis. *Nature Clinical Practice Neurology, 2,* 264.]

of the lesions within the central nervous system. While there are no randomized controlled trials regarding ADEM treatment, it is usually treated as an inflammatory disorder, with a combination of high-dose steroids, intravenous immunoglobulin, and/or plasma exchange. Outcome is usually very good, with mortality rates less than 5% in pediatric studies and ranging from 8% to 25% in adult populations (Sonneville, Klein, de Broucker, & Wolff, 2009). Behavioral and cognitive sequelae are seen in 6% to 50% of all survivors of ADEM, although these are likely underreported (Tenembaum, Chitnis, Ness, & Hahn, 2007). Recent studies suggest that even children thought to have full recovery demonstrate subtle neurocognitive deficits in attention, executive function, and behavior when evaluated more than 3 years after ADEM (Hahn, Miles, MacGregor, et al., 2003). In addition, other studies reported slower verbal processing (Jacobs, Anderson, Neale, et al., 2004). Among adults who required intensive care unit admission as a result of ADEM, 35% of the patients had persistent sensory or motor sequelae (Sonneville et al., 2009).

Immunocompromised Patients

There is a subset of neuroinfectious conditions more frequently observed among patients who are immunocompromised, including those with human immunodeficiency virus (HIV) infection and acquired immunodeficiency syndrome (AIDS) as well as patients who have recently completed chemotherapy, those with cancer, and patients on immunosuppressant medications. Numerous members of the herpes virus family are more common among immunocompromised patients in causing encephalitis. These viruses include cytomegalovirus, herpes simplex virus, and varicella-zoster virus. In addition, toxoplasmosis is more common among the immunosuppressed. These infections may present in a more generalized form with fever, malaise, and a decreased mental status, or they may present with focal neurological deficits including aphasia depending on the location of the nidus.

Progressive Multifocal Leukoencephalopathy

Progressive multifocal leukoencephalopathy (PML) is another virus that is a feared complication of AIDS and is associated with having less than 100 cells/μL of a special type of white blood cell called CD4 cells. A reactivation of the prevalent John Cunningham virus (JCV), PML may present with a subacute onset of altered mental status as well as focal symptoms that are attributable to the location of the PML lesions, including aphasia when the lesions are in the language

dominant hemisphere. Once considered fatal, aggressive treatment with combination antiretroviral therapy (cART) has improved mortality considerably (Clifford et al., 1999). If patients do survive, there are often cognitive sequelae, with AIDS patients noted to have difficulty with information processing and motor functioning (Levine, Hinkin, Ando, et al., 2008). PML has also been noted in patients with multiple sclerosis and rheumatoid arthritis who have received the immunosuppressant natalizumab to treat their symptoms. Because there is no proven treatment, PML in these patients is often fatal (Jilek, Jaquiery, Hirsch, et al., 2010).

Immune Reconstitution Inflammatory Syndrome

In addition to increased infection rates, patients who are treated with cART are also at risk for an immune reaction known as *immune reconstitution inflammatory syndrome* (IRIS). IRIS is an uncommon complication of starting cART, usually begins 4 to 8 weeks after starting medication, and is more likely to occur in patients with profound immunosuppression prior to starting therapy (McCombe, Auer, Maingat, et al., 2009). Characterized by a paradoxical worsening in the patient's clinical status, IRIS consists of an inflammatory reaction in the brain leading to swelling and neurological complications. IRIS may occur with or without a concurrent opportunistic infection and may result in elevated intracranial pressure due to the profound inflammation. Focal findings in these patients result from brain inflammation or reactivation of opportunistic infections. In the latter situation, focality will also be related to the infection location within the brain. The most common infections associated with IRIS are toxoplasmosis, CMV, and PML (Singer, Valdes-Sueiras, Commins, & Levine, 2010).

Human Immunodeficiency Virus Infection

Finally, the HIV virus alone can lead to cognitive changes. HIV-associated neurocognitive disorder (HAND) may afflict up to 45% of patients with HIV and includes those with mild deficits on neuropsychiatric testing as well as those with frank HIV-associated dementia (Grant, 2008). HAND is generally considered a subcortical-type dementia, with impairments in the areas of attention, concentration, psychomotor processing speed, executive function, and verbal memory, particularly retrieval of stored information (Heaton et al., 1995). Patients started on antiretroviral therapy have significant improvement in cognitive testing and functional status.

DISEASES THAT RELAPSE AND REMIT, THEN GENERALLY TREND DOWNWARD

Multiple Sclerosis

MS is an immune-mediated inflammatory disorder, usually considered to be part of the same family of diseases as ADEM. MS is most common among women of European descent. It is estimated to affect more than 1 million people worldwide and have a mean annual cost per patient in the United States of $47,215 (Marrie, Yu, Blanchard, et al., 2010). MS typically consists of a relapsing and remitting course with patients returning to a neurologically normal baseline between times of clinically evident disease. Most patients ultimately have a buildup of neurological deficits and may even convert into a secondarily progressive course where deficits are slowly acquired with little or no neurological recovery between exacerbations. Prior to the introduction of disease-modifying therapies, patients would progress from no disability to requiring a walker or cane for ambulation in about 15 years (Weinshenker et al., 1989). More recent natural history studies showed that in about the same time period, on average, patients progressed from no disability to having some impairments in function but still being fully ambulatory (Brex, Ciccarelli, O'Riordan, et al., 2002). Specifically, patients with MS often develop difficulty with bowel and bladder function, balance, vision, and other cranial nerve abnormalities, as well as cerebellar, sensory, and cognitive abnormalities.

Nearly 50% of MS patients demonstrate cognitive impairments, with difficulties in memory, sustained attention, information processing speed, and executive function (Bobholz & Rao, 2003). While less common, language difficulties may occur as part of these chronic cognitive changes. Kujala et al. (1996) described abnormalities in semantic and circumlocutory naming that could not be explained by other cognitive deficits. In addition, patients with MS may present with acute aphasia. This presentation is relatively rare, with estimates ranging from 0.7% to 3% of all patients with MS (Lacour, De Seze, Revenco, & Lebrun, 2004). The most common aphasic syndrome described was Broca's aphasia, with conduction, transcortical motor, global, unclassified, and alexia-agraphia all decreasing in relative frequency. Of the patients with acute onset aphasia, a complete recovery was observed in about 64% (Lacour et al., 2004).

Systemic Lupus Erythematosus

Another autoimmune disease with a relapsing and remitting course that can be associated with a language disorder is systemic lupus erythematosus (SLE). As its name suggests, it is a systemic disorder associated with arthritis, fatigue, joint pain and swelling, and a skin rash over the cheeks and bridge of the nose. In addition, approximately 22% to greater than 80% of SLE patients have some involvement of either the peripheral or central nervous system. The broad estimate of neuropsychiatric involvement is indicative of a variety of diagnostic criteria and patient selection (Muscal & Brey, 2010). Patients with SLE may experience a form of ischemic or hemorrhagic stroke that is secondary to vascular occlusions in the brain blood vessels by antibody reactions. The subsequent loss of function in the involved area of the brain leads to the language deficits that have been previously described (Rhiannon, 2008). Similar to other etiologies of strokes, these patients' deficits may improve over time and with therapy, although additional ischemic events may occur depending on the efficacy of the patient's treatment. Unfortunately, the mood, anxiety, and cognitive disorders associated with neuropsychiatric lupus may make recovery from ischemic or hemorrhagic strokes more difficult (Huizinga & Diamond, 2008).

DISEASES THAT WORSEN OVER TIME

Many neurological diseases worsen over time despite our best medical treatments and therapies. The neurodegenerative diseases are the largest collection of neurological illnesses that follow this downward trajectory. Prion diseases such as familial and sporadic Creutzfeldt-Jakob disease (CJD), new variant CJD (nvCJD), or "mad cow disease" are well known in the popular press; they are characterized by a rapid decline once symptoms develop. In addition, some primary brain tumors and many cancers that metastasize to the brain are very aggressive such that most patients ultimately succumb to their disease without remission.

Alzheimer disease (AD) and Parkinson disease (PD) are the most common neurodegenerative diseases. In patients who have had the disease for many years and display the characteristic symptoms, these illnesses can be easy to diagnose. There are numerous other neurodegenerative diseases, however, whose symptoms overlap with AD and PD. These illnesses and make up the Parkinson-plus syndromes and frontotemporal disease or frontotemporal lobar degeneration. These last two labels are used interchangeably, although there is a move to use the term *frontotemporal lobar degeneration* for the pathological diagnosis alone, and to use the term *frontotemporal disease* for a class of clinical syndromes that include the nonfluent variant primary progressive aphasia, semantic variant primary progressive aphasia, and behavioral variant frontotemporal dementia. These three clinical syndromes have much in common; they typically begin when the patient is in their mid 50s to 60s, result from asymmetric atrophy in the frontal and/or temporal lobes, and affect episodic memory and visuospatial skills relatively late. They can be caused by accumulations of tau or ubiquitin (abnormal protein) in brain cells, and are sometimes referred to as "tau-opathies" or "ubiquitin-opathies." They are closely related to two other "tau-opathies": progressive supranuclear palsy and corticobasal degeneration, described later. Among these neurodegenerative diseases, a patient may present with signs and symptoms more than one of these syndromes, making characterization, diagnosis, and prognosis difficult. Some patients may even start out with symptoms typical of one clinical syndrome, only to develop characteristics of one of the other clinical syndromes. There is a fairly close, but very imperfect, relationship between the clinical syndrome and the pathological diseases that cause them.

Alzheimer Disease

About two thirds of all dementia cases are the result of AD (Nussbaum & Ellis, 2003). It was estimated to have a prevalence of 4.5 million people in the United States in 2000 and a projected prevalence of as high as 15.4 million by 2050 (Brookmeyer, Gray, & Kawas, 1998). The clinical hallmark of the disease is the presence of slowly progressive memory impairment. In addition, patients with AD will also develop apraxia, agnosia, executive dysfunction, and aphasia. The deficits must be a decline from previous function and severe enough to affect the patient's ability to function independently, including whether they can maintain employment or volunteer positions, fulfill domestic responsibilities, or maintain relationships. Once diagnosed with AD, life expectancy is generally shorter than for persons without the disease, with patients surviving between 4 and 10 years after the diagnosis (Brookmeyer, Corrada, Curriero, & Kawas, 2002; Larson, Shadlen, Wang, et al., 2004). As the dementia advances, these patients may also develop what are considered atypical features, including parkinsonism, incontinence, and myoclonus. Behavioral difficulties are also common as part of the disease course (Kelley & Peterson, 2007).

The language disorder observed in AD is a fluent aphasia with varying degrees of circumlocution or semantic or phonemic paraphasias. There is often also a lack of specificity or paucity of specific content words. Sometimes, these patients also have pauses, hesitancy, or delayed initiation of verbal responses (Josephs, Whitwell, Duffy, et al., 2008).

Parkinson Disease

When patients with PD develop language abnormalities, these patients may have trouble processing long, complex sentences and have verb generation difficulties, impaired semantic priming, and difficulty understanding metaphoric meanings (Bastiaanse & Leenders, 2009). Executive dysfunction and other cognitive changes observed in patients with Parkinson disease dementia (PDD) may play a large role in these language abnormalities (Monetta & Pell, 2007). The cognitive deficits observed in PDD are different from those noted in AD. PDD is generally considered a more subcortical type dementia, with cognitive impairments including cognitive and motor slowing, executive dysfunction, and impaired memory retrieval. When compared with AD, patients with PDD display greater attentional, visuospatial, and executive impairments (Troster, 2008).

PDD is a common complication of PD, with approximately 32% of PD patients afflicted with the dementia and 3% to 4% of all dementia cases attributable to PDD (Aarsland, Zaccai, & Brayne, 2005). To be diagnosed with PDD, the patient must have displayed the symptoms of PD for at least 1 year prior to the onset of the cognitive problems. The three core clinical features of PD are a resting tremor, bradykinesia, and rigidity. Postural instability is a fourth feature that usually develops later in the disease course. The presence of two of the three major symptoms is required for diagnosis of parkinsonism. Similar to the other neurodegenerative disorders, the incidence of PD increases with age, with about 10 to 17 per 100,000 person-years affected with the disease in the overall population (Bower, Maraganore, McDonnell, & Rocca, 1999; Van Den Eeden, Tanner, Berstein, et al., 2003) and about 44 per 100,000 person-years affected among people over 50 years old (Van Den Eeden et al., 2003).

Primary Progressive Aphasia

Unlike patients with AD and PD, patients with primary progressive aphasia (PPA) have a prominent, isolated language deficit. Specifically, there is a gradual impairment of language production, object naming, syntax and/or word comprehension at least two years before the emergence of other cognitive and behavioral impairments (Mesulam, 2007). While other cognitive domains may eventually become affected, language remains the most impacted area and the domain in which deficits accumulate the most rapidly. Primary progressive aphasia includes: nonfluent/agrammatic variant PPA, characterized by apraxia of speech, agrammatic spontaneous speech and repetition, and relatively spared word comprehension (usually a tau-opathy); semantic variant PPA, characterized by fluent speech and repetition with limited content and poor word comprehension (typically a ubiquitin-opathy); and logopenic variant primary progressive aphasia, characterized by anomia and relatively poor repetition of sentences (most often associated with AD pathology) (Gorno-Tempini, Hillis, Weintraub, et al., 2011). Regardless of the variant of PPA, many of these patients will eventually develop additional cognitive deficits and reduced insight into their difficulties, and many develop parkinsonism and other motor symptoms and signs. In addition, patients with PPA have a higher rate of depressive symptoms than control groups (Medina & Weintraub, 2007) and this should be carefully monitored as it provides an opportunity for treatment. Finally, patients with PPA may also develop behavioral difficulties similar to patients with frontotemporal dementia (Marczinski, Davidson, & Kertesz, 2004), though these problems will usually come late in the disease.

Semantic Variant Primary Progressive Aphasia Case

A 60-year-old man presented to clinic for evaluation of difficulty with word retrieval, reading, and verbal memory. The patient had noticed these problems for about 10 years. About 3 years prior to the consultation he had noticed difficulties listening during work, and about 6 months prior to the consultation these difficulties were noticed by his wife and colleagues at the law office where he was a litigator. The mental status examination demonstrated cognitive difficulties and poor verbal memory and verbal fluency. The remainder of his neurological examination was unremarkable. His speech difficulties progressed, and over the next few months he began to have marked difficulties at work; he could no longer argue a legal case in the same manner. About a year after his initial evaluation, he reported significant trouble reading, concentrating, and with word retrieval. He was no longer serving as the primary litigator on cases. When he was examined in clinic approximately 2 years after initial presentation, he had stopped working and was on full-time disability. He was having significant difficulty with verbal expression and understanding others. He made frequent semantic paraphasias, more in naming nouns than verbs. Object knowledge was now impaired; he confused credit cards with insurance cards. He made errors on picture association tests. He was no longer able to live alone or prepare a simple meal for himself. He put on clothes that were inappropriate to the occasion or the weather and got lost in familiar places. His marked left anterior temporal lobe atrophy can be seen in the MR images in Figure 3-10.

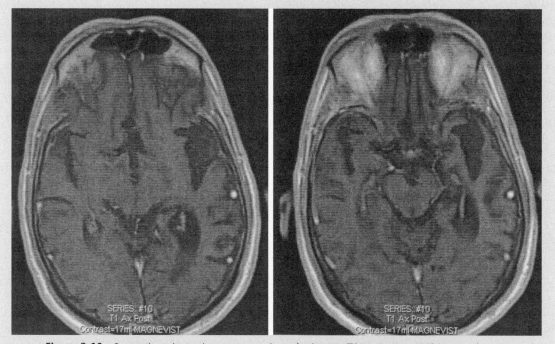

Figure 3-10   Semantic variant primary progressive aphasia case: T1 postcontrast MR images demonstrating significant left temporal atrophy.

Behavioral Variant Frontotemporal Dementia

In behavioral variant frontotemporal dementia (bvFTD), the behavioral difficulties are usually the presenting symptom. Specifically, family and clinical staff will note profound changes in personality and social conduct. These patients also present with a change in affect and lack of basic emotions such as sadness, sympathy, and empathy, and they may demonstrate repetitive, stereotyped behaviors and changes in eating habits. In addition, they have an altered response to sensory stimuli including a reduced pain response and hypersensitivity to neutral stimuli. Executive dysfunction is also a hallmark of the disease (Neary, Snowden, & Mann, 2005). In its strictest definition, bvFTD is not associated with a language disorder. However, as previously discussed, there is significant overlap amongst the neurodegenerative diseases. Some patients with many of the features of bvFTD may also demonstrate language abnormalities (Grossman, 2002).

Progressive Supranuclear Palsy

Progressive supranuclear palsy (PSP) is a closely related neurodegenerative disease, which like about half of cases of bvFTD and most cases of nonfluent variant PPA, is caused by accumulations of tau in the brain. Primary clinical features of PSP are gait instability, impairment of eye movements, spastic or "pseudobulbar" dysarthria, dysphasia, bradykinesia, rigidity, and frontal behavior changes (Golbe, 2001). Patients with PSP may also demonstrate symptoms of a nonfluent aphasia (Boeve, Dickson, Duffy, et al., 2003; Josephs, Boeve, Duffy, & Smith, 2005; Mochizuki, Ueda, Komatsuzaki, et al., 2003; Robinson, Shallice, & Cipolotti, 2006) or other cortical signs such as executive dysfunction. Most of the cognitive changes in patients with PSP, however, are subcortical with bradyphenia and poor recall predominating. In early stages or in patients with bradykinetic and rigid predominance, it may be confused with PD, but patients with PSP generally do not respond well to dopaminergic and anticholinergic medications. In addition, eye movement abnormalities, specifically an inability to look down, coupled with axial greater than appendicular rigidity is pathognomonic for the disease.

Corticobasal Syndrome

An additional syndrome that is often grouped with frontotemporal disease and PSP is corticobasal degeneration (CBD) syndrome. Classic features of this disease include limb apraxia, constructional and visuospatial difficulties, akinetic rigidity, acalculia, and frontal dysfunction. In addition, the presence of the alien limb phenomenon in which patients feel like they have lost control of a limb, or that the limb has a mind of its own, is specific to CBD. CBD is also known for a nonfluent aphasia and, in fact, these patients may present with symptoms consistent with nonfluent variant PPA (Ferrer, Hernandez, Boada, et al., 2003; Kertesz & McMonagle, 2010). Other studies have characterized the aphasia associated with CBD as more variable, with some patients with anomic, Broca's, or transcortical motor aphasias (Frattali, Grafman, Patronas, et al., 2000). Patients with CBD, like all of the patients with neurodegenerative diseases, experience a slow downward course with increasing functional deficits. Over time, most patients lose their independence and mobility (Reich & Grill, 2009).

Multiple System Atrophy

Multiple system atrophy (MSA) is a neurodegenerative disease that presents with symptoms of autonomic failure, parkinsonism, cerebellar ataxia, and pyramidal signs in varying degrees of severity depending on the subtype. MSA is a rare disease, present in about 1.9 to 4.9 cases per 100,000 people. These patients suffer from speech difficulties secondary to a high-pitched, strangled dysarthria that often develops (Wenning, Colosimo, Geser, & Poewe, 2004), but do not generally develop language disorders. However, one of the subtypes of MSA in which patients develop parkinsonian features (MSA-P) is associated with deficits in verbal fluency (Kawai, Suenaga, Takeda, et al., 2008).

Creutzfeldt-Jakob Disease

In contrast to the slow accumulation of deficits described in the neurodegenerative diseases discussed earlier, prion diseases such as Creutzfeldt-Jakob disease (CJD) are characterized by a rapid accumulation of neurological complaints. In the sporadic form of CJD, the median time from onset of symptoms to death is about 5 months and 90% of patients are dead within 1 year (Brown, Gibbs, Rodgers-Johnson, et al., 1994; Johnson & Gibbs, 1998). While the sporadic form is the most common, the familial form has a much slower progression with death occurring about 5 to 11 years after onset of symptoms. Regardless of the subtype, CJD remains very rare with about 0.5 to 1.5 cases per 1 million people per year (Johnson, 2005). The initial symptoms of patients can be divided into three primary categories: about a third of cases of sporadic CJD present with systemic complaints of fatigue, disordered sleep, and decreased appetite; another third present with behavioral or cognitive changes and the final third have focal signs including visual loss, cerebellar ataxia, aphasia, or motor deficits (Bernoulli, Masters, Gajdusek, et al., 1979). The disease then rapidly progresses, with prominent features being the cognitive decline and the development of startle-sensitive myoclonus. Interesting, highly selective aphasias at onset have been described. One patient was noted to have profoundly impaired spoken naming and word comprehension with relatively intact written naming and comprehension (Hillis & Selnes, 1999). Other authors described a patient with perseverations in his utterances as well as disjointed, stereotyped phrases. This same patient also had difficulty understanding complex syntax and repetition span was reduced to four digits. Still other patients had phonemic paraphasias with hesitant speech (Snowden, Mann, & Neary, 2002).

Brain Tumors

In contrast to the rapid clinical course of CJD, patients with primary brain tumors and metastasis to the brain progress at a variable rate depending on the cancer type, other complications, and location of the lesions within the brain. Tumors in the language dominant hemisphere frequently cause aphasia while tumors in the nondominant hemisphere result in deficits in prosody and discourse comprehension. Again, depending on the type of cancer, life expectancy and disease course vary widely, with some of the tumors having reasonably good life expectancy and others, such as glioblastoma multiforme (GBM), being uniformly fatal. Among primary brain tumors, GBM is the most common accounting for 50% to 60% of all cases. Life expectancy without any treatment is about 3 to 4 months but it has been improving in recent years with aggressive treatment (Tran & Rosenthal, 2010). Seizures and headaches are the most common initial presentations of primary brain tumors and metastasis, with subsequent evaluation revealing the mass. The accompanying clinical signs and symptoms are based on the localization of the tumor and surrounding brain edema.

DISEASES THAT ARE EPISODIC

There are three neurological diseases that are episodic in their nature. Language deficits can occur and resolve completely, in some cases even without treatment. These include TIAs, seizures, and migraines.

Transient Ischemic Attack

A TIA will appear exactly like a stroke except the patient's deficits resolve usually within a few minutes (by traditional definition, within 24 hours). Any type of language disorder, mild or severe, from any vascular territory, can result from TIA. When a deficit lasts as long as 24 hours, it is nearly always associated with a lesion on MRI and would therefore be considered a stroke (rather than TIA) by most neurologists. Current

MRI, especially diffusion-weighted imaging, is much more sensitive to small infarcts that caused transient language deficits previously referred to as TIA because no lesion was identified on CT scan. Many patients say that they have had "mini-strokes" in the past. These might refer to either TIAs (stroke symptoms with no lesion on MRI) or small lesions on MRI (which may or may not have been symptomatic). About one-third of patients with TIA have subsequent stroke, most often within the first few days after the TIA, so it is critical for individuals with TIA to be evaluated and treated quickly to reduce the risk of subsequent stroke as much as possible.

Seizures

Approximately 2% to 3% of the general population has a seizure disorder (Hauser, Annegers, & Kurland, 1993; Kobau, DiIorio, Price, et al., 2004) with the incidence of epilepsy highest among those in the first year of life and people over the age of 75 (Hauser et al, 1993). The most well known seizures are the generalized tonic-clonic type of seizures, formerly described as grand mal seizures. In this type of seizure, afflicted patients lose consciousness and shake rapidly in their upper and lower extremities in a rhythmic manner that subsequently slows. These patients are then often somnolent and slowly recover from the episode, with a postictal period lasting a few hours to as long as 24 hours depending on the patient's neurological baseline and other characteristics. In the case of these types of seizures, the postictal period may result in some focal findings, with a unilateral weakness that slowly resolves (called Todd's paralysis) or with an aphasia that slowly recovers. In other types of seizures, called partial seizures, the aphasia itself can be the outward manifestation of the seizure. That is, when a patient is having a seizure, he or she might have language comprehension or production impairment, and when the seizure stops, the language deficit will dramatically resolve. An exception occurs in the case of Landau-Kleffner syndrome (also called "acquired epileptic aphasia"), a progressive aphasia syndrome with peak age of onset between age 3 and 6 years with associated epilepsy with seizures arising from left temporal cortex. This syndrome is not an episodic disorder, but a progressive language disorder of childhood.

Migraines

Migraines are even more common, with the 1-year prevalence estimated to be at 11.7%. They are much more common in women than in men, and their peak prevalence is in middle life. While generally not dangerous, they are very debilitating. Individuals with migraine have a higher than average health care expenditures compared to those without migraine. In addition, the projected national burden of migraines is about $11.07 billion (Hawkins, Wang, & Rupnow, 2008). Classic migraine consists of a visual aura followed by intense, throbbing pain, photophobia, and phonophobia as well as nausea and sometimes even emesis. Migraine sufferers also report cognitive slowing and difficulty talking during the peak pain. Frank aphasia and hemiplegia are rare, but reported, symptoms of migraine. Resolution of the pain does not always result in eradication of the cognitive, speech, and motor deficits. In terms of diagnosis and treatment, it is important that these patients have secondary causes of migraine ruled out and that they are offered prophylactic therapy if they meet the appropriate criteria.

CONCLUSIONS

The neurological diseases that are associated with language disorders include numerous illnesses that affect the brain, particularly the cortex. These diseases include stroke and SDH, in which the patient has great potential to improve with both medical and speech therapies. The neuroinflammatory and infectious diseases also offer great potential for improvement with either antibiotic therapy or immune suppression, depending in the specific illness. While often a more subtle presentation, aphasia is also seen among illnesses that are better characterized by their waxing and waning though ultimately downward course, including multiple sclerosis. Among the neurodegenerative illnesses, most of these patients have cognitive difficulties and language abnormalities. While we currently lack any disease-modifying medical treatments, speech-language therapy can help these patients with communication impairments that develop as part of their disease. For patients with the episodic diseases of seizures and migraines, the aphasia should be brief and they should return to their neurological baseline after the postictal state or pain subsides.

REFERENCES

Aarsland, D., Zaccai, J., & Brayne, C. (2005). A systematic review of prevalence studies of dementia in Parkinson's disease. *Movement Disorders, 20*(10), 1255–1263.

Bastiaanse, R., & Leenders, K. L. (2009). Language and Parkinson's disease. *Cortex, 45*, 912–914.

Belanger, H. G., Curtiss, G., Demery, J. A., Lebowitz, B. K., & Vanderploeg, R. D. (2005). Factors moderating neuropsychological outcomes following mild traumatic brain injury: A

meta-analysis. *Journal of the International Neuropsychological Society, 11*, 215–227.

Bernoulli, C. C., Masters, C. L., Gajdusek, D. C., Gibbs, C. J., Jr., & Harris, J. O. (1979). Early clinical features of Creutzfeldt-Jakob disease (subacute spongiform encephalopathy). In: *Slow transmissible diseases of the nervous system, Vol 1: Clinical, epidemiological, genetic and pathological aspects of the spongiform encephalopathies* (pp. 229–241). New York: Academic Press.

Bershad, E. M., Farhadi, S., Suri, M. F., Feen, E. S., Hernandez, O. H., Selman, W. R., & Suarez, J. I. (2008). Coagulopathy and inhospital deaths in patients with acute subdural hematoma. *Journal of Neurosurgery, 109*(4), 664–669.

Bobholz, J. A., & Rao, S. M. (2003). Cognitive dysfunction in multiple sclerosis: A review of recent developments. *Current Opinion in Neurology, 16*, 283–288.

Boeve, B. F., Dickson, D., Duffy, J. R., Bartleson, J., Trenerry, M., & Petersen, R. (2003). Progressive nonfluent aphasia and subsequent aphasic dementia associated with atypical progressive supranuclear palsy pathology. *European Neurology, 49*, 72–78.

Bower, J. H., Maraganore, D. M., McDonnell, S. K., & Rocca, W. A. (1999). Incidence and distribution of parkinsonism in Olmsted County, Minnesota, 1976–1990. *Neurology, 52*, 1214–1220.

Brazis, P. W., Masdeu, J. C., & Biller, J. (2007). Vascular syndromes of the forebrain, brainstem, and cerebellum. In: *Localization in clinical neurology* (5th ed., pp. 521–555). Philadelphia: Lippincott Williams & Wilkins.

Brex, P. A., Ciccarelli, O., O'Riordan, J., Sailer, M., Thompson, A. J., & Miller, D. H. (2002). A longitudinal study of abnormalities on MRI and disability from multiple sclerosis. *The New England Journal of Medicine, 346*, 158–164.

Broca, P. (1865). Sur le siège de la faculté du langage articulé. *Bulletins de la Société d'anthropologie de Paris, 6*, 377–393.

Brookmeyer, R., Gray, S., & Kawas, C. (1998). Projections of Alzheimer's disease in the United States and the public health impact of delaying disease onset. *American Journal of Public Health, 88*, 1337–1342.

Brookmeyer, R., Corrada, M. M., Curriero, F. C., & Kawas, C. (2002). Survival following a diagnosis of Alzheimer disease. *Archives of Neurology, 59*, 1764–1767.

Brown, P., Gibbs, C. J., Jr., Rodgers-Johnson, P., Asher, D. M., Sulima, M. P., Bacote, A., Goldfarb, L. G., & Gajdusek, D. C. (1994). Human spongiform encephalopathy: The National Institutes of Health series of 300 cases of experimentally transmitted disease. *Annals of Neurology, 35*, 513–529.

Bullock, M. R., Chesnut, R., Ghajar, J., Gordon, D., Hartl, R., Newell, D. W., Servadei, F., Walters, B. C., & Wilberger, J. E. (2006). Surgical management of acute subdural hematomas. *Neurosurgery, 58*, S2-16–S2-24.

Carroll, L. J., Cassidy, J. D., Peloso, P. M., Borg, J., Von Holst, H., Holm, L., Paniak, C., & Pepin, M. (2004). Traumatic brain injury: Results of the WHO Collaborating Centre Task Force on Mild Traumatic Brain Injury. *Journal of Rehabilitation Medicine, Suppl. 43*, 84–105.

Chen, S. T., Tang, L. M., & Ro, L. S. (1995). Brain abscess as a complication of stroke. *Stroke, 26*, 696–698.

Clifford, D. B., Yiannoutsos, C., Glicksman, M., Simpson, D.M., Singer, E. J., Piliero, P. J., Marra, C. M., Francis, G. S., McArthur, J. C., Tyler, K. L., Tselis, A. C., & Hyslop, N. E. (1999). HAART improves prognosis in HIV-associated progressive multifocal leukoencephalopathy. *Neurology, 52,* 623–625.

Croquelois, A., Wintermark, M., Reichhart, M., Meuli, R., & Bogousslavsky, J. (2003). Aphasia in hyperacute stroke: Language follows brain penumbra dynamics. *Annals of Neurology, 54,* 321–329.

Dax, M. (1865). Lésions de la moitié gauche de l'encéphale coïncident avec l'oubli des signes de la penseé (lu à Montpellier en 1836). *Bulletin hebdomadaire de médecine et de chirurgie, 2me série, 2,* 259–62.

Dell, S. O., Batson, R., Kasdon, D. L., & Peterson, T. (1983). Aphasia in subdural hematoma. *Archives of Neurology, 40,* 177–179.

Ernestus, R. I., Beldzinski, P., Lanfermann, H., & Klug, N. (1997). Chronic subdural hematoma: Surgical treatment and outcome in 104 patients. *Surgical Neurology, 48,* 220–225.

Ewing-Cobbs, L., Brookshire, B., Scott, M. A., & Fletcher, J. M. (1998). Children's narratives following traumatic brain injury: Linguistic structure, cohesion, and thematic recall. *Brain and Language, 61,* 395–419.

Ferrer, I., Hernandez, I., Boada, M., Llorente, A., Rey, M. J., Cardozo, A., & Ezquerra, P. B. (2003). Primary progressive aphasia as the initial manifestation of corticobasal degeneration and unusual tauopathies. *Acta Neuropathologica, 106,* 419–435.

Frattali, C. M., Grafman, J., Patronas, N., Makhlouf, F., & Litvan, I. (2000). Language disturbances in corticobasal degeneration. *Neurology, 54*(4), 990–992.

Golbe, L. I. (2001). Progressive supranuclear palsy. *Current Treatment Options in Neurology, 3,* 473–477.

Goozee, J., & Murdoch, B. (2009). Encephalitis. In M. R. McNeil (Ed.), *Clinical Management of Sensorimotor Speech Disorders* (2nd ed., pp. 317–319). New York: Thieme Medical Publishers.

Gorno-Tempini, M. L., Hillis, A. E., Weintraub, S., Kertesz, A., Mendez, M., Cappa, S., Ogar, J., . . . Grossman, M. (2011). Recommendations for the classification of primary progressive aphasia and its variants. *Neurology, 76*(11), 1006–1014.

Grant, I. (2008). Neurocognitive disturbances in HIV. *International Review of Psychiatry, 20,* 33–47.

Grossman, M. (2002). Frontotemporal dementia: A review. *Journal of the International Neuropsychological Society, 8*(4), 566–583.

Hackett, M. L., & Anderson, C. S. (2000). Health outcomes 1 year after subarachnoid hemorrhage: An international population-based study. *Neurology, 55,* 658–662.

Hahn, C. D., Miles, B. S., MacGregor, D. L., Blaser, S. I., Banwell, B. L., & Hetherington, C. R. (2003). Neurocognitive outcome after acute disseminated encephalomyelitis. *Pediatric Neurology, 29,* 117–123.

Hankey, G. J. (2003). Long-term outcome after ischaemic stroke/transient ischaemic attack. *Cerebrovascular Diseases, 16*(Suppl. 1), 14–19.

Hauser, W. A., Annegers, J. F., & Kurland, L. T. (1993). Incidence of epilepsy and unprovoked seizures in Rochester, Minnesota: 1935–1984. *Epilepsia, 34,* 453–468.

Hawkins, K., Wang, S., & Rupnow, M. (2008). Direct cost burden among insured US employees with migraine. *Headache, 48,* 553–563.

Heaton, R. K., Grant, I., Butters, N., White, D. A., Kirson, D., Atkinson, H. J., . . . and the HNRC group. (1995). The HNRC 500-neuropsychology of HIV infection at different disease stages. HIV Neurobehavioral Research Center. *Journal of the International Neuropsychological Society, 1,* 231–251.

Hillis, A. E., & Selnes, O. (1999). Cases of aphasia or neglect due to Creutzfeldt-Jakob disease. *Aphasiology, 13,* 743–754.

Hillis, A. E. (2005). For a theory of rehabilitation: progress in the decade of the brain. In P. Halligan & D. Wade (Eds.), *Effectiveness of rehabilitation of cognitive deficits* (pp. 271–280). Oxford, UK: Oxford University Press.

Hillis, A. E. (2007). Aphasia: Progress in the last quarter of a century. *Neurology, 69,* 200–213.

Hough, M. (1990). Narrative comprehension in adults with right and left hemisphere brain-damage: Theme organization. *Brain and Language, 38,* 253–277.

Hoofien, D., Gilboa, A., Vakil, E., & Donovick, P. (2001). Traumatic brain injury (TBI) 10-20 years later: A comprehensive outcome study of psychiatric symptomatology, cognitive abilities and psychosocial functioning. *Brain Injury 15,* 189–209.

Huizinga, T. W., & Diamond, B. (2008). Lupus and the central nervous system. *Lupus, 17,* 76–79.

Jacobs, R. K., Anderson, V. A., Neale, J. L., Shield, L. K., & Kornberg, A. J. (2004). Neuropsychological outcome after acute disseminated encephalomyelitis: Impact of age at illness onset. *Pediatric Neurology, 31,* 191–197.

Jilek, S., Jaquiery, E., Hirsch, H. H., Lysandropoulos, A., Canales, M., Guignard, L., Schluep, M., . . . Du Pasquier, R. A. (2010). Immune responses to JC virus in patients with multiple sclerosis treated with natalizumab: A cross-sectional and longitudinal study. *Lancet Neurology, 9,* 264–272.

Johnson, R. T., & Gibbs, C. J., Jr. (1998). Creutzfeldt-Jakob disease and related transmissible spongiform encephalopathies. *New England Journal of Medicine, 339,* 1994–2004.

Johnson, R. T. (2005). Prion diseases. *Lancet Neurology, 4,* 635–642.

Josephs, K. A., Boeve, B. F., Duffy, J. R., & Smith, G. E. (2005). Atypical progressive supranuclear palsy underlying progressive apraxia of speech and nonfluent aphasia. *Neurocase, 11,* 283–296.

Josephs, K. A., Whitwell, J. L., Duffy, J. R., Vanvoordt, W. A., Strand, E. A., Hu, W. T., & Petersen, R. C. (2008). Progressive aphasia secondary to Alzheimer disease vs FTLD pathology. *Neurology, 70,* 25–34.

Kajula, P., Portin, R., & Ruutiainen, J. (1996). Language functions in incipient cognitive decline in multiple sclerosis. *Journal of the Neurological Sciences, 141,* 79–86.

Kalita, O., Kala, M., Svebisova, H., Ehrmann, J., Hlobilkova, A., Trojanec, R., . . . Houdek, M. (2008). Glioblastoma multiforme with an abscess: Case report and literature review. *Journal of Neurooncology, 88,* 221–225.

Kaminski, H. J., Hlavin, M. L., Likavec, M. J., & Schmidley, J. W. (1992). Transient neurologic deficit caused by chronic subdural hematoma. *The American Journal of Medicine, 92,* 698–700.

Kawai, Y., Suenaga, M., Takeda, A., Ito, M., Watanabe, H., Tanaka, F., . . . Sobue, G. (2008). Cognitive impairments in multiple system atrophy: MSA-C vs MSA-P. *Neurology, 70,* 1390–1396.

Kelley, B., & Petersen, R. (2007). Alzheimer's disease and mild cognitive impairment. *Neurologic Clinics, 25,* 577–609.

Kertesz, A., & McMonagle, P. (2010). Behavior and cognition in corticobasal degeneration and progressive supranuclear palsy. *Journal of Neurological Sciences, 289,* 138–143.

Kobau, R., DiIorio, C. A., Price, P. H., Thurman, D. J., Martin, L. M., Ridings, D. L., & Henry, T. R. (2004). Prevalence of epilepsy and health status of adults with epilepsy in Georgia and Tennessee: Behavioral risk factor surveillance system, 2002. *Epilepsy & Behavior, 5,* 358–366.

Koc, R., Akdemir, H., Oktem, I. S., Meral, M., & Menku, A. (1997). Acute subdural hematoma: Outcome and outcome prediction. *Neurosurgical Review, 20,* 239–244.

Kujala, P., Portin, R., & Ruutiainen, J. (1996). Language functions in incipient decline in multiple sclerosis. *Journal of the Neurological Sciences, 141,* 79–86.

Lacour, A., De Seze, J., Revenco, E., & Lebrun, C. (2004). Acute aphasia in multiple sclerosis: A multicenter study of 22 patients. *Neurology, 62,* 974–977.

Larson, E. B., Shadlen, M. F., Wang, L., McCormick, W. C., Bowen, J. D., Teri, L., & Kukull, W. A. (2004). Survival after initial diagnosis of Alzheimer disease. *Annals of Internal Medicine, 140,* 501–509.

Levine, A. J., Hinkin, C. H., Ando K., Santangelo, G., Martinez, M., Valdes-Sueiras, M., . . . Singer, E. J. (2008). An exploratory study of long-term neurocognitive outcomes following recovery from opportunistic brain infections in HIV+ adults. *Journal of Clinical and Experimental Neuropsychology, 30,* 836–843.

Mamelak, A. N., Mampalam, T. J., Obana, W. G., & Rosenblum, M. L. (1995). Improved management of multiple brain abscesses: A combined surgical and medical approach. *Neurosurgery, 36,* 76–86.

Marczinski, C. A., Davidson, W., & Kertesz, A. (2004). Longitudinal study of behavior in frontotemporal dementia and primary progressive aphasia. *Cognitive and Behavioral Neurology, 17,* 185–190.

Marrie, R. A., Yu, N., Blanchard, J., Leung, S., & Elliott, L. (2010). The rising prevalence and changing age distribution of multiple sclerosis in Manitoba. *Neurology, 74*(6), 465–471.

Mathisen, G. E., & Johnson, J. P. (1997). Brain abscess. *Clinical Infectious Diseases, 25,* 763–779.

McCombe, J. A., Auer, R. N., Maingat, F. G., Houston, S., Gill, M. J., & Power, C. (2009). Neurologic immune reconstitution inflammatory syndrome in HIV/AIDS: Outcome. *Neurology, 72,* 835–841.

Medina, J., & Weintraub, S. (2007). Depression in primary progressive aphasia. *Journal of Geriatric Psychiatry and Neurology, 20,* 153–160.

Mesulam, M. (2007). Primary progressive aphasia: A 25-year retrospective. *Alzheimer Disease Associated Disorders, 21,* S8–S11.

Millis, S., Rosenthal, M., Novack, T., Sherer, M., Nick, T. G., Kreutzer, J. S., . . . Ricker, J. H. (2001). Long-term neuropsychological outcome after traumatic brain injury. *The Journal of Head Trauma Rehabilitation, 16,* 343–355.

Mitchell, R. L., & Crow, T. J. (2005). Right hemisphere language functions and schizophrenia: The forgotten hemisphere? *Brain, 128,* 963–978.

Miyazaki, H., Ito, S., Nitta, Y., Iino, N., & Shiokawa, Y. (2004). Brain abscess following cerebral infarction. *Acta Neurochirurgica, 146,* 531–532.

Mochizuki, A., Ueda, Y., Komatsuzaki, Y., Tsuchiyak, K., Arai, T., & Shoji, S. (2003). Progressive supranuclear palsy presenting with primary progressive aphasia. *Acta Neuropathologica, 105,* 610–614.

Monetta, L., & Pell, M. D. (2007). Effects of verbal working memory deficits on metaphor comprehension in patients with Parkinson's disease. *Brain and Language, 101,* 80–89.

Mori, K., & Maeda, M. (2001). Surgical treatment of chronic subdural hematoma in 500 consecutive cases: Clinical characteristics, surgical outcome, complications, and recurrence rate. *Neurologia Medico Chirurgia, 41,* 371–381.

Moster, M. L., Johnston, D. E., & Reinmuth, O. M. (1983). Chronic subdural hematoma with transient neurological deficits: A review of 15 cases. *Annals of Neurology 14*(5), 539–542.

Muscal, E., & Brey, R. L. (2010). Neurologic manifestations of systemic lupus erythematosus in children and adults. *Neurologic Clinics, 28,* 61–73.

Nakai, K., Yamamoto, T., Yasuda, S., & Matsumura, A. (2006). Brain abscess following intracerebral haemorrhage. *Journal of Clinical Neuroscience, 13,* 1047–1051.

Neary, D., Snowden, J., & Mann, D. (2005). Frontotemporal dementia. *Lancet Neurology, 4,* 771–780.

Nussbaum, R. L., & Ellis, C. E. (2003). Alzheimer's disease and parkinson's disease. *New England Journal of Medicine, 348,* 1356–1364.

Ochfeld, E., Newhart, M., Molitoris, J., Leigh, R., Cloutman, L., Davis, C., . . . Hillis, A. E. (2009). Ischemia in Broca area is associated with broca aphasia more reliably in acute than in chronic stroke. *Stroke, 41,* 325–330.

Ogden, J. A., Mee, E. W., & Henning, M. (1993). A prospective study of impairment of cognition and memory and recovery after subarachnoid hemorrhage. *Neurosurgery, 33,* 572–587.

Parlato, C., Guarracino, A., & Moraci, A. (2000). Spontaneous resolution of chronic subdural hematoma. *Surgical Neurology, 53,* 312–317.

Qureshi, A. I., Tuhrim, S., Broderick, J., Batjer, H. H., Hondo, H., & Hanley, D. F. (2001). Spontaneous intracerebral hemorrhage. *New England Journal of Medicine, 344,* 1450–1460.

Radanovic, M., & Scaff, M. (2003). Speech and language disturbances due to subcortical lesions. *Brain and Language, 84,* 337–352.

Reich, S. G., & Grill, S. E. (2009). Corticobasal degeneration. *Current Treatment Options in Neurology, 11,* 179–185.

Rhiannon, J. J. (2008). Systemic lupus erythematosus involving the nervous system: Presentation, pathogenesis, and management. *Clinical Reviews in Allergy & Immunology, 34,* 356–360.

Robinson, G., Shallice, T., & Cipolotti, L. (2006). Dynamic aphasia in progressive supranuclear palsy: A deficit in generating a fluent. *Neuropsychologia, 44,* 1344–1360.

Ross, E. D., & Monnot, M. (2008). Neurology of affective prosody and its functional-anatomic organization in right hemisphere. *Brain and Language, 104,* 51–74.

Selnes, O., & Hillis, A. E. (2000). Patient Tan revisited: A case of atypical Global aphasia? *Journal of the History of the Neurosciences, 9,* 233–237.

Senft, C., Schuster, T., Forster, M. T., Seifert, V., & Gerlach, R. (2009). Management and outcome of patients with acute traumatic subdural hematomas and pre-injury oral anticoagulation therapy. *Neurological Research, 31,* 1012–1018.

Singer, E. J., Valdes-Sueiras, M., Commins, D., & Levine, A. (2010). Neurologic presentations of AIDS. *Neurologic Clinics, 28,* 253–275.

Snowden, J. S., Mann, D. M. A., & Neary, D. (2002). Distinct neuropsychological characteristics in Creutzfeldt-Jakob disease. *Journal of Neurology, Neurosurgery, and Psychiatry, 73,* 686–694.

Sonneville, R., Klein, I., de Broucker, T., & Wolff, M. (2009). Post-infectious encephalitis in adults: Diagnosis and management. *Journal of Infection, 58,* 321–328.

Stapf, C., Mohr, J. P., Choi, J. H., Hartmann, A., & Mast, H. (2006). Invasive treatment of unruptured brain arteriovenous malformations is experimental therapy. *Current Opinion in Neurology, 19,* 63–68.

Suarez, J. I., Tarr, R. W., & Selman, W. R. (2006). Aneurysmal subarachnoid hemorrhage. *The New England Journal of Medicine, 354,* 387–396.

Tenembaum, S., Chitnis, T., Ness, J., & Hahn, J. S.; International Pediatric MS Study Group. (2007). Acute disseminated encephalomyelitis. *Neurology, 68*(16 Suppl. 2), S23–36.

Tran, B., & Rosenthal, M. A. (2010). Survival comparison between glioblastoma multiforme and other incurable cancers. *Journal of Clinical Neuroscience, 17,* 417–421.

Troster, A. I. (2008). Neuropsychological characteristics of dementia with Lewy bodies and Parkinson's disease with dementia: Differentiation, early detection, and implications for "mild cognitive impairment" and biomarkers. *Neuropsychology Review, 18,* 103–119.

Tunkel, A. R. (2005). Acute meningitis. In: *Principles and practice of infectious disease* (6th ed., p. 1099). Philadelphia: Elsevier Churchill Livingstone.

Urbinelli, R., Bolard, P., Lemesle, M., Osseby, G. V., Thomas, V., Boruel, D., Megherbi, S. E., . . . Giroud, M. (2001). Stroke patterns in cardio-embolic infarction in a population-based study. *Neurological Research, 23,* 309–314.

Van Den Eeden, S. K., Tanner, C. M., Bernstein, A. L., Fross, R. D., Leimpeter, A., Bloch, D. A., & Nelson, L. M. (2003). Incidence of Parkinson's disease: Variation by age, gender, and race/ethnicity. *American Journal of Epidemiology, 157,* 1015–1022.

Van Gijn, J., & Rinkel, G. J. (2001). Subarachnoid haemorrhage: Diagnosis, causes and management. *Brain 124,* 249–278.

Warrington, E. K., & Shallice, T. (1984). Category specific semantic impairments. *Brain, 107,* 829–854.

Weinshenker, B. G., Bass, B., Rice, G. P., Noseworthy, J., Carriere, W., Baskerville, J., & Ebers, G. C. (1989). The natural history of multiple sclerosis: A geographically based study. I. clinical course and disability. *Brain, 112* (1), 133–146.

Wenning, G. K., Colosimo, C., Geser, F., & Poewe, W. (2004). Multiple system atrophy. *Lancet Neurology, 3,* 93–103.

Wernicke, C. (1881). *Lehrbruch der gehirnkrankheiten.* Berlin: Theodore Fisher.

Whitfield, P. C., & Kirkpatrick, P. J. (2001). Timing of surgery for aneurysmal subarachnoid haemorrhage. *Cochrane Database of Systematic Reviews, 2,* CD001697.

Whitley, R. J., & Alford, C. A., & Hirsch, M. S. (1986). Vidarabine versus acyclovir therapy in herpes simplex encephalitis. *New England Journal of Medicine, 314,* 144–149.

Whitley, R. J. (2006). Herpes simplex encephalitis: Adolescents and adults. *Antiviral Research, 71,* 141–148.

Winner, E., & Gardner, H. (1977). The comprehension of metaphor in brain damaged patients. *Brain, 100,* 717–729.

Xiao, F., Tseng, M. Y., Teng, L. J., & Tseng, H. K. (2005). Brain abscess: Clinical experience and analysis of prognostic factors. *Surgical Neurology, 63,* 442–449.

Yang, S. Y., & Zhao, C. S. (1993). Review of 140 patients with brain abscess. *Surgical Neurology, 39,* 290–296.

CHAPTER 4

Attention: Architecture and Process

CHAPTER OUTLINE   *Thomas H. Carr and Jacqueline J. Hinckley*

WHAT IS ATTENTION?

What are its component parts? What does it do, and how does it work?

Perhaps these are easy questions. In 1890 William James proclaimed that "Everyone knows what attention is. It is the taking possession by the mind in clear and vivid form of one out of what seem several simultaneous objects or trains of thought." But after 120 years and an immense amount of research, the picture has grown more complicated than James' proposal.

An Attention-Rich Scenario

Suppose you are at your desk composing an email, but at the moment you are off in some imaginary mental space, enjoying a pleasant daydream. A colleague pokes her head in your door and gently knocks on the doorframe. She says, "Hey—do you have a second?"

How, if at all, will you heed that question? Will you even notice it? Though the request seems reasonable under *these* circumstances, is it always good advice to "pay attention"? Are there times when you are better off *not* paying attention—whatever that means? What if you have trouble "paying attention"? Can anything be done? And once you are "paying attention," what does attention actually do, and how does that happen?

You say, "Sure—come in." Your colleague sits down and begins to talk. You listen, but you also try to read what you have written in the email, which you are again thinking about. You start to type the next sentence in the message. Can you succeed at this multitasking?

Your colleague asks again, "Really—can you just pay attention?" You say, "Oh—OK. What's this about?" Your colleague says, "Well, I know you don't like math, but you're the only person around and I need some help with this calculation. Here—take a look."

What do we know about attention and how it works during this scenario?

THE ATTENTION SYSTEMS OF THE HUMAN BRAIN

In 1990—100 years after James—Posner and Petersen suggested that there are multiple roles for attention to play in regulating mental life. They argued two important points about attention and how it is implemented in the brain.

Attention Is Separate

Attention is a set of mental functions separate from the rest of information processing, executed by neural systems separate from the regions of the brain that process the information to which attention is being allocated or denied. That is, specialized attentional systems exist separately from sensory, memory, language, and motor information-processing systems. The attentional systems modulate the operation of the information-processing systems.

What sort of evidence might support such a claim? Kastner, Pinsk, De Weerd, et al. (1999) as well as Corbetta and colleagues (e.g., Corbetta, Kincade, Ollinger, et al., 2000) used functional magnetic resonance imaging (fMRI) to show that different brain regions were active in response to a spatial cue telling the participant where to look for an upcoming stimulus than were subsequently active when the stimulus actually appeared and was being perceived. The latter perceptual regions were activated more strongly if the cue had correctly signaled where the stimulus would appear and hence the upcoming location had become the focus of spatial attention. Activation of the regions that processed the cue—the "attentional regions"—predicted both the activation of the perceptual regions and the speed and accuracy of the behavioral responses in the task. Thus, different brain regions appeared to be generating attentional information based on the cue, sending out control signals that then modulated the operation of the perceptual regions actually responsible for processing the stimulus. An excellent example of this type of research comes from Hopfinger (2000), whose results are shown in Figure 4-1.

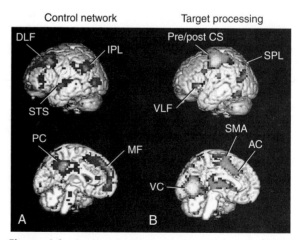

Figure 4-1 Separation of selective attention regions from information-processing regions. [From Hopfinger, J. B., Buonocore, M. H., & Mangun, G. R. (2000). The neural mechanisms of top-down attentional control. *Nature Neuroscience, 3,* 284–292.]

Attention Is Complex

Second, Posner and Petersen argued that the brain regions devoted to implementing the functions of attention are themselves hierarchically organized systems distributed across cortical and subcortical structures. Considerable evidence supports this claim, some of which we will describe.

Attentional Functions

What *are* the functions of attention? There has been much discussion of this question. For present purposes we follow the lead of Posner and Petersen (1990), distinguishing three major functions and attributing each to its own system of neural structures. System 1 is responsible for *arousal, alerting, and vigilance*. System 2 is responsible for *orienting toward and selecting sources of information*, both from the external perceivable world and from memory. System 3 is responsible for *executive control and supervision* of intentional, goal-directed task performances, and includes *working memory*.

THE ATTENTIONAL NETWORK TEST

We will elaborate on each of these systems individually, but first we consider in detail a single study that addresses all three in the same task environment. This important kind of research design obtains data on all systems at the same time from each participant, and it holds constant the stimuli, responses, and other task demands that are not directly related to identifying the attentional systems per se.

Using a procedure they called the Attention Network Test (ANT), Fan, McCandliss, Fossella, et al. (2005) combined three manipulations in a single task, one manipulation for each system. The ANT was administered in a magnetic resonance imaging (MRI) scanner, so that distributions of blood oxygen levels could be measured across the brain to indicate regional brain activation while the task was being performed. Blood oxygen levels vary in a fairly direct way with neuronal activity, so fMRI provides a good indication of where neurons are busy processing information.

The ANT, shown in Figure 4-2, required the participant to focus attention on a fixation cross that was constantly present in the middle of the field of view on a computer display projected into the scanner. On each trial a target arrow appeared either directly above or directly below the fixation cross. The participant's job was to indicate the arrow's direction as rapidly and accurately as possible by pressing a button on the left if the arrow pointed left or on the right if the arrow pointed right.

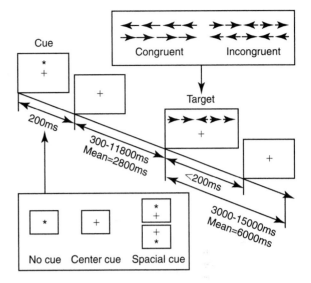

Figure 4-2 Trial time line for the Attention Network Task. [Fan, J., McCandliss, B. D., Fossella, J., Flombaum, J. I., & Posner, M. I. (2005). The activation of attentional networks. *NeuroImage, 26*, 471–479.]

The Three Manipulations

Box 4-1 summarizes the manipulations used in this study. We begin with the manipulation relevant to System 3—Executive Control and Supervision, because it is fundamental to understanding the logic of the ANT. Participants needed to respond to the direction of a target arrow, but the target arrow did not appear by itself. It occurred in the middle of a row of five arrows, two on either side, that were designated as irrelevant—the decision about direction was to be made on the basis of the middle arrow only. Thus, this task was a version of Eriksen and Hoffman's (1972) "Flanker Task." It is well established that if flanking stimuli are close enough in space to the target, they are difficult to ignore and they will get processed to some degree if attention is not focused on them very carefully. This is more likely to happen if the target stimulus is simple and easy to process and interpret (Lavie, 1995; 2006; see also Huang-Pollack, Nigg, & Carr, 2002), which of course an arrow certainly is, and of course the flanking arrows are also simple and easy to process.

These conditions create a need for executive control. When the flanking arrows point in the same direction as the target arrow (the "congruent" condition), then the participant need not succeed in focusing attention

Manipulations of Attentional Systems Used in the Attentional Network Test

System 1 Arousal, Alerting, and Vigilance: Whether an asterisk appears at the start of a trial telling participants to get ready

System 2 Orienting and Selecting (aka Selective Attention): Whether the asterisk that alerts the participant appears at the spatial location at which the target stimulus display will appear (helping to guide selective attention), or in the middle of the screen (thereby providing no information that could be used to guide selective attention)

System 3 Executive Control and Supervision: Whether distractor arrows on either side of the target arrow in the target stimulus display signaled the same response as the target arrow ("congruent" condition) or the opposite response ("incongruent" condition)

the congruent condition to those in the incongruent condition.

System 1—Arousal, Alerting, and Vigilance was manipulated by providing or withholding a warning signal, consisting of an asterisk that alerted the participant to prepare for the target display. The no-warning condition served as a baseline.

The manipulation of System 2—Orienting and Selecting added spatial information to alerting. On warning-present trials, the warning asterisk appeared in one of two locations: either in the middle of the screen, superimposed over the fixation cross that was always present (providing a warning that alerted the participant to get ready for an arrow, but no additional spatial information about where the target might occur), or in the location at which the target arrow was about to appear (providing a valid spatial cue to aid in orienting attention toward the correct location, in addition to providing an alerting cue). Thus, the manipulation of System 2—Orienting and Selecting was whether the cue that provided an alerting signal also provided spatial information that could be used to direct attention in advance of the target's actual appearance.

As with Executive Control, substractions of the appropriate reaction times and accuracies provided measures of the impact of Alerting and of Orienting and Selecting on behavioral task performance, and comparisons between the appropriate blood flow images provided maps of the brain regions whose activity was associated with the behavioral effects.

completely on the middle arrow. The directional response will be correct regardless. But if the flankiing arrows point in the opposite direction (the "incongruent" condition), then the participant must work hard enough and long enough to ultimately focus completely on the middle arrow before making his or her decision about direction.

Fan and colleagues obtained a measure of the burden that the flanking arrows placed on Executive Control by subtracting response times and accuracies in the easier congruent condition from response times and accuracies in the conflicted and therefore more demanding incongruent condition. A map of the brain regions involved in dealing with this burden was obtained by comparing blood oxygen levels in

Reaction time differences for the effects of alerting, selective attention ("orienting" in the table), and executive control ("conflict" in the table), as well as the correlations among these differences, are shown in Table 4-1. Each manipulation produced an impact. Performance was 60 ms faster (about 7.5%) when alerted, 31 ms faster (about 3.8%) when given orienting information, and 102 ms slower (about 12.5%) when dealing with the conflict created by the incongruent flankers. None of

Table **4-1** Effects of Alerting, Orienting, and Conflict Resolution on Reaction Times in the Attentional Network Task				
	Effect and SD (ms)	**Alerting**	**Orienting**	**Conflict**
Alerting	60 (34)			
Orienting	31 (34)	.258		
Conflict	102 (57)	.258	.155	
Mean reaction time	768 (118)	.556	−.180	.385

*Correlation is significant at the .05 level (two-tailed).
From Fan, J., McCandliss, B. D., Fossella, J., Flombaum, J. I., & Posner, M. I. (2005). The activation of attentional networks. *NeuroImage, 26,* 471–479.

the correlations among these difference-scores was significant, meaning that statistically, the effects were independent of one another. This is consistent with the hypothesis that they reflect the operation of independent processes, as suggested by Posner and Petersen's (1990) view of the organization of the attentional systems.

Brain activation maps were consistent with this view. The alerting effect was associated with activation of the thalamus and anterior and posterior cortical regions. The orienting effect was associated with activation in parietal regions and the frontal eye fields. The executive control effect was associated with activation of the anterior cingulate, regions in left and right prefrontal cortex, and regions in the left and right fusiform gyrus in ventral posterior cortex. Conjunction analyses seeking regions active in two or all three of the maps found very little overlap. Thus, the fMRI results indicate that the attention-relevant manipulations of the Attention Network Task activated three separate neural networks, each associated with a different attentional system.

SYSTEM 1—AROUSAL, ALERTING, AND VIGILANCE: PREPARING FOR TASK PERFORMANCE

Mental energy levels and readiness to engage with a task are important to performance. Fan and colleagues (2005) found a specific neural substrate associated with the impact of an aspect of getting ready they called alerting—of receiving a specific warning that a task stimulus was coming soon. Kahneman (1973, p. 13) called the process of getting ready "the mobilization of effort," and related it more generally to the concept of arousal—overall physiological activity level in the nervous system, reflected in measures such as heart rate, galvanic skin response, diameter of the pupil of the eye, and activity in the locus coeruleus or "reticular activating system."

Neurotransmitter-Defined Pathways of Arousal, Alerting, and Vigilance

Neurochemical studies have focused on pathways between locus coeruleus and cortex that rely on noradrenalin as the primary neurotransmitter, as well as pathways connecting basal forebrain, cortex, and thalamus that rely on acetylcholine and dopamine (Cools & Robbins, 2004; Parasuraman, Warm, & See, 1998; Ron & Robbins, 2003). It appears that pathways involving these neurotransmitter systems in anterior cingulate cortex, right prefrontal cortex, and thalamus are particularly important in modulating arousal and the ability to mobilize effort.

Arousal and the Rhythms of Performance

The neural substrates of alertness, arousal, and vigilance remain objects of intense investigation. Quite a bit is known at the cognitive/behavioral level. It is clear that readiness as measured through task performance rises and falls in predictable patterns, and this happens on at least two different time scales.

Circadian Rhythm

First, readiness varies with the circadian sleep-wakefulness cycle. Work relating this cycle to the speed and accuracy of task performance has been summarized by Hasher, Zacks, and May (1999). Some people are "morning people" and others are "evening people" or even "night owls." That is, the time of day at which people feel most energetic and prefer to engage in demanding mental or physical activity varies systematically from person to person. Such preferences are persistent and reliable enough to be measured psychometrically—for example, using Horne and Ostberg's Morningness-Eveningness Questionnaire. Hasher and colleagues reported that people tested at their preferred or optimal time of day perform faster and more accurately in a wide range of tasks than if they are tested at earlier or later times, when they say they are likely to feel tired or would prefer less strenuous activity.

Time-of-day preferences vary strikingly with age (Table 4-2). Young adults tend toward eveningness, whereas older adults tend rather strongly toward morningness. Testing younger and older adults in the evening exaggerates differences due to cognitive aging that generally favor young adults—young adults are more likely to be at or near their optimum times whereas older adults are wearing down. Testing in the morning reverses relative energy and readiness levels, with younger adults being at a down time and older adults being at or near their optimum time of day. The result is a reduction or even elimination of the age difference favoring younger adults, with the amount of reduction depending on the task.

In general, a person's task performance improves as his or her optimal time of day approaches and falls after that time is passed. This performance cycle is thought to happen because arousal and the ability to prepare for task performance—to mobilize effort—rises and falls in accord with this same circadian pattern.

Alerting

A very similar pattern can be seen on a much smaller time scale in manipulations of alerting such as used by Fan and colleagues (2005). For example, Posner and Boies (1971) conducted a same-different matching task in which a pair of letters was presented sequentially.

Table 4-2   Distribution of "Morning People" Versus "Evening People" as a Function of Age

| Group | MORNINGNESS-EVENINGNESS TYPE | | | | |
	Definitely Evening (16–30)	Moderately Evening (31–41)	Neutral (42–58)	Moderately Morning (59–69)	Definitely Morning (70–86)
Young (N = 210)					
n	15	78	105	12	0
%	7	37	50	6	0
Old (N = 91)					
n	0	0	24	45	22
%	0	0	26	50	24

Young adults ranged in age from 18 to 22 years. Old adults ranged in age from 66 to 78 years. From May, C. P., Hasher, L., & Stoltzfus, E. R. (1993). Optimal time of day and the magnitude of age differences in memory. *Psychological Science, 4*, 326–330.

The participant's job was to indicate as rapidly and accurately as possible whether the two letters were the same or different. Posner and Boies found that providing a warning signal in advance of the first letter speeded performance of the judgment.

The amount of benefit, however, depended on how much in advance the warning signal occurred. The benefit increased over the first half a second or so, reaching a maximum with an interval of 400 to 600 ms between the onset of the warning signal and the onset of the first letter. This is typical of reaction-time tasks requiring relatively simple judgments. Beyond this optimum warning interval of about half a second, benefit declines over the next few seconds, suggesting that it is difficult to maintain maximum readiness for very long (Kornblum & Requin, 1984; Thomas, 1974).

Vigilance

Extending readiness for longer periods—minutes or hours—proves to be a major problem. Failure under such demands for "vigilance" causes much human error in real-world task performance, especially when events that actually call for action are rare, or when the performer is at a nonoptimal part of the sleep-wakefulness cycle (Parasuraman et al., 1998; Thomas, Sing, Belenky, et al., 2000). Under sleep deprivation, performance becomes highly variable. Some stimuli elicit a normal response, some a very slow response, and some are missed altogether (Doran, Van Dongen, & Dinges, 2001).

We have seen so far that low levels of arousal and readiness produce poor performance and that this pattern occurs on two different time scales. What happens if the level of arousal rises above the optimal level, rather than falling below it? This can happen under conditions of extreme stimulation, whether externally induced

(for example, by consuming caffeine or amphetamines or performing in a very noisy or otherwise annoying environment) or generated internally (as in anxiety, fear, or hypermotivation from an extreme desire to perform well). Under these conditions of high rather than low arousal, performance declines from the best levels achieved at the optimal level of arousal.

Yerkes-Dodson Law

The general shape of the resulting function is reflected in what has come to be called the Yerkes-Dodson Law, which relates level of arousal to the quality of performance. As shown in Figure 4-3, *A*, there is in general an optimum level of arousal and resultant readiness at which performance of any given task is maximized. Arousal levels that are lower or higher than this result in poorer performance. As shown in Figure 4-3, *B*, the optimum level of arousal varies by complexity of the task. In the simplest tasks, high levels of arousal are helpful. As task complexity increases, high levels of arousal become harmful. Progressively lower arousal levels are required for best performance as the number of component processes increases, or larger amounts of information must be attended to or maintained in working memory.

But for any task, arousal levels substantially lower than the optimum depress performance, as do levels substantially higher than the optimum, though perhaps for different reasons. Low arousal results in sluggishness or even drowsiness, leading to poor preparation and readiness to perform. Very high arousal appears to restrict attention and interfere with executive control and decision making (for discussions of the Yerkes-Dodson function, see Anderson, 1994; Kahneman, 1973; Yerkes & Dodson, 1908).

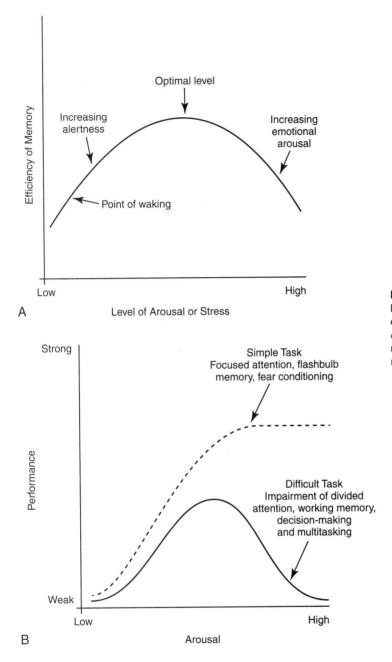

Figure 4-3 A, Generic portrayal of Yerkes-Dodson Law. **B,** Yerkes-Dodson Law as a function of task complexity. Not all "simple tasks" (*upper dotted line*) remain at the highest levels of performance as arousal increases—many do fall off, but not as rapidly as "difficult" or complex tasks.

SYSTEM 2—SELECTIVE ATTENTION: ORIENTING AND SELECTING INFORMATION

A simple fact of mental life is that more information is available in the environment than a human being can take in, notice, interpret in a meaningful fashion, act upon, or store in memory. That is the reason for studies and theories of selective attention, the processes that regulate the flow of information, give priority, reduce priority, or perhaps even produce inhibition, so that the next time the stimulus occurs, it will be harder to perceive than it was before (Dagenbach & Carr, 1994; Keele, 1973; Pillsbury, 1908; Posner & Petersen, 1990; Treisman, 1969, 1988).

As Keele (1973, p. 4) put it, "One use of the term *attention* implies that when a person is attending to one thing, he cannot simultaneously attend to something else. Typing is said to require attention because one cannot simultaneously type and participate in conversation. Walking is said to require very little attention because other tasks performed simultaneously, such as thinking, interfere very little with walking."

The Costs and Benefits of Selective Attention

Typing and walking are complicated activities extended in time. Much less complex perceptual and sensorimotor tasks show the impact of attention. One of the simplest and most widely used methods of isolating and measuring selective attention was applied in the Attentional Network Task of Fan and colleagues (2005). Stimuli could appear at two different locations in the visual environment—and even this limited variety taxed the perceiver's capacity to some extent, as was evidenced by the benefit that arose when a cue directed attention to the upcoming stimulus location. Giving the perceiver the ability to select and monitor the relevant location from which information would be arriving proved to be helpful. Fan's experiment did not measure what would have happened if the cue had been misleading—signaling and hence calling attention to a location that was *not* where the stimulus would ultimately appear. Other studies give the answer. Performance is hurt, with reaction time and/or accuracy falling below what would have been achieved with no cue at all. Both effects—the facilitation or benefit from a valid cue and the inhibition or cost from an invalid cue—are illustrated in Figure 4-4.

The Functional Architecture and Functional Anatomy of Selective Attention

Posner and Petersen (1990), using visual attention as an example, suggested that orienting and selecting a source of input is built around three component operations implemented in sequence. This is the "functional architecture" of selective attention, consisting of "disengage," "move," and "engage." Each operation is accomplished by a different region of neural tissue (the "functional anatomy" of selective attention).

Posner and Petersen hypothesized that the "disengage" operation is supported by left and right posterior parietal cortex (and, as we will see, by neighboring posterior regions of superior temporal cortex). The disengage operation implements a decision to curtail the priority being given to input from the location on which attention is currently focused. The decision to give up a source of input as a priority in order to shift to another source might be made intentionally

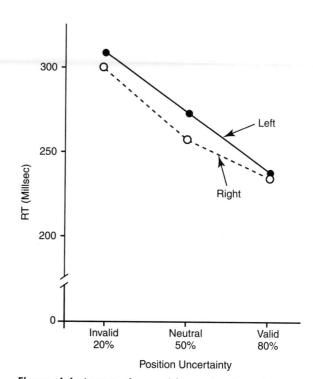

Figure 4-4 Impact of a spatial cue signaling where an upcoming stimulus is likely to occur, either accurately (valid cue, given on 805 of the trials) or inaccurately (invalid cue, given on 205 of the trials). 80% validity makes using the cue helpful, encouraging intentionally applied endogenous control. [From Posner, M. I., Snyder, C. R. R., & Davidson, B. J. (1980). Attention and the detection of signals. *Journal of Experimental Psychology: General, 109*, 163.]

by executive control processes in working memory and transmitted as a top-down goal-directed instruction to parietal cortex, or it might arise from bottom-up signals driven by the sudden onset of a new, high-intensity, or potentially important stimulus in the environment. This difference between top-down or *endogenous* control and bottom-up and stimulus-driven *exogenous* control was not explicitly built into Posner and Petersen's anatomical model, but it is necessary to the story. Exogenous control is also called automatic or reflexive attention capture and has been the topic of considerable research (Folk, Remington, & Johnston, 1992; Folk, Remington, & Wright, 1994; Schriej, Owens, & Theeuwes, 2008; Yantis, 1995).

In either case, implementing a shift of attention from its current focus to a new one begins with disengaging from the current focus. But after disengagement, where is attention going and how does it get there? The second operation is "move," implemented via interactions between posterior parietal cortex and superior colliculus, both of which contain topographic maps of environmental space. Single shifts of attention appear to be the responsibility of more inferior regions of parietal cortex and neighboring temporal cortex interacting with superior colliculus, whereas a planned sequence of attentional foci, moving systematically from one location to another, appears to recruit additional parietal regions that are more superior (Corbetta, Shulman, Miezen, & Petersen, 1993).

Once the focus of attention arrives at its new location, it must "engage" with the new source and give priority to input coming from that location. "Engaging" is critically dependent on portions of the thalamus, in particular the pulvinar nucleus.

Since 1990, the functional anatomy of the "posterior attention system," as Posner and Petersen called this network of regions responsible for selective attention, has grown more elaborate. Figure 4-5, borrowed from a widely used textbook in cognitive neuroscience (Gazzaniga, Ivry, & Mangun, 2009), assigns a larger array of attention-relevant functions to posterior anatomical regions in accord with this elaboration.

Auditory Selective Attention

Effects much like those observed in vision are obtained in studies of audition. A cue to the location from which sounds or speech will come facilitates detection and identification. A misleading cue that causes perceivers to orient attention to the wrong location harms detection and identification (Mondor & Zatorre, 1995).

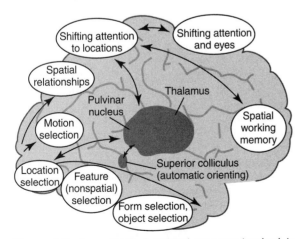

Figure 4-5 Approximate functional anatomy involved in System 2. Selective Attention: Orienting and selecting sources of information. [From Gazzaniga, M. S., Ivry, R. B., & Mangun, G. R. (2009). *Cognitive neuroscience: The biology of the mind* (3rd ed., p. 522). New York: Norton.]

There is a tight relationship between visual and auditory attention. Studies by Driver and Spence (e.g., 1994, 1998) show that visual cues attract auditory attention and vice versa, though these cross-modality cues may not be as powerful as within-modality cues. Cross-modal costs and benefits suggest a partially overlapping hierarchical organization, such that each sensory modality has to some degree its own dedicated piece of the attentional system, but these dedicated components in turn feed into and are modulated by a more general system that serves multiple modalities.

Cross-Modal Attention and Speech

Cross-modal interactions are particularly important in speech perception. Visual information from lip configurations impacts the identification of spoken syllables and words—congruent information in which the lip configuration corresponds to the sound that is heard facilitates identication, whereas incongruent lip configuration and auditory informaton impedes identification. This is called the "McGurk Effect" (McGurk & McDonald, 1976; see also, e.g., Jones & Callan, 2003; Rosenblum, Yakel, & Green, 2000). In a study that required selective repetition of one of two auditory messages—one presented from the left side of space and the other from the right—Driver and Spence (1994) found that a video of the to-be-repeated speaker helped more if it was presented on the same side as the message was coming from. Thus, being able to align spatial attention in the visual and auditory modalities facilitates integration of the information.

How Does Selection Work? Biasing Activation among Representations

The mechanics of how attention intervenes to modulate information processing have been debated for a long time. In 1995 Desimone and Duncan (see also Duncan, 2004) proposed that attention operates directly on pathways of information flow and representations of information, adding activation to a pathway or representation in order to give it priority over others. According to this hypothesis, pathways that are irrelevant to the goal being served are ignored by attention and therefore left to their own devices. They may or may not become activated, but if they do, they are unlikely to become more active than the ones biased by the boost supplied from attention. Some might, however, which creates a mechanism for exogenous control of attention—the unintended reflexive shifts of attention discussed earlier. These "hyperactivating" stimuli include newly appearing stimuli with sudden onsets (Klein, 2004; Yantis, 1995), familiar stimuli with a long history of importance (Cherry, 1953; Treisman, 1969;

Carr & Bacharach, 1976), as well as stimuli with properties that make them very easily recognizable as relevant
to a current task goal, such as a particular color or shape
(Folk, Remington, & Johnson, 1992; Folk, Remington,
& Wright, 1994; Schreij, Owens, & Theeuwes, 2008).

Deploying and Directing Attention During Language Processing and Communicative Interactions

One of the most important communicative uses of language is to enable one person to engage the attention
of another, so that they can exchange information via
conversation, share a perceptual experience, or plan
and collaborate in a joint action. A number of features
of language facilitate such interactions. It is almost as if
language were designed to capture attention and entrain
the cognitive processes of conversational partners.

Signals from the Speaker Call the Listener's Attention to Language

Of course speech is an auditory signal that can attract
attention. However, once speech begins, internal features further moderate the listener's attention. Hesitations during otherwise fluent speech serve to orient
attention to the subsequent word. In a study involving
ERPs, Collard, Corley, MacGregor, and Donaldson
(2008) manipulated spoken sentences that ended with
either a predictable or unpredictable word. In half of
the cases, the sentence-final word was preceded by a
hesitation, "er." The ERP results suggested that the
hesitations helped to orient attention to the preceding
word, thus decreasing the novelty (P300) response
when the sentence-final word was unpredictable. This
example showcases the important role of orienting and
selective attention in understanding spoken language.

The Development of Shared Attention via Looking and Pointing

A foundation is laid early in infancy for communicative
interaction to direct attention. From birth, mothers and
fathers look at the faces of infants during many of their
interactions (though by no means all). In these face-to-
face interactions, adults will follow the gaze of the infant
and respond to it vocally, asking simple (but possibly
quite developmentally profound) questions like "Oooh—
what do you see?" Later on, adults will say things like
"Oh, look at that" and accompany the directive command with a shift of gaze and a point. By 12 to
18 months of age, infants will follow these gazes and
points, orienting head, eyes, and presumably attention in
their direction. Only slightly later, infants will themselves
look, point, and vocalize in apparently intentional ways
during social interactions, trying to direct the attention

of their interactional partner. These changes during
the first year and half of life have been researched as the
development of shared attention and joint regard. Bruner
(1975) and Bates (1976) argued that these developments
are important precursors both to the attentional powers
of language and to one of the fundamental uses of communication (for a review, see Evans & Carr, 1984).

Eye Movements Give a Real-Time View of Language Comprehension

Where the head is turned and where the eyes are looking
continue to be important indicators of attention throughout life, and have been used increasingly as real-time
indicators of language comprehension (Henderson &
Ferreira, 2004; Tanenhaus, 2007). A great boon to this
research was the invention of small and lightweight
eye-movement monitoring equipment that can be
worn like a hat while carrying out a task that might
involve reaching for objects, picking them up and moving
them around or using them in response to instructions, or
walking from one place to another (Tanenhaus,
Spivey-Knowlton, Eberhard, & Sedivy, 1995).

Imagine a task in which the participant, wearing
an eye-movement monitor, is confronted with an array
of four or five objects laid out on the floor. A verbal
instruction is played through earphones, such as "Put
the apple that's next to the knife on the plate" and the
participant's job is to carry out the instruction. Results
from such studies indicate that gaze is often fixated on
the target object, in this case the apple, within half a
second or less of the onset of the object's name in the
instruction. This means that in many cases, attention is
already moving toward the location of the target object
before the target's name has even been completely
heard. Of course, this only happens when the target's
name is unambiguous in the task environment. Suppose that there are two apples in the array, so that the
participant doesn't know for sure which one is the
target until hearing the word "knife." Under circumstances like these, possible targets are being narrowed
down. Gaze will move back and forth between the two
apples until "knife" is heard, at which point the eyes
will fix on the appropriate apple and reaching for it will
be initiated. The close time-locking of the direction of
attention as measured by eye movements provides a
powerful and versatile onto the time course of language
comprehension.

The Impact of Descriptions Measured with Memory

More generally, it is quite clear that descriptions of the
visual environment serve to direct the listener's attention. There are multiple consequences—establishment

of joint regard and correct following of instructions among them. A lasting consequence involves the memories that the hearer of a description carries away from the experience. Bacharach, Carr, and Mehner (1976) showed fifth-grade children simple line drawings, each containing two objects interacting—a bee flying near a flower, a boy holding up his bicycle, and so forth. Before each picture, an even simpler description was provided: "This is a picture of a bee," or "This is a picture of a bicycle." After the list was completed, a memory test was administered, in which pictures of single objects were shown one at a time. The child's job was to say for each object whether it had been in the objects seen in the pictures. A baseline condition with no descriptions established that all the objects were equally likely to be remembered. With a description before each picture, however, objects that had been named in the descriptions were remembered more often than baseline, whereas objects that had not been named were remembered less often.

SYSTEM 3—EXECUTIVE AND SUPERVISORY CONTROL: MANAGING GOALS AND TASKS

An easy introduction to System 3—Executive and Supervisory Control is to quote from the investigator most closely associated with the system's other name, Working Memory. As Baddeley (2000) puts it:

The term *working memory* appears to have been first proposed by Miller, Galanter, and Pribram (1960) in their classic book *Plans and the Structure of Behavior*. The term has subsequently been used in computational modeling approaches(Newell & Simon, 1972) and in animal learning studies, in which the participant animals are required to hold information across a number of trials within the same day (Olton, 1979). Finally, within cognitive psychology, the term has been adopted to cover the system or systems involved in the temporary maintenance and manipulation of information. Atkinson and Shiffrin (1968) applied the term to a unitary short-term store, in contrast to the proposal of Baddeley and Hitch (1974), who used it to refer to a system comprising multiple components. They emphasized the functional importance of this system, as opposed to its simple storage capacity. It is this latter concept of a multicomponent working memory that forms the focus of the discussion that follows.

And so it does. The topics of Working Memory and Executive Control are treated in detail in Chapters 5 and 7 of this book. Here we raise matters most relevant to issues raised later in this chapter, which include training of attention, skill acquisition, and the impact

on attention and performance of motivation, emotion, self-concept, and pressure.

The Functional Architecture and Functional Anatomy of Working Memory

The basics of the functional architecture of working memory can be seen in Figure 4-6. The pieces of mental equipment that comprise this multicomponent system are the executive controller plus three "buffers" or short-term-storage devices. One of these buffers is the "phonological loop," which maintains a small amount of verbal information for rehearsal (for example, three to nine unrelated syllables, possibly more if the sequence consists of related words that can be chunked into groups). The exact capacity is debated (e.g., Carr, 1979; Cowan, 2000; Jonides, Lewis, Nee, et al., 2008; Miller, 1956), but there is wide agreement that rehearsal is needed to keep the information active and readily available. Once attention is turned to other activities, stopping rehearsal, then the information being rehearsed either fades or is replaced by new material to which attention has been turned.

A second buffer is the "visuospatial sketchpad," which fulfills an analogous function for visual information—storing images rather than sounds, syllables, or words. An analogous debate has been waged over the capacity of the visual storage buffer, with perhaps slightly smaller estimates of capacity (Alvarez & Cavanagh, 2004; Awh, Barton, & Vogel, 2007; Jonides, Lewis, Nee, et al., 2008; Vogel & Machizawa, 2004; Xu & Chun, 2006).

The third storage subsystem, which is the main focus of the caption in Panel A, is the "episodic buffer." The episodic buffer is a late addition to the theory of

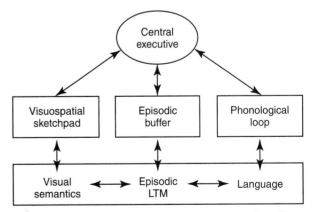

Figure 4-6 Current architectural organization of working memory. [From Baddeley, A. D. (2000). The episodic buffer: A new component of working memory? *Trends in Cognitive Sciences, 4,* 421.]

working memory (although it bears kinship to the concept of "long term working memory" described by Ericsson & Kintsch, 1995).

What is the functional anatomy or brain circuitry of working memory? Pioneering work on verbal versus spatial working memory by Smith and Jonides (1997) showed that verbal working memory was heavily left lateralized, as one might expect from the neuropsychological data on brain injury (Banich, 2004, Chapters 10 and 11). In this important study, a task requiring short-term memory for letters activated a large region of tissue in left prefrontal cortex and a smaller region in left parietal cortex. Subsequent neuroimaging research using fMRI rather than PET has been quite consistent with Smith and Jonides' early findings. In contrast to verbal working memory, visuospatial working memory is heavily right-lateralized, also as might be expected from the neuropsychology of brain injury (Banich, 2004, Chapters 7 and 10). A task requiring short-term memory for the spatial locations of a pattern of dots activated a small region of tissue in right prefrontal cortex and a larger region of tissue in right parietal cortex. One might speculate from this comparison that for dealing with verbal materials the "thinking" part (attributed to frontal cortex) is more demanding than the "storage of data" part (attributed to parietal cortex), whereas the reverse might be true when dealing with spatial materials. Storage of spatial data appears to take up lots of brain space, compared to storage of verbal data. This is only a speculation about human beings, but it does hold true for computers and smart-phones. Visuospatial materials take up a lot of storage room compared to text or speech.

It has probably not escaped you that Baddeley's diagrams of functional architecture are backward with respect to the neuroanatomy—they place the phonological loop on the right and the visuospatial sketchpad on the left. Perhaps this is no more than left-right confusion, a common affliction, but it does allow us to make an important point about inspecting diagrams of functional architecture versus diagrams of functional anatomy. Functional architecture must capture the abstract information-processing activities and the patterns of information flow and process-to-process communication, but only at the computational level. It need not directly reflect the underlying brain structures that actually perform the computations or their locations relative to one another in brain geography. In contrast, a diagram of functional anatomy should aim to be true to brain geography.

It is clear that crucial functional components of working memory reside in prefrontal cortex. The amount of prefrontal cortex in the brain varies substantially from species to species, with humans up toward the top of the distribution. Given the role of prefrontal cortex in executive control and working memory, such differences lead almost inexorably to hypotheses about the existence and origins of species differences in planfulness and in learning of complex tasks. This in turn raises questions about the role of executive control and working memory in language.

Working Memory and Language

The importance of working memory in language has been a matter of debate. Most theories of language and reading comprehension give working memory a seat at the table, though what it is supposed to do can vary from theory to theory (Caplan & Waters, 1995; Daneman & Merikle, 1996; Snowling, Hume, Kintsch & Rawson, 2008; Perfetti, 1985). Much the same holds for language production (Eberhard, Cutting, & Bock, 2005; Bock & Cutting, 1992). Gruber and Goschke (2004) argue in favor of a domain-specific and heavily left-lateralized portion of the working memory system devoted specifically to language. Baddeley (2000) reviews a variety of evidence regarding the role of working memory in language learning, acquiring a second language, and how working memory might be compromised in language disorders such as specific language impairment.

What is currently agreed about the functional anatomy of the phonological loop—the specifically verbal storage and processing component of the working memory system—is shown in Figure 4-7.

Pursuing the question of whether the phonological loop is involved in any aspect of speech production, Acheson, Hamidi, Binder, and Postle (2011) have established a direct link between verbal working memory and the phonological/articulatory demands on one act of speech production—reading aloud. Using transcranial magnetic stimulation (TMS) to temporarily scramble neural signals from highly localized subregions of the cortex. They attempted to disrupt performance in three different tasks. One of these tasks—paced reading, in which participants had to read lists of phonologically similar pseudowords aloud—was chosen because it ought to draw on the specifically phonological and articulatory resources of working memory. Acheson and colleagues predicted from previous work on the functional anatomy of working memory that TMS administered to the posterior superior temporal gyrus (a region involved in a variety of reading functions and implicated in verbal working memory and also in the phonological loop) ought to harm paced reading. As can be seen in Figure 4-8, this is exactly what they observed.

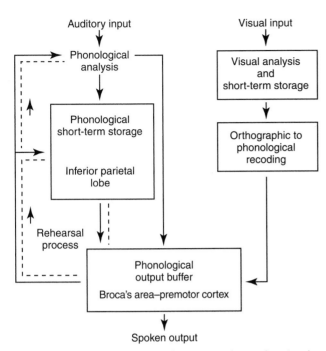

Figure 4-7 The functional architecture and gross functional anatomy of the phonological loop. [From Baddeley A. (2003). Working memory: Looking back and looking forward. *Nature Reviews Neuroscience, 4*(10). In M. S. Gazzaniga, R. B. Ivry, & G. R. Mangun, (2009). *Cognitive neuroscience: The biology of the mind* (3rd ed.). New York: Norton.]

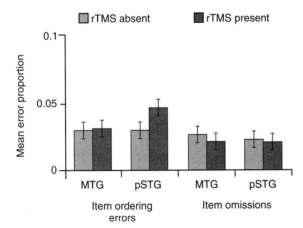

Figure 4-8 TMS stimulation to posterior superior temporal gyrus, but not another region of posterior cortex in middle temporal gyrus, lead to errors in the order of reading nonwords aloud. [From Acheson, D. J., Hamidi, M., Binder, J. R., et al. (2011). A common neural substrate for language production and verbal working memory. *Journal of Cognitive Neuroscience, 23*(6): 1358–1367.]

Conflict Monitoring and Inhibitory Regulation

In 1908, Walter Pillsbury—a black sheep who wandered off from the Pillsbury Flour family business to become a professor—contrasted two means by which attention might work. One involved facilitation of information needed to pursue a goal. The other involved inhibition—that is, attention might achieve much the same ends by inhibiting what was *not* desired. If so, then what *was* desired would be the last representations left standing (so to speak), and they would take control by default.

Pillsbury allowed that both might be at work, and this is the position taken by most current theories of attention. Sometimes inhibitory processes need not be engaged, but when conflict and confusion arise, or when the interpretation of the situation changes so that "old news" needs to be discarded in favor of new goals or new information, then inhibition comes into play. The engagement of inhibitory processes is thought to be triggered by conflict-monitoring operations that run in the background of all task performances (see Botvinick, Cohen, & Carter, 2004). Detection of conflict or ambiguity alerts the executive and supervisory control system, which slows performance so that more care can be taken, updates goals to be pursued, deletes now-irrelevant information so as to reduce "cognitive clutter" (Hasher, Zacks, & May, 1999), and allows the system to resolve the conflict or deal with the ambiguity.

A compelling and much-studied example of dealing with conflict comes from the Stroop Color-Naming Task (Cohen, Aston-Jones, & Gilzenrat, 2004; MacLeod, 1991; Stroop, 1935). This task presents words printed in different colors. One might see the word "blue" printed in blue, the word "red" printed in blue, the word "chair" printed in red or in blue, or one might simply see a patch of color. In all cases, the job is to name the color of the stimulus—*not* to read it if it is a word.

Relative to naming the color of a patch of color, which is the simplest color-naming task imaginable, any stimulus that includes a word slows performance, at least for skilled readers. It is as if just having a word available to perception creates dual-task interference in which it is difficult to ignore the word or to try to perform its automatically associated task of reading (Brown, Gore, & Carr, 2002).

What if the stimulus is a word that spells out the name of the color that must be produced ("red" printed in red), or alternatively, spelling out the name of a different color (e.g., "red" printed in blue)? These contrasting conditions produce the classic "Stroop Effect." Naming times are much slower when the word spells a different color-name than the one that must be produced, and errors are more frequent. Most errors arise from reading the word rather than naming the color in which the word is printed.

In neuroimaging studies of the Stroop Effect, an important locus of the neural activity elicited by conflict, ambiguity, and error is the anterior cingulate cortex (ACC), which consists of two large gyri running side-by-side from front to back along the bottom of prefrontal cortex in the middle of the brain. ACC communicates widely with other prefrontal regions, with motor cortex, and with the motor control and arousal/alerting pathways involving the basal ganglia.

Work on communications patterns among different brain regions—called "effective connectivity" or "functional connectivity"—shows that ACC participates in a network with other prefrontal regions and portions of parietal cortex to process conflict and also to deal with surprising stimuli, as when an unexpected or rare stimulus occurs that requires a response (Wang, Liu, Guise, et al., 2009). It appears that surprising stimuli are recognized in parietal cortex, especially the intraparietal sulcus, which signals ACC and dorsolateral prefrontal cortex (DLPFC) with the news that something unexpected requires scrutiny and possibly action. Recognizing and adjusting for conflict works in the opposite direction—ACC and DLPFC serve as sentinels and interact to determine what processing adjustments need to be made in executive and supervisory control. This prefrontal collaboration includes signaling parietal cortex about changes to be made in selective attention. Thus, parietal cortex initiates network activity in the processing of surprise stimuli, whereas ACC and DLPFC interact with each other to resolve conflict by changing the deployment of attention during task performance.

As might be expected from earlier discussion of partial modality-specificity and partial modality-overlap between visual and auditory attention, monitoring and adjusting for conflict also depends to some degree of the sensory modality in which stimuli are being processed. Roberts and Hall (2008) compared a standard visual Stroop color-naming task, as described above, to an auditory Stroop-like task with similar demands for management of conflict. The auditory Stroop task presented participants with the words "high," "low," or "day"—the neutral equivalent of a patch of color. These words were spoken in a high-pitched or a low-pitched voice. The participant's job was to indicate the pitch of the voice. Thus, the congruent condition was a high-pitched voice saying the word "high" or a low-pitched voice saying the word "low," whereas the incongruent condition eliciting conflict was the high-pitched voice

saying "low" or the low-pitched voice saying "high." Imaging data from fMRI conducted during task performance showed shared regions of activation corresponding to the basic conflict monitoring and adjustment already described, plus additional modality-specific regions appearing only in the visual Stroop task or the auditory Stroop task.

Goal-Directed Action Versus Task-Irrelevant Thought and Mindwandering

Conflict means that more than one thought is competing to be entertained or more than one action is competing to be performed. So far conflict has played out *within the functional confines of a goal-directed task performance*. What happens if mental activity strays outside the bounds of the task? This is called "task-irrelevant thought" or "mindwandering." Studies of mindwandering interrupt performance to ask for reports of on-task versus off-task thinking. The mind appears to wander off task up to 30% of the time, with wandering more likely during simple tasks or when bored (Antrobus, Singer, Goldstein, & Fortgang, 1970; Kane, Brown, McVay, et al., 2007; Smallwood & Schooler, 2006). The mind wishes to be busy.

Christoff, Gordon, Smallwood, et al. (2009) measured brain activity with fMRI during a long task in which a digit appeared every 2 seconds. If a "3" appeared, the participant needed to press a button. About once per minute, participants were probed with two questions: where was their attention just before the probe, and how aware were they of what they were attending to.

fMRI analysis compared 10-second intervals just before probes that indicated mindwandering to intervals before probes that indicated being on task. During mindwandering, error rates increased in the go/no-go task, and activation was observed in a particular network of brain regions that was not activated before probes that indicated being on task. The mindwandering regions belonged to what has been called the "default network" (Buckner, Andrews-Hanna, & Schacter, 2008; Fair, Cohen, Dosenbach, et al., 2008; Raichle & Snyder, 2007), which is a system of midline cortical regions activated when people focus on internal tasks such as envisioning the future, retrieving memories, about oneself; and trying to take someone else's mental perspective. It supports introspection, and correlates negatively with selective attention and information-processing systems that focus on perceptual input. Thus, mindwandering involves attention bouncing back and forth between attention to tasks and the external world versus introspection, attention to self, and the internal world.

TRAINING ATTENTION

On introspection, attention seems both out of our control and under it. This phenomenology mirrors the evidence for both exogenous and endogenous control discussed earlier in the chapter. Events or objects in the environment seem to grab our attention, leading us to attend to some stimuli but to ignore something or someone else in the environment. We seem to be able to direct our attention at times, but fail to control it at others. And when we do focus attention on a desired activity, we sometimes have too little capacity to carry it out, or we are too easily distracted, getting derailed onto something else. What happens when attempts are made to improve or train aspects of attention? Are all aspects of attention equally susceptible to training?

Tang and Posner (2009) define attention training as a curriculum designed to develop an aspect of executive control. Their training approaches require a degree of effort, and are linked to nonautonomic neural control systems such as working memory. Tang and Posner differentiate this type of attention training from attention *state* training, which they define as a curriculum designed to produce a relaxed mind-body state, such as meditation, mindfulness training, and integrative mind-body training. These latter techniques are correlated with changes in the autonomic system. In addition, attention state training can produce results without conscious effort after the initial stages of training are mastered (see also Raffone & Srinivasan, 2010). Figure 4-9 shows the relationships between these two types of training. Optimal performance is characterized as a balance between effortful and effortless performance. At each of the extremes, attentional effort can produce mental fatigue, whereas a lack of attentional effort might lead to poor performance and a wandering mind.

These two approaches to training produce different outcomes (Tang & Posner, 2009). Some researchers have used the Attention Network Test (ANT) described earlier in the chapter to investigate these differences. (Remember that the ANT is based on a flanker task in which participants press a key to indicate the direction of a target arrow, given particular cues on where and when the target will appear. Sometimes these cues are congruent with the target, and sometimes they are incongruent. The task generates an alerting measure, orienting measure, and conflict measure based on subtractions between the task reaction times in the various conditions.) An extremely convenient way to describe the outcomes of different kinds of training is to compare the ANT results across studies.

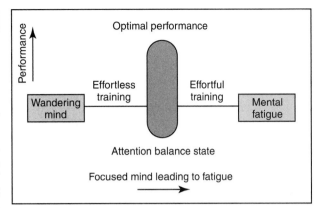

Figure 4-9 AT, AST, and performance mindwandering and mental fatigue are two extremes of the untrained mind (left and right gray rectangles). AT requires effortful control to improve performance whereas AST changes body-mind state through effortless practice. Optimal balance (attention balance state) is hypothesized to trigger the most efficient performance (middle cylinder area). [From Tang, Y.-Y., & Posner, M. I. (2009). Attention training and attention state training. *Trends in Cognitive Sciences, 13,* 225.]

Attention state training, such as meditation training, aims to generally improve the participant's ability to attend to stimuli and tasks at various levels. Thus, it might be predicted that the desired outcome of attention state training would be an observable improvement in attention performance for alertness, orientation, and executive function. One form of attention state training is relaxing or meditating in nature, and the effects of gazing at nature scenes compared to urban scenes on performance in the ANT task can be seen in all three attentional systems. Similarly, a structured, short-term mediation training improves alerting, orienting, and conflict measures on the ANT compared to simple relaxation training. Figure 4-10 shows the results of these two studies. The undergraduate participants in this study also reported improved mood and vigor as a result of training.

Attention training programs are more didactically designed. The participant practices a particular skill, usually with one or more forms of feedback, and outcomes on attention or potentially related skills are measured. The ANT has been used to assess the outcomes of an executive attention training program in preschool children (Rueda, Rothbart, McCandliss, et al., 2005). A child-oriented version of the ANT, involving swimming fish rather than arrows, was designed and used as one of the assessments following the training. A computerized training designed to focus on visual control and conflict training was

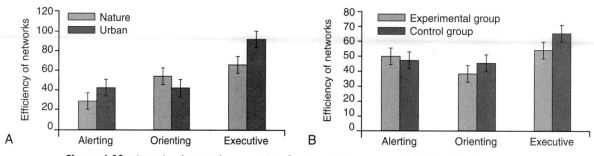

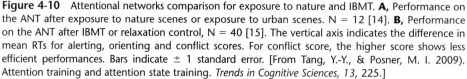

Figure 4-10 Attentional networks comparison for exposure to nature and IBMT. **A,** Performance on the ANT after exposure to nature scenes or exposure to urban scenes. N = 12 [14]. **B,** Performance on the ANT after IBMT or relaxation control, N = 40 [15]. The vertical axis indicates the difference in mean RTs for alerting, orienting and conflict scores. For conflict score, the higher score shows less efficient performances. Bars indicate ± 1 standard error. [From Tang, Y.-Y., & Posner, M. I. 2009). Attention training and attention state training. *Trends in Cognitive Sciences, 13,* 225.]

administered during five 45-minute sessions over a 2- to 3-week period. Results showed that preschoolers' post-training conflict scores on the ANT were similar to adult scores. In this example, there were no particular changes in the alerting and orienting scores. Thus, the computerized control and conflict training seemed to affect primarily executive attentional functions. Happily, these were the skills the training was intended to address.

There are other computerized activities, however, that seem to have broader effects across a range of attentional and cognitive skills. Playing video games appears to influence a number of different attentional components. For example, playing action video games is thought to require the active use of sensory detection, selective attention, task-switching, working memory, way-finding and navigation, the control of emotional arousal or threat, and the suppression of task-irrelevant stimuli (Spence & Feng, 2010). Indeed, numerous studies demonstrate that playing video games enhances a number of cognitive capabilities. For example, players of action video games tend to score higher on mental rotation tasks. A period of playing video games can so improve spatial attention that it eliminates pre-test gender differences in spatial tasks including mental rotation. Video game playing has been associated with higher scores on the useful field of view test, a measure associated with the deployment of attention over space, which has in turn been associated with performance in car-driving tasks. Action video game playing is also associated with higher performance in measures of visual conflict resolution and visual tracking, compared to playing nonaction video games (for reviews, see Green & Bavelier, 2008; Spence & Feng, 2010).

In several studies, playing action video games has been used as a training or intervention, in which

participants who did not play action video games were taught to do so. Practice amount and rate is always a critical issue when discussing any sort of training. In one study, massed practice (60 minutes of continuous practice) and distributed practice (four periods of 15 minutes each, separated by breaks between each period) rates were compared for their effect on the learning of visuomotor tasks (Studer, Koeneke, Blum, & Janke, 2010). EEGs were recorded during the training sessions and during pre- and post-testing. The two practice rates did not produce any differences in final performance on this task, but there were differences in EEG patterns. Heightened power distributions over the sensorimotor cortex occurred in the massed practice group compared to the distributed practice group, suggesting an increase in attentional demands and cognitive effort with massed practice. Thus, massed practice of this kind of skill appears to be more effortful, but with no particular benefit.

In general, attention state training such as meditation appears to produce wide-ranging effects across attentional systems. Attention training such as computerized tasks is unlikely to transfer to other attentional or cognitive skills, except for action video game playing, which seems to transfer broadly across a range of cognitive skills. Of course, not all studies have routinely measured transfer effects across all attentional systems. We turn now to some training examples in which an effect on a specific component of the attentional system was targeted.

Training that Affects System 1: Arousal, Alerting, and Vigilance

We observed earlier in the chapter that the decrement in vigilance that occurs over time is a common source of human error in a variety of performance conditions.

Few attempts to improve general vigilance in healthy individuals have been made, but two sources of training have reported effects. MacLean et al. (2010) investigated the potential effects of intensive meditation training on perceptual detection and vigilance. Participants were adults with an average age of 49 years, with no neurological impairment, all of whom had previous experience with meditation retreats and daily meditation. Before, during, and after a five-day intensive meditation retreat, attention performance was measured on computerized tasks involving identification and discrimination of line lengths. The intensive meditation was viewed as practice on sustained selective attention to breathing patterns. Results showed that the intensive meditation practice improved vigilance in the visual selective attention task immediately after practice and statistically significant improvements were sustained five months after the meditation retreat.

There have also been attempts to improve vigilance through specific practice at the task requiring vigilance, rather than attempting to provide general training that might transfer. During 30-minute practice sessions on a signal detection task, asymptomatic performance was achieved for most younger, middle-aged, and older adult participants after 20 sessions (Parasuraman & Giambra, 1991). In this study, training involved repetition of the target task and performance was measured as detection accuracy in the task. The study compared low- (15 per minute) versus high- (40 per minute) event rates and found the expected event rate effect—higher event rates correspond to faster achievement of task accuracy and maintenance of vigilance. Thus, practice of vigilance on a target task can improve vigilance in that task.

Training that Affects System 2: Orienting and Selecting

Visual selection skills can be trained, and the training transfers to nontrained object targets and backgrounds in a similar task environment (Neider, Boot, & Kramer, 2010). Older and younger adults practiced discriminating and locating pictures of real objects among similar background patterns, in camouflaged and noncamouflaged environments. Older adult participants, like the younger ones, improved their abilities and showed transfer of the training to nontrained object pictures and backgrounds. This suggests that visual search skills can be trained and improved among younger and older adults.

Elsewhere in the chapter it is observed that selective attention is impacted by perceived threat to one's self-concept—performance decrements are associated with calling attention to someone's association with a group that is thought to perform poorly on such a task, particularly when the task must be done in front of others. Given the widespread observation of this kind of phenomenon—called "stereotype threat"—across different types of individuals and different performances, there have been some efforts to determine whether a training focused on selective attention could thwart these social reactions, thus improving performance.

For example, Dandeneau, Baldwin, Baccus, et al. (2007) investigated whether training individuals to seek supportive expressions in an array of photographs could reduce performance stress and produce specific lifestyle benefits. Adults with either high or low self-esteem participated in the training, which focused on selective attention to accepting faces among an array of rejecting faces ("find-the-smile" training). Healthy adults with low self-esteem experienced reduced levels of cortisol stress reaction and self-reported stress after the training. The same kind of selective attention training yielded lower stress reports and improved exam performance among college students who typically experience exam stress. This selective attention training also improved work performance and reduced stress response among telemarketers.

The ability to selectively focus on positive faces and decrease attention on rejecting or negative facial expressions was carried one step further by Legerstee et al. (2009). These researchers wanted to know if there was an association between selective attention to positive images and treatment for anxiety disorder. They observed that children who were able to disengage from threatening pictures at pretreatment were more likely to have success in response to treatment for their anxiety disorder than those who did not. It remains to be investigated whether a pretreatment course of selective attention training would improve the outcomes of those who were unable to direct their focus prior to treatment.

Training that Affects System 3: Executive and Supervisory Control

Focused training on aspects of executive control can improve the trained skills among children and older adults. Thorel, Lindqvist, Nutley, et al. (2009) trained preschool children, using a computerized working memory program. This program required the child to remember the location and order of objects presented on the computer screen—much like the board game of "Memory." In addition, there was an inhibition control training program, based on the go/no-go and flanker tasks. Children in the experimental group played at these computerized training programs for 15 minutes per day for 5 weeks. Children in the control group also played computer games for 15 minutes per day, but these were commercially available computer games with no particular expectation of influencing either working memory or inhibition control. Training improved working memory performance and transferred to nontrained attention tasks. Similar results have been obtained by Rueda, Rothbart, McCandliss, et al. (2005)—who also demonstrated transfer to the Kaufman Brief Intelligence Test.

It seems reasonable to think that a computerized training program with multiple tasks or modules, such as this one, might produce benefit across a number of different attentional and memory skills. There may be a continuum, yet to be investigated, from more static task repetition training that has limited transfer to the playing of dynamic action video games, with broad transfer (Green & Bavelier, 2008; Spence & Feng, 2010).

Dual-task performance can also be trained, with improvements noted on the trained tasks. Bherer, Kramer, Peterson, et al. (2006) studied a group of 12 older participants (average age 70 years) and younger participants (average age 20 years). The two groups participated in a baseline assessment which involved both single-task and dual-task performance of an auditory discrimination task (choosing among tones of different frequency) and a visual selection task (choosing among different letters).

Training consisted of repetition of the tasks in single and dual-task conditions with added instructions that sometimes emphasized one task over the other in the dual-task condition. Feedback on performance was provided. Results showed that both older and younger adults improved speed and accuracy during dual-task performance as a result of the training. Whether this kind of task-specific dual-task training would generalize to other functional abilities is yet to be determined.

Beyond cognitive effects, dual-task or divided attention decrements appear to be associated with an increased risk of falls among elderly individuals. Verghese et al. (2002) observed that poor performance on a "walking while talking" task was highly associated with the likelihood of falling during the subsequent 12 months. It would be useful to know whether any kind of dual-task training could reduce this fall risk among the elderly.

Task-switching is also amenable to training. For example, adults trained on two tasks improved the cost of switching from one task to another, but a certain residual switch cost remained even after long-term training (Berryhill & Hughes, 2009). Task-switch training was remarkably durable—training effects persisted over a 10-month follow-up period without practice.

Dual-task training has neurological correlates. Erickson et al. (2007) found a decrease in the extent of brain tissue activated after dual-task training, compared to the extent of activation before training. However, there was an *increase* in activation in an area of the dorsal prefrontal cortex for the training group, and this was associated with an improvement in performance. Thus, it would appear that training shifted control of performance somewhat, while achieving an overall decrease in neural effort.

In summary, complex attention training environments that involve multiple inputs and varied responses improve performance in those particular task settings, and also seem to have broader-ranging transfer to skills that are not explicitly trained. Meditation and interactive mind-body training are examples of training programs that require the participant to selectively focus while ignoring irrelevant stimuli, while producing various other physical and mental responses simultaneously. Action video games also require attention and processing of multiple inputs with strategic analysis and varied responses. In contrast, training programs that involve the repetition of less complex tasks with the same response type seem to produce improvements in the type of attentional skill that the task was intended to improve, but nothing more. Attention training produces effects across the lifespan, from the very young to the older adult. All aspects of attention seem to be susceptible to training among neurologically healthy individuals.

SKILL ACQUISITION: CHANGES IN THE NEED FOR ATTENTION WITH INCREASES IN PRACTICE AND EXPERTISE

This chapter began with James' (1890) proclamation that attention is *selective*, giving priority to some inputs, thoughts, or choices at the expense of others. James proposed a second idea that has proven just as important. The need for attention's services, and the role that attention plays in task performance, both *change with practice*. Performances that draw heavily on attention when being done for the first time can be replaced by well-practiced habits, reducing or perhaps even eliminating the need for the guidance, temporary storage, and decision-making processes provided by the attention system that we now call working memory.

Some investigators see such a transition from attended processing to habit as widespread, even inevitable, happening in every aspect of mental life. Bargh and Chartrand (1999) suggest that people greatly overestimate the scope of attended processing—what we are aware of, choose intentionally, and control volitionally. Always the provocateur, Alfred North Whitehead (1911) wrote that "It is a profoundly erroneous truism, repeated in all copybooks and by eminent people making speeches, that we should cultivate the habit of thinking about what we are doing. The precise opposite is the case. Civilization advances by extending the number of operations we can perform without thinking about them. Operations of thought are like cavalry charges in a battle—they are strictly limited in number, they require fresh horses, and must be made only at decisive moments."

In current cognitive science, what James (1890) called "habit" and Whitehead (1911) wanted more of is likely to be called "automatic processing." Indeed, the title of Bargh and Chartrand's (1999) paper was "The unbearable automaticity of being."

Most theories of skill acquisition are built around some version of the idea that attended processing gives way to automatic processing with practice. An important class of theory, however, dissents vigorously from this idea, emphasizing instead an increase in knowledge that accompanies practice and enables the flexibility needed for very high achievement. Automaticity is viewed as a poor sister—a byproduct of practice that can be useful but is not the major contributor to becoming a fluidly performing expert in a task domain.

Five Alternatives

In this section, we consider five alternative approaches to describing how the duties and deployment of attention change with practice and expertise, four having in one way or another to do with the development of automaticity and the fifth with the development of flexible knowledge-based expertise (Box 4-2). We treat these five approaches as complementary. Each has a piece of the truth, and all are necessary to understanding the role of attention in skill acquisition and expertise. Taken together, they tell a story.

The Basic Framework: Proceduralization/ Programming Theory

Following on groundwork laid late in the nineteenth century by Bryan and Harter's (1897) pioneering study of telegraphers learning Morse Code, Fitts (1964; Fitts & Posner, 1967) originated what has become the best-known and most widely applied class of theories of skill acquisition. Over the course of practice, governance of a task's performance undergoes a transition from reliance on a process of step-by-step control orchestrated in working memory to reliance on integrated procedures, routines, or programs that can run automatically once initiated and are largely free from the need for

Box 4-2

Five Theoretical Approaches to Skill Acquisition

1. *Proceduralization/Programming Theory:* Practice automates task performance.
2. *Strategy Selection Theory:* Early in practice, people try out different strategies for performing the task, discard inefficient strategies, and settle on a one that seems to work.
3. *Consistent-Practice Theory:* Task situations in which the same stimulus always requires the same response lead to the fastest improvements and automatization with practice.
4. *Instance Retrieval Theory:* Practice creates specific episodic memories of particular performances, which are retrieved later when the task is performed again and used as guides for what to do.
5. *Expert Performance Theory:* Experience with a task, and especially with variations in that task across lots of different situations, enables the accumulation of knowledge that supports creativity and truly high levels of achievement in the task domain.

working memory's resources and oversight. Thus, novice skill execution is controlled by a *strategy* or *algorithm*—a series of self-instructions and relevant pieces of information held in working memory and attended in a sequential fashion to control task performance and move it forward. Highly practiced expert performance is "automated"—controlled by *procedural knowledge*, which can be thought of as a *program* that integrates the self-instructions and task-relevant information into a package (see, e.g., Anderson, 1982, 1987; Brown & Carr, 1989; Beilock, Wierenga, & Carr, 2003; Keele, 1968, 1981; Newell & Rosenbloom, 1981; Proctor & Dutta, 1995). This integrated package functions much like a "callable subroutine" in computer programming. Once started, it runs to completion. At that point, either the entire task has been completed if all of its steps have been compiled into the package, or if the package represents only part of the task, then the next part of the task must be initiated. Depending on the level of practice and degree of integration of the next set of component task steps, continuation might involve calling another compiled procedure or returning to the more laborious step-by-step control processes of working memory.

Obviously such a progression from attention to automaticity would satisfy Northhead's desire to add to what we can do without thinking, and it might possibly increase our overall performance capabilities by increasing the ability to multitask. If attention is not needed for a while, maybe it can get involved in something else, or perhaps two automated procedures can run simultaneously.

Automaticity and Multitasking

One demonstration of increased multitasking capability as a consequence of practicing a task to a high level comes from Brown and Carr (1989). They gave participants several sessions of practice on a sequential reaction time task. Learning the task began with memorizing six sequences of digits of varying length, each labeled with a letter. Then, on each trial of the task itself, one of the labels was presented and the participant had to tap out the associated sequence on a circular array of six buttons, each of which was labeled with a digit. At the beginning of practice and again after practice was completed, a test session compared the sequence-tapping task performed all by itself to a dual-task situation in which the participant maintained a working-memory load of eight digits while identifying the label and tapping out the associated sequence. When tapping was finished, the participant recalled the list of digits. This dual-task combination presented particular difficulties, given the potential for interference between the digit content of the memory load and the digit content of the tapping sequence. Results showed that the working-memory load task interfered substantially with both the speed and the accuracy of tapping out the sequence during the pretest—interference was not completely debilitating, but it was substantial! The amount of interference was greatly reduced in the posttest, just as would be expected from the perspective of Fitts' proceduralization/programming theory of skill acquisition.

When Not to Pay Attention

An additional and rather dramatic point about the role of attention at different levels of practice was demonstrated by Beilock, Carr, MacMahon, and Starkes (2002), who asked novice and expert golfers to take short putts on an indoor putting green, trying to make the ball stop on a target that served as a "hole" (the university would not let them drill a real hole in the laboratory floor!). Distance the ball stopped from the center of the target was the measure of putting accuracy.

Putting was done in two different dual-task situations. One involved putting while listening for a target tone that occurred occasionally among a series of tones of different frequencies played through earphones. This irrelevant extra task was intended to distract attention away from putting. The other extra task called attention specifically *to* the act of putting, rather than distracting attention away. Participants were reminded that keeping the head of the putter straight onto the ball—that is, perpendicular to the line the ball should follow to the target—is important, and they were told to monitor the straightness of the putter head and say "straight" at the moment the putter contacted the ball. One might imagine that providing a reminder about something important to do and creating a structure for being sure to do it might be helpful. And indeed, novices' putting performance was better in this "skill focus" condition than in the irrelevant dual-task condition.

In contrast, experts' performance was better in the irrelevant dual-task condition (and the same effect was found in a second experiment comparing novice and expert soccer dribbling). Similar results were obtained in pioneering work by Masters (1992), who found that distraction provided by an irrelevant extra task could help expert performers in pressure situations (a point we will return to in the last section of the chapter). Adding Beilock and colleagues' findings to those of Masters (1992) indicates that once a task is automatized, it is better not to pay attention to its step-by-step control. While not explicitly *predicted* by proceduralization/programming theory, this pattern is consistent with that framework, and it certainly deepens our understanding of the changing role of attention as practice progresses.

What Should Be Attended During Learning?

The work of Beilock and colleagues raises the question of what exactly should be attended to during learning. Paying attention to something about the task appears to help the novice, but can more be said?

Wulf (2007; Wulf, Höß, & Prinz, 1998) has accumulated a large body of evidence that where attention is focused during practice is extremely important to the rate of skill improvement. It is clear from the work of Beilock and colleagues that in complex sensorimotor skills, it is bad for an expert to attend to step-by-step control of the performance, but it might be good for novices to do so. According to Wulf, attention to components of the task would be an example of "internal focus." Internal focus could be implemented at the level of a component step of execution, as in Beilock's experiments, or in Wulf's experiments, at a more molecular level, such as the configuration of a particular body part, or a body part's rate of movement or point of transition from one configuration to another during performance. Wulf contasts "internal focus" with attention to the outcome that the performance is supposed to achieve, such as the ball stopping on the target (or falling in the hole) when putting, which Wulf calls "external focus." The difference between internal and external focus is attending to what one is *doing* (internal focus) versus attending to input from the outside world about what one is *achieving* (external focus).

Wulf's argument is that paying attention to perceptual information about whether one's actions are achieving the intended goal is a more effective deployment of attention during learning than is paying attention to controlling the individual components of the actions themselves. Powers (1978) expresses much the same view in terms of engineering control theory, arguing that control of skilled performance is best achieved by attending to and monitoring perceptual feedback from the environment about the success of goal achievement. Called "perceptual control theory," Powers' view is that task goals are best framed in terms of the perceptual feedback one would get if the goal were achieved, not in terms of the signals to be sent to information-processing and muscle-control operations to make them do one thing or another. (Powers put this point very strongly in 2008, and we cannot resist quoting from pp. xi–xii: "Human beings do not plan actions and carry them out; they do not respond to stimuli according to the way they have been reinforced. They control. They never produce any behavior except for the purpose of making what they are experiencing become more like what they intend or want to experience, and then keeping it that way even in a changing world. If they plan, they plan perceptions, not actions.") Schütz-Bosbach and Prinz (2007) agree, referring to James (1890)—a recurrent theme in the study of skill acquisition. They say that the most effective focus of attention during learning, at least for sensorimotor skills, is "goals over movement."

Putting the arguments of Beilock and colleagues (2002) and Masters (1992) together with those of Wulf (2007), Powers (1978, 2008), and Schütz-Bosbach and Prinz (2007) allows us to say several things. When performing a well-learned, possibly automated skill, it is better to attend to an irrelevant extra task than it is to attend to trying to control the steps of the skill itself—this is from the work of Beilock and of Masters. Somewhat earlier in learning, it is better to attend to perceptual evidence about outcomes than to attend to controlling steps—that is from the work of Wulf and Prinz. And even at high levels of learning, paying attention to feedback about outcome success or failure enables the greatest success—that is from the work of Powers, and both Wulf and Prinz agree. (Here is an important point to think about: In the experiments of Beilock and colleagues, and also of Masters, the extra task whose distraction helped experts was auditory—while listening for the target sounds, the eyes of the golfers or soccer players were still able to take in visual information about the success and failure of their putts or kicks. Presumably blindfolding the participants in these experiments would have hurt even the experts! This would, of course, be expected by Wulf, Prinz, and Powers.)

A question remains about just how early in learning attention to evidence of achieved outcomes rather than attention to step-by-step control becomes beneficial—bearing in mind that for novice golfers just learning to putt, Beilock found that attention to the steps of execution, which Wulf would classify as internal focus, did produce good performance. The contrast is this: The Fitts proceduralization/programming framework suggests that at the earliest stages of learning, the component steps of the task must be held in working memory and attended in sequence. Wulf argues for a focus on attention to feedback about outcomes from the very beginning. Both of these points might be correct—they are not mutually exclusive, though if both are true they would imply a kind of dual-task situation, oddly enough, in which novice performers are attending both to controlling the steps of their performances and also to perceptual feedback about what those steps are causing to happen. This combination seems sensible. Future research will tell the tale.

Strategy Selection Theory

The proceduralization/programming framework raises a number of questions that are taken up as major points of emphasis in other approaches to skill acquisition. An important question is how do you come up with a strategy to begin with? This question is addressed in a type of theory whose origins might be glimpsed in models of problem solving such as Newell and Simon (1972: Newell, Shaw, & Simon, 1957) and especially further back in work on trial-and-error learning, beginning with Thorndike's (1898) famous studies of cats learning to escape from "puzzle boxes." In 1959, Crossman, after studying how employees in a Cuban cigar factory got better at the task of rolling cigars, proposed that trial-and-error plus problem solving plus instruction enables performers to devise successively more efficient step-by-step sequences of processes for doing a task (Figure 4-11 portrays Crossman's view of the sources of strategies). These strategies can be thought of as hypotheses about how the task might be done better, faster, more accurately, or with less effort. Once a good strategy is found (or a strategy that seems good enough given the speed

Figure 4-11 Sources of the range of strategies to be tried out during the early stage of acquiring a new skill which Crossman called "variance of method." [From Crossman, E. R. F. W. (1959). A theory of the acquisition of speed skill. *Ergonomics, 2,* 164.]

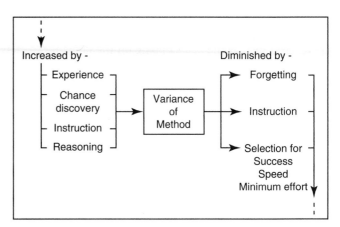

and accuracy criteria that need to be met), continued use of the chosen strategy consolidates and strengthens its execution—that is, the automatization process of Fitt's proceduralization/programming theory can set in. Crossman's practice data on cigar-rolling speed present a picture consistent with Bryan and Harter's (1897) findings from message-sending and message-receiving speed from telegraphers. A "law of diminishing returns" characterizes the benefits gained from practice, with rapid improvement early and rate of improvement per try slowing down as skill grows until performance finally reaches an asymptote beyond which it gets no faster. This is a finding of such scope across types of tasks and conditions of practice that is has come to be known as a law of learning (see Newell & Rosenbloom, 1981).

There may be a role for working memory capacity in the early period of strategy invention and try-out. Greater capacity is thought to allow more complex strategies to be constructed and maintained during performance, and might also allow more complex strategies to be grasped and attempted during instruction. A similar view about the efficacy of larger versus smaller working memory capacity has been applied with considerable success in studies of cognitive development (Case, 1985)

Consistent-Practice Theory

It is easy to suppose that settling on a single strategy might be advantageous—or even necessary—for automaticity to develop. While keeping several different strategies alive in one's repertoire might be advantageous in dealing with changing conditions, or simply in warding off boredom, it limits the practice time and number of repetitions for any one of the strategies. This notion has spawned an approach to skill acquisition that focuses on "consistent practice" of specific

stimulus-response mappings as the key to automaticity. Visual search tasks have served as the paradigm example illustrating the power of consistent practice. Shiffrin and Schneider (1977) used a search task in which one or more target stimuli—in their case letters, but similar search tasks have been conducted with many different kinds of stimuli—were sought in visual arrays containing varying numbers of nontarget stimuli and perhaps containing a target. The job of the performer was to indicate as rapidly and accurately as possible whether or not the target was present among the distracting nontargets. The presence-absence judgment is not crucial—similar results have subsequently been obtained in versions of search tasks in which every display contains a target and the job is to indicate which target it is.

When the task is new to the performer, the number of distractors makes a substantial difference—the more distractors, the slower and less accurate the search. However, if the target remains constant from trial to trial and never serves as a distractor, then performance improves with practice and eventually the number of distractors no longer matters. Search becomes "automatized." But if the target varies from trial to trial, so that sometimes a particular stimulus is a target but other times it is a distractor, performance improves very little. In particular, speed and accuracy continue to depend heavily on the number of stimuli in the array. Thus, "automatization" of search, so that the target seems to pop out without interference from the distractors, only happens with consistent stimulus-reponse mappings in which a target is always a target to be attended and a distractor is always a distractor to be ignored.

This is a powerful idea, but it is not always simple to implement. Duncan (2004) has pointed out that what will work as an effective consistent mapping is determined by how best to describe the "stimulus" and how best to describe the "response" for the particular purposes of the task. That is, what exactly the performer pays attention to and tries to map from perception to action is crucial. This point is made quite clearly in a widely cited study by Jonides and Gleitman (1972) in which search was for a target among distracting letters or distracting digits. The target was the same in all conditions—a circle—but participants were told either that they were searching for the letter "o" or the digit "zero." Search was considerably faster and less dependent on the number of distractors when the search was for the letter "o" among digits or the digit "zero" among letters—even though the target itself was identical. Thus, what participants thought about how they were doing the task and how they categorized the stimuli mattered to the mapping between stimulus and response and to the ability to separate the target stimulus from the to-be-ignored distractors.

Richards and Reicher (1978) and Wang, Cavanagh, and Green (1994), among others, have extended such findings to the role of familiarity with the stimuli in being able to discriminate targets from distractors—in particular, more familiar distractors can be more easily ignored, speeding search. Hout and Goldinger (2010) showed that if distractors remained the same, then search increased in efficiency with practice as expected, but this effect was accelerated if distractors not only remained the same stimuli, but occurred in the same spatial locations in the visual array (see also Chun & Jiang, 1998, for evidence on the impact of consistent spatial locations and repeated spatial relations among objects). Thus, consistent practice builds increasingly efficient performance, and the more factors in the task situation are remaining consistent, the more rapidly benefits accrue. Applications of these ideas have been successful in a variety of different real-world training and instructional environments (see, e.g., Dulaney, 1998; Fisk & Eboch, 2003; Verdolini, 2000).

Instance Retrieval Theory

Consistent practice's focus on overlearned stimulus-response mappings is reminiscent of James' (1890) concept of habit. Certainly there is a strong tradition in the study of habit formation in conditioned learning that focuses on the importance of associations between stimulus and response. Might such a notion apply more widely in theories of skill acquisition, particularly with respect to the nature of the representation that supports automatic processing? Thinking along these lines generated an approach that has come to be called the "instance theory" (or "exemplar theory" or "episodic memory retrieval theory") of skill acquisition, in which storing memories of specific instances of task performances is the key

to automaticity. Logan (1988, 2003, and several later papers) argues that the transition from reliance on a step-by-process in working memory (the strategy or algorithm) to automaticity is not achieved by forming a procedure, program, or "callable subroutine" representation of the task. Instead, automatic performance relies on direct retrieval of individual episodes of past performance from memory.

How is this supposed to work? Every time a task is performed, an episodic memory of that life event—the environmental context in which performance took place, the rules that define what is to be done, the stimulus that is perceived, and the action or response that is produced—gets stored in long term memory. Should the task be performed again, the context, the rules of the task, and the stimulus serve as retrieval cues, activating the memory of the past performance, which includes the action or response. This memory can circumvent or short-circuit the need to apply the algorithm to figure out what action to take—the memory supplies the information directly. The more times the task is performed, the more memories of its past performances are available to be retrieved, which means that retrieval is more likely to occur and to occur rapidly. Working memory can still plug along executing the step-by-step algorithm, but the algorithm will be slow compared to memory retrieval from a large and consistent body of performance memories.

Thus, the more practice with the task, the more probable it is that memory retrieval will beat the algorithm, speeding performance. As more and more memories accumulate, it becomes commonplace for memory retrieval to win the "race" to support performance, which eventually releases working memory from the need to engage in the algorithm at all (as long as the memories are accurate and the stimuli and the response mappings have stayed the same). This supplies a basis for multitasking—again, if working memory is not needed for the task being performed, perhaps it can be devoted to something else.

The instance retrieval approach to automaticity makes many of the same predictions and can account for many of the same phenomena as the proceduralization/programming approach. Indeed, Logan's initial argument was that retrieval of instances from episodic memory might be the basis for all automated performances, and the two approaches have generally been viewed as competitors.

However, the two approaches are not identical. The retrievable memories of instance theory are very specific life events, with their contents determined by exactly what was attended to during each performance

(Logan & Etherton, 1994). The specificity of stored instances means that retrieving and using them, like other applications of episodic memory, is constrained by the stimuli, contexts, and problems actually encountered during practice and hence stored in memory as retrievable instances. This implies that a skill supported by instance retrieval would not be easily transferable to new exemplars of a problem, except through simple processes of similarity-based stimulus generalization from stimuli that have been encountered before to quite similar new stimuli (Logan, 1988; Ericsson, 1999). Thus, exact repetition—the extreme of consistent practice—is the most effective vehicle for the transition to automaticity, and new stimuli might often require a return to the algorithm.

Such a restriction does not apply to proceduralization/programming theory, since a procedure can consist of relatively abstract stimulus descriptions and rules for generating a response that combine across the stimuli that have been encountered during training and responses that have been produced to them, rather than representing each stimulus and response pair individually (see, e.g., Singley & Anderson, 1989). This supplies a possible basis for distinguishing between the approaches. Crucial evidence might be found by analyzing the basis for transfer of acquired skill to unpracticed contexts.

Koh and Meyer (1991) used this difference in the flexibility and breadth of transfer allowed by the two theories of automatization to argue that practiced sensorimotor skills are in fact supported by procedures rather than retrieval of instances. They drew this conclusion from broad transfer functions obtained in a task specifically designed to test the mental representations underlying sensorimotor learning. In contrast, Beilock, Kulp, Holt, and Carr (2004) found that even after considerable practice at a particular type of complex mental arithmetic task, participants were no faster or more accurate on brand new problems of the same form requiring the same solution strategy than they had been at the beginning of training. On specific problems that had been encountered during training—the problems that would supply stored instances according to Logan's theory—performance was substantially improved, and in proportion to the number of times each particular problem had been encountered and solved. These results for mental arithmetic are in complete accord with instance theory.

Could it be that proceduralization/programming theory and instance theory are complementary, rather than being competitors? Comparing the properties of a variety of complex sensorimotor tasks—golf putting, soccer dribbling, volleyball serving—to those of complex mental arithmetic. Beilock, Weirenga, and Carr (2002) proposed that working-memory-demanding cognitive skills that require storage of intermediate products in between computational steps—such as mental arithmetic—automate via establishment of retrievable instances or episodes in long-term memory in accord with instance theory, whereas sensorimotor skills automate via the formation of more abstract rule-governed procedures or programs that are thought to be able to transfer more broadly. The difference in transfer results for the sensorimotor task studied by Koh and Meyer (1991) and the mental arithmetic task studied by Beilock et al. (2004) is promising for this complementarity hypothesis.

Expert Performance Theory

So far the focus has been on automatization through repetitive practice as a way to free task performance from the need to draw heavily on the limited capacities of working memory and selective attention. However, there is a danger to this progression, in that a consequence of automatization is likely to be routinization and stereotypy. With increasing amounts of practice, performance becomes more predictable and less variable, both in outcome and in execution time. This is known to happen in a wide variety of tasks, ranging from simple finger movements to reaching and grasping to many different kinds of choice reaction time tasks (see Mowbray & Rhoades, 1959; Newell & Corcos, 1993), to selecting and producing an appropriate verb in response to a noun (Raichle, Fiez, Videen, et al., 1994), and it is consistent with both the proceduralization/programming approach and the instance-retrieval approach to automaticity. Thus, the price of gaining freedom from reliance on working memory's oversight may be a loss of flexibility. Sometimes this is exactly what is wanted. Variability can be the enemy of stable and reliable performance. However, under some circumstances—particularly at the very high end of performance achievement—flexibility is needed in order to adapt to the requirements of difficult or unusual versions of the task or of the conditions under which the task is being performed.

In this light, we raise a final approach to the role of attention in skill and expertise, which emphasizes ways in which the importance of attention to the task increases rather than decreases as performance gets better. This "expert performance" approach (Ericsson, 2003) focuses not on practice as a source of automaticity, but on practice as a source of knowledge about the task domain that can be used flexibly to achieve maximum performance, and on paying careful attention to performance, especially during practice, when problems are encountered and a skill needs to be altered, fine-tuned, or improved.

The basic idea in the "expert performance approach" (Ericsson, 2003; Chase & Simon, 1973) is that the more you know the better you can perform. The most useful knowledge comes not from mere repetitive practice of the task, but from a particular kind of instructional and practice experience that has been labeled "deliberate practice" (Ericsson, 2003; Ericsson, Krampe, & Tesch-Romer, 1993). Ericsson (2006, p. 348) argues that differences in level of performance among high-level experts is no longer a function simply of the number of repetitions that have been completed (as in instance theory or proceduralization/programming theory). Instead, individual differences at the high end of skill depend on—and this quote comes from a study of musicians—"the amount of time accumulated in solitary practice—wherein musicians worked on specific, teacher-directed practice goals using methods purposely designed to improve specific aspects of their performance, including problem solving and feedback."

Thus, at high levels of skill, there are situations in which attention—very close attention—to step-by-step performance is beneficial, a notion that is not encompassed within the proceduralization/programming or instance theory frameworks. When the goal is explicitly to modify already-established performance processes in order to change execution parameters for the purpose of improving performance, or in an attempt to achieve a different performance outcome, then attention to step-by-control of performance, and also to the outcomes achieved by varying these steps, become major contributors to continued practice-based improvement.

An illustration can be found in experimental findings from Beilock, Weirenga, and Carr (2002). As described earlier, expert golfers using a regular putter—the kind on which they had practiced and developed their skills—did not fail in putting accuracy from under dual-task conditions requiring them to listen for target words. In addition, compared to novices, the experts had higher recognition memory for the words heard while putting but scantier episodic memories of specific putts. This is consistent with the experts paying less attention to putting and having more attention "left over" to devote to the extra task of monitoring auditorily presented words for a target. However, when using an S-shaped arbitrarily weighted "funny putter" designed to disrupt the practiced mechanics of skill execution, expert golfers showed decreased dual-task putting accuracy and produced extensive episodic memories of specific putts, but had trouble recognizing words from the extra monitoring task. Thus, the change in putter forced the experts to adapt their skills, changing them to accommodate the very different tool they were trying to use. The measures of attention—dual-task putting accuracy and relative memory for putting versus the stimuli of the extra task—showed a pattern much more like that of novices, who need to pay attention to step-by-step task control in order to perform well. This was not a full return to being a novice—putting accuracy by the experts with the funny putter was still significantly better than putting accuracy of novices—and it does not appear to last very long. In a subsequent study, Beilock, Bertenthal, Hoerger, and Carr (2008) found that relatively small amounts of practice with the "funny putter" returned the properties of experts' performance to "regular putter" standards.

To summarize, according to expert performance theory, the outcome of attended deliberate practice is an increase in the breadth, depth, and organization of the knowledge base that represents the performance domain in the expert's long term memory (Chase & Simon, 1973; Ericsson & Charness, 1994). Much of this knowledge base is thought to consist of patterns of past performance that can be retrieved in a new performance situation. Once retrieved, a pattern or set of patterns can either be relied upon directly to guide the new performance—a notion much like instance theory—or used more creatively in problem solving by analogy (Ericsson, 1999). In either case, performance benefits from increased rather than decreased attention. So the expert can go on autopilot when dealing with a familiar problem solved many times before—same-old, same-old, been there and done that—but has a vast knowledge base to draw upon via attended processing when a novel problem arises.

IMPACT OF ANXIETY, THREATENED SELF-CONCEPT, AND PRESSURE TO PERFORM

Let us go back to the office you were imagining at the beginning of the chapter. Your colleague had just said, "I know you don't like math, but you're the only person around and I need some help with this calculation. Here—take a look." You say to yourself, "It's way more than that. I'm scared to death of math. And lots of people think I'm not very good at it. So I'm on the spot. The pressure is on." You feel anxious, you fear that you might fail in front of your colleague—adding to your perceived public impression that you can't do math—and you want desperately to succeed. You've got something to prove. You say out loud, "All right. I'll give it a try."

In this concluding section, we return to the issues of energy, motivation, emotion, and readiness to perform that were first raised earlier in discussing arousal, alerting, and vigilance. The focus there was on mobilization of effort leading to readiness. Here the focus is on motivation, emotion, and their consequences.

Domain-Specific Anxieties as Factors in Attention

Mathematics provides an illustrative testing ground. Ashcraft and Kirk (2001) found that chronically math-anxious people evidence smaller working-memory capacities in standardized assessments than do non–math-anxious people who are otherwise comparable—but only if the working-memory assessment is computation-based, as in the Operation Span Task described in the section on executive and supervisory control. Entirely verbal working-memory measures show no systematic difference between math-anxious and non–math-anxious people. The magnitude of the decrement in working-memory capacity measured in a math environment predicts speed and accuracy of performance in a separate mental arithmetic task, especially when mental arithmetic is done as multitasking with a memory load (even one as simple and as different from numbers as a list of letters). Ashcraft and Krause (2007) reviewed these findings plus other research, and concluded that "High math anxiety works much like a dual task setting: Preoccupation with one's math fears and anxieties functions like a resource-demanding secondary task" (p. 243).

We might note that effects of anxiety or fear could impact language production in an analogous fashion—whether inner speech used in support of thinking as the situation unfolds and remembering it later, or external speech as in public-speaking situations, especially in people who are fearful of public performance. Whether these possibilities are true is still a matter under investigation, but given the established role of working memory in language comprehension and production (e.g., Bock & Cutting, 1992; Gruber & Goeschke, 2004; Waters & Caplan, 2004, 2005), they are worth pursuing.

"Pressure to Perform" as a Factor in Attention

A pressure situation generally consists of one or more of three components: rewards can be won if performance is good or lost if it is bad, other people are depending on your performance to be good, which gives you a certain amount of social responsibility, and the performance is open to public scrutiny and external evaluation, so that you can look good or bad in your own eyes and also in the eyes of others. The putt to win the golf match, the foul shot to win the basketball game, and the Scholastic Aptitude Test score to get into college are all examples.

What happens in such situations? Evidence (Beilock & Carr, 2001; Beilock, Kulp, Holt, & Carr, 2004; Markman, Maddox, & Worthy, 2006) indicates that pressure induces two changes in the executive control and selective attention systems. One is that a portion of working memory capacity is likely to be occupied with worries and concerns about the situation, its importance, and the consequences of failure—negative thoughts that might be in a sense about the task, but that do not contribute to its control or its performance. This means that the demands of a working-memory intensive task are more likely than usual to exceed the supply available during the performance. The other change is that attention is likely to be devoted in step-by-step fashion to the sequence of component information-processing operations and actions or responses required by successful performance. If the task is not automated and therefore can benefit from control at such a detailed level, then a gain in performance might be seen—except that the capacity available for such control has been reduced. If the task is automated and should no longer be explicitly controlled at such a level, then—as seen earlier in the work of Beilock et al. (2002)—performance is likely to be slower and more error-prone that it would have been under the control of a procedure/program or retrieved instances from memory.

The upshot is that pressure creates two attention-related ways to fail, with different domains of task performance susceptible to each. Working-memory–intensive tasks such as mathematical computation or novice performance of a complex sensorimotor skill might deteriorate due to reduced working memory capacity. Well-practiced sensorimotor skills might deteriorate due to attending at a grain-size of task structure that is smaller than the task's already-automatized chunks.

When High-Powered People Fail

An extremely counterintuitive outcome of these processes can occur in working-memory-intensive task domains. Beilock and Carr (2005) gave college undergraduates a series of mental arithmetic problems requiring both subtraction and division on each problem. The problems varied in complexity—defined mainly by whether the numbers involved were double-digit and whether the subtraction required borrowing. No problem was seen more than once, so each new problem was novel and could not be solved by retrieval of the answer from episodic memory.

Speed and accuracy were measured first in a relatively neutral condition described as practice, and then in a pressure condition in which participants were told that if they could improve their performance by 20% over the practice trials, then (a) they could win $5, (b) it was a "team game" in which two participants had been paired up and both had to meet the improvement criterion to receive the money—and the participant's partner had already succeeded, and (c) the performance was being videotaped for examination at an upcoming conference of professors and teachers interested in math achievement. These are the three characteristics of a pressure situation identified above: reward, social responsibility, and public scrutiny or evaluation.

Participants were also given an assessment of working memory capacity, consisting of the average score between a version of the Operation Span Test and a version of the Reading Span Test (both described earlier in the chapter). Based on these average scores, which could range from 2 to 42, participants were divided into a high-capacity group (mean 21.1) and a low-capacity group (mean 9.8). The question was then asked: which group showed the bigger impact of pressure?

In a working-memory–intensive task such mental arithmetic, it might seem that people with higher working memory capacities would be better equipped to deal with the reductions in capacity that are likely to happen in pressure situations. But the title of the publication gives away the story: "When high-powered people fail: Working memory and choking under pressure in math."

What happened? Both groups worked faster under pressure, so the arousal of the pressure situation led people to hurry up to some degree. Turning to accuracy, neither group suffered on the simpler problems. But on the more complex problems, the *high*-capacity participants dropped significantly in accuracy, whereas the low-capacity participants actually improved somewhat. The result was that the high-capacity group, which during practice had shown a substantial advantage in accuracy, was no better in the pressure condition than the low-capacity group. It was as if the high-capacity group had been gaining its advantage by using their working memory capacity to the fullest—if you've got it, flaunt it. Imposing pressure reduced their capacity to levels that would no longer support their high-powered strategies, costing them in performance. The low-capacity group did not try such complicated strategies to begin with, and perhaps the pressure situation served more to focus their attention on doing the best they could with the simpler strategies at their command. At present this might be just a story. Future research will determine if it is correct.

EPILOGUE: THE OFFICE CONVERSATION

We opened the chapter with an office conversation that involved many "attentional moments" and raised many attentional issues. At this point we can revisit that conversation and refer to some of the things we have learned. Here is how the scenario got started:

Suppose that physically you are sitting in your office. In principle you are composing an email, but in fact you are off in some imaginary mental space, enjoying a pleasant daydream.

Mindwandering is a fact of mental life, highlighting the sources of information to which attention can be devoted. Input can come from external perceptual sources, with audition, vision, somatosensation, and kinesthesis all playing important roles in language. Input can also come from internal sources. These involve long-term memory—including semantic and syntactic memory for language—and imagination, which is a working-memory-invented product that draws its raw materials from long-term memory and perception.

The distinction between external and internal sources of information highlights in turn the distinction between endogenous and exogenous control. There is an important interplay between engodenous and exogenous control in selective attention and also in working memory. This brings us to the next event in the scenario.

A colleague who wants to talk about a project pokes her head in your door and gently knocks on the doorframe. She says "Hey—earth to you! Can you pay attention for a second?"

How, if at all, are you going to heed that request? Will you even notice it?

Three perceptual inputs from the external world are calling for your attention: visual motion in the periphery, a noise with particular auditory characteristics (rapid onset and offset, short duration, and an agreed-upon social meaning), and speech. Any of these signals might gain exogenous control over the direction of your attention, eliciting an orienting response that switches attention from its internal focus on your daydream to the perceptual pathways bringing in the signal from the outside (remember Posner, Snyder, & Davidson, 1980).

It is possible that no single one of these signals is intense enough by itself to capture attention. However, since vision and audition can combine their influences when they arrive from the same location, the set of signals added together might be sufficient.

Because the speech input is extended in time and is an extremely high-value cognitive and social input in the priority structure of human information processing, it is likely to hold your attention once you have oriented toward its source, recognized it as speech, and begun to interpret it.

Of course all of this is happening rapidly and in a largely reflexive manner. Endogenous control by which you *decide* (or perhaps the better word would be *agree*) to acknowledge this set of signals as representing a person with whom to interact comes rapidly but not instantaneously.

Even if the request seems reasonable under these circumstances, is it always good advice to "pay attention"? Are there times when you are better off not paying attention— whatever that means?

These questions were an aside from the scenario itself, and they raised crucial issues. The answers covered a lot of conceptual and empirical ground, including (a) the need for selective attention when conditions are information-dense and there is lots of distracting information; (b) the need for executive control when a task is new or complicated, (c) the difficulties of multitasking and its occasional successes, which are governed in large part by practice and the development of automaticity; (c) the changing role that attention plays in task performance as practice accumulates and expertise grows; and (d) the multiple theories of automaticity and how it develops.

What if you have trouble "paying attention"? Can anything be done?

These questions were another aside—though perhaps not irrelevant to the scenario itself, if it had turned out that you never did notice your colleague even after she knocked louder, walked further into your office, and spoke again more forcefully. The section on training attention described several training success stories, suggesting that there is promise for overcoming attentional and capacity-related difficulties—even in language processing and language rehabilitation.

And once you are "paying attention," what does attention actually do, and how does that happen?

You say, "Sure—come in."

Apparently the set of calls for attention generated by your colleague did succeed in shifting your attention— a process we considered in the section on selective attention. You then exerted endogenous control by deciding to interact and in formulating an appropriate reply, a set of processes whose attention demands we considered in the section on executive and supervisory control.

Your colleague sits down and begins to talk. You listen, but you also try to read what you have written in the email, which you are again thinking about. You start to type the next sentence in the message. Can you succeed at this multitasking?

Your colleague asks again, "Really—can you pay attention for a second?"

Apparently not! This multitasking defeated you. The simple fact is that multitasking *often* proves to be too much, even when you *believe* that you can do it, and sometimes even when you believe you *are* doing it. The illusion persists until something goes wrong—perhaps dreadfully wrong. You may not notice slightly slowed performance time or small mistakes, but a *big* mistake will cause you to take notice.

Particular kinds of practice might help in getting better at multitasking. We saw in the section on skill acquisition that if a task is highly automated, then the chances increase for successfully combining that task with another task.

Chances for successful combination increase again if the specific tasks are practiced together. Spelke, Hirst, and Neisser (1976) showed that even a combination of tasks as demanding as reading for comprehension and memory, while concurrently writing down words from dictation, can be mastered with *enough* practice, though the amount was considerable. (And, to be honest, memory for the passages never did reach single-task levels.)

You say, "OK—sure. What's this about?" Your colleague says "Well, I know you don't like math, but you're the only person around and I need some help with this calculation. Here—take a look."

At this point in the scenario, two important things happen. One is that perceiving and processing your colleague's cue requires the establishment of joint regard between the two of you. "Here—take a look" is a cue that a visual stimulus is available somewhere in the environment and that your conversational companion wishes that you both should attend to it together. We considered the establishment of joint regard in the section on selective attention.

The second thing that happens is less propitious. In general you are quite willing to engage in joint attention with your fellow human beings, but mathematical calculation is not on your list of favorite activities.

You say to yourself, "It's way more than that. I'm scared to death of math. And lots of people think I'm not very good at it. So I'm on the spot. The pressure is on." You feel anxious, you fear that you might fail in front of your colleague—adding to your perceived public impression that you can't do math— and you want desperately to succeed. You've got something to prove. You say out loud, "All right. I'll give it a try."

And now we are really in the real world, where situations arise that matter, emotions are engaged, motivations to succeed come into play, and fears of failing can all too easily arise. We considered the attentional and performance consequences of emotion and motivation in the last section of the chapter.

REFERENCES

Acheson, D. J., Hamidi, M., Binder, J. R., & Postle, B. R. (2011). A common neural substrate for language production and verbal working memory. *Journal of Cognitive Neuroscience.*

Allport, A., & Wylie, G. (2000). Task-switching, stimulus-response bindings, and negative priming. In S. Monsell & J. Driver (Eds.), *Control of cognitive processes: Attention and performance XVIII*. Boston: MIT Press.

Alvarez, G. A., & Cavanagh, P. (2004). The capacity of visual short-term memory is set both by visual information load and by number of objects. *Psychological Science, 15,* 106–111.

Anderson, J. R. (1982). Acquisition of cognitive skill. *Psychological Review, 89,* 369–406.

Anderson, J. R. (1987). Skill acquisition: Compilation of weak-method problem solutions. *Psychological Review, 94,* 192–210.

Anderson, K. (1994). Impulsivity, caffeine, and task difficulty: A within-subjects test of the Yerkes-Dodson Law. *Personality and Individual Differences, 16,* 813–829.

Antrobus, J. S., Singer, J. L., Goldstein, S., & Fortgang, M. (1970). Mindwandering and cognitive structure. *Transactions of the New York Academy of Science, 32,* 242–252.

Ashcraft, M. H., & Kirk, E. F. (2001). The relationships among working memory, math anxiety, and performance. *Journal of Experimental Psychology: General, 130,* 224–237.

Ashcraft, M. H., & Krause, J. A. (2007). Working memory, math performance, and math anxiety. *Psychonomic Bulletin & Review, 14,* 243–248.

Atkinson, R. C., & Shiffrin, R. M. (1986). Human memory: A proposed system and its control processes. In K. W. Spence, & J. T. Spence (Eds.), *The psychology of learning and motivation: Advances in research and theory* (Vol. 2, pp. 742–775). New York: Academic Press.

Awh, E., Barton, B., & Vogel, E. K. (2007). Visual working memory represents a fixed number of items regardless of complexity. *Psychological Science, 18,* 622–628.

Bacharach, V. R., Carr, T. H., & Mehner, D. S. (1976). Interactive and independent contributions of verbal descriptions to children's picture memory. *Journal of Experimental Child Psychology, 22,* 492–498.

Baddeley, A. D., & Hitch, G. (1974). Working memory. In G. A. Bower (Ed.), *Recent advances in learning and motivation* (*Vol. 8,* pp. 47–90). New York: Academic Press.

Baddeley, A. D. (2000). The episodic buffer: A new component of working memory? *Trends in Cognitive Sciences, 4,* 417–423.

Banich, M. T. (2004). *Cognitive neuroscience and neuropsychology* (2nd ed.). Boston: Houghton-Mifflin.

Bargh, J. A., Chartrand, T. L. (1999). The unbearable automaticity of being. *American Psychologist, 54,* 462–479.

Bates, E. (1976). *Language and context: The acquisition of pragmatics.* New York: Academic Press.

Beek, P. J., Jacobs, D. M., Daffertshofer, A., & Huys, R. (2003). Expert performance in sport: Views from the joint perspectives of ecological psychology and dynamical systems theory. In J. L. Starkes & K. A. Ericsson (Eds.), *Expert performance in sports: Advances in research on sport expertise* (pp. 321–344). Champaign, IL: Human Kinetics.

Beilock, S. L., Bertenthal, B. I., Hoerger, M., & Carr, T. H. (2008). When does haste make waste? Expertise, speed versus accuracy, and the tools of the trade. *Journal of Experimental Psychology: Applied, 14,* 340–353.

Beilock, S. L., & Carr, T. H. (2001). On the fragility of skilled performance: What governs choking under pressure? *Journal of Experimental Psychology: General, 130,* 701–725.

Beilock, S. L., & Carr, T. H. (2005). When high-powered people fail: Working memory and "choking under pressure" in math. *Psychological Science, 16,* 101–105.

Beilock, S. L., Carr, T. H., MacMahon, C., & Starkes, J. L. (2002). When paying attention becomes counterproductive: Impact of divided versus skill-focused attention on novice and experienced performance of sensorimotor skills. *Journal of Experimental Psychology: Applied, 8,* 6–16.

Beilock, S. L., Kulp, C. A., Holt, L. E., & Carr, T. H. (2004). More on the fragility of performance: Choking under pressure in mathematical problem solving. *Journal of Experimental Psychology: General, 133,* 584–600.

Beilock, S. L., Wierenga, S. A., & Carr, T. H. (2002). Expertise, attention, and memory in sensorimotor skill execution: Impact of novel task constraints on dual-task performance and episodic memory. *Quarterly Journal of Experimental Psychology, 55A,* 1211–1240.

Beilock, S. L., Wierenga, S. A., & Carr, T. H. (2003). Skilled performance, explicit memory, and "expertise-induced amnesia." In J. Starkes & K. A. Ericsson (Eds.), *Expert performance in sports: Advances in research on sport expertise.* Champaign, IL: Human Kinetics.

Berryhill, M. E., & Hughes, H. C. (2009). On the minimization of task switch costs following long-term training. *Attention, Perception, & Psychophysics, 71,* 503–514.

Bherer, L., Kramer, A. F., Peterson, M. S., Colcombe, S., Erickson, K., & Becic, E. (2006). Testing the limits of cognitive plasticity in older adults: Application to attentional control. *Acta Psychologica, 123,* 261–278.

Bock, J. K., & Griffin, Z. M. (2000). Producing words: How mind meets mouth. In L. Wheeldon (Ed.), *Aspects of language production* (pp. 7–47). Hove, England: Psychology Press.

Bock, K., & Cutting, J. C. (1992). Regulating mental energy: Performance units in language production. *Journal of Memory and Language, 31,* 99–127.

Botvinick, M. M., Cohen, J. D., & Carter, C. S. (2004). Conflict monitoring and anterior cingulate cortex: An update. *Trends in Cognitive Sciences, 8,* 539–546.

Brown, T. L., & Carr, T. H. (1989). Automaticity in skill acquisition: Mechanisms for reducing interference during concurrent performance. *Journal of Experimental Psychology: Human Perception and Performance, 15,* 686–700.

Brown, T. L., Gore, C., & Carr, T. H. (2002). Is word recognition "automatic"?: Spatial attention and word recognition in Stroop color-naming. *Journal of Experimental Psychology: General, 131,* 220–241.

Bruner, J. S. (1975). The ontogenesis of speech acts. *Journal of Child Language, 2,* 1–19.

Bryan, W. L., & Harter, N. (1897). Studies in the physiology and psychology of the telegraphic language. *Psychological Review, 4,* 27–53.

Buckner, R. L., Andrews-Hanna, J. R., & Schacter, D. L. (2008). The brain's default network: Anatomy, function, and relevance to disease. *Annals of the New York Academy of Science, 1124,* 1–38.

Caplan, D., & Waters, G. S. (1995). On the nature of the phonological output planning process involved in verbal rehearsal: Evidence from aphasia. *Brain and Language, 48,* 191–220.

Carr, T. H. (1979). Consciousness in models of information processing: Primary memory, executive control, and input regulation. In G. Underwood & R. Stevens (Eds.), *Aspects of consciousness* (Vol. 1, pp. 123–153). London: Academic Press.

Carr, T. H., & Bacharach, V. R. (1976). Perceptual tuning and conscious attention: Systems of input regulation in visual information processing. *Cognition, 4,* 281–302.

Case, R. (1985). *Intellectual development: Birth to adulthood.* New York: Academic Press.

Chase, W. G., & Simon, H. A. (1973). The mind's eye in chess. In W. G. Chase (Ed.), *Visual information processing* (pp. 215–281). New York: Academic Press.

Chein, J. M., & Fiez, J. A. (2010). Evaluating models of working memory through the effects of concurrent irrelevant information. *Journal of Experimental Psychology: General, 139,* 117–137.

Cherry, E. C. (1953). Some experiments on the recognition of speech, with one and with two ears. *Journal of the Acoustical Society of America, 25,* 975–979.

Christoff, K., Gordon, A. M., Smallwood, J., Smith, R., & Schooler, J. W. (2009). Experience sampling during fMRI reveals default network and executive system contributions to mind wandering. *Proceedings of the National Academy of Sciences of the USA, 106,* 8719–8724.

Chun, M. M., & Jiang, Y. (1998). Contextual cueing: Implicit learning and memory of visual context guides spatial attention. *Cognitive Psychology, 36,* 28–71.

Cohen, J. D., Aston-Jones, G., & Gilzenrat, M. S. (2004). A systems-level perspective on attention and cognitive control: Guilded activation, adaptive gating, conflict monitoring, and exploitation versus exploration. In M. I. Posner (Ed.), *Cognitive neuroscience of attention.* New York: Guilford Press.

Collard, P., Corley, M., MacGregor, L. J., Donaldson, D. I. (2008). Attention orienting effects of hesitations in speech: Evidence from ERPs. *Journal of Experimental Psychology: Learning, Memory, and Cognition, 34,* 696–702.

Cools, R., & Robbins, T. W. (2004). Chemistry of the adaptive mind. *Philosophical transactions. Series A, Mathematical, Physical, and Engineering Sciences, 15,* 2871–2888.

Corbetta, M., Kincade, J. M., Ollinger, J. M., McAvoy, M. P., & Shulman, G. L. (2000). Voluntary orienting is dissociated from target detection in human posterior parietal cortex. *Nature Neuroscience, 3,* 292–297.

Corbetta, M., Miezen, F. M., Shulman, G. L., & Petersen, S. E. (1993). A PET study of visuospatial attention. *Journal of Neuroscience, 13,* 1202–1226.

Cowan, N. (2000). The magical number 4 in short-term memory: A reconsideration of mental storage capacity. *Behavioral and Brain Sciences, 24,* 87–185.

Crossman, E. R. F. W. (1959). A theory of the acquisition of speed skill. *Ergonomics, 2,* 153–166.

Dagenbach, D., & Carr, T. H. (1994). *Inhibitory processes in attention, memory, and language.* San Diego: Academic Press.

Dandeneau, S. D., Baldwin, M. W., Baccus, J. R., Sakellaropoulo, M., & Pruessner, J. C. (2007). Cutting stress off at the pass: Reducing vigilance and responsiveness to social threat by manipulating attention. *Journal of Personality and Social Psychology, 93,* 651–666.

Daneman, M., & Merikle, P. M. (1996). Working memory and language comprehension: A meta-analysis. *Psychonomic Bulletin & Review, 3,* 422–433.

Desimone, R., & Duncan, J. (1995). Neural mechanisms of selective attention. *Annual Review of Neuroscience, 18,* 193–222.

Doran, S. M., Van Dongen, H. P. A., & Dinges, D. F. (2001). Sustained attention performance during sleep deprivation: Evidence of state instability. *Archives Italiennes de Biologie, 139,* 253–267.

Driver, J., & Spence, C. J. (1994). Spatial synergies between auditory and visual attention. In C. Umilta & M. Moscovitch (Eds.), *Attention and performance, XV: Conscious and nonconscious information processing* (pp. 311–331). Cambridge, MA: MIT Press.

Driver, J., & Spence, C. J. (1998). Cross-modal links in spatial attention. *Philosophical Transactions of the Royal Society of London B Biological Sciences, 353,* 1319–1331.

Dulaney, C. L. (1998). Automatic processing: Implications for job training of individuals with mental retardation. *Journal of Developmental and Physical Disabilities, 10,* 175–184.

Duncan, J. (2004). Selective attention in distributed brain systems. In M. I. Posner (Ed.), *Cognitive neuroscience of attention* (pp. 105–113). New York: Guilford Press.

Eberhard, K. M., Cutting, J. C., & Bock, J. K. (2005). Making syntax of sense: Number agreement in sentence production. *Psychological Review, 112,* 531–559.

Erickson, K. I., Colcombe, S. J., Wadha, R., Bherer, L., Peterson, M. S., Scalf, P. E., Kim, J. S., . . . Kramer, A. F. (2007). Training-induced functional activation changes in dual-task processing: An fMRI study. *Cerebral Cortex, 17,* 192–204.

Ericsson, K. A. (1999). Creative expertise as superior reproducible performance: Innovative and flexible aspects of expert performance. *Psychological Inquiry, 10*(4), 329–333.

Ericsson, K. A. (2003). The acquisition of expert performance as problem solving: Construction and modification of mediating mechanisms through deliberate practice. In J. E. Davidson & R. J. Sternberg (Eds.), *Problem solving* (pp. 31–83). New York: Cambridge University Press.

Ericsson, K. A. (2006). Protocol analysis and expert thought: Concurrent verbalizations of thinking during experts' performance on representative task. In K. A. Ericsson, N. Charness, P. Feltovich, & R. R. Hoffman, R. R. (Eds.), *Cambridge handbook of expertise and expert performance* (pp. 223–242). Cambridge, UK: Cambridge University Press.

Ericsson, K. A. (2006). The influence of experience and deliberate practice on the development of superior expert performance. In K. A. Ericsson, N. Charness, P. Feltovich, & R. R. Hoffman, R. R. (Eds.), *Cambridge handbook of expertise and expert performance* (pp. 685–706). Cambridge, UK: Cambridge University Press.

Ericsson, K. A., & Charness, N. (1994). Expert performance: Its structure and acquisition. *American Psychologist, 49*(8), 725–747.

Ericsson, K. A., & Kintsch, W. (1995). Long-term working memory. *Psychological Review, 101*, 211–245.

Ericsson, K. A., Krampe, R. T., & Tesch-Romer, C. (1993). The role of deliberate practice in the acquisition of expert performance. *Psychological Review, 100*, 363–406.

Ericsson, K. A., & Ward, P. (2007). Capturing the naturally occurring superior performance of experts in the laboratory: Toward a science of expert and exceptional performance. *Current Directions in Psychological Science, 16*, 346–350.

Eriksen, C. W., & Hoffman, J. E. (1972). Temporal and spatial characteristics of selective encoding from visual displays. *Attention, Perception, & Psychophysics, 12,* 201–204.

Evans, M. A., & Carr, T. H. (1984). The ontogeny of description. In L. Feagans, C. Garvey, & R. Golinkoff (Eds.), *The origins and growth of communication* (pp. 297–316). Norwood, NJ: Ablex.

Fair, D. A., Cohen, A. L., Dosenbach, N. U. F., Church, J. A., Miezin, F. M., Barch, D. M., Raichle, M. E., . . . Schlaggar, B. L. (2008). The maturing architecture of the brain's default network. *Proceedings of the National Academy of Science of the USA, 105*, 4028–4032.

Fan, J., McCandliss, B. D., Fossella, J., Flombaum, J. I., & Posner, M. I. (2005). The activation of attentional networks. *NeuroImage, 26*, 471–479.

Fisk, A. D., & Eboch, M. (2003). An automatic/controlled processing theory application to training component map reading skills. *Applied Ergonomics, 20*, 2–13.

Fitts, P. M. (1964). Perceptual-motor learning. In A. W. Melton (Ed.), *Categories of human learning.* New York: Academic Press.

Fitts, P. M. & Posner, M. I. (1967). *Human performance.* Belmont, CA: Brooks/Cole.

Flegal, K. E., & Anderson, M. C. (2008). Overthinking skilled motor performance: Or why those who teach can't do. *Psychonomic Bulletin & Review, 15*, 927–932.

Folk, C. L., Remington, R. W., & Johnston J. C. (1992). Involuntary covert orienting is contingent on attentional control settings. *Journal of Experimental Psychology: Human Perception & Performance, 18*, 1030–1044.

Folk, C. L., Remington, R. W., & Wright, J. H. (1994). The structure of attentional control: Contingent attentional capture by apparent motion, abrupt onset, and color. *Journal of Experimental Psychology: Human Perception & Performance, 20*, 317–329.

Gazzaniga, M. S., Ivry, R. B., & Mangun, G. R. (2009). *Cognitive neuroscience: The biology of the mind* (3rd ed.). New York: Norton.

Green, C. S. & Bavelier, D. (2008). Exercising your brain: A review of human brain plasticity and training-induced learning. *Psychology and Aging, 23*, 692–701.

Gruber, O., & Goeschke, T. (2004). Executive control emerging from dynamic interactions between brain systems mediating language, working memory and attentional processes. *Acta Psychologica, 115*, 105–121.

Hasher, L., Zacks, R. T., & May, C. P. (1999). Inhibitory control, circadian arousal, and age. In D. Gopher & A. Koriat (Eds.), *Attention and performance, XVII. Cognitive regulation of performance: Interaction of theory and applications* (pp. 653–675). Cambridge, MA: MIT Press.

Henderson, J. M., & Ferreira, F. (Eds). (2004). *The interface of language, vision, and action: Eye movements and the visual world.* New York: Psychology Press.

Hopfinger, J. B., Buonocore, M. H., & Mangun, G. R. (2000). The neural mechanisms of top-down attentional control. *Nature Neuroscience, 3*, 284–292.

Hout, M. C., & Goldinger, S. D. (2010). Learning in repeated visual search. *Attention, Perception, & Psychophysics, 72*, 1267–1282.

Huang-Pollack, C. L., Nigg, J. T., & Carr, T. H. (2002). Development of selective attention: Perceptual load influences early versus late selection in children and adults. *Developmental Psychology, 38*, 363–375.

James, W. (1890). *Principles of psychology.* New York: Henry Holt.

Jones, J. A., & Callan, D. E. (2003). Brain activity during audio-visual speech perception: An fMRI study of the McGurk Effect. *NeuroReport, 14*, 1129–1133.

Jonides, J., & Gleitman, H. (1972). A conceptual category effect in visual search: O as letter or digit. *Perception & Psychophysics, 12*, 457–460.

Jonides, J., Lewis, R. L., Nee, D. E., Lustig, C. A., Berman, M. G., & Moore, K. S. (2008). The mind and brain of short-term memory. *Annual Review of Psychology, 59*, 193–224.

Kahneman, D. (1973). *Attention and effort.* Englewood Cliffs, NJ: Prentice-Hall.

Kane, M. J., Brown, L. H., McVay, J. C., Silvia, P. J., Myin-Germeys, I., & Kwapil, T. R. (2007). For whom the mind wanders, and when: An experience-sampling study of working memory and executive control in daily life. *Psychological Science, 18*, 614–621.

Kastner, S., Pinsk, M. A., De Weerd, P., Desimone, R., & Ungerleider, L. G., 1999. Increased activity in human visual cortex during directed attention in the absence of visual stimulation. *Neuron, 22* (4), 751–761.

Keele, S. W. (1968). Movement control in skilled motor performance. *Psychological Bulletin, 70*, 387–403.

Keele, S. W. (1973). *Attention and human performance.* Pacific Palisades, CA: Goodyear.

Keele, S. W. (1981). Behavioral analysis of movement. In V. Brooks (Ed.), *Handbook of physiology: Motor control.* Washington, DC: American Physiological Society.

Klein, R. M. (2004). On the control of visual orienting. In M. I. Posner (Ed.), *Cognitive neuroscience of attention* (pp. 29–44). New York: Guilford.

Koh, K., & Meyer, D. E. (1991). Induction of continous stimulus-response associations for perceptual-motor performance. *Journal of Experimental Psychology: Learning, Memory, and Cognition, 17*, 811–836.

Kornblum, S., & Requin, J. (Eds.) (1984). *Preparatory states and processes.* Hillsdale, NJ: Lawrence Erlbaum.

Lavie, N. (1995). Perceptual load as a necessary condition for selective attention. *Journal of Experimental Psychology: Human Perception and Performance, 21*, 451–468.

Lavie, N. (2006). The role of perceptual load in visual awareness. *Brain Research, 1080*, 91–100.

Legerstee, J. S., Joke, H. M., Tulen, V. L., Kallen, G. C., Dieleman, P. D. A., Treffers, F. C., & Verhulst, E. M. W. J. (2009). Threat-related selective attention predicts treatment success in childhood anxiety disorders. *Journal of the American Academy of Child and Adolescent Psychiatry, 48*, 196–205.

Logan, G. D. (1988). Toward an instance theory of automatization. *Psychological Review, 95,* 492–527.

Logan, G. D., & Bundesen, C. (2003). Clever homunculus: Is there an endogenous act of control in the explicit task-cueing procedure? *Journal of Experimental Psychology: Human Perception and Performance, 29,* 575–599.

Logan, G. L., & Etherton, J. L. (1994). What is learned during automatization? The role of attention in constructing an instance. *Journal of Experimental Psychology: Learning, Memory, and Cognition, 20,* 1022–1050.

MacLean, K. A., Ferrer, E., Aichele, S. R., Bridwell, D. A., Zanesco, A. P., Jacobs, T. L., King, . . . Saron, C. D. (2010). Intensive meditation training improves perceptual discrimination and sustained attention. *Psychological Science, 21,* 829–839.

MacLeod, C. M. (1991). Half a century or research on the Stroop effect: An integrative review. *Psychological Bulletin, 109,* 163–203.

Markman, A. B., Maddox, W. T., & Worthy, D. A. (2006). Choking and excelling under pressure. *Psychological Science, 17,* 944–948.

Masters, R. S. W. (1992). Knowledge, knerves, and know-how: The role of explicit versus implicit knowledge in the breakdown of a complex motor skill under pressure. *British Journal of Psychology, 83,* 343–358.

May, C. P., Hasher, L., & Stoltzfus, E. R. (1993). Optimal time of day and the magnitude of age differences in memory. *Psychological Science, 4,* 326–330.

McGurk, H., & MacDonald, J. W. (1976). Hearing lips and seeing voices. *Nature, 264,* 746–748.

Miller, G. A. (1956). The magical number seven, plus or minus two: Some limits on our capacity for processing information. *Psychological Review, 63,* 81–97.

Miller, A., Galanter, E., and Pribaum K. H. (1960). *Plans and the structure of behavior.* New York: Holt, Rinehart, & Winston.

Mondor, T. A., & Zatorre, R. J. (1995). Shifting and focusing auditory spatial attention. *Journal of Experimental Psychology: Human Perception and Performance, 21,* 387–409.

Mowbray, G. H. & Rhoades, M. V. (1959). On the reduction of choice reaction times with practice. *Quarterly Journal of Experimental Psychology, 11,* 16–23.

National Safety Council, 2010. National Safety Council estimates that at least 1.6 million crashes each year involve drivers using cell phones and texting. Retrieved from: www.nsc.org/pages/NSCestimates1.6millioncrashescausedbydriversusingcellphonesandtexting/aspx.

Neider, M. B., Boot, W. R., & Kramer, A. F. (2010). Visual search for real world targets under conditions of high target-background similarity: Exploring training and transfer in younger and older adults. *Acta Psychologica, 134,* 29–39.

Newell, A., & Rosenbloom, P. (1981). Mechanisms of skill acquisition and the law of practice. In J. R. Anderson (Ed.), *Cognitive skills and their acquisition.* Hillsdale, NJ: Erlbaum.

Newell, A., & Simon H. H. A. (1972). *Human problem solving.* Englewood Cliffs, NJ: Prentice-Hall.

Newell, A., Shaw, J. C., & Simon, H. A. (1957). Problem solving in humans and computers. *Carnegie Technical, 21*(4), 35–38.

Newell, K. M., & Corcos, D. M. (Eds.) (1993). *Variability and motor control.* Champaign, IL: Human Kinetics.

Olton, D. S. (1979). Mazes, maps, and memory. *American Psychologist, 34,* 583–596.

Perfetti, C. A. (1985). *Reading ability.* New York: Oxford.

Parasuraman, R., & Giambra, L. (1991). Skill development in vigilance: Effects of event rate and age. *Psychology and Aging, 6,* 155–169.

Parasuraman, R., Warm, J. S., & See, J. E. (1998). Brain systems of vigilance. In R. Parasuraman (Ed.), *The attentive brain* (pp. 221–256). Cambridge, MA: MIT Press.

Pillsbury, W. B. (1908). *Attention.* New York: Macmillan.

Posner, M. I., & Boies, S. J. (1971). Components of attention. *Psychological Review, 78,* 391–408.

Posner, M. I., & Petersen, S. E. (1990). The attention system of the human brain. *Annual Reviews of Neuroscience, 13,* 25–42.

Posner, M. I., Snyder, C. R. R., & Davidson, B. J. (1980). Attention and the detection of signals. *Journal of Experimental Psychology: General, 109,* 160–174.

Powers, W. T. (1978). Quantitative analysis of purposive systems: Some spadework at the foundations of scientific psychology. *Psychological Review, 85,* 417–435.

Powers, W. T. (2008). *Living control systems, III: The fact of control.* New Canaan, CT: Benchmark Publications.

Proctor, R. W., & Dutta, A. (1995). *Skill acquisition and human performance.* Thousand Oaks, CA: Sage.

Raffone, A., & Srinivasan, N. (2010). The exploration of meditation in the neuroscience of attention and consciousness. *Cognitive Processing, 11,* 1–7.

Raichle, M. E., Fiez, J. A., Videen, T. O., MacLeod, A.-.M. K., Pardo, J. V., Fox, P. T., & Petersen, S. E. (1994). Practice-related changes in human brain functional anatomy during nonmotor learning. *Cerebral Cortex, 4,* 8–26.

Raichle, M. E., & Snyder, A. Z. (2007). A default mode of brain function: A brief history of an evolving idea. *NeuroImage, 37,* 1083–1090.

Richards, J. T., & Reicher, G. M. (1978). The effect of background familiarity in visual search: An analysis of underlying factors. *Perception & Psychophysics, 23,* 499–505.

Roberts, K. L., & Hall, D. A. (2008). Examining a supramodal network for conflict processing: A systematic review and novel functional magnetic resonance imaging data for related visual and auditory Stroop tasks. *Journal of Cognitive Neuroscience, 20,* 1063–1078.

Ron, M., & Robbins, T. W. (Eds.) (2003). *Disorders of mind and brain 2.* Cambridge, UK: Cambridge University Press.

Rose, M., Schmid, C., Winzen, A., Sommer, T., & Buchel, C. (2005). The functional and temporal characteristics of top-down modulation in visual selection. *Cerebral Cortex, 15,* 1290–1298.

Rosenblum, L. S., Yakel, D. A., & Green, K. P. (2000). Face and mouth inversion effects on visual and audiovisual speech perception. *Journal of Experimental Psychology: Human Perception and Performance, 26,* 806–819.

Rueda, M. R., Rothbart, M. K., McCandliss, B. D., Saccomanno, L., & Posner, M. I. (2005). Training, maturation, and genetic influences on the development of executive attention. *Proceedings of the National Academy of Sciences of the USA, 102,* 14931–14936.

Schriej, D., Owens, C., & Theeuwes, J. (2008). Abrupt onsets capture attention independent of top-down control settings. *Attention, Perception, & Psychophsyics, 70,* 208–218.

Schütz-Bosbach, S., & Prinz, W. (2007). Perceptual resonance: Action-induced modulation of perception. *Trends in Cognitive Sciences, 11*(8), 349–355.

Shiffrin, R. M., & Schneider, W. (1977). Controlled and automatic human information processing: II. Perceptual learning, automatic attending, and a general theory. *Psychological Review, 84,* 127–190.

Singley, M. K., & Anderson, J. R. (1989). *The transfer of cognitive skill.* Cambridge, MA: Harvard University Press.

Smallword, H., & Schooler, J. W. (2006). The restless mind. *Psychological Bulletin, 132,* 946–958.

Smith, E. E., & Jonides, J. (1997). Working memory: A view from neuroimaging. *Cognitive Psychology, 33,* 5–42.

Snowling, M., J., Hume, C., Kintsch, W., & Rawson, K. A. (2008). Comprehension. In M. J. Snowling & C. Hume (Eds.), *The science of reading.* Wiley Online Library doi:10.1002/9780470757642.ch12

Spelke, E., Hirst, W., and Neisser U. (1976). Skills of divided attention. *Cognition, 4,* 215–230.

Spence, I., & Feng, J. (2010). Video games and spatial cognition. *Review of General Psychology, 14,* 92–104.

Stroop, J. R. (1935). Studies of interference in serial verbal reactions. *Journal of Experimental Psychology, 18,* 643–662.

Studer, B., Koeneke, S., Blum, J., & Janke, L. (2010). The effects of practice distribution upon the regional oscillatory activity in visuomotor learning. *Behavioral and Brain Functions, 6,* doi:10.1186/1744-9081-6-8

Tanenhaus, M. K. (2007). Eye movements and spoken language processing. In R. P. G. van Gompel, M. H. Fischer, W. S. Murray, & R. L. Hill (Eds.), *Eye movements: A window on mind and brain* (pp. 443–469). Oxford, UK: Elsevier.

Tanenhaus, M. K., Spivey-Knowlton, M., Eberhard, K., & Sedivy, J. (1995). The interaction of visual and linguistic information in spoken language comprehension. *Science, 268,* 1632–1634.

Tang, Y.-Y., & Posner, M. I. (2009). Attention training and attention state training. *Trends in Cognitive Sciences, 13,* 222–227.

Thomas, E. A. C. (1974). The selectivity of preparation. *Psychological Review, 81,* 442–464.

Thorel, L. B., Lindqvist, S., Nutley, S. B., Bohin, G., & Klingberg, T. (2009). Training and transfer effects of executive functions in preschool children. *Developmental Science, 12,* 106–114.

Thomas, M., Sing, H., Belenky, G., Holcomb, H., Mayberg, H., Dannals, R., Wagner, H. Jr., . . . Redmond, D. (2000). Neural basis of alertness and cognitive performance impairments during sleepiness. I. Effects of 24 h of sleep deprivation on waking human regional brain activity. *Journal of Sleep Research, 9,* 335–352.

Thorndike, E. L. (1898). Animal intelligence: An experimental study of the associative processes in animals. *Psychological Monographs, 2* (Issue 8).

Treisman, A. M. (1969). Strategies and models of selective attention. *Psychological Review, 76,* 282–299.

Treisman, A. M. (1988). Features and objects: The fourteenth Bartlett Memorial Lecture. *Quarterly Journal of Experimental Psychology A: Human Experimental Psychology, 40A,* 201–237.

Verdolini, K. (2000). Principles of skill acquisition applied to voice training. In *The vocal vision: Views on voice by 24 leading teachers, coaches, and directors* (Chapter 8). Milwaukee, WI: Applause Books.

Verghese, J., Buschke, H., Viola, L., Katz, M., Hall, C., Kustansky, G., & Lipton, R. (2002). Validity of divided attention tasks in predicting falls in older individuals: A preliminary study. *Journal of the American Geriatrics Society, 50,* 1572–1576.

Virginia Tech Transportation Institute. (2009, July 27). New data from VTTI provides insight into cell phone use and driving distraction. Press releases. http://www.vtti.vt.edu/whats-new.html

Vogel, E. K., & Machizawa, M. G. (2004). Neural activity predicts individual differences in visual working memory capacity. *Nature, 426,* 748–751.

Wang, L., Liu, X., Guise, K. G., Knight, R. T., Ghajar, J., & Fan, J. (2009). Effective connectivity of the fronto-parietal network during attentional control. *Journal of Cognitive Neuroscience, 22,* 543–553.

Wang, Q., Cavanagh, P., & Green, M. (1994). Familiarity and pop-out in visual search. *Perception & Psychophysics, 56,* 495–500.

Waters, G. S., & Caplan, D. (2004). Verbal working memory and on-line syntactic processing: evidence from self-paced listening. *Quarterly Journal of Experimental Psychology. A, Human Experimental Psychology, 57,* 129–163.

Waters, G. S., & Caplan, D. (2005). The relationship between age, processing speed, working memory capacity, and language comprehension. *Memory, 13,* 403–413.

Whitehead, A. N. (1911). *An introduction to mathematics.* Oxford, England: Oxford University Press.

Wulf, G. (2007). *Attention and motor skill learning.* Champaign, IL: Human Kinetics.

Wulf, G., Höß, M., & Prinz, W. (1998). Instructions for motor learning: Differential effects of internal versus external focus of attention. *Journal of Motor Behavior, 30,* 169–179.

Xu, Y. D., & Chun, M. M. (2006). Dissociable neural mechanisms supporting visual short-term memory for objects. *Nature, 440,* 91–95.

Yantis, S. (1995). Attentional capture in vision. In A. F. Kramer, M. G. H. Coles, & G. D. Logan (Eds.), *Converging operations in the study of visual selective attention* (pp. 45–76). Washington, DC: American Psychological Association.

Yerkes, R. M., & Dodson, J. D. (1908). The relation of strength of stimulus to rapidity of habit formation. *Journal of Comparative Neurology, 18,* 459–482.

CHAPTER 5

The Role of Memory in Language and Communication

Language comprehension requires the ability to construct linguistic dependencies between nonadjacent constituents. For example, a subject must agree with its verb, but the two are often separated by several words, phrases, or even clauses, as in *The athlete(s) in the training program run(s) every day* or *The athlete(s) in the training program that was designed by an Olympic gold-medal winner run(s) every day*. At the same time, research in verbal memory has long recognized that our ability to actively attend to and concurrently process information is severely limited. This constraint leads to a functional requirement for the language comprehension system: comprehenders must *retrieve* items that have already been processed in order to fully integrate new information into an evolving interpretation. Naturally then, limitations on memory storage and retrieval are important determinants of language performance. In addition, language systems must interact with linguistic and conceptual knowledge in order to create meaning. For example, native speakers of English will immediately perceive the unacceptability of *Sam uncrossed the street, while Sam uncrossed his arms* is perfectly acceptable. This points to a second functional requirement: the need to retrieve passively held lexical and conceptual knowledge about meanings of words and when particular grammatical devices (here "un") may be applied. These two requirements demonstrate the close dependence of language processes on memory, suggesting that a thorough understanding of language processing, and acquired language disorders, will benefit from an understanding of the healthy

memory system. It is the goal of the current chapter to provide a brief review of this literature.

TYPES OF MEMORY

Ever since the early days of psychology, when the discipline was more akin to philosophy than science, thinkers who concerned themselves with the phenomenon of memory found cause to make distinctions based on the *type* of information held in that memory. For example, the French philosopher Maine de Biran proposed three distinct memories, which he referred to as mechanical, sensitive, and representative, each depending on different mechanisms and characterized by different properties (Maine de Biran, 1804/1929). According to Biran, mechanical memory involved the acquisition of motor and verbal habits and operates unconsciously; sensitive memory involves feelings and affect and also operates unconsciously; and representative memory involves the conscious recollection of ideas and events. A second early distinction was made by William James in his seminal text *Principles of Psychology* (1890), where he focused on temporal properties of particular memories, contrasting elementary memory (also called primary memory) and secondary memory. He wrote:

> Elementary memory makes us aware of . . . the just past. The objects we feel in this directly intuited past differ from properly recollected objects. An object which is recollected, in the proper sense of the term, is one which has been absent from consciousness

altogether, and . . . is brought back . . . from a reservoir in which, with countless other objects, it lay buried and lost from view. But an object of primary memory is not thus brought back; it never was lost; its date was never cut off in consciousness from that of the immediately present moment. In fact it comes to us as belonging to the rearward portion of the present space of time, and not to the genuine past. (pp. 646–647)

Distinctions such as these have remained relevant even to the present day, with the field of memory research being divided into those that characterize memory based on separate *systems*, largely aligned to the type of information they contain, or else based on separate *processes*, which focuses on mechanisms of retrieval and forgetting. Both approaches are discussed later.

Multiple Memory Systems

The multiple memory systems approach focuses on identifying functionally and anatomically distinct systems, which differ in their "methods of acquisition, representation, and expression of knowledge" (Tulving, 1985, p. 3). There are a number of different versions of this approach. For example, Squire (2004; Squire & Zola-Morgan, 1988) suggested that the most fundamental distinction is between declarative and nondeclarative memories. Declarative memory is what is usually meant by the term *memory* in ordinary language, and is the kind of memory impaired in amnesia, that relating to the conscious recollection of facts and events. For this reason it has also been termed explicit memory. It provides a representational vocabulary for modeling the external world, and the resulting models can be evaluated as either true or false with respect to the world. It is typically assessed by tests of recall, recognition, or cued recall. In contrast, nondeclarative memory is actually a catch-all term referring to a variety of other memories, including most notably *procedural* memory. Nondeclarative (or *implicit*) memories have in common that they are expressed through action rather than recollection. As such, they are not true or false, but rather reflect qualities of the learning experience. Strong evidence in support of this distinction comes from studies of amnesic patients from as early as Milner (1962), who demonstrated that patient H. M. could learn a mirror drawing task (invoking procedural memory), but displayed no memory of actually having practiced the task before (a declarative memory). Additional demonstrations have shown normal rates of learning in a variety of skills without conscious awareness that the learning has taken place (cf. Squire, 1992, for a review).

Studies from brain damaged patients and animal models point to medial temporal lobe structures, including the hippocampal region and the adjacent entorhinal, perirhinal, and the parahippocampal cortices as crucial for establishing new declarative memories (Buckner & Wheeler, 2001; Squire, Stark, & Clark, 2004). These structures are significant because they receive multi-modal sensory input via reciprocal pathways from frontal, temporal, and parietal areas, enabling them to consolidate inputs from these regions (Alvarez & Squire, 1994; McClelland, McNaughton, & O'Reilly, 1995). A hallmark of damage to the medial temporal lobe is profound forgetfulness for any event occurring longer than 2 seconds in the past (Buffalo, Reber, & Squire, 1998), regardless of sensory modality (e.g., Levy, Manns, Hopkins, et al., 2003, Milner, 1972; Squire, Schmolck, & Stark, 2001). In addition, impairment in recollection of declarative memories can occur despite intact perceptual abilities and normal performance on intelligence tests (Schmolck, Kensinger, Corkin, & Squire, 2002; Schmolck, Stefanacci, & Squire, 2000), lending support to the idea that declarative memory may constitute a separable memory system. Over time, however, memories become largely independent of the medial structures, and more dependent on neocortical structures, especially in the temporal lobes.

In contrast, there is no specific brain system related to establishing nondeclarative memories, as the category includes a variety of different types of memories. For example, creation of memories via classic conditioning depends on the cerebellum and amygdala (e.g., Delgado, Jou, LeDoux, & Phelps, 2009; Thompson & Kim, 1996), while procedural learning depends on the basal ganglia, especially the striatum (e.g., Packard, Hirsh, & White, 1989; Poldrack, Clark, Pare-Blagoev, et al., 2001; Salmon & Butters, 1995; Ullman, 2004). Figure 5-1 provides a summary of the subtypes of memory falling under each of these two distinctions, together with the primary brain structures that have been shown to support these memories in humans and experimental animals.

A second frequently cited taxonomy of memory systems is that developed by Tulving and colleagues (Schacter & Tulving, 1994; Tulving, 1983). This approach is particularly concerned with establishing a distinction between two subtypes of declarative memory: semantic and episodic memory, distinguished by the relation of a particular piece of knowledge to a particular individual. For example, the knowledge that pizza is made with cheese and tomato sauce would reside in semantic memory, and would be shared by everyone, while the knowledge that Andrew had two slices of mushroom

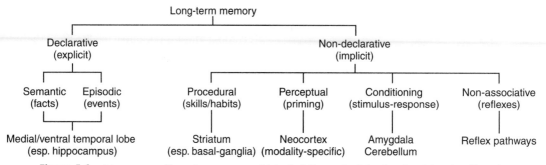

Figure 5-1   A taxonomy of long-term memory. Note that the ventro-lateral prefrontal cortex (Broca's area and its right homologue) have been implicated in semantic, episodic, and procedural memories). Brain regions supporting the perceptual representation system depend on the perceptual modality; the ventral occipital-temporal region is claimed to store word forms. [Adapted from Squire, L. R. (2004). Memory systems of the brain: A brief history and current perspective. *Neurobiology of Learning and Memory, 82,* 171–177.]

pizza and a soda for lunch would reside in episodic memory and be held only by Andrew and those who ate together with him. In addition to these two separate memory systems, these researchers have argued for the functional and neurological distinctness of three others: perceptual representation system (PRS), procedural memory, and working memory (WM). These first two would be considered nondeclarative memories under the taxonomy suggested by Squire and colleagues, and WM would be considered as a separate memory system all together according to this approach. We discuss the behavioral and neurological properties of each of these five systems in turn.

Semantic Memory

Semantic memory is generally assessed through object naming ("This is a picture of a ____"), and queries that require access to world knowledge (i.e., the Pyramids and Palm Trees test (Howard & Patterson, 1992) in which individuals must decide what type of tree is most associated with an Egyptian pyramid. Synonym generation tasks, in which patients are asked to name as many exemplars of a provided category in 1 minute, have also been used to evaluate fluency and speed of accessing categories of information. In addition to storing facts about the world, semantic memory is the repository for linguistic knowledge about words, including phonological (e.g., that the word *night* rhymes with *kite*), morphological (e.g., that *taught* is the past tense of *teach*), grammatical (e.g., that *hit* takes a direct object), and semantic properties (that *sleep* and *snooze* are synonyms). This knowledge has been referred to as the *mental lexicon* (Ullman, 2004; see also Chapter 6).

Cognitive psychology has long been interested in the organization of the mental lexicon, especially its semantic aspects, and the means through which it supports comprehension and communication (cf. Murphy, 2002, for a review). That knowledge is *organized* has been demonstrated experimentally in numerous studies observing correlations between reaction times to verify relationships between concepts and their degree of relation. For example, the early study of Collins and Quillian (1969) found that participants took less time to verify the statement "A canary is a bird" compared to "A canary is an animal." They interpreted this result as evidence for a hierarchical representation of concepts, such as that presented in Figure 5-2, where relationships between categories are represented by solid lines and properties of individual objects are represented by dashed lines. Since the concept *canary* is closer to *bird* than to *animal,* they reasoned that the faster reaction time was possible because there were fewer links to traverse in order to verify the statement. Later research revealed a situation not so simple as this, as statements about items that are more *typical* of a category, such as "A robin is a bird" were judged more quickly than atypical exemplars, such as "An ostrich is a bird," despite the fact that they are both located at the same level of the conceptual hierarchy (Rips, Shoben, & Smith, 1973; Rosch & Mervis, 1975). With this result, it became clear that knowledge organization reflects not just static or logical relationships between concepts, but also an individual's experience with the world.

There is now a substantial amount of evidence from neuroimaging techniques (e.g., PET, fMRI) that experience with the world determines how the mental lexicon is stored in the brain. For example, reading action words that are semantically related to different body parts (e.g., "kick," "pick," "lick") activates regions of the motor and premotor cortex responsible for controlling

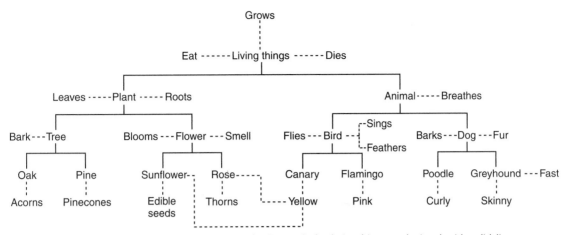

Figure 5-2 Hierarchical semantic network. Categorical relationships are depicted with solid lines between concepts, properties of individual concepts are depicted as dashed lines. Note that properties may apply to multiple concepts, and certain category members need not inherit all properties from its category (e.g., ostriches are birds but don't fly). Prototypical members of a category will inherit most of the properties of that category, however. [Adapted from Collins, A. M., & Quillian, M. R. (1969). Retrieval time from semantic memory. *Journal of Verbal Learning and Verbal Behavior, 8,* 240–247.]

those body parts (Aziz-Zadeh, Wilson, Rizzolatti, & Iacoboni, 2006; Hauk, Johnsrude, & Pulvermuller, 2004; Pulvermuller, 2005; Tettamanti, Buccino, Saccuman, et al., 2005). Similarly, reading or naming words associated with tool actions (e.g., hammer) activate a network of sensorimotor regions also engaged when perceiving and using tools (Chao, Haxby, & Martin, 1999). In addition to the influence of embodiment, a variety of other properties of objects in the world appear to have dedicated temporal lobe regions in which they are processed, and accessing words associated with these properties activates adjacent brain regions. For example, color and motion perception are associated with separate regions in the left ventral and medial temporal lobe, respectively (Corbetta, Miezin, Dobmeyer, et al., 1990; Zeki, Watson, Lueck, et al., 1991). In a study in which participants were shown achromatic pictures of objects (e.g., line drawing of a pencil), and asked to generate color words (e.g., "yellow") and action words (e.g., "write") related to these objects, Martin, Haxby, Lalonde, et al. (1995) found that regions just anterior to the ventral and medial lobe regions just mentioned were active. Similar findings have been observed for size and sounds of objects (Kellenbach, Brett, & Patterson, 2001), as well as grammar related properties such as the animate/inanimate distinction (Chao, Haxby, & Martin, 1999). Taken together, these results suggest that knowledge in the mental lexicon is represented by a distributed network of features processed primarily in the temporal lobes, with different object categories

eliciting different patterns of activation among relevant features (Martin & Chao, 2001; McClelland & Rogers, 2003). In addition to these temporal regions, neuroimaging suggests that the retrieval and selection of information in the mental lexicon is managed by the left ventrolateral prefrontal cortex, corresponding to the inferior frontal gyrus (including Broca's area) and Brodmann's areas 44, 45, and 47 (cf. Bookheimer, 2002; Thompson-Schill, 2003, for reviews). These areas will also become relevant later in the discussion of the interaction of memory and syntactic processing.

Episodic Memory
The existence of a separate episodic memory system appears to receive strong motivation from data from amnesic patients, who have specific deficits in episodic memory with very few, if any, deficits in the other memory systems. Such pathology suggests that episodic memories should be dissociable from other types of memories, and may occupy a neurologically distinct region in the brain (Tulving, 2002, p. 12). Assessment of episodic memory proves difficult, however, since the personal nature of these memories limits the ability of experimenters to manipulate them and evaluate the correctness of responses. Consequently, many studies investigating episodic memory utilize list-learning paradigms, which give experimenters complete control over properties of the to-be-remembered stimuli. Participants are presented with a list of words (or visual items such as faces or patterns) and asked to report on

various incidental properties of them during an encoding phase (e.g., whether presented in upper or lower case letters, in particular colors, with a particular other word, or even whether it occurred at all). The subsequent retrieval phase then asks them to make judgments about whether items have been seen before (recognition) or to produce the item or its associates (recall), and sometimes to specify whether they consciously remember learning the word during the study phase or not (remember/know judgment). These paradigms enable experimenters to directly examine the conditions that lead to the successful creation of memories. For example, a group of studies have investigated "subsequent memory effects" in which sets of items that have been identified via post-hoc memory tests as having been successfully remembered are contrasted with those that have not been remembered (e.g., Rugg, Otten, & Henson, 2002; Wagner, Koutstaal, & Schacter, 1999). The goal was to uncover brain regions specifically involved in task-invariant episodic encoding, however such a region has so far resisted identification. Instead, the main result from these studies is that the pattern of brain activation associated with a particular memory differs depending on the type of processing engaged during study (e.g., Kelley, Miezin, McDermott, et al., 1998; McDermott, Buckner, Petersen, et al., 1999; Otten & Rugg, 2001; Wagner, Poldrack, Eldridge, et al., 1998). Thus, words encoded via a semantic task (i.e., judging whether a word is animate) activate areas of the medial prefrontal cortex and in the dorsal part of the left inferior frontal gyrus, which has been linked to semantic WM (e.g., Buckner & Koutstaal, 1998; Gabrieli, Poldrack, & Desmond, 1998; Wagner et al., 1998). Words encoded via a syllable counting task, on the other hand, failed to activate any prefrontal areas, and instead showed activations in bilateral parietal and fusiform regions and in the left occipital cortex, areas that have been implicated in phonological processing tasks (e.g., Mummery, Patterson, Hodges, & Price, 1998; Poldrack, Wagner, Prull, et al., 1999; Price, Moore, Humphreys, & Wise, 1997).

Such task-specific activations are consonant with the idea that a memory for a particular stimulus includes a variety of incidental information about the context in which it was remembered—even including subjective factors such as mood or cognitive state. Thus, episodic memories—like semantic memories—are represented in the brain as distributed networks of activation, pointing to the need for a more refined explanation of episodic amnesia than simply to look for the region that houses them. One approach is the idea that damage must be specific to the mechanism through which these ideas are reactivated (wherever they may be

stored), and not the means through which they are stored. Indeed, Tulving and Pearlstone (1966) pointed out that much of what we commonly view as memory loss—a memory no longer being *available*—is in fact more properly viewed as a failure in *accessibility*. Subsequently, Tulving (1979) formulated the *encoding specificity principle*, which states "[t]he probability of successful retrieval of the target item is a monotonically increasing function of information overlap between the information present at retrieval and the information stored in memory" (p. 408). Indeed, a recent survey of neuroimaging research concludes that the same brain areas are active both at encoding and retrieval (Danker & Anderson, 2010). One demonstration of this idea is the classic study by Thomson and Tulving (1970), who observed the expected result when no associate for the target word *flower* was present during the study phase: a strong associate presented at test (*bloom*) elicited recall of *flower* better than no associate or than a weak associate (*fruit*) presented at test. But when the weak associate is presented during the study phase, the presence of this same weak associate at test produces markedly better recall than when the strong associate is presented (73% versus 33% correct recalls). Thus, the effectiveness of even a longstanding cue, drawn from semantic memory, depends crucially on the processes that occurred when particular episodic memories are created.

While the foregoing discussion has centered around studies of memory per se, evidence for the role of encoding context and its interaction with the information available at retrieval has also been observed in studies of language comprehension. In order to isolate the importance of encoding versus retrieval operations, Van Dyke and McElree (2006) manipulated the cues available at retrieval during sentence processing while keeping the encoding context constant. We tested grammatical constructions in which a direct object has been displaced from its verb by moving it to the front of the sentence (e.g., *It was the boat that the guy who lived by the sea sailed in two sunny days*). Here, when the verb *sailed* is processed, a retrieval must occur in order to restore the noun phrase *the boat* into active memory so that it can be integrated with the verb. We manipulated the encoding context by asking participants to remember a three-word memory list prior to reading the sentence (e.g., TABLE-SINK-TRUCK); this memory list was present for some trials (Load Condition) and not for others (No Load Condition). The manipulation of retrieval cues was accomplished by substituting the verb *fixed* for *sailed*, creating a situation where four nouns stored in memory (i.e., table, sink, truck, boat) are suitable direct objects for the verb *fixed* (Matched

Condition), while only one is suitable for the verb *sailed* (Unmatched Condition). The results of reading times on the manipulated verb are shown in Figure 5-3; when there was no load present, there was no difference in reading times, however the presence of the memory words led to increased reading times when the verb was Matched as compared to when it was Unmatched. Thus, as predicted by encoding specificity, the overlap between retrieval cues generated from the verb (e.g., cues that specify "find a direct object that is fixable/sailable") and contextual information was a strong determinant of reading performance. We note, however, that an important difference between this study and the Thomson and Tulving (1970) study is that here, the match between the cues available at retrieval and the encoding context produced a *detrimental* effect. This is because the similarity between the context words and the target word (i.e., table, sink, truck, and boat are all fixable) created *interference* at retrieval. We will discuss the role of interference in memory and language further in the section on forgetting. The important point here, however, is that encoding context has its effect *in conjunction with* the retrieval cues used to reaccess the encoded material.

An important unresolved question pertains to the relationship between episodic memories and semantic memories. From the perspective of the multiple memories approach, these two types of memories are considered to be separate *systems*; however, the criteria by which a system is determined had been criticized as indecisive (e.g., Surprenant & Neath, 2009). Much of the support for separate systems comes from functional and neurological *dissociations*, such that tasks that are diagnostic of System A, or brain regions implicated in the healthy functioning of System A are different from those tapping into the function of System B. While dissociations are common, a number of researchers have published papers questioning their logic as a means for identifying separate brain systems (e.g., Ryan & Cohen, 2003; Van Orden, Pennington, & Stone, 2001). For example, Parkin (2001) notes that apparent dissociations observed in amnesic patients, who show unimpaired performance on standardized tests of semantic memory, but intense difficulty recalling episodic events such as a recently presented word list or lunch menu, are confounded by test difficulty. In the face of the temporally graded nature of amnesia, in which more recently acquired memories are the most susceptible to loss, the key problem with these assessments of semantic memory is that they test information that was acquired by early adult life. When semantic memory tests are carefully controlled so as to test more recently acquired semantic memories, the relative sparing of one system over the other is less apparent.

While the debate on whether episodic and semantic memories are distinct systems will likely continue, from the point of view of language, it is at least helpful to distinguish autobiographical episodic memories, which are not fundamentally related to language processing, from other contextually anchored memories (e.g., Conway, 2001). The relationship between the latter type of episodic memories and semantic memory seems intrinsic—no scientist has ever claimed that individuals are *born* knowing the conceptual knowledge that comprises the meaning of words in the mental lexicon.[1] These must be learned through experience with the world and with language. There is now a considerable body of evidence suggesting that the meaning—and grammatical usage—of individual words is learned (even by infants) through repeated learning episodes (e.g., Harm & Seidenberg, 2004; Mirković, MacDonald, & Seidenberg, 2005; Sahni, Seidenberg, & Saffran, 2010). Fewer learning episodes appears to produce low quality lexical representations, characterized by variable and

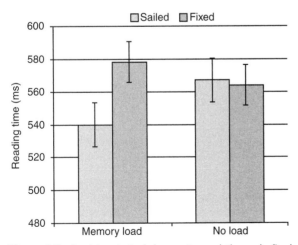

Figure 5-3 Participants took longer to read the verb *fixed* when it was preceded by a memory list of *fixable* words. The same memory list did not affect reading times for *sailed*. [Results from Van Dyke, J. A., & McElree, B. (2006). Retrieval interference in sentence comprehension. *Journal of Memory and Language, 55*, 157–166.]

---

[1] In contrast, there *have* been prominent proposals within linguistic theory that children are born with knowledge of grammar—a so-called Universal Grammar (e.g., Chomsky, 1986; Crain & Thornton, 1998), through which they can deduce the rules of grammar specific to their own native language. Some theories of language assign these rules to procedural memory (discussed later); the statistical learning approaches discussed here offer an important alternative to this approach.

inconsistent phonological forms, and more shallow meaning representations, incomplete specification of grammatical function, and (for reading) underspecified orthographic representations (Perfetti, 2007). The process of consolidating individual learning events into efficiently accessed long-term memory (LTM) representations has been attested in the domain of reading by neuroimaging studies showing that repeated exposures to a word results in *reduced* activation in reading-related brain regions, especially areas of the ventral occipital-temporal region thought to contain visual word forms (cf. McCandliss, Cohen, & Dehaene, 2003, for a review), and in the inferior frontal gyrus (e.g., Katz, Lee, Tabor, et al., 2005; Pugh, Frost, Sandak, et al., 2008). This reduction is consistent with studies of perceptual and motor skill learning in which initial (unskilled) performance is associated with increased activation in task-specific cortical areas, to be followed by task-specific *decreases* in activation in the same cortical regions after continued practice (e.g., Poldrack & Gabrieli, 2001; Ungerleider, Doyon, & Karni, 2002; Wang, Sereno, Jongman, & Hirsch, 2003).

Although episodic and semantic memories—both declarative memories—are generally characterized as explicit memories, in that they are accessible to conscious reporting, the process of learning that binds the two is not conscious. The ability to learn via repeated exposures engages the brain's ability to extract statistical regularities across examples, which occurs gradually over time without conscious awareness (Perruchet & Pacton, 2006; Reber, 1989; Reber, Stark, & Squire, 1998; Squire & Zola, 1996). A number of recent studies have shown that infants as young as 8 months old are sensitive to the statistical regularities that exist in natural languages and can use them, for example, to identify word boundaries in continuous speech (Saffran, Aslin, & Newport, 1996; Sahni, Seidenberg, & Saffran, 2010) and to learn grammatical and conceptual categories (Bhatt, Wilk, Hill, & Rovee-Collier, 2004; Gerken, Wilson, & Lewis, 2005; Shi, Werker, & Morgan, 1999). Computational models that implement this learning process over a distributed representation of neuronlike nodes (i.e., *connectionist* models) have demonstrated that the resulting networks produce humanlike performance in language acquisition and language comprehension (e.g., Seidenberg & MacDonald, 1999), including the same types of performance errors common to children learning language and adults processing ambiguous sentences.

Nondeclarative Memory

In contrast to the earlier discussion, the traditional taxonomy depicted in Figure 5-1, suggests a clear separation between explicit and implicit memories. Historically,

this reflected the need to account for certain cases of amnesia (e.g., patient H.M., Scoville & Milner, 1957) in which patients displayed increasing improvement on complex cognitive skills (i.e., game playing) with no ability to recall ever having learned to play the game or even playing it previously. The explanation afforded was that while damage to the medial temporal lobe structures destroyed the ability to access declarative memory, these patients' nondeclarative memory (especially procedural memory), which does not depend on these brain regions was intact. This memory is characterized as *implicit* because patients are unaware of the learning that has taken place.

A second type of implicit memory that has observed in amnesic patients with an inability to access semantic memory is the preservation of priming effects. That is, these patients display improved performance in recognition tasks for target items following the previous presentation of the same object or some other object that is identical to the target on some perceptual dimension (e.g., sound, shape, etc.). Notably, patients need not be aware that the primed object occurred in order for these effects to occur, and in many cases primes are presented extremely quickly or extremely faintly, so as to be below the threshold of conscious perception.

Schacter and Tulving (1994) proposed two separate memory systems to account for these results: the procedural memory system (discussed later) and the PRS, comprised of a collection of domain-specific modules, which was responsible for priming results (Schacter, Wagner, & Buckner, 2000). The visual word form area, noted earlier, has been offered as one of the modules comprising the PRS (Schacter, 1992), based mainly on evidence from aphasics who show normal priming effects for the surface form of novel words, which consequently could not be stored in semantic memory (e.g., Cermak, Verfaellie, Milberg, et al., 1991; Gabrieli & Keane, 1988; Haist, Musen, & Squire, 1991; Bowers & Schacter, 1992). In addition, it has been observed that some amnesic patients can read irregularly spelled or unknown words, despite having no apparent contact with their meaning (e.g., Funnel, 1983; Schwartz, Saffran, & Marin, 1980). This has been interpreted as support for a separate word form representation independent of meaning.

Procedural Memory

Of the implicit memory systems, procedural memory—memory for *how* to do something—has received the most attention, both in the memory and in the language domain. It has been claimed to support the learning of new, and the control of established, sensorimotor and cognitive habits and skills, including riding a bicycle and skilled game playing. As with all implicit memory systems, learning is gradual and unavailable to conscious description, however in the procedural system the outcome of learning is thought to be *rules*, which are rigid, inflexible, and not influenced by other mental systems (Mishkin, Malamut, & Bachevalier, 1984; Squire & Zola, 1996). Neurologically, the system is rooted in the frontal lobe and basal ganglia, with contributions from portions of the parietal cortex, superior temporal cortex and the cerebellum. The frontal lobe, especially Broca's area and its right homologue, is important for motor sequence learning (Conway & Christiansen, 2001; Doyon, Owen, Petrides, et al., 1996) and especially learning sequences with abstract and hierarchical structures (Dominey, Hoen, Blanc, & Lelekov-Boissard, 2003; Goschke, Friederici, Kotz, & van Kampen, 2001). The basal ganglia have been associated with probabilistic rule learning (Knowlton, Mangels, & Squire, 1996; Poldrack, Prabhakaran, Seger, & Gabrieli, 1999), stimulus-response learning (Packard & Knowlton, 2002), sequence learning (Aldridge & Berridge, 1998; Boecker, Dagher, Ceballos-Baumann, et al., 1998; Doyon, Gaudreau, Laforce, et al., 1997; Graybiel, 1995, Peigneux, Maquet, Meulemans, et al., 2000; Willingham, 1998), and real-time motor planning and control (Wise, Murray, & Gerfen, 1996).

From the perspective of language, one prominent proposal (Ullman, 2004) suggests that the procedural memory system should be understood as the memory system that subserves grammar acquisition and use. Implicit in this proposal is an understanding of grammar as fundamentally rule-based; an idea with a long (and controversial) history in linguistic theory (e.g., Chomsky, 1965, 1980; Marcus, 2001; Marcus, Brinkmann, Clahsen, et al., 1995; Marcus, Vijayan, Bandi, et al., 1999; Pinker, 1991). A frequently cited example is the rule that describes the past tense in English, namely, verb stem + *ed*. This rule allows for the inflection of novel words (e.g., *texted*) and accounts for the phenomenon of overgeneralizations in toddlers (e.g., Daddy goed to work). According to this view, the language-related functions of the neurological structures that support procedural memory are expected to be similar to their nonlanguage function. Thus, the basal ganglia and Broca's area (especially BA 44) are hypothesized to govern control of hierarchically structured elements in complex linguistic representations and assist in the learning of rules over those representations.

This approach is incompatible with the connectionist approach, discussed earlier, in which regularities in language are represented in distributed networks extracted through the process of statistical learning. In these models there are no rules, and indeed, one connectionist implementation specifically demonstrated that such a model could capture the rule-based behavior of past-tense assignment in a system without any rules (Rumelhart & McClelland, 1986). A number of heated exchanges between scientists on both sides of this debate have been published (e.g., Seidenberg, MacDonald, & Saffran [2002] versus Peña, Bonatti, Nespor, & Mehler [2002]; Seidenberg & Elman [1999] versus Marcus et al. [1999]; Keidel, Kluender, Jenison, & Seidenberg [2007] versus Bonatti, Peña, Nespor, & Mehler [2005]) with each side pointing to significant empirical results in support of their position. What is important for our current purpose is the conclusion that there need not be a separable declarative memory system to support grammar processing, as viable non–rule-bound systems have demonstrated that statistical learning over examples held in declarative memory can produce a network with the necessary knowledge held in a distributed representation. Even Ullman (2004) seems to acknowledge the difficulty of distinguishing between the separate declarative and procedural systems he proposes, as he states that the same or similar types of knowledge can in some cases by acquired by both systems. What appears to be more critical, as revealed by the statistical learning approach, and especially studies of language acquisition (e.g., Saffran et al., 1996), is the ability to identify and make use of *cues* in order to learn about the regularities in language. Indeed, a central claim of the connectionist approach is that the cues that facilitate language acquisition in infants become the *constraints* that govern language comprehension in adults (Seidenberg & MacDonald, 1999). As we discuss the memory mechanisms that support comprehension in the sections later, cues will again arise as an important determinant of successful language use.

Working Memory

The construct of WM as a separate store for temporarily held information is an outgrowth of the two-store memory taxonomy, which has been termed the Modal Model (Murdock, 1974) after the statistical term *mode*, because its influence became so pervasive during the last half of the twentieth century. Indeed, even in 2010 it figures prominently in many cognitive and introductory psychology textbooks. This model featured a short-term memory (STM) store characterized by a limited capacity in which verbal information could be held for very short durations, but only if constantly *rehearsed* via active articulation. This is in contrast to the LTM store, which corresponds roughly to the semantic, episodic and procedural memory systems discussed earlier, which is assumed to have an unlimited capacity and duration, so long as appropriate retrieval cues are present to restore passive memories into conscious awareness. The most frequently cited presentation of this model is that of Atkinson and Shiffrin (1968), illustrated in Figure 5-4, which also included a third store for sensory information, subdivided into separate registers for visual, auditory, and haptic information. The modal model emphasized both the qualitative differences between different memory types but also the *processing* mechanisms of each and the way they interact. Inspired by the nascent computer metaphor of the 1950s, this model embodied a specific algorithm through which fleeting sensory information was transformed into a lasting memory. In particular, research demonstrating the highly limited duration of sensory information (1–3 seconds; Sperling, 1960) suggested that it was necessary for information to be verbally *recoded*, and also *rehearsed*, in order to be maintained, and this occurred in the short-term store. Once information had received a sufficient amount of rehearsal in STM, it would move into LTM, where it would reside in a passive state until *retrieved* back into STM where it would be restored into consciousness. Thus, STM is the gateway to and from LTM—any information entering LTM must go through STM and whenever information is retrieved it must again enter STM. (It should be noted that original information is not really transferred, but rather *copied* from one store to another.) At the same time, STM represented a considerable bottleneck for cognitive activity, as it too was found to have a limited storage capacity, made memorable by George Miller's (1956) famous report entitled "The Magical Number Seven, Plus or Minus Two." Miller arrived at this estimate after reviewing data from a number of different paradigms in which individuals were presented with the task of learning new information, only to show highly limited recall on lists containing more than 8 items. Thus, as new information entered STM, some old information becomes lost through displacement—especially information that was not actively rehearsed. Further research revealed that it was possible to expand the capacity of STM via a process called *chunking*, in which meaningful pieces of information are grouped together into a single unit (i.e., the numbers 1, 4, 9, and 2 are remembered as the single unit 1492); however, a limit on the number of chunks that could be actively maintained remains restricted to 3–5 items (cf. Cowan, 2001, for a detailed review).

The centrality of STM motivated the development of models that more precisely articulate how information is brought in and out of consciousness during the performance of cognitive tasks. It is this workspace of active information that has been termed Working Memory—the most influential version of which is the model proposed by Alan Baddeley and colleagues (e.g., Baddeley & Hitch, 1974; reviewed in Baddeley, 2003), depicted in Figure 5-5.[2] The Working Memory model fractionated STM into a set of systems that separately characterized processing and storage; in fact, it was evidence from neuropsychological damage that emphasized the problems with a unitary STM, as patients with severe damage to STM nevertheless retained the ability to access LTM during complex cognitive tasks (Shallice & Warrington, 1970). The key and, ironically, least understood component of the Working Memory model is the Central Executive, which is the controlling mechanism through which information from three subsidiary "slave" storage systems (depicted as gray boxes in Figure 5-5) is brought in and out of the focus of attention (Baddeley, 2003). It is responsible for (at least) updating, shifting, and inhibiting information (Miyake et al., 2000) and has its neurological locus in the frontal lobes, especially dorsolateral prefrontal regions (BA 9/46) and inferior frontal regions (BA 6/44), with some parietal extension into (BA 7/44) (e.g., Braver et al., 1997; Cohen et al., 1997).

The three slave systems can be distinguished by their type of encoding, or the type of information they process. The visuospatial sketchpad is responsible for visuospatial information (e.g., images, spatial configuration, color, shape) and is fractionated into the visual cache (storage) and the inner scribe (rehearsal) components. The more recently postulated episodic buffer (Baddeley, 2000) is responsible for allowing information from LTM to interact with the other two slave systems to create multimodal *chunks* that are open to conscious examination. This buffer should not be confused with episodic memories, discussed earlier, as those are part of LTM while chunks created in Baddeley's episodic buffer are merely temporary associations between different types of information simultaneously manipulated by the central executive. A limit on the amount of information held in this buffer comes from the computational complexity of combining multiple types of codes into a single representation (Hummel, 1999).

---

[2] The Baddeley model is only one of many different formulations of working memory; however, it is the one that has received the most attention. The volume edited by Miyake and Shah (1999) provides a summary of 10 different models of working memory, including several with computational implementations, together with a compare and contrast discussion.

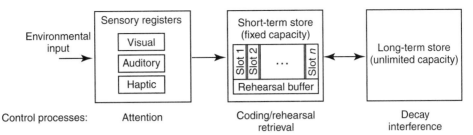

Figure 5-4 Modal Model based on Atkinson and Shiffrin, 1968. Information flow begins with processing information in sensory registers, which have an extremely short duration (<3 seconds). Attentional processes move information from sensory stores into short-term memory, where it is encoded and maintained via rehearsal. Related information may be brought out of the long-term store during encoding. Sufficiently encoded and rehearsed information transfers to long-term store and remains indefinitely, but may become inaccessible due to decay and/or interference. [From Atkinson, R. C., & Shiffrin, R. M. (1968). Human memory: A proposed system and its control processes. In K. W. Spence (Ed.), *The psychology of learning and motivation: Advances in research and theory* (Vol. 2, pp. 89–195). New York: Academic Press.]

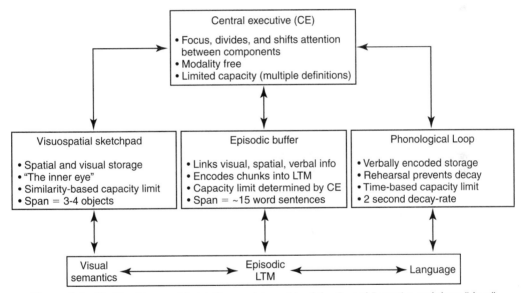

Figure 5-5 Working Memory Model. The model consists of the Central Executive and three "slave" systems, which it directs. The phonological loop is further fractionated into the "articulatory control system" which serves as the "inner voice" and the "phonological store" which serves as the "inner ear". Similarly, the visualspatial sketchpad is fractionated into the "inner scribe" and the "visual cache". The episodic buffer is a recent addition to the model (Baddeley, 2000) and is not as well developed as the other components. [From Baddeley, A. D. (2000). The episodic buffer: A new component of working memory? *Trends in Cognitive Science, 4,* 417–423, and Baddeley, A. (2003). Working memory: Looking back and looking forward. *Nature Reviews Neuroscience, 4,* 829–839.]

The third "slave system," the phonological loop, is the most theoretically developed and experimentally attested. It is responsible for phonological encoding and rehearsal—the means through which verbal information is maintained in an active state. The psychological reality of this process was demonstrated in a number of important early experiments (e.g., Baddeley, 1966; Conrad, 1964; Wickelgren, 1965). For example, Murray (1967) developed a technique to prevent participants from utilizing inner speech to recode information, which became known as *articulatory suppression.* While given a list of words to remember, participants were required to say the word "the" over and over, out loud. When words in the list were similar sounding (i.e., man, mad, cap, can, map) recall errors in the memory condition *without* articulatory supression reflected acoustic confusions: participants were more likely to incorrectly recall items that sounded like the target items but that were not actually in the memory list. With articulatory suppression, on the other hand, acoustic errors were no longer more likely, suggesting that the speaking task prevented participants from recoding, or rehearsing, the memory words using inner speech. These results suggest that not only is information encoded acoustically, but that the amount of information that can be maintained is limited by the ability to actually articulate it—as the number of items to remember increases, some will be forgotten because they cannot be rehearsed. The exact capacity limit for the phonological loop has been quoted as being the amount of information that can be articulated in about 2 seconds (Baddeley, 1986; Baddeley, Thomson, & Buchanan, 1975). Neurologically, lesion studies and neuroimaging methods implicate the left temporoparietal region in the operation of the phonological loop, with BA 40 as the locus of the storage component of the loop and Broca's area (BA 6/44) supporting rehearsal (reviewed in Vallar & Papagno, 2002, and Smith & Jonides, 1997).

WORKING MEMORY AND LANGUAGE COMPREHENSION

The notion that WM capacity is fixed has had a huge influence on theories of language processing. For example, it is a well-replicated finding that sentences in which grammatical heads are separated from their dependents are more difficult to process than when heads and dependents are adjacent (e.g., Grodner & Gibson, 2005; McElree, Foraker, & Dyer, 2003). This is true of unambiguous sentences (e.g., *The book ripped.* versus *The book that the editor admired ripped.*) and of ambiguous sentences (e.g., *The boy understood the man was afraid.* versus *The boy understood the man who was swimming near the dock was afraid.*), where reanalyses prove more difficult as the distance between the ambiguity and the disambiguating material is increased (e.g., Ferreira & Henderson, 1991; Van Dyke & Lewis, 2003). A number of prominent theories have attempted to account for these results by invoking WM capacity, with the common assumption being that capacity is exhausted by the need to simultaneously "hold on to" the unattached constituent (the grammatical subjects *book* and *man* in these examples) while processing the intervening material until the main verb (*ripped* or *was afraid*) occurs. The chief question is taken to be "how much

is too much" intervening material before capacity is exhausted; some have suggested that the relevant metric is the number of words (Ferriera & Henderson, 1991; Warner & Glass, 1987) or discourse referents (Gibson, 1998; 2000). Others have focused on the hierarchical nature of dependencies, suggesting that difficulty depends on the number of embeddings (Miller & Chomsky, 1963), or the number of incomplete dependencies (Abney & Johnson, 1991; Gibson, 1998; Kimball, 1973).

This focus on capacity has also spawned a large body of research seeking to demonstrate that sentence comprehension suffers when capacity is reduced either experimentally through the use of dual-task procedures (e.g., Fedorenko, Gibson, & Rohde, 2006, 2007) or clinically, as when poorly performing participants also score poorly on tests of WM capacity, compared with those who do well. For example, King and Just (1991) found that college-level readers with "low" WM capacity showed worse comprehension and slower reading times on syntactically complex sentences than those with "high" or "middle" capacity levels. Similarly, MacDonald, Just, and Carpenter (1992) found that low capacity individuals from the same population had more difficulty interpreting temporarily ambiguous constructions than those with larger capacities. They suggested that this was because a larger WM capacity enabled readers to maintain all possible interpretations for longer, while the smaller capacity readers could only maintain the most likely interpretation. In cases where the ultimately correct interpretation was not the most likely one, low capacity readers would fail to comprehend because the correct interpretation had been "pushed out" of memory.

Studies of reading development also point to an association between low WM capacity and poor comprehension. In a longitudinal study of children with normal word-level (i.e., decoding) skills, Oakhill, Cain, and Bryant (2003) found that WM capacity predicted significant independent variance on standardized measures of reading comprehension at age 7–8 and again 1 year later. Further, Nation, Adams, Bowyer-Crane, and Snowling (1999) found that 10–11 year old poor comprehenders had significantly smaller verbal WM capacity (though not spatial WM capacity) than normal children matched for age, decoding skill, and nonverbal abilities. Likewise, reading disabled children have been found to score in the lowest range on tests of WM capacity (e.g., Gathercole, Alloway, Willis, & Adams, 2006; Swanson & Sachse-Lee, 2001), and these scores are significant predictors of standardized measures of both reading and mathematics attainment.

In all these studies, the standard means of measuring WM capacity is via tests referred to as complex span tasks (e.g., Turner & Engle, 1989; Daneman & Carpenter, 1980).[3] The Reading/Listening Span version of these tasks requires participants to read or listen to an increasingly large group of sentences, and report back only the last words of each sentence in the set. The task of processing the sentence (and in some cases answering questions about it) provides a processing component that, together with the requirement to store the last words, is thought to provide an assessment of the efficiency with which the central executive can allocate resources to both maintain and process linguistic information. Indeed, the task mirrors the functional demand of processing complex linguistic constructions (e.g., long-distance dependencies) mentioned earlier, where substantial information is situated in between two linguistic constituents that must be associated. A meta-analysis of 77 studies found that the Reading Span task predicted language comprehension better than simple span tasks (e.g., digit span) in which participants simply had to remember and report back lists of words (Daneman & Merikle, 1996).

While the impact of the Working Memory model on the study of language processing is undeniable, a close examination of the model reveals that it is not well matched to the functional demands of language comprehension (Lewis, Vasishth, & Van Dyke, 2006). For example, to process the types of sentences discussed earlier (*The book that the editor admired ripped.*), it is argued that the noun phrase *the book* must be held active in WM while the subsequent information is processed, and the difficulty associated with this is what makes the sentence difficult to process. Yet it seems clear that, even when not processing intervening information (*The book ripped.*), there would simply be no time to actively rehearse previously processed constituents during real-time comprehension, where grammatical associations must be made within a few hundred milliseconds (Rayner, 1998). In addition, it seems logical that language comprehension in patients with brain damage should be significantly limited when WM spans are reduced, yet such a relation has failed to materialize, whether span is measured in terms of traditional serial recall measures (Caplan & Hildebrandt, 1988; Martin & Feher, 1990) or in terms of reading span (Caplan & Waters, 1999). Moreover, the emphasis on Reading/Listening span as an index of WM capacity further complicates the issue, as the format of the task in which participants must switch between list maintenance and language comprehension evokes conscious executive processes that are not part of normal comprehension. Consequently, it is unclear whether a participant classified as having a "Low Working Memory Span" actually has a smaller memory capacity, a slower processing speed, difficulty with attention switching, or some combination of these. Next, we discuss further problems with the capacity view itself and then return to the issue of the type of memory model that might better support language processing.

Problems with the Capacity View

Despite its wide acceptance, the empirical support for a separate, fixed-capacity temporary storage system (either STM or WM) is weak. The main evidence in support of separable systems comes from neuropsychological double dissociations, where patients who show severely impaired LTM present with apparently normal STM, and vice versa (e.g., Cave & Squire, 1992; Scoville & Milner, 1957; Shallice & Warrington, 1970). At issue is the role of the medial temporal lobes (MTL) in STM tasks. Recall from our previous discussion that these structures are crucial for the creation and retrieval of long-term declarative memories, so if LTM were entirely distinct from STM, then the prediction is for no MTL involvement in creating STMs or in performing STM tasks. A number of studies have recently cast doubt on whether the double dissociation actually exists, however, showing MTL involvement in short-term tasks (Hannula, Tranel, & Cohen, 2006; Nichols, Kao, Verfaellie, & Gabrieli, 2006; Ranganath & Blumenfeld, 2005; Ranganath & D'Esposito, 2005).

Another source of evidence raising questions about the separability of the two types of memory is data suggesting that representations assumed to be in WM are not retrieved in a qualitatively different manner than those in LTM. Recent fMRI studies indicate that the retrieval of items argued to be within WM span recruit the same brain regions as retrieval from LTM, notably the left inferior frontal gyrus (LIFG) and regions of the medial temporal lobe (MTL) (Öztekin, Davachi, & McElree, 2010; Öztekin, McElree, Staresina, & Davachi, 2008). These imaging results align with behavioral investigations of experimental variables diagnostic of the nature of retrieval process, such as manipulations of recency and the size of the memory set (Box 5-1).

---

[3] One indication of how influential these tests have been is the number of citations they have received. The original Daneman and Carpenter (1980) paper describing the Reading/Listening span task has been cited 1712 times according to ISI Web of Knowledge. The article had 125 citations in 2009 and 74 as of July 2010. The Turner and Engle (1989) paper describing the nonlanguage version of the task (i.e., Operation span) has been cited 501 times since publication: 49 times in 2009 and 29 as of July 2010. A second indication of their influence is their presence on the Web. A Google search for "individual differences and Sentence Span" received 2.2 million hits (103,000 on Google Scholar) and the same search for "individual differences and operation span" received 485,000 hits (366,000 on Google Scholar) as of July 2010.

Box 5-1

Important Concepts

Connectionism/connectionist models: A computational model of cognition in which knowledge is stored in connections among a set of "nodes" which are assumed to operate like neurons in the brain (i.e., propagating activation to other nodes when they themselves have attained a sufficient level of activation). Knowledge is acquired in these models through a process of supervised learning, wherein the strength of connections between nodes is adjusted over a series of learning episodes. These strengths modulate the rate at which activation is propagated throughout the system, allowing for certain nodes to be "tuned" to particular properties of a stimulus, yielding more activation in certain contexts.

Hierarchical embedding: Grammatical relationships may be either *linear* or *hierarchical.* Hierarchical relationships require retrieval of previous encountered material. For example, in a relative clause, such as *The teacher who gave the difficult test called the principal.* the noun phrase *the teacher* must be retrieved in order to be associated with *called.* In contrast, this retrieval is not required in the following construction, which contains linear relationships: *The teacher gave the difficult test and the teacher called the principal.*

Long-distance/nonadjacent dependency: Refers to grammatical constructions in which two elements that should be associated together are non-adjacent. For example, the simple sentence *The teacher called* becomes a long distance dependency when additional information is inserted between the subject and the verb, as in *The teacher who gave the very difficult test during English class called.* In such a case, the subject *the teacher* would need to be retrieved in order to be associated with the verb *called.* This retrieval would not be necessary in the simple case, when the two words are adjacent. A variety of constructions fall into this category, in addition to the relative clause example discussed earlier, viz.: wh-questions (*Which teacher did you say called our house yesterday?*) where *teacher* is retrieved to be associated with *called;* cleft constructions (*It was the phone that the startled lady realized was ringing.*) where *phone* must be retrieved to be associated with *ringing;* and verb-phrase ellipsis (*The lady heard the phone ring, and the toddler did too.*) where the verb associated with *toddler* has been omitted, and must be retrieved from the previous clause.

Proactive/Retroactive interference: Two separate types of interference, distinguished by the position of the distracting information vis-à-vis the retrieval target, have been identified. For example in the series $[x_1\ x_2\ x_3\ A\ y_1\ y_2\ y_3\ B]$, if we consider that A is the retrieval target and B is the retrieval cue, then each of the x's create *proactive* interference for retrieving A, while each of the y's create *retroactive* interference for retrieving A. Recent research (Öztekin & McElree, 2007) in the memory domain suggests that proactive interference has its effect primarily on assessments of stimulus familiarity, such as those that yield "know" judgments in the Remember/Know task (cf. Box 3). Recent research in the language domain suggests that retroactive interference is more detrimental than proactive interference for resolving long-distance dependencies (Van Dyke & McElree, in press).

Pronoun resolution: The process of identifying the semantic content of a pronoun by matching it with elements from the previous discourse. For example, if the previous sentence in a text reads *The mother and the baby sat in the waiting room.* a following sentence like *She cried.* has two possible interpretations.

DIAGNOSING THE MECHANISMS OF RETRIEVAL

A number of retrieval mechanisms with quite different computational properties may be available to aid in the recovery of stored information, and empirical research is required to determine if and when each is employed. For example, retrieval may occur through a serial search process in which each item in memory must be checked until the desired item is found (Sternberg, 1966). An alternative process, discussed in the text, is content-addressable retrieval, which operates via direct association between the information available at retrieval-time (cues) and the content of stored memories. An easily understood example of this kind of retrieval is a search in a dictionary for the word "memory": A content-addressable mechanism could go directly to the page containing the words beginning "mem . . . ," while a serial search mechanism would have to begin at "A" and check each item. The chief diagnostic for distinguishing these mechanisms is the retrieval speed for a variety of set sizes and positions in the set. If retrieval occurs via serial search, then the time to access an item will depend on the number of items that must be examined prior to the target. For example, if the dictionary is quite large, then the time for a serial search mechanism to get to the *M*'s will be longer than if the dictionary is abridged. Similarly, a serial search mechanism will take less time to find a word beginning with "D" than it will to find one beginning with "M" because of their respective order in the alphabet. On the other hand,

---

Box 5-1

Important Concepts—cont'd

if retrieval is direct, then speed will be invariant across all set-sizes or serial positions, assuming the cues available at retrieval-time are sufficient to uniquely identify the target.

A considerable body of research has investigated set-size and serial position effects in the memory domain using a variety of methods (reviewed in McElree, 2006) and there is broad consensus over the conditions requiring direct access versus serial retrieval mechanisms. As reviewed in the text, direct access retrieval occurs when content must be retrieved, however if relational (or order) information is necessary, then serial search processes have been attested (e.g., Gronlund et al., 1997; McElree & Dosher, 1993). Research of this sort in the language domain is more recent, however the evidence points to direct access as the prominent retrieval mechanism. Manipulations that have attempted to duplicate the conditions of set-size by increasing the amount of information, and the amount of interference, between dependencies have consistently found no effects on retrieval speed (e.g., McElree, Foraker, & Dyer, 2003; Van Dyke & McElree, in press).

Contra long-standing claims that information in WM is retrieved with specialized operations (e.g., Sternberg, 1975), the retrieval profiles observed have consistently shown the signature pattern of a direct-access operation, the same type of retrieval operation thought to underlie LTM retrieval. In this type of operation, memory representations are "content-addressable," enabling cues in the retrieval context to make direct contact to representations with overlapping content, without the need to search through irrelevant representations. We take up this discussion further later.

Thus, while it is well documented that our ability to concurrently process different types of information is extremely limited (e.g., Broadbent, 1958), the evidence noted sheds doubt on whether this necessitates the existence of a temporary storage system (be it STM or WM) distinct from LTM. Indeed, there is long strain of research that has challenged the multi-store view, in favor of a unitary-store model, where the information that multi-store models would ascribe to STM/WM is characterized as just the temporarily active portion of LTM (e.g., Anderson et al., 2004; Cowan, 1988, 1995, 2001; Crowder, 1976; McElree, 2001, 2006; Oberauer, 2002; Verhaeghen, Cerella, & Basak, 2004). While these models differ in a variety of details, Cowan's (2001) model can serve as an example (Figure 5-6).

This model suggests that there is only one representation of known information—that in LTM. These representations vary in activation strength, determined by such variables as recency and frequency of occurrence, and representations of increased strength are more available for retrieval when required, but remain in passive memory until such retrievals occur. One type of evidence in support of a unitary-store architecture comes from precise measures of retrieval speed: information in

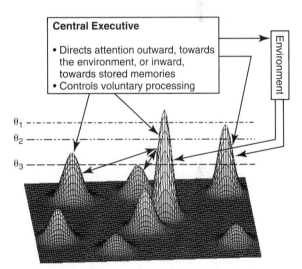

Figure 5-6 Unitary store model. Memories have various levels of activation within the same store. Activation is triggered by cues from the environment or from deliberate attentional processes. Activation may also increase due to associations between items in memory. Dashed lines represent possible threshold levels, θ, by which the size of activated memory would be determined. The most restrictive theories claim that active memory contains only the single item that is in the focus of attention, corresponding to the highest threshold, θ_1; others suppose a lower threshold, such that active memory may contain as many as 4 items.

WM should have a privileged status compared to that in LTM, and so should be accessed more quickly. Based on this reasoning, it would be expected to find a "breakpoint" between the speed of accessing the items that have just been processed (i.e., that are in the focus of attention) and then another "breakpoint" between items that are active in WM and those in LTM. This is not the pattern that has been observed, however. As reviewed in McElree (2006), direct measures of the speed and accuracy of memory retrieval across a broad range of tasks requiring the retention of sequentially presented information have consistently shown that items predicted to be within WM span do *not* exhibit privileged access, but rather are retrieved with the same speed as items well beyond the assumed WM span.

These tasks include item recognition, paired-associate recognition, judgments of recency, rhyme and synonym judgments, and the n-back task (Box 5-2). Across all these tasks, there is unequivocal evidence that information being actively processed at test time—typically, the last item studied when there is no distracting activity between study and test—exhibits privileged access, with responses being 30%–50% faster than responses to items outside focal attention.

Box 5-2

Memory Research Methods

RECOGNITION TASKS

Recognition tasks can be distinguished by the overt presence of the very item participants are being asked to remember. As such, participants are generally better at recognition tasks compared to recall tasks (discussed later), making them a more sensitive test of the contents of memory. Participants will often do well in a recognition test even when they fail a recall test for the same item. Specific examples of these tasks are given:

Item recognition: Participants are presented with a memory set, typically containing letters or words, and asked to memorize them during a study phase. At test, participants are presented either with an item which occurred in the memory set, or with an item they had never seen before, and they are required to make a yes/no judgment about whether the item occurred in the memory set. Variable amounts of time may occur between the study and test phases, although studies using this method to examine short-term memory processes typically have the test immediately following the study phase.

Paired-associate recognition: A variation on the item recognition task in which the memory set contains two items (e.g., letters or words) that have been previously studied as a pair. When the pair is presented at test, the participant must verify whether they studied it previously (as a pair). In this paradigm, it may also be of interest to present participants with a pair containing one (or both) item(s) previously studied, but with different partners. This condition forces participants to distinguish specific learning episodes where the two items are paired, from a general feeling of familiarity with the individual members of the pair.

Recency judgments: A variation on the test phase of the item recognition paradigm in which participants are asked to judge which of two items occurred more recently in the study list. Hence, this task requires participants to remember not only whether particular items were seen previously, but also in what order they occurred.

Rhyme/Synonym judgments: Variations of the test phase of the item recognition paradigm in which participants are asked to judge whether two items rhyme or mean the same. These tests can be used to force participants to focus on content-related aspects of the studied items, in contrast to simple item recognition tests which may not require deep processing of the studied material.

Remember/Know judgments: Variation of the test phase of the item recognition paradigm in which participants must indicate whether they actually have a conscious recollection of the item's occurrence in the study list, or whether they have a more diffuse intuition that it was there (they "just know it"). This procedure is useful for distinguishing memories that may be present as the result of explicit retrieval processes versus implicit memories based on quick assessments of familiarity based on sensory or perceptual features of the stimulus.

N-back task: A test of continuous working memory in which participants are presented with a stream of stimulus items and told to indicate (e.g., press a button) when the current stimulus item matches one that appeared n items earlier in the sequence. The variable n represents the load factor, which determines the task difficulty. For example, if n = 2, then participants report on every other stimulus; if n = 4 then participants report on the content of every fourth stimulus, remembering whether it matched the item occurring three trials previous.

Box 5-2

Memory Research Methods—cont'd

RECALL TASKS

Free recall: Participants reproduce material just learned, without any prompts are cues. As the task is quite difficult, it is common to encourage participants to recall as much of the information as possible. Guessing may also be encouraged, as a means of accessing subconscious (implicit) memory traces.

Serial recall: A variation of free recall with the added constraint that participants must recall the information learned in the same order it was learned. The addition of this constraint typically increases difficulty.

Cued recall: A variation of free recall in which partial information is given in order to aid memory. For example, when the memory list contained a list of words, a cued recall test may supply the first letter of each of the memory words. Another frequent example is for a single item of a studied pair to be presented, in order to prompt recall its associate.

IMPLICATIONS FOR LANGUAGE PROCESSING

In principle, language processing might use different memory operations than what has been observed in these basic memory tasks or even use a specialized memory system—for example, Caplan and Waters (1999) suggested that it might draw upon separate WM resources. However, studies investigating the real-time memory operations involved in the processing of linguistic dependencies have yielded results indicating that a dependant constituent is retrieved from memory with the same type of retrieval mechanism described earlier. A range of dependencies have been explored, including verb-argument dependencies (McElree, 2000; McElree, Foraker, & Dyer, 2003), subject-verb dependencies (McElree et al, 2003), verb-phrase ellipsis (Martin & McElree, 2008; 2009), and pronoun resolution (Foraker & McElree, 2007). The crucial studies have used adaptations of the speed-accuracy tradeoff procedure (Dosher, 1979; Wickelgren, 1977; Reed, 1973, 1976) to conjointly measure the speed and accuracy of interpreting an expression with a nonadjacent dependency as a function of 'distance,' viz., the amount of material interpolated between the dependant constituents.

For example, McElree et al. (2003) contrasted the speed of resolving subject-verb dependencies with no material intervening, such as *The editor laughed*, to sentences in which one or two subject- or object relative clauses intervened between the subject and verb. They found that interpretation of the subject-verb dependency occurred at an exceptionally fast rate when the dependent elements were adjacent to one another. However, the speed of accessing a distant noun phrase (NP) to bind as subject to the final verb was constant for each of the nonadjacent constructions, which contain varying numbers of intervening words, discourse items,

and hierarchically embedded constituents. These results mirror those found in basic memory studies in two key respects. First, there was a "breakpoint" in processing speed for the most recent item processed and all other items, marking the distinction between items being actively processed and those that require retrieval to be restored to active processing. Second, retrieval speed was invariant across linear distance, as well as other types of metrics such as level of embedding or the number of incomplete dependencies. This is the signature pattern of a direct-access operation, in which associative retrieval cues provide direct access to the content of stored representations. It is not the pattern expected if retrieval required a search (either forward or backward) through the hierarchical parse-tree in a step-by-step fashion in order to identify the correct grammatical dependent (McElree, 2006).

At first blush, it might appear that a processing architecture eschewing a traditional 3-4 item WM storage buffer may be too restrictive to subserve sentence processing. However, Lewis, Vasishth, and Van Dyke (2006; see also Lewis & Vasishth, 2005) described a computational model of sentence processing that requires maintaining only the most recently parsed item in active memory. The model's memory consists of chunks representing the syntactic structure built so far, together with predictions for constituents licensed by the current state of the parse. These chunks are not actively held in memory and decay as a function of time and prior retrievals. The only access to these items is via a retrieval buffer with the capacity to hold a single chunk. This affords the model the minimum capacity required to create new linguistic relations—the item waiting to be integrated into the parse, and the chunk that licenses it. The item that is waiting is in the focus of attention and does not need to be retrieved. The chunk that licenses it is retrieved via the cues derived from the features of the waiting item. Critically, it is this cue-based retrieval process, which occurs via direct access, that provides the computational power necessary to create dependencies in real time. Mathematical analyses of reaction time distributions (Ratcliff, 1978) and evidence from the Speed-Accuracy Tradeoff (SAT) paradigm (McElree, 2001) suggest that humans can restore items into active memory in approximately 80–90 ms. Retrieval speeds that are this fast enable the parsing mechanism to compensate for the severe limit on the size of active memory, while still enabling parsing decisions to be made in about 200 ms, which is typical for real-time language processing.

Forgetting

Lost memory is perhaps the most vexing problem human beings face. Even in a nonclinical setting, the phenomenon is a constant reminder that even our highly evolved brains have inescapable limits. We noted earlier in our discussion of episodic memory that the primary account of forgetting long-held information relates to an inability to retrieve the information—that is, the information becomes *inaccessible,* but nevertheless remains in memory and can be reactivated if only suitable retrieval cues are supplied (Tulving, 1979). The usefulness of reminders and mnemonic devices seems to fit naturally with this account, and gives intuitional support to the body of evidence that weighs against other explanations based on failure to store memories in the first place (e.g., Crowder, 1982; Keppel, 1984; Quartermain, McEwen, & Azmitia, 1972).

From the perspective of language processing, the crucial question is what causes forgetting over the short term, since we are interested in the processing that occurs over the span of a paragraph, or even a sentence. This has been a question of great debate in the memory literature, centering around the role of *decay* (e.g., Nairne, 2002; Lewandowsky, Duncan, & Brown, 2004). As discussed earlier, limited-capacity multistore models have traditionally favored decay, or displacement, as the mechanism that controls forgetting; any information that is not maintained via some mechanism of active maintenance (e.g., rehearsal) will be lost. Alternative unitary-store models relinquish a separate maintenance mechanism for a fast cue-based retrieval mechanism that can restore information into active memory as needed. From this perspective, information is lost because retrieval cues are insufficient to uniquely identify the necessary information. This occurs when the presence of similar items in memory creates a condition of *cue-overload*, where retrieval cues are associated with multiple items in memory, making them inadequate

discriminators (e.g., Öztekin & McElree, 2007; Nairne, 2002; Watkins & Watkins, 1975). The result is *interference*, where unwanted items are retrieved instead of the target item. Interference can come in two varieties: the case where similar items *precede* the target, creating *proactive interference*, and the case were similar items *follow* the target, creating *retroactive interference*.

Despite its popularity as a component of multistore models, and its intuitive appeal, the evidence supporting decay is weak. Even from the early days of memory theorizing, decay came under fire as a logically inadequate explanation: John McGeoch (1932) pointed out that just as iron rusts over time, memories are forgotten over time, but in neither case is time the causal agent. While oxidation is the mechanism through which rust forms, similarly, the mechanism through which forgetting arises must be stated. McGeoch proposed that interference is the most likely candidate.

One of the chief problems with evaluating the decay hypothesis is that it is nearly impossible to rule out interference as an alternative explanation. For example, the classic Brown-Peterson studies (Brown, 1958; Peterson & Peterson, 1959) used articulatory suppression to block rehearsal during a memory task where participants were supposed to remember a 3-consonant trigram (TWF). They found that correct recall was reduced as the length of the suppression task increased from 3 to 18 seconds (increasing the delay between study and test), until only about 10% of studied trigrams could be recalled. The apparent conclusion is that without the ability to rehearse, information will be almost completely lost within about 18 seconds. However, two follow-up studies make it clear that this conclusion is incorrect. Waugh & Norman (1965) varied the presentation rate for a study list of 16 digits, so that in the fast condition only 4 seconds passed during which decay could occur, while in the slow conditions (digits presented 1 per second) 16 seconds passed. Following the study list, a target digit was presented, and participants were asked to recall the digit that followed this target. Contrary to the prediction that a longer amount of time should produce more forgetting, they found no difference between the two presentation rate conditions. A further challenge to the decay account of the Brown-Peterson studies came from Keppel and Underwood (1962), who conducted a modified analysis of data produced via the Brown-Peterson method. The prediction of an interference account is that trials from the beginning of the experiment should be more easily recalled than those from the later part of the experiment because earlier trials will have less prior buildup of interfering material (i.e., less proactive interference).

By analyzing individual trials—something that was not done in the original studies—they found exactly this; accuracy on trial 1 was nearly 100% even after 18 minutes of delay time, but begins to reduce after this with each trial getting successively worse as more information in memory builds up. This finding directly contradicts the original study, suggesting that those results were obtained only because the experimenters aggregated data over individual trials, causing them to miss observing the buildup of proactive interference.

While it has proved difficult to disentangle decay and interference in memory studies, Van Dyke and Lewis (2003) presented data suggesting that both are at work in the domain of language processing. They manipulated the distance between two grammatically dependent constituents (*man* and *was paranoid* in this example) by comparing a sentence with no intervening distance (*1. The frightened boy understood that the man was paranoid about dying.*) with a sentence with an intervening clause (*2. The frightened boy understood that the man who was swimming near the dock was paranoid about dying.*) They also manipulated the amount of interference present in the intervening region by comparing the long sentence in (2) with the sentence (*3. The frightened boy understood that the man who said the townspeople were dangerous was paranoid about dying.*) The amount of interference is measured with respect to the retrieval cues set by the verb phrase *was paranoid*. This verb phrase is assumed to contain retrieval cues that will identify a grammatical subject with which it can be associated so that it can be integrated into a coherent interpretation of the sentence. Thus, sentence (3) is considered to have more interference than sentence (2) because the intervening noun phrase *the townspeople* shares its grammatical encoding with the target constituent; they are both grammatical subjects. The retrieval cues from the verb will therefore match to both *the townspeople* and *the man* as potential subjects. In contrast, sentence (2) is a low interference condition because it does not have a subject intervening between the verb phrase and the target noun phrase; the intervening noun phrase *the dock* is the object of a prepositional phrase. Note that sentences (2) and (3) are matched on the distance dimension; both have 6 intervening words. Thus, the contrast between (1) and (2) provides an estimate of the distance effect, while the contrast between (2) and (3) provides an estimate of the additional interference effect. The left panel of Figure 5-7 shows the results for acceptability judgments; an identical pattern of results was found for reading times on the verb phrase itself. Interference (2 versus 3) had a significant effect, but distance (1 versus 2)

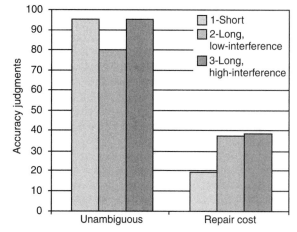

Figure 5-7 Participants had to judge whether sentences were grammatical. Repair cost was calculated by subtracting accuracy scores to unambiguous sentences from the ambiguous version of the same sentence. The interference manipulation (2 versus 3) had an effect on procedures associated with integrating the separated subject and verb, but this did not affect repair cost. Distance (1 versus 2), on the other hand, *did* affect repair cost. [Results from Van Dyke, J. A., & Lewis, R. L. (2003). Distinguishing effects of structure and decay on attachment and repair: A retrieval interference theory of recovery from misanalyzed ambiguities. *Journal of Memory and Language, 49*, 285–413, Experiment 3.]

did not. This is consistent with the view that the critical factor for making constituents unavailable for retrieval is not the *amount* of information, but rather *how similar* the intervening information is to the target.

A further manipulation of ambiguity, created by removing the *that* in the earlier conditions, enabled Van Dyke and Lewis to investigate effects of decay because the less preferred interpretation is not pursued. For example, in the ambiguous version of (1), given here as (*4. The frightened boy understood the man was paranoid about dying.*) the verb *understood* can be interpreted either as a verb that takes a direct object (cf. *The boy understood the question and answered it*) or as a verb that takes a sentential complement (cf. *The boy understood the question was difficult*). Van Dyke and Lewis designed the experiment to include a large number of direct object sentences as filler items, so as to strongly bias the reader toward taking the direct object interpretation initially. The assumption was that the ultimately correct sentential complement interpretation of *understood* would not be pursued, causing the syntactic features licensing the sentential complement to decay because of disuse. Thus, in the ambiguous version of

(2), given here as (5. *The frightened boy understood the man who was swimming near the dock was paranoid about dying*), the initial interpretation could be consistent with the sentence *The boy understood the man who was swimming near the dock and smiled at him.*[4] A similar relationship between understood and the man would be adopted prior to the occurrence of was paranoid for the ambiguous version of the high interference sentence (3), given here as (6. *The frightened boy understood the man who said the townspeople were dangerous was paranoid about dying.*) Crucially, at the point when *was paranoid* must be processed, the sentential complement features must be reactivated in order to integrate the verb phrase into the sentence. The prediction was that any difficulty in reactivating the sentential complement features arises as a result of how much these features decayed while the incorrect interpretation was pursued. Consistent with this view, the distance effect on the ability reanalyze the ambiguous sentence was significant (cf. right panel of Figure 5-7), suggesting the decay of the less preferred interpretation. There was no additional effect of interference during reanalysis, however, consistent with the fact that the interfering material in the unambiguous sentences is identical to that in the ambiguous sentences.

These results have strong implications for the type of memory system thought to underlie sentence comprehension. As discussed earlier, the dominant capacity approach has suggested that sentences such as (2) and (3) are difficult to process because *the man* must be "held" in WM while processing the intervening material, which expends memory resources because of its length (e.g., Gibson, 1998, 2000). Contra this, Van Dyke and Lewis found that only particular types of intervening constructions—those containing syntactically similar material—produced difficulty. Thus, the distance effects that were previously thought to occur because of decay, or because of a lack of memory resources, can be attributed to retrieval interference. Decay, on the other hand, seems to have its effect only on the ability to re-retrieve information after it has been completely abandoned—and notably, without any new retrieval cues that would guide the retrieval mechanism in doing so.

While the Van Dyke and Lewis study investigated interference arising from syntactically similar distractors, other types of interference effects have also been observed in sentence comprehension. For example, in an extension of the study just described, Van Dyke (2007) showed that interference could arise from *semantically* similar distractors, even when not in a syntactically similar position. Thus, (2) was easier than the same sentence with the word *dock* replaced with the word *girl*, which fits the semantic cues of the verb phrase (i.e., a *girl* can be paranoid but a *dock* cannot). Still another type of interference—referential interference—was observed by Gordon and colleagues (Gordon, Hendrick, & Johnson, 2001; 2004) who investigated the role of various noun phrase types appearing as the second (underlined) noun in subject relative clauses (e.g., The banker that praised the barber climbed the mountain) and object relative clauses (e.g., The banker that the barber praised climbed the mountain). The greater difficulty of the object relative as compared with the subject relative construction has been repeatedly documented (e.g., King & Just, 1991; Staub, 2010; Traxler, Morris, & Seely, 2002), with the dominant explanation focusing on different demands each construction makes on memory. Gordon et al. sought to pinpoint the contribution of interference to this contrast by manipulating the referential status of the second noun phrase. In several experiments, they contrasted the sentences earlier with identical sentences except for substituting a pronoun (*you* or *everyone*) or a proper name (*Joe*) for *barber*, and found that the advantage for subject-relative clauses over object-relative clauses was reduced or eliminated. Common nouns like *barber* and *banker* refer indirectly by virtue of their description, while pronouns and proper names refer directly, singling out specific entities in the current discourse context. Thus, similarity-based interference arises in a variety of linguistic contexts in the presence of syntactic, semantic, and referentially similar distractors.

The appearance of interference effects—a classic memory phenomenon—in language comprehension weighs against the proposal of a language-specific memory capacity (Caplan & Waters, 1999) and points to a unification of memory mechanisms operating both over the short- and long-term temporal periods, and both in the memory and language domains. Support for this parsimonious approach is apparent in neuroimaging research that has attempted to identify the brain regions responsible for memory retrieval. We have already noted fvMRI evidence suggesting that retrieval of recent items recruits the same brain regions as retrieval from LTM, notably the left inferior frontal gyrus (LIFG) (Öztekin et al., 2008, 2010). The LIFG has also been repeatedly implicated in neuroimaging studies of memory interference resolution (reviewed in Jonides & Nee, 2006).

---

[4] The continuation *and smiled at him* is included here only to emphasize that *the man* is interpreted as the direct object of *understood*. The experiment did not include continuations such as these.

Additionally, patient work (e.g., Thompson-Schill et al., 2002) and repetitive transcranial magnetic stimulation investigations (e.g., Feredoes, Tononi, & Postle, 2006) have provided converging evidence for a direct role of LIFG in successful interference resolution. This is exciting because this same region, which includes Broca's area, has also had a long history of being associated with language (especially syntactic) processing (Rogalsky & Hickock, 2010, for a review). In particular, the subregions of BA 44 and 45 in LIFG have been been repeatedly implicated in the processing of syntactically interfering sentence constructions as in (3) earlier (e.g., Cooke et al., 2001; Fiebach, Vos, & Friederici, 2004; Makuuchi, Bahlmann, Anwander, & Friederici, 2009; Stowe et al., 1999). Likewise, a recent fMRI study following on Van Dyke (2007) has found semantic interference effects in the pars triangularis region of BA 45 (Guo, Martin, Van Dyke, & Hamilton, 2010). Recent attempts to further specify the functional role of the subregions of LIFG during memory retrieval comport well with the language processing results, as they point to a unique role of the pars triangularis region (BA 45) in tasks requiring selection among competing alternatives (Badre & Wagner, 2007; Badre, Poldrack, Paré-Blagoev, et al., 2005). Taken together, these separate streams of research in the memory and language domains appear to converge on the idea that the ability to manage retrieval interference may be at the root of memory and language deficits in both clinical and nonclinical populations. Indeed, a number of researchers have already suggested that differences in susceptibility to interference (Hasher & Zacks, 1988; Stoltzfus, Hasher, & Zacks, 1996) provide more veridical characterizations of age-related changes and individual differences in memory ability. Current approaches to language deficits in clinical populations have also moved toward explanations that implicate interference. For example, comprehension deficits in patients with Parkinson's disease have been linked to deficits in cognitive flexibility and the ability to inhibit irrelevant information (Hochstadt, Nakano, Lieberman, & Friedman, 2006).

CONCLUSIONS

A long history of research in neuropsychology, psycholinguistics, and cognitive psychology has attempted to characterize the relationship between memory and language. While advances have been made, a number of stumbling blocks have been encountered due to the adoption of memory models that were developed to account for memory phenomenon unrelated to the task of language processing. The advent of connectionism

and statistical learning theory has led to a number of important advances, but there is still much to understand about how the two systems interact. This review has emphasized areas where it would be fruitful to examine the extent to which the memory system and the language processing system rely on (at least functionally) the same mechanisms. Namely, a growing body of evidence now suggests that language processing is supported by a memory architecture that emphasizes a unitary store and a fast cue-based retrieval mechanism, which is susceptible to retrieval interference (e.g., Lewis, Vasishth, & Van Dyke, 2006). The central issue in determining how clinical variables resulting from brain damage and aging affect this system will be to develop a further understanding into the mechanisms necessary for identifying and using cues, both as a means through which new linguistic knowledge is learned and as the engine that drives comprehension. Although this issue is understudied at present, it has gained increased attention in recent years. The data available so far suggest that individuals do vary in their capacity for statistical learning and that these differences are correlated with differences in language and reading performance (Ahissar et al., 2006, Ahissar, 2007; Conway, Bauernschmidt, Huang, & Pisoni, in press; Evans, Saffran, & Robe-Torres, 2009). Additional research into the neural basis for cue-based learning and retrieval will be important in order to gain a more complete understanding of the interaction of memory and language processes.

ACKNOWLEDGMENTS

Preparation of this chapter was supported by NIH/NICHD grant R21-HD-058944 to Haskins Laboratories (Van Dyke, PI), NIH/NICHD grant R01-HD-040353 to Haskins Laboratories (Shankweiler, PI), and by NIH/NICHD grant R01-HD-056200 to New York University (McElree, PI).

REFERENCES

Abney, S. P., & Johnson, M. (1991). Memory requirements and local ambiguities of parsing strategies. *Journal of Psycholinguistic Research, 20*, 233–250.

Ahissar, M. (2007). Dyslexia and the anchoring-deficit hypothesis. *Trends in Cognitive Sciences, 11*(11), 458–465.

Ahissar, M., Lubin, Y., Putter-Katz, H., & Banai, K. (2006). Dyslexia and the failure to form a perceptual anchor. *Nature Neuroscience, 9*, 1558–1564.

Aldridge, J. W., & Berridge, K. C. (1998). Coding of serial order by neostriatal neurons: A "natural action" approach to movement sequence. *Journal of Neuroscience, 18*(7), 2777–2787.

Alvarez, P., & Squire, L. R. (1994). Memory consolidation and the medial temporal lobe: A simple network model. *Proceedings of the National Academy of Sciences USA, 91*, 7041–7045.

Anderson, J. R., Bothell, D., Byrne, M. D., Douglass, S., Lebiere, C., & Qin, Y. (2004). An integrated theory of mind. *Psychological Review, 111*, 1036–1060.

Atkinson, R. C., & Shiffrin, R. M. (1968). Human memory: A proposed system and its control processes. In K. W. Spence (Ed.), *The psychology of learning and motivation: Advances in research and theory* (Vol. 2, pp. 89–195). New York: Academic Press.

Aziz-Zadeh, L., Wilson, S. M., Rizzolatti, G., & Iacoboni, M. (2006). Congruent embodied representations for visually presented actions and linguistic phrases describing actions. *Current Biology, 16*(18), 1818–1823.

Baddeley, A. D. (1966). Short-term memory for word sequences as a function of acoustic, semantic and formal similarity. *The Quarterly Journal of Experimental Psychology, 18*, 362–365.

Baddeley, A. D. (1986). *Working memory.* Oxford, UK: Clarendon Press.

Baddeley, A. D. (2000). The episodic buffer: A new component of working memory? *Trends in Cognitive Science, 4*, 417–423.

Baddeley, A. (2003). Working memory: Looking back and looking forward. *Nature Reviews Neuroscience, 4*, 829–839.

Baddeley, A. D., & Hitch, G. (1974). Working memory. In G. H. Bower (Ed.), *The psychology of learning and motivation: Advances in research and theory* (Vol. 8, pp. 47–89). New York: Academic Press.

Baddeley, A. D., Thomson, N., & Buchanan, M. (1975). Word length and the structure of short-term memory. *Journal of Verbal Learning and Verbal Behavior, 14*, 575–589.

Badre, D., Poldrack, R. A., Paré-Blagoev, E. J., Insler, R., & Wagner, A. D. (2005). Dissociable controlled retrieval and generalized selection mechanisms in ventrolateral prefrontal cortex. Neuron, 47, 907–918.

Badre D., & Wagner, A. D. (2007). Left ventrolateral prefrontal cortex and the control of memory. *Neuropsychologia, 45*, 2883–2901.

Bhatt, R. S., Wilk, A., Hill, D., & Rovee-Collier, C. (2004). Correlated attributes and categorization in the first half-year of life. *Developmental Psychobiology, 44*, 103–115.

Boecker, H., Dagher, A., Ceballos-Baumann, A. O., Passingham, R. E., Samuel, M., Friston, K. J., Poline, J., . . . Brooks, D. J. (1998). Role of the human rostral supplementary motor area and the basal ganglia in motor sequence control: Investigations with H2 150 PET. *Journal of Neurophysiology, 79*(2), 1070–1080.

Bookheimer, S. (2002). Functional MRI of language: New approaches to understanding the cortical organization of semantic processing. *Annual Review of Neuroscience, 25*, 151–188.

Bonatti, L. L., Peña, M., Nespor, M., & Mehler, J. (2005). Linguistic constraints on statistical computations: The role of consonants and vowels in continuous speech processing. *Psychological Science, 16*, 451–459.

Bowers, J. S., & Schacter, D. L. (1992). Priming of novel information in amnesia: Issues and data. In P. Graf & M. E. J. Masson (Eds.), *Implicit memory: New directions in cognition, neuropsychology, and development.* New York: Academic Press.

Braver, T. S., Cohen, J. D., Nystrom, L. E., Jonides, J., Smith, E. E., & Noll, D. C. (1997). A parametric study of prefrontal cortex involvement in human working memory. *NeuroImage, 5*, 49–62.

Broadbent, D. E. (1958). *Perception and communication.* London: Pergamon Press.

Brown, J. (1958). Some tests of the decay theory of immediate memory. *Quarterly Journal of Experimental Psychology, 10*, 12–21.

Buckner, R. L., & Koutstaal, W. (1998). Functional neuroimaging studies of encoding, priming, and explicit memory retrieval. *Proceedings of the National Academy of Sciences USA, 95*, 891–898.

Buckner, R. L., & Wheeler, M. E. (2001). The cognitive neuroscience of remembering. *Nature Reviews Neuroscience, 2*(9), 624–634.

Buffalo, E. A., Reber, P. J., & Squire, L. R. (1998). The human perirhinal cortex and recognition memory. *Hippocampus, 8*(4), 330–339.

Caplan, D., & Hildebrandt, N. (1988). *Disorders of syntactic comprehension.* Cambridge, MA: MIT Press/Bradford Books.

Caplan, D., & Waters, G. S. (1999). Verbal working memory and sentence comprehension. *Behavioral and Brain Sciences, 22*, 77–94.

Cave, C. B., & Squire, L. R. (1992). Intact and long-lasting repetition priming in amnesia. *Journal of Experimental Psychology: Learning, Memory, and Cognition, 18*(3), 509–520.

Cermak, L. S., Verfaellie, M., Milberg, W., Letourneau, L., & Blackford, S. (1991). A further analysis of perceptual identification priming in alcoholic Korsakoff patients, *Neuropsychologia, 29*, 725–736.

Chao, L. L., Haxby, J. V., & Martin, A. (1999). Attribute-based neural substrates in temporal cortex for perceiving and knowing about objects. *Nature Neuroscience, 2*(10), 913–919.

Chomsky, N. (1965). *Aspects of the theory of syntax.* Cambridge, MA: MIT Press.

Chomsky, N. (1980). *Rules and representations.* New York: Columbia University Press.

Chomsky, N. (1986). *Knowledge of language: Its nature, origin, and use.* New York: Praeger.

Cohen, J. D., Perlstein, W. M., Braver, T. S., Nystrom, L. E., Noll, D. C., Jonides, J., & Smith, E. E. (1997). Temporal dynamics of brain activation during a working memory task. *Nature, 386*, 604–608.

Collins, A. M., & Quillian, M. R. (1969). Retrieval time from semantic memory. *Journal of Verbal Learning and Verbal Behavior, 8*(2), 240–247.

Conrad, R. (1964). Acoustic confusion in immediate memory. *British Journal of Psychology, 55*, 75–84.

Conway, C., & Christiansen, M. (2001). Sequential learning in non-human primates. *Trends in Cognitive Sciences, 5*(12), 539–546.

Conway, C. M., Bauernschmidt, A., Huang, S. S., & Pisoni, D. B. (2010). Implicit statistical learning in language processing: Word predictability is the key. *Cognition, 114*(3), 356–371.

Conway, M. A. (2001). Sensory-perceptual episodic memory and its context: Autobiographical memory. *Philosophical Transactions of the Royal Society of London, B356*, 1375–1384.

Cooke, A., Zurif, E. B., DeVita, C., Alsop, D., Koenig, P., Detre, J., Gee, J., . . . Grossman, M. (2001). Neural basis for sentence comprehension: Grammatical and short-term memory components. *Human Brain Mapping, 15*(2), 80–94.

Corbetta, M., Miezin, F. M., Dobmeyer, S., Shulman, G. L., & Petersen, S. E. (1990). Attentional modulation of neural processing of shape, color, and velocity in humans. *Science, 248*, 1556–1559.

Cowan, N. (1988). Evolving conceptions of memory storage, selective attention, and their mutual constraints within the human information processing system. *Psychological Bulletin, 104*, 163–191.

Cowan, N. (1995). *Attention and memory: An integrated framework.* Oxford, UK: Oxford University Press.

Cowan, N. (2001). The magical number 4 in short-term memory: A reconsideration of mental storage capacity. *Behavioral and Brain Sciences, 24*, 87–185.

Crain, S., & Thornton, R. (1998). *Investigations in universal grammar.* Cambridge, MA: MIT Press.

Crowder, R. G. (1976). *Principles of learning and memory.* Hillsdale, NJ: Erlbaum.

Crowder, R. G. (1982). General forgetting theory and the locus of amnesia. In L. S. Cermak (Ed.), *Human memory and amnesia.* Hillsdale, NJ: Erlbaum.

Daneman, M. E., & Carpenter, P. A. (1980). Individual differences in working memory and reading. *Journal of Verbal Learning and Verbal Behavior, 19*, 450–466.

Daneman, M. E., & Merikle, P. M. (1996). Working memory and language comprehension: A meta-analysis. *Psychonomic Bulletin & Review, 3*(4), 422–433.

Danker, J. F., & Anderson, J. R. (2010). The ghosts of brain states past: Remembering reactivates the brain regions engaged during encoding. *Psychological Bulletin, 136*(1), 87–102.

Delgado, M. R., Jou, R. L., LeDoux, J. E., & Phelps, E. A. (2009). Avoiding negative outcomes: Tracking the mechanisms of avoidance learning in humans during fear conditioning. *Frontiers in Behavioral Neuroscience, 3*, 1–9. doi:10.3389/neuro.08.033.2009

Dominey, P. F., Hoen, M., Blanc, J. M., & Lelekov-Boissard, T. (2003). Neurological basis of language and sequential cognition: Evidence from simulation, aphasia, and ERP studies. *Brain and Language, 83*, 207–225.

Dosher, B. A. (1979). Empirical approaches to information processing: Speed-accuracy tradeoff or reaction time. *Acta Psychologica, 43*, 347–359.

Doyon, J., Gaudreau, D., Laforce, R., Castonguay, M., Bedard, P. J., Bedard, F., & Bouchard, J. P. (1997). Role of the striatum, cerebellum, and frontal lobes in the learning of a visuomotor sequence. *Brain and Cognition, 34*(2), 218–245.

Doyon, J., Owen, A. M., Petrides, M., Sziklas, V., & Evans, A. C. (1996). Functional anatomy of visuomotor skill learning in human subjects examined with positron emission tomography. *European Journal of Neuroscience, 8*(4), 637–648.

Evans, J. L., Saffran, J. R., & Robe-Torres, K. (2009). Statistical learning in children with specific language impairment. *Journal of Speech, Language, and Hearing Research, 52*, 321–335.

Fedorenko, E., Gibson, E., & Rohde, D. (2006). The nature of working memory capacity in sentence comprehension: Evidence against domain specific resources. *Journal of Memory and Language, 54*(4), 541–553.

Fedorenko, E., Gibson, E., & Rohde, D. (2007). The nature of working memory in linguistic, arithmetic and spatial integration processes. *Journal of Memory and Language, 56*(2) 246–269.

Feredoes, E., Tononi, G., and Postle, B. R. (2006). Direct evidence for a prefrontal contribution to the control of proactive interference in verbal working memory. *Proceedings of the National Academy of Sciences USA, 103*(51), 19530–19534.

Ferreira, F., & Henderson, J. M. (1991). Recovery from misanalyses of garden-path sentences. *Journal of Memory and Language, 30*(6), 725–745.

Fiebach, C. J., Vos, S. H., & Friederici, A. D. (2004). Neural correlates of syntactic ambiguity in sentence comprehension for low and high span readers. *Journal of Cognitive Neuroscience, 16*, 1562–1575.

Foraker, S., & McElree, B. (2007). The role of prominence in pronoun resolution: Availability versus accessibility. *Journal of Memory and Language, 56*(3), 357–383.

Funnell, E. (1983). Phonological processes in reading: New evidence from acquired dyslexia. *British Journal of Psychology, 74*, 159–180.

Gabrieli, J. D. E., & Keane, M. M. (1988). Priming in the patient H. M.: New findings and a theory of intact and impaired priming in patients with memory disorders. *Society for Neuroscience Abstracts, 14*, 1290.

Gabrieli, J. D. E., Poldrack, R. A., & Desmond, J. E. (1998). The role of left prefrontal cortex in language and memory. *Proceedings of the National Academy of Sciences USA, 95*, 906–913.

Gathercole, S. E., Alloway, T. P., Willis, C., & Adams, A. M. (2006). Working memory in children with reading disabilities. *Journal of Experimental Child Psychology, 93*, 265–281.

Gerken, L., Wilson, R., & Lewis, W. (2005). Infant can use distributional cues to form syntactic categories. *Journal of Child Language, 32*, 249–268.

Gibson, E. (2000). The dependency locality theory: A distance-based theory of linguistic complexity. In A. Marantz (Ed.), *Image, language, brain: Papers from the first mind articulation project symposium* (pp. 94–126). Cambridge, MA: MIT Press.

Gibson, E. A. (1998). Linguistic complexity: Locality of syntactic dependencies. *Cognition, 68*, 1–76.

Gordon, P. C., Hendrick, R., & Johnson, M. (2001). Memory interference during language processing. *Journal of Experimental Psychology: Learning, Memory, and Cognition, 27*(6), 1411–1423.

Gordon, P. C., Hendrick, R., & Johnson, M. (2004). Effects of noun phrase type on sentence complexity. *Journal of Memory and Language, 51*, 97–114.

Gordon, P. C., Hendrick, R., & Levine, W. H. (2002). Memory-load interference in syntactic processing. *Psychological Science, 13*, 425–430.

Goschke, T., Friederici, A., Kotz, S. A., & van Kampen, A. (2001). Procedural learning in Broca's aphasia: Dissociation between the implicit acquisition of spatio-motor and phoneme sequences. *Journal of Cognitive Neuroscience, 13*(3), 370–388.

Graybiel, A. M. (1995). Building action repertoires: Memory and learning functions of the basal ganglia. *Current Opinion in Neurobiology, 5,* 733–741.

Grodner, D., & Gibson, E. (2005). Consequences of the serial nature of linguistic input. *Cognitive Science, 29,* 261–290.

Gronlund, S. D., Edwards, M. B., & Ohrt, D. D. (1997). Comparison of retrieval of item versus spatial position information. *Journal of Experimental Psychology: Learning, Memory, and Cognition, 23,* 1261–1274.

Guo, Y., Martin, R., Van Dyke, J., & Hamilton, C. (2010). Interference effects in sentence comprehension: An fMRI study. In S. Ohlsson & R. Catrambone (Eds.), *Proceedings of the 32nd Annual Conference of the Cognitive Science Society.* Austin, TX: Cognitive Science Society.

Haist, F., Musen, G., & Squire, L. R. (1991). Intact priming of words and nonwords in amnesia. *Psychobiology, 19,* 275–285.

Hannula, D. E., Tranel, D., & Cohen, N. J. (2006). The long and the short of it: Relational memory impairments in amnesia, even at short lags. *The Journal of Neuroscience, 26*(32), 8352–8359.

Harm, M. W., & Seidenberg, M. S. (2004). Computing the meanings of words in reading: Cooperative division of labor between visual and phonological processes. *Psychological Review, 111,* 662–720.

Hasher, L., & Zacks, R. T. (1988). Working memory, comprehension, and aging: A review and a new view. In G. H. Bower (Ed.), *The psychology of learning and motivation* (Vol. 22, pp. 193–225). New York: Academic Press.

Hauk, O., Johnsrude, I., & Pulvermuller, F. (2004). Somatotopic representation of action words in human motor and premotor cortex. *Neuron, 41,* 301–307.

Hochstadt, J., Nakano, H., Lieberman, P., & Friedman, J. (2006). The roles of sequencing and verbal working memory in sentence comprehension deficits in Parkinson's disease. *Brain & Language, 97,* 243–257

Howard, D., & Patterson, K. (1992). *Pyramids and palm trees: A test of semantic access from pictures and words.* Thames Valley: Bury St Edmunds.

Hummel, J. (1999). The binding problem. In R. A. Wilson & F. C. Keil (Eds.), *The MIT encyclopedia of cognitive sciences* (pp. 85–86). Cambridge, MA: MIT Press.

James, W. (1890). *The principles of psychology.* New York: Henry Holt and Company.

Jonides, J., & Nee, D. E. (2006). Brain mechanisms of proactive interference in working memory. *Neuroscience, 139,* 181–193.

Katz, L., Lee, C. H., Tabor, W., Frost, S. J., Mencl, W. E., Sandak, R., Rueckl, J., & Pugh, K. R. (2005). Behavioral and neurobiological effects of printed word repetition in lexical decision and naming. *Neuropsychologia, 43,* 2068–2083.

Keidel, J., Kluender, K., Jenison, R., & Seidenberg, M. (2007). Does grammar constrain statistical learning? *Psychological Science, 18,* 922–923.

Kellenbach, M. L., Brett, M., & Patterson, K. (2001). Larger, colorful, or noisy? Attribute- and modality-specific activations during retrieval of perceptual attribute knowledge. *Cognitive and Affective Behavioral Neuroscience, 1,* 207–221.

Kelley, W. M., Miezin, F. M., McDermott, K. B., Buckner, R. L., Raichle, M. E., Cohen, N. J., Ollinger, J. M., . . . Petersen, S. E. (1998). Hemispheric specialization in human dorsal frontal cortex. *Neuron, 20,* 927–936.

Keppel, G. (1984). Consolidation and forgetting theory. In H. Weingartner & E. S. Parker (Eds.), *Memory consolidation: Psychobiology of cognition.* Hillsdale, NJ: Erlbaum.

Keppel, G., & Underwood, B. J. (1962). Proactive-inhibition in short-term retention of single items. *Journal of Verbal Learning and Verbal Behavior, 1,* 153–161.

Kimball, J. (1973). Seven principles of surface structure parsing in natural language. *Cognition, 2,* 15–47.

King, J., & Just, M. A. (1991). Individual differences in syntactic processing: The role of working memory. *Journal of Memory and Language, 30*(5), 580–602.

Knowlton, B. J., Mangels, J. A., & Squire, L. R. (1996). A neostriatal habit learning system in humans. *Science, 273,* 1399–1402.

Levy, D. A., Manns, J. R., Hopkins, R. O., Gold, J. J., Broadbent, N. J., & Squire, L. R. (2003). Impaired visual and odor recognition memory span in patients with hippocampal lesions. *Learning and Memory, 10,* 531–536.

Lewandowsky, S., Duncan, M., & Brown, G. D. A. (2004). Time does not cause forgetting in short-term serial recall. *Psychonomics Bulletin Review, 11,* 771–790.

Lewis, R. L., & Vasishth, S. (2005). An activation-based model of sentence processing as skilled memory retrieval. *Cognitive Science, 29,* 375–419.

Lewis, R. L., Vasishth, S., & Van Dyke, J. A. (2006). Computational principles of working memory in sentence comprehension. *Trends in Cognitive Science, 10*(10), 447–454.

MacDonald, M. C., Just, M. A., & Carpenter, P. C. (1992). Working memory constraints on the processing of syntactic ambiguity. *Cognitive Psychology, 24,* 56–98.

Maine de Biran, F. P. G. (1929/1804). *The influence of habit on the faculty of thinking.* Baltimore: Williams & Wilkins.

Makuuchi, M., Bahlmann, J., Anwander, A., Friederici, A. D. (2009). Segregating the core computational faculty of human language from working memory. *Proceedings of the National Academy of Sciences USA, 106*(20), 8362–8367.

Marcus, G. F. (2001). *The algebraic mind: Integrating connectionism and cognitive science.* Cambridge, MA: MIT Press.

Marcus, G. F., Brinkmann, U., Clahsen, H., Wiese, R., & Pinker, S. (1995). German inflection: The exception that proves the rule. *Cognitive Psychology, 29,* 189–256.

Marcus, G. F., Vijayan, S., Bandi Rao, S., & Vishton, P. M. (1999). Rule learning by seven-month-old infants. *Science, 283,* 77–80.

Martin, A., & Chao, L. L. (2001). Semantic memory and the brain: Structure and processes. *Current Opinion in Neurobiology, 11,* 194–201.

Martin, A., Haxby, J. V., Lalonde, F. M., Wiggs, C. L., & Ungerleider, L. G. (1995). Discrete cortical regions associated with knowledge of color and knowledge of action. *Science, 270,* 102–105.

Martin, A., & McElree, B. (2008). A content-addressable pointer mechanism underlies comprehension of verb-phrase ellipsis. *Journal of Memory and Language, 58*(3), 879–906.

Martin, A. E., & McElree, B. (2009). Memory operations that support language comprehension: Evidence from verb-phrase ellipsis. *Journal of Experimental Psychology: Learning Memory & Cognition, 35,* 1231–1239.

Martin, R. C., & Feher, E. (1990). The consequences of reduced memory span for the comprehension of semantic versus syntactic information. *Brain and Language, 38,* 1–20.

McCandliss, B., Cohen, L., & Dehaene, S. (2003). The visual word form area: expertise for reading in the fusiform gyrus. *Trends in Cognitive Sciences, 7(7),* 293–299.

McDermott, K. B., Buckner, R. L., Petersen, S. E., Kelley, W. M., & Sanders, A. L. (1999). Set- and code-specific activation in frontal cortex: an fMRI study of encoding and retrieval of faces and words. *Journal of Cognitive Neuroscience, 11,* 631–640.

McClelland, J. L., McNaughton, B. L., & O'Reilly, R. C. (1995). Why there are complementary learning systems in the hippocampus and neocortex: Insights from the successes and failures of connectionist models of learning and memory. *Psychological Review, 102(3),* 419–457.

McClelland, J. L., & Rogers, T. T. (2003). The parallel distributed processing approach to semantic cognition. *Nature Reviews Neuroscience, 4,* 1–13.

McElree, B. (2000). Sentence comprehension is mediated by content-addressable memory structures. *Journal of Psycholinguistic Research, 29,* 111–123.

McElree, B. (2001). Working memory and focal attention. *Journal of Experimental Psychology: Learning, Memory & Cognition, 27,* 817–835.

McElree, B. (2006). Accessing recent events. In B. H. Ross (Ed.), *The psychology of learning and motivation* (Vol. 46). San Diego: Academic Press.

McElree, B., & Dosher, B. A. (1989). Serial position and set size in short-term recognition: Time course of recognition. *Journal of Experimental Psychology: General, 118,* 346–373.

McElree, B., Foraker, S., & Dyer, L. (2003). Memory structures that subserve sentence comprehension. *Journal of Memory and Language, 48,* 67–91.

McGeoch, J. (1932). Forgetting and the law of disuse. *Psychological Review, 39,* 352–370.

Miller, G. (1956). The magical number seven, plus or minus two: Some limits on our capacity for processing information. *Psychological Review, 63,* 81–97.

Miller, G. A., & Chomsky. N. (1963). Finitary models of language users. In D. R. Luce, R. R. Bush, & E. Galanter (Eds.), *Handbook of mathematical psychology* (Vol. II). New York: John Wiley.

Milner, B. (1962). Les troubles de la memoire accompagnant des lesions hippocampiques bilaterales. In *Physiologie de l'hippocampe* (pp. 257–272). Paris: Centre National de la Recherche Scientifique. English translation: B. Milner & S. Glickman (Eds.). Princeton: Van Nostrand, 1965 (pp. 97–111).

Milner, B. (1972). Disorders of learning and memory after temporal lobe lesions in man. *Clinical Neurosurgery, 19,* 421–466.

Mirković, J., MacDonald, M. C., & Seidenberg, M. S. (2005). Where does gender come from? Evidence from a complex inflectional system. *Language and Cognitive Processes, 20,* 139–168.

Mishkin, M., Malamut, B., Bachevalier, J. (1984). Memories and habits: Two neural systems. In G. Lynch, J. L. McGaugh, & N. W. Weinburger (Eds.), *Neurobiology of learning and memory* (pp. 65–77). New York: Guilford Press.

Miyake, A., Friedman, N., Emerson, M., Witzki, A., Howerter, A., & Wager, T. (2000). The unity and diversity of executive functions and their contributions to complex "frontal lobe" tasks: A latent variable analysis. *Cognitive Psychology, 41,* 49–100.

Miyake, A., & Shah, P. (1999). *Models of working memory: Mechanisms of active maintenance and executive control.* Cambridge University Press: Cambridge.

Mummery, C. J., Patterson, K., Hodges, J. R., & Price, C. J. (1998). Functional neuroanatomy of the semantic system: divisible by what? *Journal of Cognitive Neuroscience, 10,* 766–777.

Murdock, B. B., Jr. (1974). *Human memory: Theory and data.* Hillsdale, NJ: Erlbaum.

Murphy, G. L. (2002). *The big book of concepts.* Cambridge, MA: MIT Press.

Murray, D. J. (1967). The role of speech responses in short-term memory. *Canadian Journal of Psychology, 21,* 263–276.

Nairne, J. S. (2002). Remembering over the short-term: The case against the standard model. *Annual Review of Psychology, 53,* 53–81.

Nation, K., Adams, J. W., Bowyer-Crane, C. A., & Snowling, M. J. (1999). Working memory deficits in poor comprehenders reflect underlying language impairments. *Journal of Experimental Child Psychology, 73,* 139–158.

Nichols, E. A., Kao, Y-C., Verfaellie, M., & Gabrieli, J. D. E. (2006). Working memory and long-term memory for faces: Evidence from fMRI and global amnesia for involvement of the medial temporal lobes. *Hippocampus, 16,* 604–616.

Oakhill, J. V., Cain, K., & Bryant, P. E. (2003). The dissociation of word reading and text comprehension: Evidence from component skills. *Language and Cognitive Processes, 18(4),* 443–468.

Oberauer, K. (2002). Access to information in working memory: Exploring the focus of attention. *Journal of Experimental Psychology: Learning, Memory, & Cognition, 28,* 411–421.

Otten, L. J., & Rugg, M. D. (2001). Task-dependency of the neural correlates of episodic encoding as measured by fMRI. *Cerebral Cortex, 11(12),* 1150–1160.

Öztekin, I., Davachi, L., & McElree, B. (2010). Are representations in working memory distinct from those in long-term memory? Neural evidence in support of a single store. *Psychological Science, 21(8),* 1123–1133.

Öztekin, I., & McElree, B. (2007). Retrieval dynamics of proactive interference: PI slows retrieval by eliminating fast assessments of familiarity. *Journal of Memory and Language, 57,* 126–149.

Öztekin, I., McElree, B., Staresina, B. P., & Davachi, L. (2008). Working memory retrieval: Contributions of left prefrontal cortex, left posterior parietal cortex and hippocampus. *Journal of Cognitive Neuroscience, 21,* 581–593.

Packard, M. G., Hirsh, R., & White, N. M. (1989). Differential effects of fornix and caudate nucleus lesions on two radial maze tasks: Evidence for multiple memory systems. *Journal of Neuroscience, 9,* 1465–1472.

Packard, M., & Knowlton, B. (2002). Learning and memory functions of the basal ganglia. *Annual Review of Neuroscience, 25*, 563–593.

Parkin, A. J. (2001). The structure and mechanisms of memory. In B. Rapp (Ed.), *The handbook of cognitive neuropsychology: What deficits reveal about the human mind.* (pp. 399–422). Philadelphia: Psychology Press.

Peigneux, P., Maquet, P., Meulemans, T., Destrebecqz, A., Laureys, S., Degueldre, C., Delfiore, G., . . . Cleeremans, A. (2000). Striatum forever, despite sequence learning variability: A random effect analysis of PET data. *Human Brain Mapping, 10*, (4), 179–194.

Peña, M., Bonatti, L. L., Nespor, M., & Mehler, J. (2002). Signal-driven computations in speech processing. *Science, 298*, 604–607.

Perfetti, C. (2007). Reading ability: Lexical quality to comprehension. *Scientific Studies of Reading, 11*:357–383.

Perruchet, P., & Pacton, S. (2006). Implicit learning and statistical learning: One phenomenon, two approaches. *Trends in Cognitive Sciences, 10*, 233–238.

Peterson, L. R., & Peterson, M. J. (1959). Short-term retention of individual verbal items. *Journal of Experimental. Psychology, 58*, 193–198.

Pinker, S. (1991). Rules of language, *Science, 253*, 530–535.

Poldrack, R. A., Clark, J., Pare-Blagoev, J., Shohamy, D., Creso Moyano, J., Myers, C., & Gluck, M. A. (2001). Interactive memory systems in the human brain. *Nature, 414*, 546–550.

Poldrack, R. A., & Gabrieli, J. D. E. (2001). Characterizing the neural mechanisms of skill learning and repetition priming: Evidence from mirror reading. *Brain, 124*, 67–82.

Poldrack, R. A., Prabhakaran, V., Seger, C. A., & Gabrieli, J. D. (1999). Striatal activation during acquisition of a cognitive skill. *Neuropsychology, 13*, 564–574.

Poldrack, R. A., Wagner, A. D., Prull, M. W., Desmond, J. E., Glover, G. H., & Gabrieli, J. D. E. (1999). Functional specialization for semantic and phonological processing in the left inferior prefrontal cortex. *NeuroImage, 10*, 5–35.

Price, C. J., Moore, C. J., Humphreys, G. W., & Wise, R. J. S. (1997). Segregating semantic from phonological processes during reading. *Journal of Cognitive Neuroscience, 9*, 727–733.

Pugh, K. R., Frost, S. J., Sandak, R., Landi, N., Rueckl, J. G., Constable, R. T., Seidenberg, M. S., . . . Mencl, W. E. (2008). Effects of stimulus difficulty and repetition on printed word identification: A comparison of nonimpaired and reading-disabled adolescent cohorts. *Journal of Cognitive Neuroscience, 20*, 1146–1160.

Pulvermuller, F. (2005). Brain mechanisms linking language and action. *Nature Reviews Neuroscience, 6*, 576–582.

Quartermain, D., McEwen, B. S., & Azmitia, E. C., Jr. (1972). Recovery of memory following amnesia in the rat and mouse. *Journal of Comparative and Physiological Psychology, 76*, 521–529.

Ranganath, C., & Blumenfeld, R. S. (2005). Doubts about double dissociations between short- and long-term memory. *Trends in Cognitive Science, 9*, 374–380.

Ranganath, C., & D'Esposito, M. (2005). Directing the mind's eye: Prefrontal, inferior and medial temporal mechanisms for visual working memory. *Current Opinion in Neurobiology, 15*(2), 175–182.

Ratcliff, R. (1978). A theory of memory retrieval. *Psychological Review, 85*, 59–108.

Rayner, K. (1998). Eye movements in reading and information processing: 20 years of research. *Psychological Bulletin, 124*(3), 372–422.

Reber, A. S. (1989). Implicit learning and tacit knowledge. *Journal of Experimental Psychology: General*, 118, 219–235.

Reber, P. J., Stark, C., & Squire, L. R. (1998). Contrasting cortical activity associated with category memory and recognition memory. *Learning and Memory, 5*, 420–428.

Reed, A. V. (1973). Speed-accuracy trade-off in recognition memory. *Science, 181*, 574–576.

Reed, A. V. (1976). The time course of recognition in human memory. *Memory and Cognition, 4*, 16–30.

Rips, L. J., Shoben, E. J., & Smith, E. E. (1973). Semantic distance and the verification of semantic relations. *Journal of Verbal Language and Verbal Behavior, 12*(1), 1–20.

Roediger, H. L., Buckner, R. L., & McDermott, K. B. (1999). Components of processing. In J. K. Foster & M. Jelicic (Eds.), *Memory: Systems, process, or function?* (pp. 31–65). Oxford, UK: Oxford University Press.

Rogalsky, C., & Hickock, G. (2010). The role of Broca's area in sentence comprehension. *Journal of Cognitive Neuroscience, 23*(7), 1664–1680.

Rosch, E., & Mervis, C. B. (1975). Family resemblances: Studies in the internal structure of categories. *Cognitive Psychology, 7*(4), 573–605.

Rugg, M. D., Otten, L. J., & Henson, R. N. A. (2002). The neural basis of episodic memory: Evidence from functional neuro-imaging. *Philosophical Transactions: Biological Sciences, 357*, 1097–1110.

Rumelhart, D. E., & McClelland, J. L. (1986). On learning the past tenses of English verbs. In D. E. Rumelhart, J. L. McClelland, & the PDP Research Group (Eds.), *Parallel distributed processing: Explorations in the microstructure of cognition. Vol. 2: Psychological and biological models* (pp. 216–271). Cambridge, MA: MIT Press.

Ryan, J. D., & Cohen, N. J. (2003). Evaluating the neuropsychological dissociation evidence for multiple memory systems. *Cognitive, Affective & Behavioral Neuroscience, 3*, 168–185.

Saffran, J. R., Aslin, R. N., & Newport, E. L. (1996). Statistical learning by 8-month-old infants. *Science, 274*, 1926–1928.

Sahni, S. D., Seidenberg, M. S., & Saffran, J. R. (2010). Connecting cues: Overlapping regularities support cue discovery in infancy. *Child Development, 81*, 727–736.

Salmon, D. P., & Butters, N. (1995). Neurobiology of skill and habit learning. *Current Opinion in Neurobiology, 5*, 184–190.

Schacter, D. L. (1992). Priming and multiple memory systems: Perceptual mechanisms of implicit memory. *Journal of Cognitive Neuroscience, 4*(3), 244–256.

Schacter, D. L., & Tulving, E. (1994). What are the memory systems of 1994? In D. L. Schacter & E. Tulving (Eds.), *Memory systems 1994* (pp. 1–38). Cambridge, MA: MIT Press.

Schacter, D. L., Wagner, A. D., & Buckner, R. L. (2000). Memory systems of 1999. In E. Tulving & F. I. M. Craik (Eds.), *The Oxford handbook of memory* (pp. 627–643). New York: Oxford University Press.

Schmolck, H., Kensinger, E., Corkin, S., & Squire, L. R. (2002). Semantic knowledge in patient H. M. and other patients with bilateral medial and lateral temporal lobe lesions. *Hippocampus, 12,* 520–533.

Schmolck, H., Stefanacci, L., & Squire, L. R. (2000). Detection and explanation of sentence ambiguity are unaffected by hippocampal lesions but are impaired by larger temporal lobe lesions. *Hippocampus, 10,* 759–770.

Schwartz, M. F., Saffran, E. M., & Marin, O. S. M. (1980). Fractionating the reading process in dementia: Evidence for word-specific print-to-sound associations. In M. Coltheart, K. Patterson, & J. C. Marshall, (Eds.), *Deep dyslexia* (pp. 259–269). London: Routledge and Kegan Paul.

Scoville, W. B., & Milner, B, (1957). Loss of recent memory after bilateral hippocampal lesions. *Journal of Neurology, Neurosurgery, and Psychiatry, 20,* 11–21.

Seidenberg, M. S., & Elman, J. L. (1999). Networks are not "hidden rules." *Trends in Cognitive Science, 3,* 288–289.

Seidenberg, M. S., & MacDonald, M. C. (1999). A probabilistic constraints approach to language acquisition and processing. *Cognitive Science, 23*(4), 569–588.

Seidenberg, M. S., MacDonald, M. C., & Saffran, J. R. (2002). Does grammar start where statistics stop? *Science, 298,* 553–554.

Shallice, T., & Warrington, E. K. (1970). Independent functioning of verbal memory stories: A neuropsychological study. *The Quarterly Journal of Experimental Psychology, 22,* 261–273.

Shi, R., Werker, J. F., & Morgan, J. L. (1999). Newborn infants' sensitivity to perceptual cues to lexical and grammatical words. *Cognition, 72,* B11–B21.

Smith, E. E., & Jonides, J. (1997). Working memory: A view from neuroimaging. *Cognitive Psychology, 33,* 5–42.

Sperling, G. (1960). The information available in brief visual presentations. *Psychological Monographs: General and Applied, 74*(11), (Issue 498), 1–29.

Squire, L. R. (1992). Declarative and nondeclarative memory: Multiple brain systems supporting learning and memory. *Journal of Cognitive Neuroscience, 4*(3), 232–243.

Squire, L. R. (2004). Memory systems of the brain: A brief history and current perspective. *Neurobiology of Learning and Memory, 82,* 171–177.

Squire, L. R., Schmolck, H., & Stark, S. (2001). Impaired auditory recognition memory in amnesic patients with medial temporal lobe lesions. *Learning and Memory, 8,* 252–256.

Squire, L. R., Stark, C. E. L., & Clark, R. E. (2004). The medial temporal lobe. *Annual Review of Neuroscience, 27,* 279–306.

Squire, L. R., & Zola, S. M. (1996). Structure and function of declarative and nondeclarative memory systems. *Proceedings of the National Academy of Sciences of the USA, 93,* 13515–13522.

Squire, L. R., & Zola-Morgan, S. (1988). Memory: Brain systems and behavior. *Trends in Neurosciences, 11*(4), 170–175.

Staub, A. (2010). Eye movements and processing difficulty in object relative clauses. *Cognition, 116,* 71–86.

Sternberg, S. (1975). Memory-scanning: New findings and current controversies. *Quarterly Journal of Experimental Psychology, 27,* 1–32.

Stoltzfus, E. R., Hasher, L., & Zacks, R. T. (1996). Working memory and aging: Current status of the inhibitory view. In J. T. E. Richardson, W. W. Engle, L. Hasher, R. H. Logie, E. R. Stoltzfus, & R. T. Zacks (Eds.), *Working memory and human cognition* (pp. 66–88). Oxford, UK: Oxford University Press.

Stowe, L. A., Paans, A. M. J., Wijers, A. A., Zwarts, F., & Vaalburg, G. M. W. (1999). Sentence comprehension and word repetition: a positron emission tomography investigation. *Psychophysiology, 36,* 786–801.

Surprenant, A., & Neath, I. (2009). *Principles of memory.* New York: Psychology Press.

Swanson, H. L., & Sachse-Lee, C. (2001). Mathematical problem solving and working memory in children with learning disabilities: Both executive and phonological processes are important. *Journal of Experimental Child Psychology, 79,* 294–321.

Tettamanti, M., Buccino, G., Saccuman, M. C., Gallese, V., Danna, M., Scifo, P., Ferruccio, F., . . . Perani, D. (2005). Listening to action-related sentences activates fronto-parietal motor circuits. *Journal of Cognitive Neuroscience, 17*(2), 273–281.

Thompson, R. F., & Kim, J. J. (1996). Memory systems in the brain and localization of a memory. *Proceedings of the National Academy of Sciences USA, 93*(24), 13438–13444.

Thompson-Schill, S. (2003). Neuroimaging studies of semantic memory: Inferring "how" from "where." *Neuropsychologia, 41,* 280–292.

Thompson-Schill, S. L., Swick, D., Farah, M. J., D'Esposito, M., Kan, I. P., & Knight, R. T. (1998). Verb generation in patients with focal frontal lesions: A neuropsychological test of neuroimaging findings. *Proceedings of the National Academy of Sciences, 95,* 15855–15860.

Thomson, D. M., & Tulving, E. (1970). Associative encoding and retrieval: Weak and strong cues. *Journal of Experimental Psychology, 86*(2), 255–262.

Traxler, M., Morris, R. K., & Seely, R. E. (2002). Processing subject and object relative clauses: Evidence from eye movements. *Journal of Memory and Language, 47,* 69–90.

Tulving, E. (1979). Relation between encoding specificity and levels of processing. In L. S. Cermak & F. I. M. Craik (Eds.), *Levels of processing in human memory* (pp. 405–428). Hillsdale, NJ: Erlbaum.

Tulving, E. (1983). *Elements of episodic memory.* Oxford, UK: Clarendon Press.

Tulving, E. (1985). Memory and consciousness. *Canadian Psychology, 26,* 1–12.

Tulving, E. (2002). Episodic memory: From mind to brain. *Annual Review of Psychology, 53,* 1–25.

Tulving, E., & Pearlstone, Z. (1966). Availability versus accessibility of information in memory for words. *Journal of Verbal Learning and Verbal Behavior, 5*(4), 381–391.

Turner, M. L., & Engle, R. W. (1989). Is working memory capacity task dependent? *Journal of Memory and Language, 28,* 27–154.

Ullman, M. T. (2004). Contributions of memory circuits to language: The declarative/procedural model. *Cognition, 92,* 231–270.

Ungerleider, L. G., Doyon, J., & Karni, A. (2002). Imaging brain plasticity during motor skill learning. *Neurobiology of Learning and Memory, 78,* 553–564.

Vallar, G., & Papagno, C. (2002). Neuropsychological impairments of verbal short-term memory. In A. D. Baddeley, M. D. Kopelman, & B. A. Wilson (Eds.), *Handbook of memory disorders* (pp. 249–270). Chichester: Wiley.

Van Dyke, J. A. (2007). Interference effects from grammatically unavailable constituents during sentence processing. *Journal of Experimental Psychology: Learning, Memory, and Cognition, 33*(2), 407–430.

Van Dyke, J. A., & Lewis, R. L. (2003). Distinguishing effects of structure and decay on attachment and repair: A retrieval interference theory of recovery from misanalyzed ambiguities. *Journal of Memory and Language, 49*, 285–413.

Van Dyke, J. A., & McElree, B. (2006). Retrieval Interference in Sentence Comprehension. *Journal of Memory and Language, 55*, 157–166.

Van Dyke, J. A., & McElree, B. (in press). Cue-dependent interference in comprehension. *Journal of Memory and Language*, doi:10.1016/j.jml.2011.05.002

Van Orden, C. G., Pennington, B. F., & Stone, G. O. (2001). What do double dissociations prove? *Cognitive Science, 25*, 111–172.

Verhaeghen, P., Cerella, J., & Basak, C. (2004). A working memory workout: How to expand the focus of serial attention from one to four items in 10 hours or less. *Journal of Experimental Psychology: Learning, Memory, & Cognition, 30*, 1322–1337.

Wagner, A. D., Koutstaal, W., & Schacter, D. L. (1999). When encoding yields remembering: Insights from event-related neuroimaging. *Philosophical Transactions: Biological Sciences, 354*, 1307–1324.

Wagner, A. D., Poldrack, R. A., Eldridge, L. L., Desmond, J. E., Glover, G. H., & Gabrieli, J. D. E. (1998). Material-specific lateralization of prefrontal activation during episodic encoding and retrieval. *NeuroReport, 9*, 3711–3717.

Wang, Y., Sereno, J. A., Jongman, A., & Hirsch, J. (2003). fMRI evidence for cortical modification during learning of Mandarin lexical tone. *Journal of Cognitive Neuroscience, 15*, 1019–1027.

Warner, J., & Glass, A. L. (1987). Context and distance-to-disambiguation effects in ambiguity resolution: Evidence from grammaticality judgments of garden path sentences. *Journal of Memory and Language, 26*, 714–738.

Warrington, E. K., & Shallice, T. (1984). Category specific semantic impairments. *Brain, 107*(3), 829–853.

Watkins, O. C., & Watkins, M. J. (1975). Build-up of proactive inhibition as a cue overload effect. *Journal of Experimental Psychology: Human Learning and Memory, 104*, 442–452.

Waugh, N. C., & Norman, D. A. (1965). Primary memory. *Psychological Review, 72*, 89–104.

Wickelgren, W. A. (1965). Short-term memory for phonemically similar lists. *The American Journal of Psychology, 78*, 567–574.

Wickelgren, W. (1977). Speed-accuracy tradeoff and information processing dynamics. *Acta Psychologica, 41*, 67–85.

Willingham, D. B. (1998). A neuropsychological theory of motor skill learning. *Psychological Review, 105*(3), 558–584.

Wise, S. P., Murray, E. A., & Gerfen, C. R. (1996). The frontal cortex-basal ganglia system in primates. *Critical Reviews in Neurobiology, 10*(3–4), 317–356.

Zeki, S., Watson, J. D., Lueck, C. J., Friston, K. J., Kennard, C., & Frackowiak, R. S. (1991). A direct demonstration of functional specialization in human visual cortex. *Journal of Neuroscience, 11*, 641–649.

CHAPTER 6

Linguistic and Psycholinguistic Foundations

CHAPTER OUTLINE   *Josée Poirier and Lewis P. Shapiro*

As speakers (or signers), we select words that match what we want to say, combine them appropriately, and hope our message gets through. As comprehenders, we are presented with a complex string of sounds, signs or letters and must reconstruct their associated meaning. Yet, every day, we speak/write and hear/read sentences that have never been produced before. Moreover, producing or comprehending language is fast and relatively effortless (at least in one's native language), but language itself is tremendously complex. How do we manage the intricate knowledge we have about our language and smoothly use it to communicate?

These are core issues in psycholinguistics, the study of the psychological underpinnings of language. In this chapter we first introduce linguistic concepts that describe the complexity of language structure. Crucially, these concepts allow us to study and then detail the mental operations involved in language processing (normal and disordered). With this toolkit under our belts, we next turn to sentence processing and sentence comprehension in particular. We examine sentence comprehension from different viewpoints to explore various ways language could be represented and processed. Our aim is for the reader to acquire descriptive tools and to gain exposure to a variety of cognitive processes so that a critical and rigorous study of language processing can be perused.

LINGUISTICS TOOLKIT

The goal of this section is to describe the features (or properties) of verbs, with an eye toward sentence processing. Why verbs? Because:

- Their properties help determine the syntax of the sentences in which they are inserted.
- They have features that constrain the semantics of sentences.
- They are the "motor" of the proposition expressed in the sentence.

Before we begin our tutorial about verbs, there are some important preliminaries. We begin with the following assumption: **The sentence is the basic unit of analysis in language processing.** Our intuitions tell us this must be so. After all, we seem to speak in sentences (embedded in discourse), and we are all amazed when young children begin to sequence words into what appear to be sentence-like units. But there are also some very simple facts that suggest that this assumption must be correct. For example, consider the following:

1. John kissed Mary.
2. Mary was kissed by John.
3. It was Mary who John kissed.

These three sequences of words seem to express the same proposition (kissed: John, Mary), yet the order of the words is distinct in each case. Moreover, in the 1950s (considered to be the time when the "modern era" in linguistics and psycholinguistics began) George Miller and his colleagues conducted several experiments that showed that the accurate perception of words in noise significantly increases when the words are strung together into sentences. Thus, at the very least, the sentence holds a privileged role in perception and production, and it will turn out, in comprehension as well.[1]

Yet it is obvious that words, too, play a critical role. Here, we assume that humans are equipped with a mental dictionary or **Lexicon.** The Lexicon, in an abstract sense, is the depository of knowledge about words. This knowledge includes, at least, lexical category information (part-of-speech), phonology (the sound structure of the word), meaning, and grammatical constraints. As a brief example of the latter, consider the verb *kiss* again. We can say, "John kissed Mary" (sentence (1), above), but if we say, "John kissed," it somehow feels incomplete. Yet it is perfectly OK to say, "John slept." These simple facts suggest that there are restrictions or constraints on what types of sentences in which a verb can be inserted. The verb *kiss* seems to require two objects (here, *John* and *Mary*) expressed in the sentence, while the verb *sleep* is perfectly happy acting with just a single object (*John*). Thus verbs are selective; they choose their syntactic and semantic partners. Our view of the lexicon, then, is that its primary role is to support well-formed sentences. That is, our ability to use words to refer to the world is not independent of the sentences in which those words are contained. This fact suggests that investigations of word-level processing, including research into word-finding difficulties and treatment of such difficulties, must eventually make contact with sentence processing. Given the primary role of the sentence, we now continue with some syntax, and how words are put together into sentences.

Merge and Phrase Structure

Words are not just linked up sequentially to form sentences; instead, sentences are formed from the hierarchical ordering of words. To see what we mean, consider a headline from the news:

4. Seven Foot Doctors Sue Hospitals

A brief consideration of this sentence reveals an ambiguity: It can mean that some very tall doctors have sued hospitals; alternatively and more likely, it can mean that seven Podiatrists sued the hospitals. This ambiguity is **structural,** as can be seen in the following:

5a. [NP[Seven foot] [doctors]] sue hospitals.
5b. [NP[Seven] [foot doctors]] sue hospitals.

Using labeled bracketing to describe the natural divisions (i.e., **constituents**) in the sentences, in (5a) the subject noun phrase (NP) is structured such that [Seven foot] forms a constituent and so does [doctors], and the combination of the two yields a complex NP, *Seven foot doctors*. In (5b), [Seven] forms a single constituent, and when combined with [foot doctors] yields the complex NP that serves as the subject of the sentence. Note that this ambiguity does not arise from any lexical ambiguity (as in, for example, "Child's stool is great for use in garden!"). Instead, the ambiguity arises because of two possible structures, with each structure governing a particular interpretation.

Another way of describing or viewing this structural ambiguity is through the use of **hierarchical tree structures.** Consider again (5a) and (5b) but represented graphically as depicted in Figure 6-1.

In (a), the word *Seven* forms a single constituent, while *foot* and *doctors* join to form a higher order constituent (at the intersection of the two branches), and when these are joined together we have *Seven* "foot doctors." In (b), the words *Seven* and *foot* combine to form a constituent, which then joins *doctors* to form the entire phrase, and hence we have *Seven foot doctors*. These representations are the tree structure analogues of the bracketing found in (5a) and (5b). The take-home message here is that there is no way to describe this ambiguity without making reference to the structure of the phrase, and that structure is hierarchical and not simply a linear string of words.

In fact, what we have done in Figure 6-1 is compute an approximation of **phrase structure,** which describes the phrasal geometry of sentences. These are node-labeled tree structures with hierarchical ordering. There are lexical nodes, which refer to lexical categories (i.e., parts-of-speech), like N (Noun), V (Verb), and P (Preposition). These lexical categories form the **heads** of the higher-order phrases to which they project.[2] So, the Verb is the head of the Verb Phrase (VP), the

---

[1]For an excellent discussion of the classical evidence for the sentence as the primary unit of analysis, see Townsend and Bever, 2001, Chapter 2.

[2]There are also intermediate nodes, those that occur between the lexical and phrasal levels, but for present purposes we will ignore this.

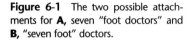

Figure 6-1 The two possible attachments for **A,** seven "foot doctors" and **B,** "seven foot" doctors.

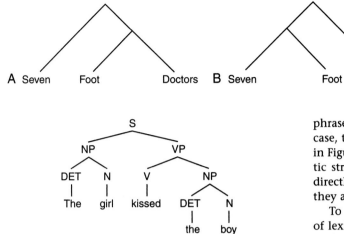

Figure 6-2 Simplified syntactic tree for "The girl kissed the boy."

Preposition the head of the Prepositional Phrase (PP), and so on. Consider Figure 6-2.

The syntactic component of the grammar includes an operation, **MERGE,** which takes two categories as input and then outputs a single, merged, category. So, in Figure 6-2, the Determiner and Noun merge to form a higher-order NP; the Verb and NP merge to form a higher-order VP, and the VP and subject NP merge to form the Sentence.

Continuing, and keeping with the focus of this section, we now consider only the VP. VPs expand to include several possibilities; Figure 6-3 shows only three. In (a), the verb *sleep* has no complements; that is, it has nothing that comes after it. In (b), the verb *kiss* takes an NP complement. Thus, the V merges with an NP and yields the VP (or alternatively, we can say that the VP expands to include an NP complement). Finally, the verb *say* merges with a complement

phrase/sentential clause (S) to form the VP. In this case, the embedded S would, itself, expand (as shown in Figure 6-2). So, each verb selects a particular syntactic structure. In this way, we have shown that verbs directly influence the syntax of the sentences in which they are contained.

To generate a sentence, we begin by enabling a set of lexical items (technically, a numeration) and then use successive merger operations. For example, beginning with the numeration: [Kiss; V; girl, boy], we would merge the Verb *kiss* with its NP (*boy*) to form the VP (see (8b)). We then select *girl*, which is an NP, and merge this with the previously formed VP, to yield the Sentence Node (see Figure 6-2 for more details). Note that the successive merger operations are not intended to mimic real-time processing of sentences (if it did, we would be parsing sentences backward!); instead, Merge is considered a linguistic operation. It remains for empirical work to discover if Merge has psycholinguistic consequences (and indeed, as we shall show shortly, there is such evidence).

We now consider another example, with the verb *think* [thinks, V; girl, boy] substituting for the verb *kiss*. So, in Figure 6-4, we go through successive merger operations (i.e., DET merges with N to form an NP, V merges with NP to form VP, NP and VP merge to form an S) to **derive** the sentence: "The girl thinks the boy." Of course, our intuitions strongly suggest

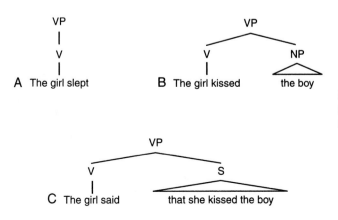

Figure 6-3 Syntactic trees for **A,** an intransitive verb and **B,** transitive verbs taking a direct object or **C,** a sentence as complements.

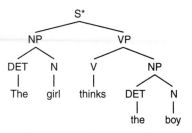

Figure 6-4 Ungrammatical sentence formed by Merge alone.

a distinction between the output of Merge in (see Figure 6-3, *B*) relative to the output in (see Figure 6-4); the former is well-formed or grammatical ("the girl kisses the boy"), while the latter is ill-formed or ungrammatical (*"the girl thinks the boy," with * signifying a sentence is ungrammatical). Merge seems to be too powerful as we have used it here—it generates both grammatical and ungrammatical sentences. Thus we need a way to restrict the output of Merge to include only well-formed sentences. The solution turns out to involve verb properties; these will allow the theory to form only grammatical sentences. We turn to this solution in subsequent sections.

Argument Structure

Consider the following verbs and the sentences in which they are contained:

6a. The boy disappeared.
6b. *The girl disappeared the boy.
7a. The girl kissed the boy.
7b. *The girl kissed.
8a. The girl put the boy in the closet.
8b. *The girl put the boy.

Each verb needs partners to describe an event or activity. The verb *disappear* requires one participant as shown in (6a); the verb *kiss*, shown in Figure 6-4 as well as in (7a), needs two participants; and the verb *put* requires three as shown in (8a). To see that this is true, consider the (b) versions above, which are all ungrammatical. That is, *disappear* cannot occur in a sentence with two participants; *kiss* cannot appear in a sentence with only one participant; and *put* cannot appear in a sentence with two participants (or even one, as in *the girl put). Thus, verbs, again, are said to select their sentence environments.

One way to describe the restrictions on a verb's environments is through **predicate-argument structure.** Borrowing from logic, we can say that sentences are composed of a verb (i.e., **predicate**) and a set of **arguments.** A verb denotes an activity or event, and an argument denotes a participant in the event. Thus, the verb *disappear* is a one-place predicate because it selects for a single argument (played by the NP *the boy* in (6a)). The verb *kiss* is a two-place predicate because it selects two arguments, both a subject NP and an object NP (7); and the verb *put* requires three arguments (8a). The maximum number of arguments that can appear with any given verb seems to be three. The minimum number is one, though there is a class of verbs that appear to express an event without any arguments; that is, they can stand on their own. This class is *weather* verbs (e.g., It is *raining*, It is *snowing*, etc.). Here, the subject (*It*, a pleonastic pronoun) carries no semantics and is not considered an argument of the verb.

Thematic Roles

Semantics also plays an important role in argument structure. Consider the following examples[3]:

9. Dillon ran.
10. Joelle laughed.
11. Philip yelled.

In (9)–(11), the verb combines with an expression that plays the role of **Agent** of the proposition; the Agent is essentially the "causer" or instigator of the event described by the verb. Hence, the NPs *Dillon*, *Joelle*, and *Philip* are all Agents of their respective verbs. This contrasts with the following examples:

12. Dillon collapsed.
13. Joelle disappeared.
14. Philip fell.

In these cases, the verb combines with an expression that undergoes some change-of-state or position; we will call this the **Theme** of the proposition. Hence, the NPs in (12)–(14) are all Themes of their respective verbs. Thus, predicates subclassify the kinds of expressions they need into different semantic types or thematic roles. We can define **thematic role** in the following way:

Thematic Role: The semantic type played by an argument in relation to its predicate.

There is a limited set of thematic roles. Though linguists are not particularly concerned with details of the roles themselves, there are some major ones that bear mention; once again, let's revisit the simple sentence:

15. The girl kissed the boy.
    AGENT THEME

---

[3]This section owes some of its organization to two texts: David Adger's *Core Syntax: A Minimalist Approach* (2003), and Andrew Radford's *Minimalist Syntax* (2004).

In (15) the subject NP, *the girl*, plays the role of the Agent of the event, and *the boy*, the Theme.

16. Mitzi loves cats.
    EXPERIENCER   THEME

In (16) the subject NP, *Mitzi*, plays the role of **Experiencer.** Roughly, the Experiencer role describes an entity experiencing some psychological or mental state.

17. The girl put the boy in the closet.
    AGENT   THEME   LOCATIVE
18. The girl gave the prize to the boy
    AGENT   THEME   GOAL

In (17) there are three thematic roles, owing to the fact that the verb *put* requires three arguments. The subject argument filled by the NP *the girl* plays the role of Agent of the event, the direct object argument filled by the NP *the boy* plays the role of Theme, and the indirect object filled by the argument *the closet* plays the **Locative** role. The Locative role describes the place in which something is situated or takes place. In (18), the third argument filled by *the boy* plays the role of the **Goal,** which is roughly defined as the entity towards which something moves.

Lexical Entries

Let's assume that these properties are represented with the verb as part of its entry in the Lexicon. Consider again the verb *kiss* and its predicate argument structure (PAS) and thematic role features (presented in Table 6-1).

Table **6-1**	Partial Lexical Entry for the Verb "Kiss"	
	PAS	**Thematic Roles**
kiss, V	X	AGENT
	Y	THEME

Table **6-2**	Checking Off Theme Role	
	PAS	**Thematic Roles**
kiss, V	X	AGENT
	Y	THEME ✓

Table **6-3**	Checking Off Agent Role	
	PAS	**Thematic Roles**
kiss, V	X	AGENT ✓
	Y	THEME ✓

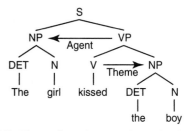

Figure 6-5 Theta-role assignment in a simple, transitive sentence.

The lexical entry table shows that *kiss*, a verb, requires two arguments, designated by X and Y. The two arguments have particular thematic roles that need to be assigned (AGENT, THEME). Let's assume that thematic roles are essentially features that need to be "checked off" for the sentence to be grammatical. Consider then Figure 6-5.

We have already discussed how the verb (V; *kissed*) merges with an NP (*the boy*) to form the VP (*kissed the boy*). We will also assume here that the V assigns a thematic role (THEME) to its NP complement, and thus we have the result appearing in Table 6-2.

Once we have assigned the thematic role to the argument position, we check-off the thematic role. As we have also discussed previously, the VP merges with the subject NP (*the girl*). As part of this Merge operation, the VP assigns the thematic role of Agent to the subject argument and thus we have the final result in Table 6-3.

That is, as each thematic role is assigned, the feature is checked-off in the lexical entry. When there is a match between the argument structure of the verb and the number of arguments in the sentence, including the set of thematic roles to be assigned, then the result is a well-formed sentence, with thematic roles describing "who did what to whom." In this way, then, the lexical properties of the verb are said to project to the sentence.

Given the lexical entry for any particular verb, if there are not enough argument positions in the sentence for the thematic roles to be assigned, or if there are too many argument positions given the number of thematic roles, then the derivation of the sentence will "crash" and the result will be an ungrammatical sentence. To see what we mean, consider Table 6-4.

The verb *put* requires three arguments. Given the sentence:

19. *The girl put the boy

Table 6-4	Partial Lexical Entry for the Verb "Put"	
	PAS	**Thematic Roles**
put, V	X	AGENT
	Y	THEME
	Z	GOAL

Table 6-5	Checking Off Two of Three Required Thematic Roles	
	PAS	**Thematic Roles**
put, V	X	AGENT ✓
	Y	THEME ✓
	Z	GOAL

Only two arguments are active in the sentence (the subject and object NPs, *the girl* and *the boy*, respectively). Thus, when thematic roles are assigned to these argument positions, there is one thematic role left in the lexical entry that has not been checked-off (Table 6-5).

Because there is a mismatch between the number of arguments required by the verb (see Table 6-4) and the number of arguments active in the sentence (see (19)), the features of the verb are not satisfied in the sentence, and hence the sentence is ungrammatical. Recall in the previous section that the Merge operation, by itself, is too powerful; it generates grammatical as well as ungrammatical sentences. Once we assume that the features of the verb (in this case, the argument structure and thematic role representations) must be accommodated in the sentence, the output of Merge will then be constrained to form only grammatical sentences.

Complex Arguments

On some accounts, not only are NPs arguments of the verb, but so too are more complex embedded sentential clauses or Complement Phrases (CPs) (Grimshaw, 1977; Shapiro, Zurif, & Grimshaw, 1987, Shetreet, Palti, Friedmann, & Hadar, 2007). Consider the following three verbs:

20a. Yosef knows [NP the time].
20b. Yosef knows [CP that the girl kissed the boy].
20c. Yosef knows [CP who the girl kissed].
21a. Yosef asked [NP the time].
21b. *Yosef asked [CP that the girl kissed the boy].
21c. Yosef asked [CP who the girl kissed].
22a. *Yosef wonders [NP the time].
22b. *Yosef wonders [that the girl kissed the boy].
22c. Yosef wonders [who the girl kissed].

As can be seen in (20)–(22), the verbs *know, ask,* and *wonder* have distinct selectional requirements; *know* and *ask* select for an NP argument while *wonder* does not, and all three select for a complement phrase (CP). Notice that the CP takes two different forms, one where it is headed by the complementizer *that*, as in (20b), while another is headed by the complementizer *who*, as in (20c)–(22c). These phrases are associated with complex semantic types (Grimshaw, 1977):

23a. Yosef knows [NP the time]
     THEME
23b. Yosef knows [CP that the girl kissed the boy]
     PROPOSITION
23c. Yosef knows [CP who the girl kissed]
     INTERROGATIVE

Those headed by a *that*-phrase are typically **Propositions,** while those headed by a *wh*-phrase are typically Interrogatives (there are additional semantic types, such as **Exclamations** and **Infinitives;** see Shetreet et al., 2007). Notice that these complex arguments have internal structure. Taking (23b) as an example, the argument playing the role of Proposition can be further divided into an AGENT THEME structure, where the embedded subject argument, *the girl*, is assigned the AGENT role and the embedded object argument, *the boy*, is assigned the THEME role.

Thus, a complex sentence with an embedded clause must satisfy the lexical requirements of two verbs. This can be seen in Figure 6-6.

As shown in Figure 6-6, when the embedded V (*kiss*) is merged with its NP complement (*the boy*), the THEME role is assigned (and checked-off) and a VP is formed. Moving up the tree, when the resulting VP is merged with the subject NP (*the girl*), the AGENT role is assigned and a CP is formed. Continuing, when the embedded clause (CP; *the girl kissed the boy*) is merged with the main verb (*know*), the PROPOSITION is assigned and a VP is formed. Finally, when the resulting main VP (*knows (that) the girl kissed the boy*) is merged with the

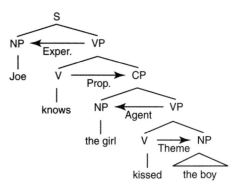

Figure 6-6 Assignment of theta-roles in a complex sentence.

main subject NP (*Joe*), the EXPERIENCER role is assigned and the S is formed[4,5].

Syntactic Features of Arguments

Notice that the syntactic form of an argument is not predictable from its thematic properties. For example, an embedded complement phrase (CP) can take the semantic form of a Proposition or Interrogative, as shown in (23). Furthermore, we began this exercise about argument structure showing that even simple NPs that appear to be in subject position can be assigned an Agent, a Theme, or an Experiencer role. These facts suggest that verbs select for their syntactic environments as well as thematic roles. Consider the following examples:

24. The girl ran.
    run: __∅
25. The girl pushed [NP the boy].
    push: __NP
26. The girl gave [NP the prize] [PP to the boy].
    give: __NP PP
27. The girl thought [CP that the prize was nice].
    think: __CP

As shown in (24)–(27), the verb *run* has no complements (for now, consider a complement as the syntactic form of the argument selected by the verb); the verb *push* takes an NP complement; the verb *give*, an NP PP complement; and the verb *think*, a CP complement. Notice that complements do not include the subject position; both the subject and complements act as the

---

[4]Note that the subject NP is not technically assigned a thematic role by the verb; instead it is assigned its role through the VP itself, as shown in Figure 6-5.

---

[5]We have greatly simplified the representation of phrasal geometry in this chapter. From our description thus far, it appears that there are only two levels to each phrase (a lexical node, and its corresponding phrasal node), as shown in Figure 6-5, for example. However, research in linguistics discovered decades ago (e.g., Chomsky, 1970; Jackendoff, 1977) that intermediate categories—falling in between the lexical and phrasal levels—must be postulated to explain the structure of the sentence. Furthermore, all arguments of the verb are said to originate within the VP, and the subject 'moves' upward in the tree for theory-internal reasons. Since arguments are associated with the verb, it makes sense to have the arguments originate within the verb phrase. There are also additional layers above the VP that we have ignored. There is the Inflectional Phrase (IP), which is used to check features of Tense and Agreement, and the Complement Phrase (CP). The CP is, in fact, the phrasal category of what we typically call the 'sentence' (or S). This account, called **X-bar theory,** allows for a uniform specification of structure across all types of phrases.

verb's arguments, as we discussed above when describing argument structure.

The formal name for the verb's syntactic properties is *syntactic subcategorization*, also known as C-selection (Complement Selection). That is, the verb is said to subcategorize for various types of phrasal complements. Now, consider a more fully established lexical entry as in Table 6-6.

The entry shown in Table 6-6 describes the following properties of the verb *discover*: It has a two-place argument structure; the second (Y) argument can C-select either an NP or a CP. If there is a direct object NP argument active in the sentence, it will be assigned the Theme role; if that argument is, syntactically, an embedded clause (CP), then it will be assigned either a PROPOSITION or an INTERROGATIVE. The lexical properties of the verb will thus yield the following example sentences:

28a. Richard [discovered [NP the fish]]
28b. Richard [discovered [CP that the fish was in the soup]]
28c. Richard [discovered [CP where the fish was hiding]]

In (28a), the VP, discovered the fish, includes an NP argument playing the Theme role. In (28b), the CP argument is assigned the PROPOSITION role, and in (28c), it is assigned the INTERROGATIVE role.

Movement and Copy-and-Delete

A pervasive fact about languages is that they allow an element in a sentence to be displaced from one position in the sentence to another position, yet grammaticality and interpretation remain relatively stable. Consider the following pair:

29. The girl kissed the boy
30. Which boy did the girl kiss?

It is clear that (29) and (30) are related; they both satisfy the lexical requirements of the verb *kiss* (it requires two arguments), and they have the same subject NP, *the girl*. The two sentences also have very similar objects (*the boy* in (29) and *which boy* in (30)). Thus we can say that in both cases, the Agent role is assigned to the subject position and the Theme is applied to the object position of the verb *kissed*. Yet, in (30) the object NP has been **displaced** (or **moved**) from its canonical

Table 6-6 Partial Lexical Entry for the Verb "Discover"

	PAS	Thematic Roles	C-Selection
discover, V	X	AGENT	NP
	Y	THEME	NP
		PROPOSITION/ INTERROGATIVE	CP

position occurring after the verb (as in (29)), to a position occurring well before the verb.

Skipping many syntactic details, when an element moves, it leaves behind a movement **trace** (from earlier work in the 70s and 80s) or leaves behind an unpronounced **copy** of itself (from more recent work in the 90s). The copy must be deleted before the sentence is interpreted; otherwise the sentence will be ungrammatical and the derivation will **crash** (*Which boy did the girl kiss which boy?). By convention, we use <angled brackets> to signify a copy, and ~~strikethrough~~ to signify deletion of that copy:

31a. Did the girl kiss [which boy]$_i$

31b. Which boy did the girl kiss ~~<which boy>~~$_i$

Thematic roles are assigned to the base grammatical positions during the derivation of the sentence. That is, Theme is assigned to the object NP position, occupied by *which boy* as in (31a). Then the object NP is moved to a position earlier in the sentence, which leaves behind a copy, and the copy is subsequently deleted (31b). Because the copy and its moved counterpart are the same object, all features of the copy are shared with its moved counterpart, and hence the Theme role is transferred to the moved NP.

The type of movement characterized in (31) is called **wh-movement,** and it is also responsible for the derivation of **clefts** and **relative clauses:**

32. It was [the boy]$_i$ [who]$_i$ the girl kissed ~~<who>~~$_i$

33. The father disliked [the boy]$_i$ [who]$_i$ the girl kissed ~~<who>~~$_i$

Like in (31), in both (32) and (33) the object NP (*who*) is displaced from its canonical position occurring after the verb *kissed* (its **base position**), and leaves a copy, which is subsequently deleted during the derivation of the sentence. Also similar to (31), the object receives the Theme role while residing in its base position. Unlike (31) however, in both (32) and (33) the head of the relative clause—the NP *the boy*—co-refers to the relative pronoun *who* (signified by co-indexation), and hence gets its reference (and thematic role) from the pronoun.

Argument Structure, Copies, and Sentence Processing

Given its contributions to the syntax and semantics of sentences, it should not be too surprising that verb representations have played a significant role in accounts of sentence processing. In perhaps the first attempt to examine how verbs influence sentence processing, Fodor, Garrett, and Bever (1968) found that sentences that contained verbs that accommodated two possible syntactic configurations—an NP or CP (S) complement—were more difficult to process than

sentences containing verbs that accommodated only a single configuration—an NP complement. They found this to be so even though the sentences to be processed took the simplest form and were syntactically identical NP-V-NP transitive constructions. Thus, it was the verb's potential to accommodate different syntactic structures (i.e., their implicit lexical representations), and not the surface realization of one or the other of these structures, that appeared to contribute to sentence processing performance. Fodor et al. (1968) used paraphrase and anagram tasks to discover the relation between the complexity of verb representations and sentence processing performance. Similar findings were reported by Holmes & Forster (1972) using rapid serial visual presentation (RSVP) and by Chodorow (1979) using time-compressed speech.

In a related series of experiments, Shapiro and colleagues (e.g., Shapiro, Zurif, & Grimshaw, 1987, 1989; Shapiro, Brookins, Gordon, & Nagel, 1991) discovered the relation between the number of argument structure configurations and sentence processing complexity, using a cross-modal lexical interference task (Box 6-1). Briefly, verbs accommodating different numbers of argument structures were inserted in sentences with similar, simple, surface forms. These sentences were presented to normal listeners, who had to complete a secondary task that was presented in the immediate temporal vicinity of the verb. Verbs that entailed more argument structure possibilities yielded greater processing load relative to verbs that entailed fewer possibilities, suggesting that once the verb is encountered in a sentence, all of its possible argument structure arrangements are activated. One reason for such exhaustive activation is that it allows for on-line thematic role assignment, as we discussed earlier. That is, once the verb is encountered and activated, so too are its argument structure and thematic roles, setting the stage for further operations of the sentence processor (see, for example, Clifton, Speer, & Abney, 1991; Pritchett, 1988; Boland, Tanenhaus, & Garnsey, 1990).

Also, our foray into the syntax of movement has important implications for sentence processing. As we shall show shortly, when a listener who is attempting to understand a sentence encounters a direct object position that is "empty"—where the direct object NP has been displaced to a position that occurs before the verb—the listener appears to activate that NP, even though it is not heard or seen at the post-verb position. This is a remarkable finding, and suggests that linguistic theory does have something to offer those of us who are interested in how the brain comprehends language. Furthermore, constructions with movement turn out to be particularly problematic for some individuals with aphasia,

Box 6-1

Experimental Techniques

OFFLINE QUESTIONNAIRES

Participants are given all the time they need to indicate their judgments, ratings, classifications, sentence completion, or selection of alternative interpretations by writing.

SELF-PACED READING

A sentence is presented one segment at a time on a screen. Participants read the first segment, press a button to move on to the next segment and have the current one disappear, and so on until the end of the sentence. Reading times for each segment (between two button presses) is recorded. Longer reading times reflect more difficult or additional processing.

CROSS-MODAL INTERFERENCE

A string of letters is briefly flashed on a screen at a specific point of interest during the presentation of an auditory sentence. Reaction times to deciding whether the string forms a word of English or not (called a lexical decision task) are compared between two sentences forming a minimal pair. Longer reaction times index a heavier processing load.

CROSS-MODAL PRIMING

Participants perform a lexical decision on a string of letters briefly flashed on a screen at a specific point of interest during the otherwise uninterrupted presentation of an auditory sentence. Visual words (probes) are either related to a noun of interest in the sentence or unrelated to the sentence completely, but participants are unaware of this relationship. The semantic relatedness between the noun of interest (the prime) and the probe facilitates the decisions on the related compared to the unrelated visual words. This priming effect is interpreted as reflecting the automatic activation of the noun of interest at the specific point in time.

EYE-TRACKING (READING, VISUAL WORLD)

In reading, a sentence appears on a screen while eye movements are recorded. In listening, related and distracting visual objects appear on display. Eye movements over the visual display are recorded as an auditory sentence unfolds. Eye-movement recordings allow experimenters to calculate a myriad of data and determine how much time is spent on an element (a word or an object), when an element is looked at, and when and how often comprehenders return to previously-processed elements. This technique provides very detailed information on the moment-by-moment processes underlying comprehension.

EVENT-RELATED POTENTIALS

Participants wear an electrodes-bearing head cap during listening or reading tasks. Electrical activity is recorded over time with millisecond precision for many sentences forming minimal pairs. The activity for each sentence type is compared, revealing differences in amplitude and/or timing between sentences. These relative differences are then interpreted with respect to the distinct properties of the sentences and/or cognitive processes underlying their comprehension. This neuroimaging technique provides very detailed temporal information, but with careful analysis techniques can also indicate the brain regions from where the activity differences may arise.

as Chapter 10 reveals. With these linguistic preliminaries out of the way, we now turn to sentence processing.

COMPREHENSION

How do we go from a series of sounds or visual letters, identify words and phrases, and extract complex meaning from them? At what point in time during the comprehension process are different types of information (syntactic, probabilistic, world knowledge, etc.) taken into account when constructing an interpretation? These are central questions in the study of language comprehension. First, we will discuss how words are organized in and retrieved from our mental lexicon. Next, we will discuss how and when information can guide the interpretation of a sentence.

What's a Word?

A word or *lexical entry* is a verbal label for a concept. Many types of information are bundled under this label: the word's written or phonological form (e.g.: dog or /dɔg/), its syntactic category (noun, verb, preposition), its number (singular or plural), its gender (feminine, masculine, neutral), its argument structure, and of course, the concept it refers to (a four-legged animal that barks and fetches objects), and others.

Psychologically, all this information, for each word, has to be easily retained and retrieved from memory. How a word's information is encoded is referred to as the *mental representation* of the word, while the access of a word's mental representation is referred to as *lexical retrieval or access*. While the types of information composing a word are largely agreed upon, there is little consensus on the nature of a word's mental representation.

Possibly, a word's representation is the psychological counterpart of a *dictionary entry*: under its form (written or phonological), a word's detailed information could be automatically retrieved as a block. A word would be a unit that is used as a building block by the comprehension system. This view tends to be assumed by modularist, form-based accounts of sentence comprehension, which we will discuss below.

Another possibility is that words are not mentally stored as wholes, but rather as *groups of properties*. That is, each type of information would be encoded independently of the word and it would be the combination of specific attributes (e.g., a noun, written form "dog," "singular," "four-legged animal," "that barks," etc.) that would come together to form the word entry "dog." This view tends to be associated with connectionist, constraint-based accounts of sentence comprehension, though it is by no means accurate to suggest that only connectionist accounts can accommodate bundles of properties.

These two views of word representation also differ on the nature of syntactic constraints, the rules governing the combination of words. For form-based accounts, these rules exist independently from word representations. For constraint-based accounts, syntactic rules do not exist on their own; rather, information on how a word can be used in a sentence is integrated into each word's lexical entry. The special status attributed to independent syntactic rules forms a cornerstone of form-based models of sentence processing, as we will see later.

Word Access

During comprehension, the listener/reader begins by identifying the sounds/letters, then by recognizing words embedded in the input. This process, *word recognition*, is robust (few errors are made) and very efficient,

taking place within about 250 ms. This is particularly impressive considering that the target word must be selected from an average lexicon of 65,000 entries!

First, it is important to note that *visual word recognition* (VWR) is different from *auditory word recognition* (AWR). In VWR, the word is visible in its entirety, earlier parts of the word can be re-read as necessary, the input is constant (meaning the signal will not fluctuate while recognition is taking place) and each letter's form is uninfluenced by its neighbors (the letter /t/ is written the same way, regardless of context). A visual word is identified when a match is found in the lexicon.

By contrast, in AWR, the word is presented piecemeal, one phoneme at a time, with each phoneme becoming inaccessible after its occurrence (e.g., the first syllable cannot be re-heard while the rest of the word is being heard). The signal changes over time, from the first to the last phoneme, which requires continuous, gradual processing of the word. Finally, phonemes may be difficult to identify, since their articulation may vary by context (coarticulation, assimilation). An auditory word is recognized via an elimination process that takes place over time: each phoneme heard activates all possible matches in the lexicon, until the next phoneme narrows down the set of candidates, and so on, until only one candidate remains.

The *recognition point* of a word refers to the moment a lexical entry is selected as matching the input (visual or auditory). Once a word is recognized, its lexical entry can be accessed in the lexicon. Regardless of modality, many factors influence the rapidity and accuracy of the word retrieval process: frequency, lexical similarity (i.e., number of words that differ by one letter/phoneme from the target word, its *neighbors*), word length, semantic priming (a word is processed more easily if a semantically-related word preceded it) and uniqueness point (point at which a word is uniquely compatible with one entry in the lexicon). This point may be after a word's uniqueness point, in case of poor listening/reading conditions, where more time is needed to confirm the selection. The properties that optimize word retrieval are listed in Box 6-2.

Once lexical access has taken place, the process of combining words, or syntactic processing, starts.

Why do we need to move on from word-level processing to understand language comprehension? We have already discussed in the Linguistic Toolkit why sentences are considered the basic unit in comprehension: we speak in sentences, not isolated words, and the same proposition (*kissed: John, Mary*) can be conveyed using different word orders that bring about subtle nuances in interpretation. These observations are backed

Box 6-2

Factors Resulting in Faster and More Accurate Lexical Access

High frequency
Small neighborhood density
Low-frequency neighbors
Shorter words
Semantic relatedness to context
Early uniqueness point

by experimental studies on perception, beginning with the seminal work of George Miller and colleagues. Miller & Selfridge (1950) first showed the relevance of sentence structure by showing that memory for word sequences is best when the sequences mimic English regularities. In other words, structure helps processing individual words. Structure does so even before words are recognized: accurate perception of words in noise significantly increases when the words are strung together into sentences (Miller, Heise, & Lichten, 1951; Miller & Isard, 1963). In fact, words are better perceived even in sentences that make no semantic sense (in strings of random, semantically unrelated words), strongly suggesting that syntactic structure can influence word perception (Miller & Isard, 1963). Together, these studies demonstrated that sentences are a telling, essential unit in language processing. Without further ado, then, we move on to the topic of sentence comprehension or the exploration of how meaning is extracted from a structured input.

Sentence Comprehension Models

An initial assumption when considering the time-course of sentence comprehension is that processing is incremental and immediate. That is, decisions are made at each and every possible point during the unfolding of the sentence; on most accounts the parser does not wait for additional material. What material does the parser take into consideration when making those decisions? A sentence's interpretation can be computed by drawing upon many types of information or constraints. Depending on the model of sentence comprehension, different types of information will be considered at distinct points in time. We will consider three views of how sentence processing proceeds: (1) by blindly applying syntactic rules; (2) by computing the most likely interpretation, considering all information available; (3) by assuming the least costly option (in computational resources).

Blindly Applying Syntactic Rules: Form-Based Accounts

Recall that form-based accounts (FBA) view the word much like a dictionary entry: once the form is located (written or auditory), all information pertaining to this form is retrieved. Out of all this information, a word's syntactic category (noun, verb, adverb, etc.) is the element that seems most important for parsing the input for FBA accounts—at least at first. The comprehension system integrates words into a sentential structure by following phrasal rules. As seen earlier, syntactic rules define how lexical heads (Ns, Vs, etc.) and phrases (NPs, VPs, etc.) can be merged. The comprehension system thus has to know what category the words are, so as to know how to combine them.

FBAs, such as Frazier's Garden-Path Model (1987), are mostly serial, two-stage models. These accounts are serial because they assume that one process takes place before another one starts. In a first stage, a syntactic structure is constructed based on phrasal rules. It is thus the form that blindly guides all parsing; combinations initially rely on words' categories to build a syntactic skeleton of the sentence, with little consideration for content. In the case where multiple rules could apply (syntactic ambiguity), one is selected following principles of economy (to minimize structure and processing costs). Note that the syntactic structure might need to be revised at a later point, if the intended interpretation was not the least costly. Quickly after words are combined and new structure is projected, a second stage integrates all other types of information that may reveal that the initial parse was incorrect, and induce re-analysis. Hence, it is only after syntax-guided combinations have taken place that other types of information (semantics, plausibility, world knowledge) can influence the final interpretation. It is typically assumed that a detailed, complete representation of the entire sentence (i.e., the whole syntactic tree) is available at the end of the parse (one exception proposes that shallow, incomplete local representations are dominant at different points in time during processing: the *Good-Enough Approach*, see Ferreira, Bailey, & Ferraro, 2002).

Processing a Simple Sentence

Let's illustrate the processes at play with a simple example:
    34. The policeman sings.
When *The* is heard, its lexical entry is retrieved. Importantly, the fact that it is a Determiner is immediately used by the comprehension system, which will begin constructing a syntactic structure. Upon recognizing *policeman*, all its associated lexical information is retrieved: human, male, law enforcement agent, third

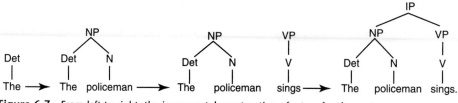

Figure 6-7   From left to right, the incremental construction of a tree for the sentence: *The policeman sings.*

person singular, and so on. *Policeman* then projects as a noun and merges with the Det to form an NP. Similarly, the verb's lexical entry is retrieved (active, third person singular, present tense, to make musical sounds with one's voice, etc.) and its syntactic category immediately serves to project a verb phrase (VP). The comprehension system then merges these phrases according to the appropriate phrasal rule (IP → DP VP) (Figure 6-7).

As soon as the two phrases are joined, the semantic detail about *policeman* and *sings* is integrated into the structure, and it is understood that the law enforcement agent is making musical sounds with his voice. In this basic example, no complications arise at the first or second stage, as there are no ambiguities. However, ambiguities are ubiquitous in language and must be dealt with very efficiently by the comprehension system.

Resolving Lexical Ambiguities

A first type of ambiguity comes from polysemy:

35. The man was not surprised when he found several spiders, roaches and other bugs in the corner of the room.

The word "bug" can have two meanings, for example, an insect or a surveillance device. Despite one meaning being much more frequent (insect) than the other, there is considerable evidence to suggest that listeners activate both potential meanings automatically upon identifying "bug," even after a biasing context such as (35) (Swinney, 1979). Two Ns are thus made available to the comprehension system, which builds two potential structures (one for each NP/meaning) in the first stage of processing. In this case, both phrasal trees will be identical, as the ambiguity lies in the semantics of the word itself, not in the way it attaches to other phrases (i.e., it is a lexical ambiguity and not a structural one). It is in the second stage when context, probability, frequency, etc. are considered and where one of the trees will be selected as the final interpretation for the sentence (in example (35), context indicates that the insect meaning was intended).

Resolving Syntactic Ambiguities

In many instances, the structure of the sentence and consequently, its interpretation, is unclear. Consider:

36. The spy saw the man with binoculars.

There are two interpretations for this sentence: either the spy used binoculars to watch the man, or the man was holding the binoculars. This global structural ambiguity arises because the prepositional phrase (PP) *with binoculars* can attach either to the verb (*saw*) or to the noun phrase (*the man*). How the PP is attached determines how the sentence is interpreted: either the binoculars were used to see the man (verb attachment) or the binoculars were held in hand by the man (noun attachment). The comprehension system thus has to choose which of the two phrase structures ([VP → V PP] or [NP → N PP]) should apply (Figure 6-8).

For FBAs, this choice is guided by principles of economy, which will favor the least costly option. For example, in the Garden-Path Model (Frazier, 1987; see also Frazier & Clifton, 1996), one of these principles is *Minimal Attachment*: Attach the PP so as to minimize the number of nodes required. By comparing the trees of the two potential interpretations, it can be seen that there are fewer nodes or levels associated with attaching the PP to the VP (i.e., the spy has the binoculars) compared to the NP.

Indeed, comprehenders seem to prefer this interpretation overall. However, the assumed structure of the tree may not correspond to the correct interpretation, if it turns out that the man held the binoculars. Similarly, lexical information could provide information constraining the interpretation. Consider *The*

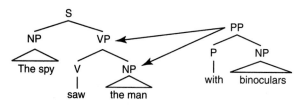

Figure 6-8   A PP attachment ambiguity: The PP can modify the verb phrase or the noun phrase.

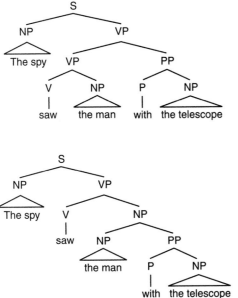

Figure 6-9   Minimal (*top*) and non-minimal (*bottom*) attachments of a PP.

spy saw the man [with nuclear weapons]$_{PP}$. According to this account, in the first processing stage, the same syntactic structure as in Figure 6-9 would be assumed (PP attaches to VP$_{saw}$) because this structure is the most economical. It is in the second stage that the semantic information that "one cannot see with nuclear weapons" will force the conclusion that the initial parse was incorrect. The system will subsequently re-parse the sentence and correctly attach the PP to NP$_{man}$.

In summary, in the case of form-driven accounts, syntactic constraints exist independently of individual words. These syntactic rules have precedence over all other types of constraints such as semantic plausibility, frequency or context. These latter constraints are only considered in a later stage, after syntactic form and/or principles guided a first-pass analysis (or parse) of the input. In the case where the initial parse is incorrect, a reanalysis considering all available information takes place to fix the structure.

Computing the Most Likely Interpretation: Constraint-Based Accounts

In contrast with FBAs, constraint-based accounts (CBAs) do not recognize the existence of independent syntactic rules. Rather, syntactic constraints on how words may merge are specified in a word's lexical entry. Recall that FBAs tend to think of words as "blocks" that exist and are stored as units. By contrast, CBAs (of which the Constraint Satisfaction Model (MacDonald, Pearlmutter, & Seidenberg, 1994) is the most influential) consider that words are not stored as entities but emerge from the unique pattern of activation of features. In their view, syntactic restrictions are thus one of the many properties making up a word. Because there are no rules to apply, syntactic processing in CBAs amounts to matching words that share (syntactic) properties.

Another distinction between FBAs and CBAs is that the latter are typically parallel, one-stage models. In CBAs, all types of information are considered simultaneously to compute the most likely interpretation—there is no priority for syntax. A second stage also becomes superfluous since semantics, plausibility, world knowledge, etc. are already integrated in the determination of an interpretation. Further, the system evaluates all possibilities allowed by the individual words' features and constraints, and ranks these possible interpretations based on likelihood or probability (because these multiple computations take place all at once, the system is said to be working in parallel). As the sentence unfolds, these alternatives are activated to different degrees, with activation levels proportionate to their likelihood of being the correct one. These rankings can fluctuate over the time-course of processing, as more and more constraints need to be satisfied. By sentence's end, it is the most likely option (if not unique) that will be selected as the correct interpretation.

Processing a Simple Sentence
Let's return to example (34) (in (37), below) to see how sentence comprehension takes place under CBAs' approach:

37. The policeman sings.

When *policeman* is encountered in the input, its associated X-bar structure (an NP), which is an integral element of the word's entry, is activated, as are its semantics, its argument structure and all of its possible thematic roles. Because its semantics (animate, human, etc.) are more compatible with an agent role, the representation of the Agent thematic role will be more active than any other role (theme, goal, experiencer, etc.). Already, multiple interpretations for the input have begun (i.e., with *policeman* being interpreted as an agent or a theme or a goal, etc.) and ranked (*policeman* as agent: first, as theme: second, and so on).

Next, the verb is recognized and its properties, including its thematic grids and argument structures ([VP → V] and [VP → V NP]), are activated. The verb *sings* is associated with multiple thematic grids (<agent>, <agent, theme>), both of which are activated to degrees proportionate to their relative frequency and to contextual constraints. The system then needs to compute a relation between the two words: it must determine how their X-bar structures connect and which thematic role is assigned to *policeman*. Considering frequency of argument structure and/or thematic grids, frequency of *policeman* as an agent or theme, plausibility, and other constraints, the system settles on a single argument structure and thematic grid for the verb. In doing so, the theta-role of agent becomes available and is assigned to *policeman*.

Resolving Lexical Ambiguities

In CBAs, much like in FBAs, all of the multiple meanings of a polysemous word, such as *bugs* in (38), are simultaneously activated (recall that the word "bug" is ambiguous between the insect and the surveillance device interpretations):

> 38. The man was not surprised when he found several spiders, roaches and other bugs in the corner of the room.

However, CBAs and FBAs deal differently with this exhaustive access of a word's meanings. The latter assume that all interpretations are equally activated until a later point in time, the second parsing stage, when context and other types of information will guide the selection of the correct alternative. In CBAs, by contrast, every possible meaning is activated but at different levels. These levels or rankings reflect the probability of being the correct interpretation given all constraints (semantic, plausibility, frequency, etc.).

Resolving Syntactic Ambiguities

Syntactic ambiguity arises when a phrase may modify more than one other phrase. For example, in (39), the prepositional phrase (PP) *with binoculars* may specify with which instrument the spy saw the man or may provide additional information about the man seen by the spy.

> 39. The spy saw the man with binoculars.

For FBAs, the ambiguity arises from having two phrase structure rules to attach the PP (one to the verb, the other to the noun). From a CBA standpoint, there are no syntactic rules; thus, syntactic ambiguity does not result from having to choose among multiple phrase structure rules. Rather, syntactic ambiguity is a type of lexical ambiguity, one in which a word has multiple sets of syntactic properties or X-bar structures. The resolution of this ambiguity is identical to that of polysemy: all alternatives (in the case of syntactic ambiguity, all sets of syntactic properties) are activated and immediately ranked.

Consider (39): The verb *saw* can present with the thematic grid of a simple transitive verb (< theme >) or of a modified transitive verb (< theme, instrument >). Both grids get activated and ranked, following frequency of usage and other constraints. Similarly, the noun and then the preposition activate and rank their lexical/syntactic properties. The preposition, for instance, may assign the thematic roles of attribute (providing more semantic information on the noun) or instrument (specifying which tool was used to perform the action). Frequency of usage will influence the ranking of these possible thematic grids, but so will the constraints (semantics, plausibility, world knowledge, etc.) introduced by the context. These contextual constraints include the presence of an action verb that can be performed with an instrument (one can see with something) and a noun describing an object that can serve as a tool. Eventually, the logical relation between a telescope's use and the action of seeing favors the parse that the telescope is used as an instrument by the spy.

To sum up, syntactic constraints are encoded in lexical entries as permissible usages of a word. When a word is processed in the input, its syntactic properties (phrasal structure, argument structure, thematic grid, etc.) are activated. If multiple possibilities exist for a type of information (semantic or syntactic), the alternatives are ranked and their activation level, modulated by their rank. The ranking reflects the frequency of usage of each option, weighted by how well an alternative satisfies the constraints established by the context. Since contextual constraints are introduced word-by-word, the ranking varies as the sentence unfolds until a single interpretation is retained as the most likely to be correct. If this choice turns out incorrect, an alternative interpretation (that had been considered less likely to be correct) is recovered.

Assuming the Least Costly Option: Resource-Based Accounts

The two first families of accounts we have discussed mainly describe how language is represented (words as blocks or as bundles of features, syntax as phrase structure rules or as constraints within the lexical entry) and how/when different types of information influence sentence comprehension. That is, although these two approaches diverge on their view of the language system, they both aim to explain how linguistic information serves the computation of an interpretation. A third, more heterogeneous group of accounts is less concerned with the linguistic characterization of the comprehension process and more interested in understanding its computational realization. The central assumption of such accounts is that understanding a sentence requires usage of cognitive resources—may they be mnemonic, attentional, or undefined—and that processing difficulty results from greater consumption of these resources. Resource-based accounts (RBAs) thus tend to compare two sentences varying in comprehension difficulty (slower reaction times and higher error rates are taken as indices of a more difficult sentence) and link extra processing costs to specific characteristics of sentences.

For example, a framework has been proposed in which comprehension is a cue-based memory retrieval mechanism (Lewis, Vasishth, & Van Dyke, 2006). In this view, when a word is processed, some of its properties are encoded into working memory (e.g., "dog": *noun, singular . . .*) along with features of the lexical item or phrase it is expected to join (e.g., *a verb, third personal singular, of which "dog" will be the subject*).

40. The dog with a brown spot jumped over the fence.

Dog:	**Jumped:**
Noun	Verb
Singular	Past tense
Subject of: *Unspecified*	Subject: *Unspecified*
verb, 3ps	*noun*

The representations of these features remain in memory until they are retrieved at the verb. At that point, some features of "jumped" (*verb, third personal singular*), and its requested item (i.e., *a subject*) serve as cues that trigger the retrieval of "dog." The verb is then integrated by association with *dog* and the preceding structure. In this model, there is no syntactic parsing; words get associated through mnemonic processes on a feature-by-feature basis. The level of difficulty in comprehending a sentence in this view is proportionate to the difficulty in maintaining the representations in memory or retrieving them from memory, especially in the face of interference.

Another model explains processing difficulty in terms of *surprisal*, that is, how unlikely a word is given the context (Hale, 2003; Levy, 2008). As in a CBA framework, multiple interpretations are computed in parallel and ranked following their likelihood. The surprisal account holds that a word's processing difficulty is proportionate to the (memory) resources required to re-rank these interpretations after this word is integrated. Therefore, a word that fits well in the context and is consistent with a highly ranked interpretation will be easy to process and cost little. In contrary, a word that is inconsistent with a high-ranked interpretation and consistent with a lower ranked one will force a re-ranking, costing much resources to the system. For this reason, comprehending the sentence will become costlier at the point where this word has to be integrated.

To sum up, RBAs aim to explain how cognitive resources are used during comprehension, and how their allocation relates to processing difficulty. In these accounts, the detailing of how linguistic characteristics lead to an interpretation takes a backseat to the description of the demands an interpretation puts on the cognitive system. This "resource complexity" approach to sentence processing is particularly present in the study of disordered language, where deficits are often said to arise from an insufficiency in cognitive resources (see Chapter 10).

In conclusion, there is a myriad of sentence comprehension accounts, with as many views on the structure of a word or the interplay of the many processes involved. Every model is supported by some experimental data and challenged by other data. Extant models are constantly refined and new frameworks are regularly proposed. Certainly, sentence comprehension is fast and incremental, and taps into many processes and/or types of information to converge onto an interpretation for what is heard or seen (Box 6-3 and Box 6-4).

Box 6-3

Terminology

Many terms are commonly used to refer to sentence comprehension. Processing can be **serial,** or **parallel** (see main text), and be restricted or unrestricted. An account is **restricted** if it limits the types of information that are considered at certain points in time. Therefore, form-based accounts, which prevent any information other than syntax from influencing the initial parse, are said to be restricted. Because the first parse is uninfluenced by nonsyntactic factors, the comprehension system is considered **modular,** that is, that assumes the existence of an independent cognitive module for syntax. On the other hand, constraint-based accounts, which argue for the immediate consideration of all types of constraints (semantic, syntactic, probabilistic . . .) are referred to as **unrestricted.** In this nonmodular view, there is no module specializing in the processing of a given type of information. Moreover, these accounts typically have a **connectionist** architecture, meaning that all representations and processes are encoded in features and distributed over the brain. By contrast, modular models are typically associated with **localizationism,** the view that a cognitive process/representation "lives" in a specific region of the brain (however, modularity does not necessarily imply a one-to-one relation between cognitive modules and brain regions).

Box 6-4

Methodology

Psycholinguistics benefits from a vast choice of **techniques** to study the cognitive mechanisms underlying language processing. Yet, many theoretical debates are sparked and fueled by results tied to specific methodologies or are difficult to replicate across techniques. It is elemental to assess the strengths and limitations of a technique in order to understand the theoretical impact of a given set of results. Sentence comprehension is particularly subject to methodological disputes and counter-arguments because of the central importance of **timing** for theoretical models. Indeed, methodologies differ in their ability to characterize or tap into cognitive processes as they take place, in real time. The techniques that are sensitive to the moment-by-moment unfolding of processes are classed as **online** techniques; by contrast, those that reveal the end-product of the interpretation process are referred to as **offline** techniques. The temporal sensitivity of a technique is not the sole methodological factor that can influence experimental results. For instance, several paradigms use **discontinuous** presentations, meaning only one word or phrase is presented at a time (compared to continuous presentations in which the entire sentence is heard/shown at once). These segmented stimuli diverge from the type of language that is typically heard or read in everyday life since it incorporates extra time periods between words/phrases. This additional time might yield comprehenders to put an unnatural emphasis on individual segments and/or alter the normal time-course of processing. It also remains to be determined if, how, and to what extent **modality** influences processing: the manner in which a stimulus is received by the processor differs between modalities (auditory or visual, see Section B2) and may implicate distinct parsing mechanisms and strategies (beyond modality-specific processes).

PSYCHOLINGUISTICS OF SENTENCE COMPREHENSION

We now turn to empirical evidence on how sentences are comprehended. Typically, experimental data are used to test a model's predictions and offer direct support for an account, while sometimes offering disconfirming evidence for alternative accounts. For our purposes, we will focus on the cognitive processes implicated in understanding a sentence, as well as on the relative contributions of distinct types of information (syntactic, semantic, world knowledge). Recall from our presentation of different accounts that the central issue is not whether context, frequency, plausibility, etc. affect sentence processing. The question is when, during the processing stream, do these factors come into play (e.g., immediately, or after a syntax-only analysis, for example). In order to determine how a given factor (for example, semantic plausibility) affects comprehension, language scientists often compare the processing of **minimal pairs,** that is, of two constructions that differ in only the factor of interest (e.g., a semantically plausible versus a semantically implausible sentence). Thus, a difference in the dependent measure—reaction times, accuracy levels, etc.—between the two elements will be attributed to the factor of interest. To conduct this work properly, scientists must understand the linguistic and nonlinguistic properties of the lexical items and sentences that will be manipulated.

Thus, scientists exploit the detailed properties of sentences to test for influences of given factors on processing or tap into specific mental operations that take place during comprehension (see Gap-Filling below for an example). It is important to realize that these sentence types offer psycholinguists a precious tool, a means to "trick" the processor and observe its inner workings. That is, it is not the particular sentence types that are of interest, but rather, it is the processing operations that are used to understand them.

In this section we will present experimental evidence from the processing of two different types of constructions: syntactically ambiguous sentences and long-distance dependencies. In the former, an ambiguous phrase or element within the phrase poses a dilemma for the processor by offering, initially, (at least) two possible analyses. These sentences are used to test whether certain factors can favor a given analysis at an early point in time. In long-distance dependencies, an element in the sentence can only be interpreted by referring back to a previously encountered element. Because several words, phrases, or even clauses can intervene between these nonadjacent elements, sentence context, semantics, and even memorial processes can influence comprehension.

Syntactically Ambiguous Sentences

In our previous discussion of sentence comprehension models, we introduced one type of structural ambiguity, prepositional phrase attachment: *The spy saw the man with binoculars*. We pointed out that the preposition phrase (*with binoculars*) can modify *the man* or the verb *saw*, and detailed how Form-Based Accounts (FBAs) and Constraint-Based Accounts (CBAs) predict the initial parse or analysis of an ambiguous segment. For FBAs, minimal attachment (syntactic simplicity) is favored initially and if the analysis turns out to be incorrect, reanalysis must occur. For CBAs, nonsyntactic information helps determine the interpretation that is most likely to be correct.

The prepositional phrase attachment example is one that remains ambiguous at the end of processing (it is thus a **global ambiguity**): comprehenders sometimes understand *with binoculars* to be attached to *saw*, sometimes to *the man*. This double reading is much like the case of a **relative clause attachment ambiguity,** such as in *The cowboy shot the servant of the actress who was on the balcony.* The relative clause *who was on the balcony* can attach to *the servant* or to *the actress*. The listener or reader, when facing the relative pronoun "who," can build two structures, one for each possible interpretation. How the choice is made (using what type(s) of information) and at what point in time (earliest or later) are two issues that discriminate opposing theoretical accounts. For example, an online and offline preference for low attachment (to *the actress*) has been documented in English (Cuetos & Mitchell, 1988; Frazier & Clifton, 1996) and other languages (for e.g.: Brazilian Portuguese; Miyamoto, 1998). The low attachment preference is consistent with a strategy favoring minimal structure, as predicted by FBA accounts. Interestingly, however, the opposite preference has been found for many languages including Spanish, French and German (Cuetos & Mitchell, 1988; Zagar, Pynte & Rativeau, 1997; Konieczny, Hemforth, Scheepers, & Strube, 1997). These data are not readily accounted for by a minimal structure strategy and cast doubt on the language-universality of the process. Since psycholinguistics attempt to describe how the brain processes language in general, more research needs to be done to better understand how this type of ambiguity is interpreted. The case of relative clause attachment ambiguities demonstrates that comprehenders have preferences when it comes to multiple interpretation alternatives. The processing explanation for this preference is still debated.

In contrast to relative clause attachment ambiguities, other types of structural ambiguities must be resolved online in order for the sentence to be interpreted (these are **temporary structural ambiguities**). That is, these are sentences that present with more than one analysis at some point during the computation of an interpretation, but there is only one correct analysis for the sentence to be grammatical. Consider, then, the NP-CP ambiguity:

41a. I suppose the girl knows <u>the answer</u> to the physics problem.

41b. The girl knows <u>the answer</u> to the physics problem was correct.

41c. The girl knows that the answer to the physics problem was correct.

The NP, *the answer*, is temporarily ambiguous in both (41a) and (41b): At the point where it is encountered, it can be analyzed as either the direct object of the verb *know* (as in (41a)), or as the subject of the embedded clause (as in (41b)). This ambiguity is due to the multiple complement frames allowed by the verb *know*; it selects for either an NP or a CP. According to the garden-path theory (a form-based account), when a post-verb NP is encountered, it should be initially analyzed as a direct object (because fewer nodes need to be postulated relative to the case where the NP turns out to be the sentential subject). This assumption turns out to be incorrect in (41b), which should then result in processing difficulty.

In an eye-tracking study (Frazier & Rayner, 1982; see also Rayner & Frazier, 1987), sentences much like those in (41) were presented to readers, and reading times and eye-movements were recorded. Results showed that average reading time per letter was longer for sentences like (41b) compared to (41a). There was also a higher probability of making a regressive eye movement in (41b) relative to (41a); that is, the eyes of the participants who were reading the sentences tended to move from a point of current focus to a point in the sentence that was previously read and that formed the initial ambiguity (e.g., the initially encountered verb phrase, *knows the answer*). Finally, it took longer to read the segment *the answer* in (41b) relative to the corresponding segment in (41c), which was disambiguated by the relative pronoun *that*. These patterns, then, confirmed that the ambiguous NP is initially attached as the direct object of the verb, causing readers to slow down and then regress back in the sentence to revise the initial analysis, if it turns out to be incorrect (as in (41b)).

Later findings from eye-tracking and self-paced reading supported the claim that the garden-path effect could be mitigated by the plausibility of the NP as a direct object. The idea here is that some verbs prefer direct objects while others prefer sentential complements, and it is this lexical preference that could dictate the initial analysis of a sentence (Garnsey, Pearlmutter, Myers, & Lotocky, 1997; Shapiro, Nagel, & Levine, 1993; Trueswell et al., 1993). This issue was revisited by Pickering, Traxler, & Crocker (2000) who argued that the stimuli in previous experiments suffered from insufficient control over plausibility in interpretation. Their eye-tracking results showed that readers adopted the direct object analysis even when the verb was biased toward the sentential analysis. Further, plausibility affected processing differently over time (see also Pickering & Traxler, 1998): More difficulty was reported for sentences with implausible direct objects in the ambiguous segment, consistent with the view that an analysis other than the NP-complement was dispreferred. Similarly, indications of more difficulty were found for sentences with plausible direct objects in the disambiguated segment, suggesting it is harder and more costly for the processor to stray away from the preferred NP-complement analysis when it is a viable possibility. For FBAs, the preference for NP- over S-complements is explained by the simpler sentence structure of the former. For CBAs, this preference should have been reversed with S-complement-biased verbs. Pickering and colleagues further offered a novel explanation for the NP preference, proposing this reading is generally more informative in that it can be verified as correct or incorrect more quickly than the S-complement reading. In their view, the parser does not always choose the most likely option, but instead chooses the one that can be confirmed more rapidly. At any rate, the findings of Pickering and colleagues indicate that the initial parse of an ambiguous segment is unaffected by preference or relative frequency of subcategorization frames. Indeed, the processor seems to strongly prefer the NP-complement parse even if it is not the most likely interpretation.

Further evidence also suggested that syntax plays a privileged role in initial parsing decisions. Consider another temporary structural ambiguity, **reduced relative clauses:**

42a. The defendant examined by the lawyer turned out to be unreliable.

42b. The evidence examined by the lawyer turned out to be unreliable.

When *examined* is encountered in (42a) the processor faces an ambiguity: *examined* could be analyzed as a main verb or as a past participle. (Note again, that the ambiguity disappears in full relatives, where a relative pronoun forces clarification: *The defendant who was examined by the lawyer* . . . .) Yet, sentence (42a) does not have two interpretations: it can ultimately only be understood as meaning that "the lawyer examined the defendant." Therefore, the ambiguity at the verb is temporary and gets resolved well before the sentence's end. How does the processor determine the correct analysis in this case? Either the simplest structure is initially assumed and revised if necessary (FBAs' view), or nonsyntactic information such as animacy favors the selection of a given structural analysis (CBA's view).

Consider (42b): its structure is identical to (42a) but its subject (*evidence*) is an inanimate object (versus an animate person in (42a)). Constraint-based accounts suggest that semantic factors such as animacy should mitigate or even eliminate the garden-path effects predicted by form-based accounts. That is, an animate NP can be considered to be a "good Agent" of a given verb, while an inanimate NP should be considered a "good Theme" of the same verb. On the other hand, form-based accounts suggest that it is only the phrase structure of the sentence (its form or syntax) that matters to initial parsing decisions, and that extra-syntactic information has its influence only after syntax has run its course. And, indeed, another study of eye-movements during sentence comprehension revealed that these sentences are equally difficult to process compared to full relatives (those containing the disambiguating relative pronoun *who*), regardless of the animacy of the first NP (Ferreira & Clifton, 1986). These results suggest that 1) the absence of a relative pronoun (*who*) incites the processor to incorrectly assume a main verb interpretation, initially; and 2) semantic constraints (the subject's animacy and the verb's preference for an animate subject) do not guide the processor into avoiding an incorrect analysis, otherwise an inanimate subject would likely have hinted that "examined" was a past participle.

However, in a follow-up eye-tracking study, Trueswell, Tanenhaus & Garnsey (1994), using stricter constraints and novel data analyses, re-evaluated whether semantic constraints could help ambiguity resolution. They found that first-pass reading times (the time taken to read a segment before leaving that segment) for the "by"-phrase (*by the lawyer*) region were longer for (42a) than for (42b). These findings indicate that the presence of an animate subject in (42a) prompts the processor to consider "examined" as a main verb. The subsequently encountered by-phrase then forces the processor to revise this assumption and reanalyze "examined." Importantly, the inanimate subject in (42b) cued that "examined" is likely not a main verb, but a past participle (since inanimate nouns make poor agents of main verbs). Thus, no revision was necessary in (42b). Moreover, the cost of a revision in sentences like (42a) was claimed to be proportional to the strength of the constraint introduced by the subject; the better an agent of the verb (and the worse a theme) a subject is, the more likely a garden-path would be subsequently encountered in structures like reduced relative clauses. These findings contradict the null results of Ferreira & Clifton, who may have failed to observe an effect that existed. The Trueswell et al. study has been regarded as robust evidence for immediate effects of nonsyntactic information (namely, semantic fit of noun as agent of a main verb) on parsing, in support of CBAs. It also argues that constraints are not of the all-or-none type: there is a gradient in how restricting semantic constraints are, and in how strongly they can influence the processor.

Aside from semantics and context, another information source might help resolve structural ambiguity: prosody. There is evidence to suggest that the prosodic contour underlying sentences may disambiguate temporary structural ambiguities. Consider the following sentences (from Nagel, Shapiro, Tuller, & Nawy, 1996):

43. The company owner promised <u>the wage increase</u> to the workers.
44. The company owner promised <u>the wage increase</u> would be substantial.

We have already met this temporary structural ambiguity. Going "left-to-right" in the speech stream, when the post-verb NP *the wage increase* is encountered, it can be analyzed as either the direct object of the verb *promised*, as in (43), or it can be analyzed as the subject of the embedded clause, as in the reduced complement sentence (44). FBAs such as the garden-path theory suggest that the simplest route (via the minimal attachment strategy) is always taken, while CBAs suggest that the path taken depends on the statistical properties or preferences of the verb for its various complement options.

Based on evidence from some previous off-line work (e.g., Beach, 1991; Price, Ostendorf, Shattuck-Hufnagel, & Fong, 1991), Nagel and colleagues (1996) surmised that differences in prosodic information (e.g., pitch and duration) could help listeners disambiguate such structural ambiguities. First, they discovered that the duration of the verb was longer, the pitch contour over the verb was steeper, and there was a significantly longer pause after the verb when it was followed by a sentential complement (sentence (44)) relative to when it was followed by a direct object (sentence (43)). These patterns suggest that there is information in the speech stream that could, in principle, be used by listeners to help determine subsequent structure. However, it is unknown, based on this study, whether/when comprehenders use this information. For instance, is prosody a type of information that can influence parsing decisions? If so, is it immediately taken into account when disambiguating a parse? Or is prosodic information only integrated at a later stage, perhaps after a syntax-only parse?

To examine the role of prosody during online processing, Nagel and colleagues (1996) next ran a series of psycholinguistic experiments that manipulated prosodic cues and structure and discovered that listeners indeed use such cues—those that are available prior to the disambiguation point—to predict upcoming structure. These researchers and others have suggested that prosodic information, much like syntax, is based on "form" and thus offers support for a form-based approach to sentence processing. Other research has found similar effects (e.g., Engelhardt, Ferreira, & Patsenko, 2010; Speer, Kjelgaard, & Dobroth, 1996), though it remains to be determined whether there are unambiguous acoustic cues underlying various sentence constructions found in spontaneous speech (see, for example, Ito & Speer 2006; Schafer, Speer, Warren, & White, 2000). Future research will also tell if prosodic information <u>must</u> be used during comprehension, i.e., if/which information types can override prosody and vice versa.

Long-Distance Dependencies

We now turn to evidence from the comprehension of long-distance dependencies, and what that evidence suggests about sentence processing. We begin with the processing of anaphora, also known as co-reference processing:

45. The boxer told the skier that the doctor for the team would blame himself/him for the recent injury.

Linguistic theory captures the intuitions that when the reflexive pronoun is used (e.g., *himself*), it must co-refer with a previously mentioned entity (or **antecedent**) that is close by (e.g., *doctor*). In linguistic terms, the reflexive pronoun and its antecedent must be located within the same clause and thus reflexive pronouns are said to be **locally bound.** When the personal pronoun (e.g., *him*) is used, it must co-refer with an antecedent that cannot be locally bound (e.g., *skier* or *boxer*). That is, the antecedent must either be in a clause not containing the pronoun, or else it can be mentioned in the discourse, without explicit mention in the sentence (e.g., *Bill said that John likes him*, where *him* refers to someone other than *Bill*).

To see whether these linguistic principles are respected by the sentence processing system, Nicol (1988; see also Nicol & Swinney, 1989) presented sentences like (45) to normal listeners and used the cross-modal lexical priming (CMLP) task to measure antecedent activation. When the reflexive pronoun was used, priming for probes related to *doctor* but not for *boxer* and *skier* was observed at the point where the reflexive was encountered in the speech stream; when the personal pronoun was used, priming for both *skier* and *boxer*, but not *doctor*, was found at the pronoun. These patterns suggest that the linguistic principles describing anaphor-antecedent relations are indeed respected by the sentence processing system.

There is another type of long-distance dependency that has garnered much attention in the psycholinguistic literature: Filler-gap dependencies. Consider:

46. The cop saw *the boy* that the crowd at the party accused [*t*] of the crime.

The verb *accused* takes two arguments, a subject and an object. In (46) its subject (*the crowd at the party*) is in its canonical position, immediately preceding the verb. However, no overt object appears in the canonical post-verb position; instead, the object (*the boy*) appears in a position earlier in the sentence. Yet, the sentence is grammatical and it is clearly understood that "the boy is accused by the crowd." How did "the boy" get associated with "accused"?

It has been suggested in linguistic theory that in such constructions the object argument is displaced from its canonical, post-verb position to a position occurring well before the verb (recall "Movement, and Copy-and-Delete" for some linguistic details). As part of displacement, a silent placeholder (a *trace* or a silent copy of 'boy') is located in the typical post-verb position. This placeholder is automatically linked to the displaced overt NP and thus the two positions are said to co-refer (much like a pronoun and its antecedent co-refer). In processing terms, the position from where the NP moved is called the **gap,** and the NP that moved is called the **filler.** Two important questions have been investigated with respect to the comprehension of these **filler-gap dependencies.** First, does the linking between the verb and its displaced object ("the boy") take place immediately, or at the end of the sentence? Second, how does the processor know which NP in the sentence is the correct filler for the gap?

The answer to the first question is now clear: The processor does not wait until the end of the sentence. As soon as it encounters a verb that requires an object argument, and a position that is "empty" (that is, does not contain an explicit representation of the argument), a **gap-filling** process is triggered, by which the semantics of the filler ("the boy") is linked to the empty position. A very convincing demonstration of the gap-filling mechanism comes from a Cross-Modal Priming study by Swinney and colleagues (reported in Nicol & Swinney, 1989; see also Balogh et al., 1998; Love & Swinney, 1996). The authors tracked the activation of the filler by looking for priming effects at two points in the sentence: right before the verb (*1*) and immediately after the verb (at the gap, *2*).

47. The cop saw the boy that the crowd at the party *1* accused *2* of the crime.

A significant priming effect was found only at the gap for the filler (*2*). In other words, the filler was not activated at discernible levels right before the verb; yet, immediately when the gap was encountered, the filler was *re*activated. Furthermore, the reverse pattern was obtained for *crowd*, which was activated at the preverbal position, but not at the gap. The gap-filling process is thus restricted to the syntactically-defined filler (to the NP that is linked to the trace), and does not imply a memory search through all previously encountered NPs (or else priming for "the crowd" would have been obtained at the gap).

If syntax constrains gap-filling, is it the case that nonsyntactic information can, too? This possibility was investigated by testing for gap-filling in cases where the filler was an implausible object for the verb:

48. The crowd saw <u>the enormous heavyweight boxer</u> that the small boy had so badly *1* beaten *2* yesterday.

The syntactically appropriate filler (underlined in (48)) is an implausible object of the verb in this example (a small boy is unlikely to beat an enormous heavyweight boxer, much less so than the other way around). The hypothesis was that if plausibility could influence gap-filling, it would prevent the reactivation of the correct but implausible NP and/or trigger the reactivation of the most plausible NP (even if syntactically incorrect). In another Cross-Modal Priming study, significant priming was found at the gap (*2) for *boxer* but not for *boy* (Osterhout & Swinney, 1993). Therefore, (im)plausibility did not obstruct the reactivation of the syntactically legitimate NP nor did it coerce the processor to reactivate an incorrect NP. Plausibility could, however, be argued to be too weak of a constraint to influence gap-filling. In effect, our knowledge of the world tells us that it is conceivable that "a boy could beat a boxer" (perhaps under special circumstances). If this interpretation is possible, then the processor should not refrain from computing it, even if it is likely incorrect. In other words, plausibility might be too weak a constraint to influence gap-filling, but a stronger constraint might block the computation of an interpretation that would be impossible in the real world. Consider, then, the real-world possibility of sentence (49):

49. The police captain said that <u>the cop from his precinct</u> that the soup in the bowl had eaten *1* was going to give a talk on public service.

In this sentence, the NP the cop from his precinct (underlined) is the object of the verb, the filler. However, it is impossible for "soup to eat people" in the real world. If a strong plausibility constraint could alter the immediate parsing decision to re-activate the filler, cop should not be primed for at the gap (*1*). Yet still, priming for cop was obtained (Swinney, 1991). The world knowledge that "people eat soup" (and not the other way around) and the fact that "soup" is very frequently the object of the verb did not suffice to eliminate gap filling for the syntactically displaced NP cop. Taken together, these results clearly demonstrate that gap-filling takes place as the sentence unfolds and is guided by syntactic constraints. This process is fast, automatic and uninfluenced by even strong constraints such as semantic impossibility or high probabilities. These characteristics are those of a **modular** system (Fodor, 1983), a central assumption of FBAs.

Now, what about ambiguous cases of gap-filling, such as in sentences (50) and (51)?

50. That's <u>the general</u> that the soldier killed enthusiastically for [*t*] during the war in Korea.
51. That's <u>the cat</u> that the dog worried about [*t*] after going to the vet because of an injury.

In these examples, a relative pronoun (*that*) identifies an NP—*general, cat*—as a filler to be linked to a later-appearing gap. The NP is thus held in memory until its co-dependent is found (event-related potential data support this premise, as we will see below). However, the relative pronoun is not enough to indicate to which gap the NP filler should be associated. Thus, in both sentences, the gap location is temporarily ambiguous. In (50) a gap could occur after the verb *killed* (as in, "the soldier killed the general") or after the preposition *for*. In (51) the gap could be after the verb *worried* (as in "the dog worried the cat") or after the preposition *about*. As the sentence unfolds, the processor must resolve the ambiguity of the location of the gap (that is, to which element the filler attaches). Here again, two theories oppose on the mechanisms underlying ambiguity resolution.

One approach (generally associated with FBAs) stipulates that the processor always posits a filler-gap dependency if the verb takes an object complement (**First-resort** or **Active Filler** strategies; Clifton & Frazier, 1989; Pickering, 1993). Another view postulates that the filler will be linked to the gap if the verb takes an object complement and that complement is its most frequent subcategorization or complementation frame (a view typical of certain CBAs). These theories make differential predictions for the processing of (50) and (51); both verbs (*killed* and *worried*) can take object complements, but only "killed" appears most frequently with an NP complement (*worried* tends to take a prepositional phrase as a complement, as in *to worry about*). A first-resort-type strategy would suggest that the processor tries to assign the filler to both verbs and their gaps immediately (the correct linkage to the preposition *about* is made later on in this view). The other possibility is that the NP filler gets associated to the verb "killed" (in (50)) but not to "worried" (in (51)), following the relative frequency

of their subcategorization frames. The idea is that the processor guesses, based on this frequency, that the filler is not an object of the verb but rather a complement of another element (in (51), of the preposition *about*). Self-paced reading times and eye-tracking evidence show that the NP filler is initially linked to the verb, regardless of subcategorization preferences (Pickering & Traxler, 2001, 2003). These results demonstrate that the processor attempts to resolve the dependency as quickly as possible, perhaps due to its memory cost (we will return to this idea soon). However, the processor might not posit a gap in cases where the filler is an implausible object of the verb, perhaps because the verb requires an animate object and the NP is inanimate; that is, NPs might only attach to a verb if it passes a basic semantic feature check (perhaps on animacy) to ensure a minimal probability for the NP to indeed be an argument of the verb (Pickering & Traxler, 2001, 2003).

An often-overlooked factor seems to have an even stronger influence on dependency resolution: prosody. In effect, prosody could provide the processor with cues it can use to determine where gaps are. Consider these ambiguous gap-filling constructions:

52. <u>Which doctor</u> did the supervisor call *1* [t] to get help for his youngest daughter?
53. <u>Which doctor</u> did the supervisor call *1* to get help for [t] during the crisis?

These sentences are similar to (50) and (51) in that the filler (underlined) could initially be taken to be the object of the verb (*call*). It turns out that these sentences have distinct prosodic contours: the duration of the verb is longer and its fundamental frequency declines more steeply in (52) in which the verb is immediately followed by a gap, than in (53), where the actual gap appears later in the sentence (after the preposition *for*). Thus, prosodic information can indicate the position of a gap, but does the processor use this information to disambiguate the sentence? In fact, it does: in a Cross-Modal Priming study, priming for *doctor* was found after the verb only in (52) (Nagel et al., 1994). In other words, the processor posits a gap only if the verb's prosodic contour signals one. Note that this conclusion is not necessarily contradictory with the findings that the processor forms a dependency as soon as possible (recall sentences (52) and (53): this evidence comes from reading, in which prosody plays no role). It thus appears that in the absence of disambiguating prosody, the processor has no choice but to test each potential gap.

Taken together, the evidence from gap-filling shows that the processor prefers to postulate the filler-gap dependency as quickly as possible, even if it is likely incorrect. The process of linking an NP and its theta-role assigner (a verb or a preposition) is fast, precise and quite robust against influence from nonsyntactic factors. On the other hand, the processor appears to efficiently integrate prosodic information to ensure successful gap-filling.

It turns out that gap-filling constructions are particularly problematic for some individuals with aphasia, and thus the results from neurologically healthy adults described above serve as a baseline in which to test sentence comprehension in aphasia (see Chapter 10).

Complexity

Intuitively, we know that ambiguous sentences are more difficult to ultimately comprehend than unambiguous ones. Similarly, gap-filling constructions are harder to understand than basic, active sentences. Why is this so? This is not as simple a question as it sounds. In fact, as we discussed earlier, there is a host of sentence processing models that specifically attempt to **operationalize** (define) complexity. So there is no clear consensus on what complexity means; yet our theories of language processing all hinge upon it insofar as models are built from empirical evidence that associates processing costs and complexity to psycholinguistic factors. Perhaps even more significant is the concept of complexity in the study of language disorders, where deficits have been proposed to arise from insufficient resources to process complex sentences (see Chapter 10).

It is beyond the scope of this chapter to fully address the question of complexity. Still, it is crucial that you think of complexity critically whenever you study language and its disorders and/or assess language functions in a clinical setting. In this section, we briefly present some definitions of complexity as implicitly or explicitly assumed in the scientific literature.

Let's begin by contrasting two (gap-filling) sentences that have been extensively studied:

54. The dog watched <u>the boy</u> who [*t*] kissed the girl. Subject Relative
55. The dog watched <u>the girl</u> who the boy kissed [*t*]. Object Relative

In both sentences, "the boy kissed the girl." However, *the dog watched* either *the boy* (the subject in the **Subject Relative,** (54)) or *the girl* (the object in the **Object Relative,** (55)). To specify which boy (or girl) the dog watched, the appropriate NP is relativized, that is, is followed by a relative clause (*who kissed the girl* in (54)) that provides additional information on the NP. The trace and the relativized NP (underlined) co-refer, which means the filler of the gap is the relativized NP (via the pronoun) and the person being watched is also

the same person kissing (or being kissed). Thus, it is understood from (54) that the dog watched the boy, and that the same boy kissed the girl.

Now, we have already seen that these constructions involve gap-filling, a process that does not apply in sentences without gaps. Hence, relative sentences are generally considered more difficult than others that do not require this additional parsing operation. Further, relative sentences are not equivalently complex: object relatives are harder to process than subject relatives in English (Ford, 1983; King & Just, 1991, and many others). This finding was replicated using various methodologies (self-paced reading, eye-tracking, event-related potentials) and utilized as the basis of a very large number of functional magnetic resonance imaging studies of syntactic processing.

Despite its well-established existence, this complexity effect is not clearly understood. First, it is not a universal phenomenon: although object-relatives (ORs) are harder than subject-relatives (SRs) in many languages (French, Spanish, German, Dutch), recent studies suggest that the opposite is true in Chinese, Korean, Japanese and Basque (Hsiao & Gibson, 2003; Kwon, Polinsky & Kluender, 2006; Ishizuka, 2005; Carreiras et al., 2010; inter alia). Any explanation of the processing difference between ORs and SRs must then refer to sentence properties that also differ between these languages.

Many hypotheses have been formulated to explain the OR/SR complexity effect, some expecting language-universal effects without appealing to sentential structure whereas several other hypotheses appeal to structure in their definition of complexity. Proposals without recourse to structural properties include an Accessibility hierarchy (Keenan & Comrie, 1977; Dowty, 1991) and the Perspective Shift Hypothesis (see MacWhinney, 2008 for a recent iteration). The first claims that grammatical functions and/or thematic roles are ranked in terms of their accessibility, the higher position of subjects in the hierarchy makes them more salient—and easier to process—than objects. By extension, SRs are less difficult and less complex than ORs. The Perspective Shift Hypothesis attributes a processing cost to every switch in perspective within a sentence. In *The dog watched the boy who kissed the girl*, the focus moves away from the dog (in the main clause) toward the boy (in the relative clause). This switch is costly, but less so than the two switches implicated in ORs (from *dog* to *boy* to *girl* in (55)).

A more varied set of proposals set their complexity explanations in structural terms. For instance, the processing load for working memory would be higher for ORs than SRs because the filler must be maintained in memory over a longer period in (49) than in (48). Event-related studies have repeatedly reported an enhanced sustained left anterior negativity (an electrical waveform) following the filler in ORs compared to SRs (see Callahan, 2008 for an extensive review). This evidence suggests that verbal working memory resources are required to store a filler until it can be linked to its gap and interpreted (a need to limit resource expenditure might explain why the processor is so keen to posit gaps when a filler is held in memory). Then, starting some 300–500 ms after the onset of the word following the gap, the filler is retrieved and integrated into the sentential context. This integration, along with memory storage, is one source of processing cost according to the Syntactic Prediction Locality Theory (SPLT; Gibson, 1998). Simply put, a cost is imputed for each new discourse referent (e.g., a newly introduced NP) processed while a syntactic dependency remains unresolved. In other words, the longer a dependency (e.g., a filler "looking for" a gap) has to be kept in memory, the greater is the memory cost; the greater the distance between the gap and the word that attaches to it, the greater the integration cost. Distance is here defined in this case as the number of syntactic categories between two elements (memory cost) and as the number of new referents to build into the structure (integration cost). As you can see, although both types of costs (and hence, the complexity of a sentence) depend on notions of distance, the calculation of distance differs according to the type of cost being computed. Moreover, these definitions of distance and its relationship to processing costs are not the only possible ones: distance could be linearly quantified as the number of words between two elements; distance effects could reflect activation levels (decay in memory) or number of similar NPs intervening between two elements (creating memory interference; recall the Lewis and colleagues cue-based memory retrieval model from earlier).

However defined, ORs and SRs do not solely differ in terms of filler-gap distance. We have already discussed a possible hierarchy of syntactic roles (subject/agents over object/themes) and of perspective switches within a sentence. In ORs, the relativized NP is associated with two thematic roles: "boy" is the theme of "watched" and the agent of "kiss." In contrast, in SRs, the relativized NP is always associated with the theme role (the girl is the one being watched and kissed). It remains to be determined whether a "double role" or "role-switching" contributes to processing difficulty. Further, the expectations may diverge between ORs and SRs from a very early point on: an eye-tracking study has shown that the processing difficulty for ORs could be

greatly reduced by manipulating the animacy of the sentential subject (underlined):

56a. The <u>director</u> that watched the movie received a prize at the film festival. SR

56b. The <u>director</u> that the movie pleased received a prize at the film festival. OR

56c. The <u>movie</u> that pleased the director received a prize at the film festival. SR

56d. The <u>movie</u> that the director watched received a prize at the film festival. OR

In a series of eye-tracking studies, Traxler and colleagues (2002, 2005) replicated the OR/SR complexity effect in relatives with animate subjects (*director*). In sentences with inanimate subjects (*movie*), ORs were still more difficult than SRs, but the OR/SR difference was much less pronounced. Because the filler-gap distance remained the same for sentences with animate or inanimate subjects, the processing difficulty can be partly attributed to the animacy of the subject. Importantly, these findings demonstrate that syntactic complexity itself is quite complicated and that multiple factors probably contribute to it.

This enumeration of complexity aspects is by no means exhaustive, and is sure to be elaborated upon in future research. Many other factors involving sentence properties (word order, number of co-indexations, semantic constraints) and/or processing concepts (competition and interference among co-activated items, divergence from probabilistic or surprisal level) may also contribute to complexity. Also, these notions are not mutually exclusive—a combination of these factors (some language-universal, some language-specific) is highly likely to yield what we think of as "processing complexity." Finally, a good description of "complexity" will only take us so far without a careful account of what "cognitive resources" are, and how they relate to processing difficulty.

SUMMARY OF PSYCHOLINGUISTICS OF SENTENCE COMPREHENSION

In this section, we reviewed experimental evidence on the psycholinguistics of sentence comprehension. We discussed various exemplars of syntactically ambiguous and gap-filling constructions and the underlying processes involved in their comprehension. Importantly, we argued that these constructions could be used to test predictions by theoretical models on the processing of all sentence types.

Indeed, the empirical evidence we reviewed is restricted and summarized, but sufficient to demonstrate a fundamental aspect of (psycholinguistic) research: There is limited consensus on how the brain/mind goes about comprehending an input. Thus, there are numerous studies speaking to each issue presented in this section (and others we have not discussed). Experimental findings sometimes support, sometimes challenge, form-based accounts (FBAs), constraint-based accounts (CBAs) and resources-based accounts (RBAs). Psycholinguists' job is to assess the support for each model and modify them as necessary to better account for the available data. New findings are reported in the scientific literature every day, so the state of affairs today will have changed in a couple of years. This section aimed to provide you with a general framework and the conceptual tools to insightfully follow (or revisit) this literature and its evolution.

What are the take-home messages from the psycholinguistics we discussed? To begin, two key aspects sentence processing stand out from our discussion of the empirical evidence: 1) the crucial importance of timing in the computation of an interpretation; 2) the central role of verbs in processing and interpretation. On the one hand, it is unequivocal from experimental data that sentence comprehension takes place over time, thus the interest in the moment-by-moment detailing of the mental operations that take place during the computation of an interpretation. Certain processes, such as syntactic ambiguity resolution and gap-filling, require fast and timely execution to ensure successful comprehension. In fact, alterations to the normal time-course may hinder comprehension (see Chapter 10 for examples from slow speech input in disordered language). On the other hand, the main discordance between theoretical models regards the exact point in time at which information types are integrated. Hence, our understanding of the sentence processing system hinges on timing issues, and consequently on the use of appropriate techniques to investigate both online and offline processing (this also holds true for disordered language).

A second, striking aspect is the fundamental role of verbs in processing and interpretation. Verb properties not only define "who does what to whom" in a sentence, they are the cause or motivation for many processes. The evidence showed, for example, that: when a verb is encountered in a sentence, its argument structure configurations (or complementation frames) are activated; a verb's subcategorization frames may give rise to structural ambiguity; a verb's semantic constraints impose a thematic fit on its arguments (such as animacy or plausibility), resulting in processing difficulty if nonrespected and; a verb's displaced argument must rapidly be integrated with the verb, triggering gap-filling. The satisfaction of verb constraints is thus a driving force of sentence comprehension.

Taken together, the findings reviewed in this section also pointed to interactions between information types. For instance, syntax identifies an NP as a filler while prosody guides the processor in determining where the associated gap is located; a structural ambiguity is resolved considering prosodic contours and/or a verb's constraints on plausible objects. It can thus be extremely difficult to single out one process or the individual contribution of an information type, especially if the timing of these effects differs. This particularity may be one of the reasons sentence complexity and processing difficulty are still relatively poorly understood. It also remains to be seen to what extent context can influence the processes underlying comprehension, although promising research—particularly using the visual world paradigm with eye-tracking (see Box 6-1)—already hints to the influence of nonlinguistic factors.

CONCLUSIONS

Language processing is an intricate cognitive function that appears to be sensitive to different sorts of information, some linguistic, some not. It interacts with other cognitive functions, such as attention and memory, and on some accounts these cognitive functions are embedded into language processing itself. It is also exquisitely sensitive to time, such that on some accounts, certain information types are used early in the processing stream, and others used later. The revelations about language processing are based on measurements that we make during particular tasks, and since there are a wide variety of such tasks, we often end up with disparate results across studies. This, of course, is true of any scientific endeavor and only further work will help clear up these disparities. Furthermore, because we are attempting to understand a system that emerges from the intricacies of the neurological system, we are essentially building theories of the inherently unobservable by using observable phenomena (e.g., speaker intuitions, reaction times, reading times, etc.). Thus, we can never be completely sure if our hypotheses and theories are correct, and this is also true of any science. Even so, these roadblocks do not stop us from trying to penetrate such a complex system, and the more we try, the more we learn. Finally, it turns out that the more we learn about a system that is working under optimal conditions, the more we can use that knowledge to understand disordered systems, and hence bridge the basic and clinical sciences.

REFERENCES

Adger, D. (2003). *Core syntax: A minimalist approach.* Oxford University Press.

Balogh, J., Zurif, E., Prather, P., Swinney, D., & Finkel, L. (1998). Gap-filling and end-of-sentence effects in real-time language processing: implications for modeling sentence comprehension in aphasia. *Brain and Language, 61*(2), 169–182. doi:10.1006/brln.1997.1917

Beach, C. M. (1991). The interpretation of prosodic patterns at points of syntactic structure ambiguity: Evidence for cue trading relations. *Journal of Memory and Language, 30*(6), 644–663. doi:10.1016/0749-596X(91)90030-N

Boland, J. E., Tanenhaus, M. K., & Garnsey, S. M. (1990). Evidence for the immediate use of verb control information in sentence processing. *Journal of Memory and Language, 29*(4), 413–432. doi:10.1016/0749-596X(90)90064-7

Callahan, S. M. (2008). Processing anaphoric constructions: Insights from electrophysiological studies. *Journal of Neurolinguistics, 21*(3), 231–266. doi:10.1016/j.jneuroling.2007.10.002

Carreiras, M., Duñabeitia, J. A., Vergara, M., de la Cruz-Pavía, I., & Laka, I. (2010). Subject relative clauses are not universally easier to process: Evidence from Basque. *Cognition, 115*(1), 79–92. doi:10.1016/j.cognition.2009.11.012

Chodorow, M. S. (1979). *Time-compressed speech and the study of lexical and syntactic processing. Sentence processing.* Hillsdale, NJ: Erlbaum.

Chomsky, N. (1970). Remarks on nominalization. In R. Jacobs & P. Rosenbaum (Eds.), *Reading in English transformational grammar* (pp. 184–221). Waltham, MA: Ginn.

Clifton, C., & Frazier, L. (1989). Comprehending sentences with long-distance dependencies. In G. Carlson & M. Tanenhaus (Eds.), *Linguistic structure in language processing.* (pp. 273–317). Boston: Springer.

Clifton, C., Speer, S., & Abney, S. P. (1991). Parsing arguments: Phrase structure and argument structure as determinants of initial parsing decisions. *Journal of Memory and Language, 30*(2), 251–271. doi:10.1016/0749-596X(91)90006-6

Cuetos, F., & Mitchell, D. C. (1988). Cross-linguistic differences in parsing: Restrictions on the use of the Late Closure strategy in Spanish. *Cognition, 30*(1), 73–105. doi:10.1016/0010-0277(88)90004-2

Dowty, D. (1991). Thematic proto-roles and argument selection. *Language, 67*(3), 547–619. doi:10.2307/415037

Engelhardt, P. E., Ferreira, F., & Patsenko, E. G. (2010). Pupillometry reveals processing load during spoken language comprehension. *Quarterly Journal of Experimental Psychology, 63*, 639–645.

Ferreira, F., Bailey, K. G., & Ferraro, V. (2002). Good-enough representations in language comprehension. *Current Directions in Psychological Science, 11*(1), 11–15. doi:10.1111/1467-8721.00158

Ferreira, F., & Clifton, C. (1986). The independence of syntactic processing. *Journal of Memory and Language, 25*(3), 348–368. doi:10.1016/0749-596X(86)90006-9

Fodor, J. (1983). *The modularity of mind: An essay on faculty psychology.* Cambridge, MA: MIT Press.

Fodor, J. A., Garrett, M., & Bever, T. G. (1968). Some syntactic determinants of sentential complexity, II: verb structure. *Perception and Psychophysic, 3*, 453–460.

Ford, M. (1983). A method for obtaining measures of local parsing complexity throughout sentences. *Journal of Verbal Learning and Verbal Behavior, 22*(2), 203–218. doi:10.1016/S0022-5371(83)90156-1

Frazier, L. (1987). Sentence processing: A tutorial review. In *Attention and performance, XII: The psychology of reading.* Hillsdale, NJ: Lawrence Erlbaum Associates.

Frazier, L., & Clifton, C. (1996). *Construal.* Cambridge, MA: MIT Press.

Frazier, L., & Fodor, J. D. (1978). The sausage machine: A new two-stage parsing model. *Cognition, 6*(4), 291–325. doi:10.1016/0010-0277(78)90002-1

Frazier, L., & Rayner, K. (1982). Making and correcting errors during sentence comprehension: Eye movements in the analysis of structurally ambiguous sentences. *Cognitive Psychology, 14*(2), 178–210. doi:10.1016/0010-0285(82)90008-1

Garnsey, S. M., Pearlmutter, N. J., Myers, E., & Lotocky, M. A. (1997). The contributions of verb bias and plausibility to the comprehension of temporarily ambiguous sentences. *Journal of Memory and Language, 37*(1), 58–93. doi:10.1006/jmla.1997.2512

Gibson, E. (1998). Linguistic complexity: locality of syntactic dependencies. *Cognition, 68*(1), 1–76. doi:10.1016/S0010-0277(98)00034-1

Grimshaw, J. B. B. (1977). English wh-constructions and the theory of grammar. Electronic Doctoral Dissertations for UMass Amherst. Paper AAI7803835. http://scholarworks.umass.edu/dissertations/AAI7803835

Hale, J. (2003). The information conveyed by words in sentences. *Journal of Psycholinguistic Research, 32*(2), 101–123.

Holmes, V., & Forster, K. (1972). Perceptual complexity and underlying sentence structure. *Journal of Verbal Learning and Verbal Behavior, 11*(2), 148–156. doi:10.1016/S0022-5371(72)80071-9

Hsiao, F., & Gibson, E. (2003). Processing relative clauses in Chinese. *Cognition, 90*(1), 3–27. doi:10.1016/S0010-0277(03)00124-0

Ishizuka, T. (2005). Processing relative clauses in Japanese. *UCLA Working Papers in Linguistics, 13*, 135–157.

Ito, K., & Speer, S. (2006). Using interactive tasks to elicit natural dialogue. In P. Augurzky & D. Lenertova (Eds.), *Methods in empirical prosody research* (pp. 229–257). New York: Mouton de Gruyter.

Jackendoff, Ray (1977). *X-bar-syntax: A study of phrase structure.* Linguistic Inquiry Monograph 2. Cambridge, MA: MIT Press.

Keenan, E. L., & Comrie, B. (1977). Noun phrase accessibility and universal grammar. *Linguistic Inquiry, 8*(1), 63–99.

King, J., & Just, M. A. (1991). Individual differences in syntactic processing: The role of working memory. *Journal of Memory and Language, 30*(5), 580–602. doi:10.1016/0749-596X(91)90027-H

Konieczny, L., Hemforth, B., Scheepers, C., & Strube, G. (1997). The role of lexical heads in parsing: Evidence from German. *Language and Cognitive Processes, 12*(2), 307–348.

Kwon, N., Polinsky, M., & Kluender, R. (2006). Subject preference in Korean. In *Proceedings of WCCFL, 25*, 1–14.

Levy, R. (2008). Expectation-based syntactic comprehension. *Cognition, 106*(3), 1126–1177. doi:10.1016/j.cognition.2007.05.006

Lewis, R. L., Vasishth, S., & Van Dyke, J. A. (2006). Computational principles of working memory in sentence comprehension. *Trends in Cognitive Sciences*, *10*(10), 447–454. doi:10.1016/j.tics.2006.08.007

Love, T., & Swinney, D. (1996). Coreference processing and levels of analysis in object-relative constructions; demonstration of antecedent reactivation with the cross-modal priming paradigm. *Journal of Psycholinguistic Research*, *25*(1), 5–24.

MacDonald, M. C., Pearlmutter, N. J., & Seidenberg, M. S. (1994). The lexical nature of syntactic ambiguity resolution [corrected]. *Psychological Review*, *101*(4), 676–703.

MacWhinney, B. (2008). How mental models encode embodied linguistic perspectives. In R. Klatzky, B. MacWhinney, & M. Behrmann (Eds.), *Embodiment, ego-space, and action* (pp. 369–410). Mahwah: Lawrence Erlbaum.

Miller, G. A., Heise, G. A., & Lichten, W. (1951). The intelligibility of speech as a function of the context of the test materials. *Journal of Experimental Psychology*, *41*(5), 329–335. doi:10.1037/h0062491

Miller, G. A., & Isard, S. (1963). Some perceptual consequences of linguistic rules. *Journal of Verbal Learning and Verbal Behavior*, *2*(3), 217–228. doi:10.1016/S0022-5371(63)80087-0

Miller, G. A., & Selfridge, J. A. (1950). Verbal context and the recall of meaningful material. *The American Journal of Psychology*, *63*(2), 176–185. doi:10.2307/1418920

Miyamoto, E. T. (1998). A low attachment preference in Brazilian Portuguese relative clauses. Architecture and Mechanisms of Language Processing (AMLaP), Friburg, September 24–26.

Nagel, H. N., Shapiro, L. P., & Nawy, R. (1994). Prosody and the processing of filler-gap sentences. *Journal of Psycholinguistic Research*, *23*(6), 473–485.

Nagel, H. N., Shapiro, L. P., Tuller, B., & Nawy, R. (1996). Prosodic influences on the resolution of temporary ambiguity during on-line sentence processing. *Journal of Psycholinguistic Research*, *25*(2), 319–344.

Nicol, J. L. (1988). Coreference processing during sentence comprehension. Electronic Doctoral Dissertations for Massachusetts Institute of Technology. http://hdl.handle.net/1721.1/14421

Nicol, J., & Swinney, D. (1989). The role of structure in coreference assignment during sentence comprehension. *Journal of Psycholinguistic Research*, *18*(1), 5–19.

Osterhout, L., & Swinney, D. A. (1993). On the temporal course of gap-filling during comprehension of verbal passives. *Journal of Psycholinguistic Research*, *22*(2), 273–286.

Pickering, M. (1993). Direct association and sentence processing: A reply to Gorrell and to Gibson and Hickok. *Language and Cognitive Processes*, *8*(2), 163–196.

Pickering, M. J., & Traxler, M. J. (1998). Plausibility and recovery from garden paths: An eye-tracking study. *Journal of Experimental Psychology: Learning, Memory, and Cognition*, *24*, 940–961.

Pickering, M. J., & Traxler, M. J. (2001). Strategies for processing unbounded dependencies: Lexical information and verb-argument assignment. *Journal of Experimental Psychology: Learning, Memory, and Cognition*, *27*(6), 1401–1410.

Pickering, M. J., & Traxler, M. J. (2003). Evidence against the use of subcategorization frequency in the processing of unbounded dependencies. *Language and Cognitive Processes*, *18*(4), 469–503.

Pickering, M. J., Traxler, M. J., & Crocker, M. W. (2000). Ambiguity resolution in sentence processing: Evidence against frequency-based accounts. *Journal of Memory and Language*, *43*(3), 447–475.

Price, P., Ostendorf, M., Shattuck-Hufnagel, S., & Fong, C. (1991). The use of prosody in syntactic disambiguation. *Journal of the Acoustical Society of America*, *90*(6), 2956–2970.

Pritchett, B. L. (1988). Garden path phenomena and the grammatical basis of language processing. *Language*, *64*(3), 539–576.

Radford, A. (2004). *Minimalist syntax: Exploring the structure of English*. Cambridge, UK: Cambridge University Press.

Rayner, K., & Frazier, L. (1987). Parsing temporarily ambiguous compléments. *Quarterly Journal of Experimental Psychology*, *39A*, 657–673.

Schafer, A. J., Speer, S. R., Warren, P., & White, S. D. (2000). Intonational disambiguation in sentence production and comprehension. *Journal of Psycholinguistic Research*, *29*(2), 169–182.

Shapiro, L. P., Brookins, B., Gordon, B., & Nagel, N. (1991). Verb effects during sentence processing. *Journal of Experimental Psychology: Learning, Memory, and Cognition*, *17*(5), 983–996.

Shapiro, L. P., Nagel, H. N., & Levine, B. A. (1993). Preferences for a verb's complements and their use in sentence processing. *Journal of Memory and Language*, *32*, 96–114.

Shapiro, L. P., Zurif, E., & Grimshaw, J. (1987). Sentence processing and the mental representation of verbs. *Cognition*, *27*(3), 219–246.

Shapiro, L. P., Zurif, E. B., & Grimshaw, J. (1989). Verb processing during sentence comprehension: Contextual impenetrability. *Journal of Psycholinguistic Research*, *18*(2), 223–243.

Shetreet, E., Palti, D., Friedmann, N., & Hadar, U. (2007). Cortical representation of verb processing in sentence comprehension: Number of complements, subcategorization, and thematic frames. *Cerebral Cortex*, *17*(8), 1958.

Speer, S., Kjelgaard, M., & Doborth, K. (1996). The influence of prosodic structure on the resolution of temporary syntactic closure ambiguities. *Journal of Psycholinguistic Research*, *25*(2), 249–271. doi:10.1007/BF01708573

Swinney, D. A. (1979). Lexical access during sentence comprehension:(Re) consideration of context effects. *Journal of verbal learning and verbal behavior*, *18*(6), 645–659.

Townsend, D. J., & Bever, T. G. (2001). *Sentence comprehension: The integration of habits and rules*. Cambridge, MA: MIT Press.

Traxler, M. J., Morris, R. K., & Seely, R. E. (2002). Processing subject and object relative clauses: evidence from eye movements. *Journal of Memory and Language*, *47*(1), 69–90.

Traxler, M. J., Williams, R. S., Blozis, S. A., & Morris, R. K. (2005). Working memory, animacy, and verb class in the processing of relative clauses. *Journal of Memory and Language*, *53*(2), 204–224.

Trueswell, J. C., Tanenhaus, M. K., & Kello, C. (1993). Verb-specific constraints in sentence processing: Separating effects of lexical preference from garden-paths. *Journal of Experimental Psychology: Learning, Memory and Cognition*, *19*, 528–553.

Trueswell, J. C., Tanenhaus, M. K., & Garnsey, S. M. (1994). Semantic influences on parsing: use of thematic role information in syntactic ambiguity resolution. *Journal of Memory and Language*, *33*(3), 285–318. doi:10.1006/jmla.1994.1014

Zagar, D., Pynte, J., & Rativeau, S. (1997). Evidence for early closure attachment on first pass reading times in French. *The Quarterly Journal of Experimental Psychology Section A*, *50*(2), 421–438.

CHAPTER 7

The Executive Functions in Language and Communication

CHAPTER OUTLINE

Alfredo Ardila

DEFINING EXECUTIVE FUNCTIONS

The understanding of the role of the prefrontal cortex in behavior and cognition and the concept of executive functions have been developed through a series of progressive historical steps.

During the late nineteenth and early twentieth centuries, clinical investigators documented diverse behavioral disorders in cases of prefrontal lobe pathology. It was observed that prefrontal pathology did not result in any evident sensory or motor disturbance, but behavioral/personality changes were frequently found. Phineas Gage has become the most typical illustration of frontal lobe dysfunction and has significantly contributed to the understanding of the role of the frontal lobes in behavior. Harlow (1868) described Phineas Gage as a responsible foreman for a railroad company who suffered a tragic accident in which a tampering rod was projected through his frontal lobes. After this accident, profound personality changes were evident, and he was described as "no longer Gage" by associates who perceived his behavior as "profane," "irascible," and "irresponsible." It was of interest to Harlow that cognitive functions (i.e., memory, language, etc.) remained intact, whereas personality (manner of behaving) was so greatly altered. Phineas Gage has become one of the best known classical cases in the history of the neurosciences, and different papers have been devoted to its analysis (e.g., Damasio, Grabowski, Frank, et al., 1994; Macmillan, 2000, 2008).

In 1880 Herman Oppenheim coined the term *witzelsucht*, which was demonstrated by childishness and joking with "alleged" cheerfulness (Oppenheim, 1890, 1891). The term *moria* (reflecting "stupidity" and a jocular attitude) was part of the change they observed associated with damage in the prefrontal regions of the brain. Oppenheim's patients all had tumors involving right frontal areas, frequently invading the mesial and basal areas. Jastrowitz (1888) further noted unconcern and "inappropriate cheerfulness" associated with right frontal pathology.

The term "executive functions" is a relatively new term in the neurosciences, and until recently, the preferred term was "frontal lobe functions" (or "prefrontal functions"). "Frontal lobe syndrome" was conceptualized by Feuchtwanger in 1923. He correlated frontal lobe pathology to behaviors that were not related to overt speech, memory, or sensorimotor deficits. He emphasized the personality changes in motivation, affective dysregulation, and the incapacity to regulate and integrate other behaviors. During the following years, particularly during the 1980s and 1990s, a diversity of books specifically devoted to the analysis of frontal lobe syndrome were published (e.g., Fuster, 1989; Levin, Eisenberg & Benton, 1991; Miller & Cummings, 1998; Perecman, 1987; Pribram & Luria, 1973; Stuss & Benson, 1986).

Luria (1980) can be regarded as the direct antecessor of the term "executive functions." He distinguished three functional units in the brain: (1) arousal-motivation (limbic and reticular systems); (2) receiving, processing, and storing information (postrolandic cortical areas); and (3) programming, controlling, and verifying activity (frontal lobes). Luria mentions that this third unit has an executive role. Lezak (1983) used the term "executive functions" to discriminate cognitive functions from the "how" or "whether" of human behaviors. Lezak emphasized the fluid nature of executive functioning and how dependent the cognitive and emotional aspects of functioning were on the "executive." Baddeley (1986) grouped these behaviors into cognitive domains that included problems in planning, organizing behaviors, disinhibition, perseveration, reduced fluency, and initiation. Baddeley also coined the term "dysexecutive syndrome."

The definition of executive function is encompassed by actions fueled by conceptualizations, such as the ability to filter interference; control attention; engage in goal-directed behaviors; abstracting; problem-solving; metacognition; anticipate the consequences of one's actions; program motor behavior; inhibit immediate responses; regulate behavior verbally; reorient behavior according to behavioral consequences; perform temporal integration of behavior, personality integrity, and consciousness; and the adaptive concept of mental flexibility (Denckla, 1996; Fuster, 2001; Goldberg, 2001; Grafman, 2006; Luria, 1969, 1980; Miller & Cummings, 1998; Stuss & Benson, 1986; Stuss & Knight, 2002). The concept of morality, ethical behaviors, self-awareness, and the idea of the frontal lobes as manager and programmer of the human psyche are also included. Elliott (2003) defines executive functioning as complex processing requiring the coordination of several subprocesses to achieve a particular goal. Intact frontal processes, although not synonymous with executive functioning, are integral to its function.

Although executive functions depend on extended dynamic networks including different brain areas (Koziol & Budding, 2009), it is assumed that the prefrontal cortex plays a major controlling and monitoring role. Neuroimaging results have also implicated posterior, cortical, and subcortical regions in executive functioning (Roberts, Robbins, & Weiskrantz, 2002). Most importantly, the prefrontal cortex does not only participate in those classically recognized executive operations (sequencing, alternating, inhibiting, etc.), but it also plays a core role in coordinating cognition and emotion (Mitchell & Phillips, 2007). Interestingly, most of the disturbances reported in Phineas Gage (and in many cases of prefrontal syndromes) refer to behavioral/emotional disturbances; or more precisely, disturbances in coordinating cognition and emotion/motivation. As noted by Harlow (1868) cognitive functions in Phineas Gage remained intact. The prefrontal lobe has extensive connections to subcortical and limbic system areas (Barbas, 2006; Damasio & Anderson, 2003), and even its orbital portion could be regarded as an extension of the limbic system. Stuss and Alexander (2000) suggest that the most important role of the frontal lobes includes affective responsiveness, social behavior, and personality development. The frontal lobes, particularly the right lobe, have also been related with empathy in general and with "theory of mind"—the ability to attribute mental states to others—in particular (Platek, Keenan, Gallup, & Mohamed, 2004; Stuss, Gallup, & Alexander, 2001).

Currently, frontal lobe function research is utilizing functional brain imaging techniques to pool collateral findings, look at antecedents, and use a large sample size to eliminate spurious variables; thus, brain regions that contribute to dysexecutive syndromes may prove to be more multifunctional (Lloyd, 2000). Functional imaging has demonstrated that adults and children with focal, especially frontal right-hemispheric, lesions display similar behaviors such as attentional deficits, inability to inhibit a response, and impersistence of activity (Filley, Young, Reardon, & Wilkening, 1999).

Typically, executive functions are analyzed in experimental conditions using diverse research strategies, such as solving diverse problems, finding similarities between two words, providing an answer that requires inhibiting another, etc. A paradigm is created, and the subject is required to solve it. Brain activity can be recorded simultaneously, using brain electrical activity or recording the regional level of activation (e.g., Osaka, Osaka, Mondo, et al., 2004). Alternatively, executive functions are analyzed in brain-damaged populations in order to find the contribution of different brain systems (e.g., Jacobs, Harvey, & Anderson, 2007). This last approach represents the classical neuropsychological method. Executive functions, however, are rarely analyzed in natural ecological conditions.

The Anatomy of the Frontal Lobes

Anatomically, the frontal lobes are the largest lobes of the brain. Laterally, they are anterior to the Rolandic fissure and superior to the Sylvian fissure. Medially, they extend forward from the Rolandic fissure and the corpus callosum. The frontal lobes include (a) the posterior regions of the frontal cortex (agranular frontal cortex), associated with motor activity. They correspond to the primary motor area (Brodmann's area—BA—4, or the precentral gyrus), on one hand; and the premotor area (or motor association area: BA6, 8—frontal eye field, and BA44—Broca's area), on the other. And (b) the prefrontral cortex (or granular frontal cortex), corresponding to BA9, 10, 11, 12, 24, 32, 45, 46, and 47, as illustrated in Figure 7-1. The prefrontal cortex is usually subdivided into the dorsolateral, mesial, and orbital regions. The limbic components of the frontal lobe include the anterior cingulum and the posterior section of the frontal orbital cortex (Damasio & Anderson, 2003; Fuster, 2008; Mesulam, 2002).

The frontal lobe increases in size throughout phylogenetic evolution. Given the overall size of the human brain, the entire frontal lobe of humans is approximately as large as expected for a primate brain (Semendeferi, Lu, Schenker, & Damasio, 2002), yet two portions of the frontal lobe (the primary motor and premotor areas) are significantly smaller; consequently, the prefrontal area is larger than expected (Schoenemann, 2006). The human prefrontal cortex is much larger than that in pongids (chimpanzees, gorillas, and orangutans): 12.7% of total brain volume, compared with an average of 10.3% for pongid species. Differences are observed in the white matter rather than in the gray matter. Comparing humans (brain size about 1350 cm^2) with chimpanzees (brain size about 311 cm^2), prefrontal gray volumes are 4.8 times larger in humans, whereas nonprefrontal gray volumes are only 4.2 times larger. However, prefrontal white volumes are about 5.0 times larger in humans, whereas nonprefrontal white volumes are only 3.3 times larger (Schoenemann, Sheehan, & Glotzer, 2005).

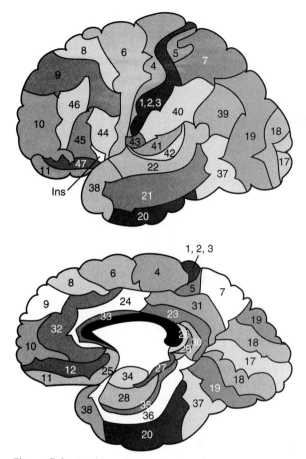

Figure 7-1 Brodmann's areas. Prefrontal cortex corresponds to areas 9, 10, 11, 12, 24, 32, 45, 46, and 47. [Adapted from Bernal, B., & Perdomo, J. (2009). *Brodmann's interactive atlas 1.1.* http://www.fmriconsulting.com/brodmann/]

The prefrontal areas of the frontal lobes can be regarded as association areas or intrinsic cortical areas. Luria (1980) considers that the prefrontal regions correspond to tertiary areas (which participate in processing information of various types) of the cerebral cortex. The prefrontal lobes maintain extensive connections, particularly with other cortical areas, the limbic system, the cortical and subcortical motor areas, and the sensory cortex.

Intracortical Connections

The major cortical connections are established with the visual, auditory, and somatosensory cortexes. The prefrontal cortex is also connected with the premotor cortex, and through this, with the primary motor cortex. Some projections are unidirectional (e.g., the caudate nucleus and the putamen); and others appear to be bidirectional (e.g., the dorsomedial nucleus of the thalamus) (Damasio & Anderson, 2003). There are multiple intracortical connections, including the superior longitudinal fasciculus—the main bundle of fibers between the posterior and anterior regions of the cerebral cortex. The uncinate fasciculus connects the anterior temporal lobe with the frontal lobe. The orbitofrontal limbic and mesial frontal cortexes receive projections from the superior temporal gyrus, and the orbitofrontal region receives projections from the inferior temporal cortex. The cingulum connects the frontal lobe with the parahippocampal gyrus. The arcuate fasciculus borders the insula and connects the inferior frontal and medial gyri with the temporal lobe. The occipitofrontal fasciculus extends posteriorly from the frontal lobe to the temporal and occipital lobes (Figure 7-2).

Subcortical Connections

According to Damasio and Anderson (2003), it is possible to distinguish the following types of fronto-subcortical connections:

Projection from the Hypothalamus

Although no direct connections between the hypothalamus and the prefrontal cortex seem to exist, there have been signs of indirect connections, particularly through the thalamus.

Projections from the Amygdala and Hippocampus

There have been signs of some projections toward the mesial aspects of the frontal lobe, particularly to the gyrus rectus and the subcallosal and anterior portions of the cingulum.

Projections from the Thalamus

The projections from the thalamus are primarily directed from the dorsolateral nucleus of the thalamus toward the orbital frontal cortex. Other additional connections have been discrete, as is the projection from the medial pulvinar nucleus to BA8.

Projections to the Amygdala and Hippocampus

Direct connections exist as do indirect connections through the cingulum and the uncinate fasciculus.

Projections to the Thalamus

These projections move toward the dorsal medial nucleus, the intralaminar nuclei, and the pulvinar.

Projections to the Hypothalamus

These projections are nuclear, probably through the mesencephalon and the periaquaductal gray matter.

Projections to the Striatum

Projections to the caudate nucleus and putamen have been identified. Especially important are the projections from the cingulum and the supplementary motor area (SMA), which are related to the motor control system of the brain.

Projections to the Claustrum, Subthalamic Region, and Mesencephalon

These projections go through the uncinate fasciculus and the external capsule. They originate primarily in the orbital and inferior dorsolateral regions.

In summary, the prefrontal cortex has extensive connections with the rest of the cerebral cortex, as well as with the limbic system, the basal ganglia, the thalamus, and other brain areas.

Some disagreement exists around the question of whether or not there is a single unitary factor accounting for the diversity of executive functions (e.g., Grafman, 2006; Kimberg, D'Esposito, & Farah, 1997; Stuss & Alexander, 2007). Friedman and colleagues (2008) found that executive functions are highly correlated, suggesting a common factor that goes beyond general intelligence. These authors concluded that executive functions represent one of the most heritable psychological traits. It is not evident, however, what the particular unitary factor saturating the different executive function tests could be. Some different proposals and interpretations have been presented during recent years.

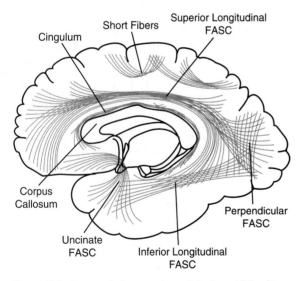

Figure 7-2 Intracortical connections of the frontal lobe. [From Gray, H., Standring, S., et al. (2005). *Gray's Anatomy: The Anatomical Basis of Clinical Practice.* (39th ed.) Edinburgh: Elsevier/Churchill Livingstone Ltd.]

Behavior inhibition has been considered as a potential candidate for the single factor responsible for successful performance in different executive tests (Barkley, 1997) alone or in combination with working memory (Pennington & Ozonoff, 1996). Salthouse (1996, 2005), on the other hand, suggested that reasoning and perceptual speed represent the underlying factors related to all executive functions. Salthouse (2005) observed that performance on two common tests of executive functioning, the Wisconsin Card Sorting Test and the Controlled Oral Word Association Test, were strongly correlated with reasoning ability and perceptual speed.

Other researchers challenge the existence of such a unitary factor. Thus, some authors have emphasized that certain frontal lobe patients perform well on some tests purported to assess executive abilities but not on others (Godefroy, Cabaret, Petit-Chenal, et al., 1999). Furthermore, it has been reported that correlations among different executive tests are frequently moderate or low and very often lack statistical significance (Salthouse, Atkinson, & Berish, 2003).

Some other investigators have taken an intermediate position. For instance, Miyake, Friedman, Emerson, et al. (2000) studied three often-postulated aspects of executive functions (shifting, updating, and inhibition) and concluded that, although these functions are clearly distinguishable, they do share some underlying commonality. Based on the results of their study, the authors stated that executive functions are "separable but moderately correlated constructs" thus suggesting both unitary and nonunitary components of the executive system. By the same token, several authors have suggested different subcomponents of executive functions (e.g., Anderson, 2001; Delis, Kaplan, & Kramer, 2001; Denckla, 1994; Elliott, 2003; Hobson & Leeds, 2001; Lafleche & Albert, 1995; Piguet, Grayson, Browe, et al., 2002). Thus, Stuss and Alexander (2007) refer to three separate frontal attentional processes within the executive category: energization (superior medial), task setting (left lateral), and monitoring (right lateral). Clinical and experimental research has converged to indicate the fractionation of frontal subprocesses and the initial mapping of these subprocesses to discrete frontal regions (Stuss & Levine, 2002). Factor analysis has also supported that executive functions include several subcomponents (Mantyla, Carelli, & Forman, 2007; Stout, Ready, Grace, et al., 2003).

Major Dysexecutive Syndromes: Normal and Abnormal Conditions

Most frequently, three different prefrontal syndromes associated with specific disturbances in executive functions are separated (Box 7-1).

Box 7-1

Three Major Prefrontal Syndromes

DORSOLATERAL SYNDROME
Impaired set shifting (stuck-in set perseveration)
Depression
Rigidity
Concreteness
Verbal-action dissociation
Impersistence
Verbal dysfluency (left)
Design dysfluency (right)
Poor problem-solving abilities
Poor motor programming
Poor planning
Working memory deficits
Spontaneous recall poorer than recognition

MEDIODORSAL SYNDROME
Mutism
Apathy
Slowness
Amotivation
Poor task maintenance
Abulia/decreased motor activity
Transcortical motor aphasia (left)
Aspontaneity
Impaired generative cognition
Reduced affect
Poor humor appreciation (right)
Akinetic mutism (bilat)

ORBITOFRONTAL SYNDROME
Sensitivity to interference
Euphoria/mania
Poor decision making
Impulsiveness
Theory of mind deficits
Disinhibition
Social and moral reasoning impairment
Jocularity
Stuck-in-set perseveration (on object alternation)
Irresponsibility
Inappropriateness
Tactlessness
Impaired social judgment

Adapted from Chayer, C., & Freedman, M (2001). Frontal lobe functions. *Current Neurology and Neuroscience Reports, 1,* 547–552.

Dorsolateral Syndrome

Cummings (1993) indicated that the dorsolateral circuit is the most important to executive functioning. The most noted deficit is an inability to organize a behavioral response to novel or complex stimuli. Symptoms are on a continuum and reflect the capacity to shift cognitive sets, engage existing strategies, and organize information to meet changing environmental demands. Dysfunction in this region disrupts essential component cognitive processes, including working memory and inhibitory control (Anderson & Tranel, 2002). Various researchers, including Luria (1969), have noted preservation, stimulus-bound behavior, echopraxia, and echolalia. According to Fuster (1997, 2002), the most general executive function of the lateral prefrontal cortex is temporal organization of goal-directed actions in the domains of behavior, cognition, and language. Lateral differences are observed: whereas left prefrontal damage is more directly associated with cognitive processes, right damage is associated with both restriction of affect and emotional dyscontrol and defects in the perception or comprehension of emotional information. Anosognosia, impaired empathy, and defects in the appreciation of humor (Shammi & Stuss, 1999) are also found. Following lesion to the right dorsolateral area, a transcortical motor aprosodia is expected, whereas a left-sided dorsal lesion will produce a decline in verbal fluency on word-generation tasks and so-called extrasylvian (transcortical) motor aphasia.

A hierarchical model of prefrontal function has been proposed in which dorsolateral and frontopolar regions are serially recruited in a reasoning or memory task that requires evaluation of internally generated information: whereas the dorsolateral prefrontal cortex is involved when externally generated information is being evaluated, the frontopolar area becomes recruited when internally generated information needs to be evaluated (Christoff & Gabrieli, 2000).

Medial Frontal Lobe

The anterior cingulate is the origin of the anterior cingulate-subcortical circuit. Goldman-Rakic and Porrino (1985) identified input from BA24 to the ventral striatum, which includes the ventromedial caudate, ventral putamen, nucleus accumbens, and olfactory tubercle. Damage to these circuits causes apathy or abulia (a severe form of apathy). Acute bilateral lesions in the medial frontal area can cause akinetic mutism, in which the individual is awake and has self awareness but does not initiate behaviors. These patients demonstrate diminished drive. The spectrum can range to the extreme following bilateral lesions (i.e., patients can be profoundly apathetic, may rarely move, may be incontinent, may eat only when fed, and may speak only in monosyllables when questioned). They are not emotionally reactive, even with painful stimuli, and appear completely indifferent (Damasio & Damasio, 1989). Subcortical deficits, as seen with Parkinson disease and Huntington disease as well as thalamic lesions, may cause apathy if the anterior cingulate is affected.

Orbitofrontal Syndrome

Orbitofrontal syndrome has been associated with disinhibition, inappropriate behaviors, irritability, mood lability, tactlessness, distractibility, and loss of import to events. Affect may become extreme with *moria* (an excited affect) or *Witzelsucht* (the verbal reiteration of caustic or facetious remarks), first noted by Oppenheim (1890, 1891). Individuals with this syndrome are unable to respond to social cues, and they are stimulus bound. Cummings (1993) noted that automatic imitation of the gestures of others may occur with large lesions. Interestingly, it has been noted that these patients have no difficulty with card-sorting tasks (Laiacona et al., 1989). Eslinger and Damasio (1985) coined the term "acquired sociopathy" to describe dysregulation that couples both a lack of insight and remorse regarding these behaviors. Much of this may reflect the stimulus-bound nature of this disorder. The orbitofrontal cortex appears to be linked predominantly with limbic and basal forebrain sites. The orbital prefrontal cortex may have the ability to maintain its own level of functional arousal due to its cholinergic innervation from the basal forebrain (Mesulam, 1986). According to Fuster (2002), the ventromedial areas of the prefrontal cortex are involved in expression and control of emotional and instinctual behaviors.

The three major prefrontal syndromes could be grouped into two. Ardila (2008) suggested that the prefrontal lobe participates in two closely related but different executive function abilities: (1) "metacognitive executive functions": problem solving, planning, concept formation, strategy development and implementation, controlling attention, working memory, and the like, which are related with the activity of the dorsolateral prefrontal cortex; and (2) "emotional/motivational executive functions": coordinating cognition and emotion/motivation (that is, fulfilling biological needs according to some existing conditions), which are related with the orbitofrontal and medial frontal cortexes. Ardila (2008) suggested that "metacognitive" and "emotional/motivational" executive functions may have presented different evolutionary patterns during human phylogeny; and while primates and hominids may possess the second, the first one is only observed in recent human evolution.

In the prefrontal cortex, as in other cortical areas, lateralization is observed. Language-related disturbances (such as extrasylvian or transcortical motor aphasia) are more frequently found in cases of left frontal pathology, whereas social, spatial, and, in general, non–language-related disturbances are usually associated with right hemisphere damage. Goldberg (2001) describes two types of cognitive control: one guiding behavior by internal cues and the other by external cues. Normally operating in concert, damage to the frontal lobes can result in perseveration (disinhibited repetition) due to the following: diminished ability to switch behaviors in response to changing demands and environmental dependency, and inability to generate behaviors that are guided and personal. The left prefrontal system is thought to subserve the guiding of cognitive selection by working memory and internal contingencies, whereas the right prefrontal area mediates guiding cognitive selection by external environmental contingencies.

Even though executive dysfunction that follows focal brain injury most often occurs (or is most severe) following frontal lobe injury, not all executive processes are exclusively sustained by the frontal cortex (Andres & Van der Linden, 2002). Lesions in nearly any part of the brain have been associated with executive dysfunction (Hausen, Lachmann, & Nagler, 1997). Contemporary research even finds strategy operations in the occipital cortical neurons on visual tasks (Super, Spekreijse, & Lamme, 2001). Andres (2003) analyzed two executive processes: inhibition and dual-task management. He concluded that (1) executive processes involve links between different brain areas, not exclusively with the frontal cortex, (2) patients with no evidence of frontal damage may present with executive deficits, and (3) patients with frontal lesions do not always show executive deficits.

Communication Disorders in Frontal Lobe Pathology

A diversity of disorders in communication ability can be observed in cases of frontal lobe pathology including dysarthria, aphasia, language pragmatic disturbances, metalinguistic skill abnormalities, and verbal reasoning impairments. Complex and conceptual verbal abilities may be significantly impaired (Novoa & Ardila, 1987). Most frequently these disorders are found in cases of left hemisphere pathology. The idiosyncrasies of the disorders depend on the specific location and extension of the damage. Alexander, Benson, and Stuss (1989) proposed a comprehensive classification of communication disorders observed in frontal lobe pathology (Table 7-1).

Left Hemisphere Pathology
Aphemia
Aphemia was the initial name used by Broca to refer to the impairment in language production associated with left posterior frontal damage (Broca, 1861), but this name was later replaced with aphasia by Trousseau in 1864. The term aphasia prevailed and aphemia was forgotten. During the following decades, the term aphemia appeared from time to time in the neurological literature to refer to the articulatory defects associated with Broca's aphasia. Schiff, Alexander, Naeser, and Galaburda published an influential paper in 1983 reacquiring the term aphemia to name the dysarthria following the appearance of left frontal-lobe lesion, including the pars opercularis, inferior prerolandic gyrus (cortical dysarthria), or the white matter deep to those regions. Today, this is the most frequent use of the term aphemia: Aphemia is the spastic dysarthria observed in cases of damage of the upper motor neuron in the pyramidal system. This dysarthria is usually associated with Broca's aphasia, and it is also observed in cases of damage involving the internal capsule.

Table **7-1** Communication Disorders Associated with Frontal Lobe Pathology

	LEFT HEMISPHERE	RIGHT HEMISPHERE
Lower motor cortex and posterior operculum	Aphemia	Dysprosody
Full operculum plus lower motor cortex	Broca's area aphasia	Dysprosody
Dorsolateral frontal	Transcortical motor aphasia	Defective pragmatic discourse
Medial frontal	Mutism	Decreased output
Prefrontal	Reduced formulation; impoverished discourse	Disordered formulation; tangential discourse; confabulation

Adapted from Alexander, M. P., Benson, D. F., & Stuss, D. T. (1989). Frontal lobes and language. *Brain and Language, 37*, 656–691.

In cases of damage of the lower motor cortex and the posterior operculum, the observed clinical syndrome is quite consistent. Initially, the patient is mute and often hemiparetic, but both conditions rapidly improve. Lower facial paresis may persist. Language function is intact or minimally impaired. Speech is slow and effortful, and dysarthria is observed. Long-term sequelae are variable, but most often language recovers to a normal status though dysarthria remains.

Broca's Aphasia

Broca's aphasia (named by Luria as efferent or kinetic motor aphasia) is characterized by nonfluent expressive language that is poorly articulated and consists of short phrases that are agrammatical and produced with great effort. The expressive language basically consists of nouns with a marked deficiency or absence of syntactic structure and affixes (agrammatism). The motor-articulatory defect has been called a variety of names, but the most frequently used term is apraxia of speech.

The level of language comprehension is always superior to verbal production, although never normal, especially in relation to grammatical comprehension. Patients with Broca's aphasia easily identify objects or body parts, but if they are asked to name multiple objects or body parts in a particular order, the patients only manage to do so at a level of about two or three words. Similarly, they produce obvious errors in the comprehension of grammatical structures of language. However, the deficit in grammatical production is more severe than their defect in comprehension.

Language repetition is inadequate, and there is a presence of phonetic deviations, phonologic paraphasias, simplifications of syllabic groups, and iterations. Despite this difficulty, repetitive language may be superior to spontaneous language. Interestingly, there is a selective defect seen in the repetition of grammatical structure also absent in spontaneous language. For example, when a patient is asked to repeat, *"the boy walks on the street,"* he/she may only be able to repeat, *"boy walk street,"* omitting the elements with a purely grammatical function. Occasionally, the patient only manages to repeat nominative elements (e.g. *"boy, street"*).

The production of automatic series (counting, days of the week, etc.) is superior to spontaneous language. Singing also frequently improves verbal production in these patients; nevertheless, there is little generalization between singing or automatic language and spontaneous production.

Pointing and naming are always deficient though pointing is superior to naming. If syntactic comprehension is excluded, (*"the dog bites the cat," "the cat bites the dog"*), linguistic comprehension can occasionally appear practically normal. During naming, however, it is common to find articulatory difficulties (phonetic deviations) that can appear as phonological paraphasias, as well as omissions and phonological simplifications. The presentation of phonological cues can help initiate articulation. Similarly, the completion of high-probability phrases (*"I write with a ____"*) can lead to a correct production of the desired name.

It is usually recognized that Broca's aphasia has two different distinguishing characteristics: (a) a motor-articulatory component (lack of fluency, disintegration of speech kinetic melodies, verbal-articulatory impairments, etc.) that is usually referred to as *apraxia of speech*; and (b) agrammatism (e.g., Benson & Ardila, 1996; Berndt & Caramazza, 1980; Goodglass, 1993; Kertesz, 1985; Luria, 1976). Indeed, a large part of the frontoparietotemporal cortex has been observed to be involved with syntactic-morphological functions (Bhatnagar, Mandybur, Buckingham, & Andy, 2000). Apraxia of speech has been specifically associated with damage in the left precentral gyrus of the insula (Dronkers, 1996; but see Hillis, Work, Barker, et al., 2004).

Noteworthy, it seems evident that the lesions limited strictly to Broca's area are not sufficient to cause the complete syndrome; in the case of injuries limited specifically to Broca's area, usually one can observe only slight defects in articulatory agility, a certain "foreign accent," grammatical simplifications with sporadic grammatical errors, the use of short phrases in the expressive language, and a reduced ability to find words. Hemiparesis is usually minimal. This restricted form of Broca's aphasia could also be named *Broca's area aphasia* (or *minor Broca's aphasia*, or *type I Broca's aphasia*). The extensive form or the complete syndrome of Broca's aphasia is observed only if the damage extends additionally to the opercular region, the precentral gyrus, the anterior insula, and the paraventricular (at the side the ventricles) and periventricular (around the ventricles) white matter. This form of Broca's aphasia can be called *extended Broca's aphasia* (or *type II Broca's aphasia).*

Transcortical (Extrasylvian) Motor Aphasia

Different names have been applied to nonfluent aphasia with preserved repetition and good comprehension, including dynamic aphasia (Luria, 1980) and anterior isolation syndrome (Benson & Geschwind, 1971), but the most frequent name is transcortical (or extrasylvian) motor aphasia. However, the term transcortical motor aphasia has been used to refer to two different language disorders: lack of verbal initiative associated with left prefrontal pathology (Luria's dynamic aphasia) and defects in language initiation observed in cases of damage in the left SMA (Ardila & Lopez, 1984). The initial mutism observed in cases of medial frontal pathology can be followed by language initiation disturbances associated with nearly normal repetition. This language defect corresponds to the aphasia of the left SMA (Alexander et al., 1989).

Transcortical motor aphasia associated with dorsolateral lesions could be interpreted as "dysexecutive aphasia" and will be analyzed later in this chapter.

Mutism

Mutism refers to the inability or unwillingness to speak. Akinetic mutism is a variety of mutism characterized by an inability to both speak and to carry out purposeful movements, regardless if the patient lies with eyes open. Mutism has been related with frontal mesial pathology involving the cingulate gyrus. Paresis may occur, and weakness is greater in the leg than in the arm. Sometimes, unilateral akinesia or hypokinesia may be observed.

Reduced Verbal Production

Reduced verbal production can be considered one of two distinctive elements of left prefrontal lesions, and it is characterized by a loss or reduction of spontaneous language, difficulty organizing expressive language (i.e., converting ideas or intentions in expressive language), poor verbal generation, and defects in verbal reasoning. More exact defects of the paralinguistic type have been found, impairing the way in which language is formulated, controlled, and structured.

Nevertheless, lesions limited to the polar region are not associated with apparent defects in language; instead, they are associated with personality changes, including apathy and irritability.

Right Hemisphere Pathology
Dysprosody

Damage in the right lower motor cortex and the posterior operculum results in so-called affective motor dysprosody, characterized by difficulties in using the melodic contours in verbal output (Ross, 1981). Speech is flat and is without the appropriate prosodic quality. This difficulty can be observed not only when speaking but also when singing. Patients may have difficulties in conferring the emotional background of communication: sadness, irony, sarcasm, happiness, etc.

Defective Pragmatic Discourse

Disturbances in the pragmatic aspects of communication are found in cases of extensive right frontal dorsolateral lesions. These patients may have a significant difficulty in organizing a coherent narrative. Irrelevant and tangential comments are frequent, and they often speak using a free-ideas association (Ardila, 1984). They have difficulties interpreting analogies, ironies, and general, figurative language. These patients may have a concrete, blunt, and impolite discourse.

Decreased Output

Patients with lesions limited to the medial right frontal lobe (including the SMA) have a reduction in language production. Prosody is also frequently reduced. According to Alexander et al. (1989), the main difference between patients presenting left and right mesial lesions is quantitative rather than qualitative. In both cases there is a reduction in verbal output, but the reduction is mild to moderate in cases of right lesions and significant in cases of left frontal lesions. However, in cases of right damage, prosody is also affected.

Disordered Verbal Formulation

Extensive right medial frontal damage is associated with significant behavioral abnormalities: emotional flattening, inappropriate and frequently vulgar behavior, apathy, and confabulation. These patients have difficulties in selecting a socially acceptable language. They tend to impulsively respond to their first associations; perseveration is not unusual, and confabulation associated with disorganized narrative in discourse is frequently observed (Alexander et al., 1989).

Frontal Lobe Language Areas: Contemporary Neuroimaging Studies

Contemporary neuroimaging studies have significantly advanced our understanding of the role of the frontal lobe in language. These studies have supported the notion that language areas in the human brain involve a network of regions, not only in the frontal lobe, but also in the temporal and parietal lobes of the left hemisphere (e.g., Binder, Frost, Hammeke, et al., 1997; Calandra-Buonaura, Basso, Gorno-Tempini et al., 2002). Evidently, the frontal lobe has a major and controlling role in language, and using fMRI and PET techniques, it has been observed that the performance of a diversity of verbal tasks results in changes of the activation level in different frontal areas. These functions are described next following the organization of Brodmann's areas (see Figure 7-1).

Brodmann's Area 6 (Lateral Premotor Cortex Area, Including the Supplementary Motor Area)

According to functional studies, Brodmann's area 6 (BA6) participates in a diversity of functions. Its basic function, however, seems to be motor sequencing and planning movements (Schubotz & von Cramon, 2001). Damage in the lateral premotor area results in kinetic apraxia. The SMA portion is related with movement initiation; the left SMA also participates in language initiation and maintenance of voluntary speech production (Basho, Palmer, Rubio, et al., 2007; De Carli, Garreffa, Colonnese, et al., 2007). Linguistic functions of left BA6 are diverse, but a major function evidently is speech motor programming (Fox, Ingham, Ingham, et al., 2000; Shuster & Lemieux, 2005); Broca's area indeed corresponds to a subdivision of the premotor cortex, and some of the linguistic functions of the lateral premotor area are probably the result of an extended activation of the frontal languages areas. Participation of BA6 in memory, attention, and executive functions (Burton, Noll, & Small, 2001; Fincham, Carter, van Veen, et al., 2002) may be due to the activation of an extended brain network, which sometimes involves BA6. The existence of mirror neurons that activate when observing (and imagining) actions plays an important role in understanding, thinking, and planning (Morin & Grèzes, 2008).

Brodmann's Area 44 (Broca's Area, Inferior Frontal Gyrus, Pars Opercularis)

From the traditional point of view, Broca's area corresponds to BA44, but several contemporary authors also include BA45 (e.g., Foundas, Eure, Luevano & Weinberger, 1998).

Different proposals have been presented to explain language disturbances in so-called Broca's aphasia; several hypotheses have attempted to postulate a core BA44 function, including binding the elements of the language, selecting information among competing sources, generating/extracting action meanings, sequencing motor/expressive elements, acting as a cognitive control mechanism for the syntactic processing of sentences, constructing higher parts of the syntactic tree in speech production, and participating in verbal working memory (Ardila, 2010). Although the core functions of BA44 remain elusive, fluency and sequencing may potentially account for many of the functions in which BA44 participates (Abrahams, Goldstein, Simmons, et al., 2003; Amunts, Weiss, Mohlberg, et al., 2004; Heim, Eickhoff, & Amunts, 2008).

The suggestion that BA44 includes mirror neurons for expressive movements is particularly provocative and may enlighten the question of inner speech (e.g., internally generated language) (Lawrence, Shaw, Giampieto, et al., 2006; Lotze et al., 2006; Manthey, Schubotz, & von Cramon, 2003). Unfortunately, just a few studies have analyzed the clinical disturbances associated with right BA44 from the perspective of the lesional model (Ardila, 2004). Functional studies have also disclosed the participation of BA44 in a diversity of tasks that are difficult to interpret with our current understanding of the brain, such as pain anticipation, perception of tactile stimulation, motion after-effect,

object manipulation, smelling familiar odors, and music enjoyment; in those cases, BA44 activation is just an additional element in a complex brain network. It may be suggested that some internal verbalization can account for BA44 involvement in these unexpected activities. Its participation in working memory (Rämä, Martinkauppi, Linnankoski, et al., 2001) may also reflect the internal rehearsal of the information.

Brodmann's Area 45 (Broca's Area, Inferior Frontal Gyrus, Pars Triangularis)

According to contemporary neuroimaging studies, the functions of BA45 are significantly coincidental with the functions of BA44 (see http://www.fmriconsulting.com/brodmann/), supporting the proposal that they both, at least partially, correspond to a single brain system. Nonetheless, BA45 seems to be involved in relatively more complex verbal functions, for instance, processing of metaphors (Rapp, Leube, Erb, et al., 2004; Shibata, Abe, Terao, & Miyamoto, 2007) and reasoning processes (Goel, Gold, Kapur, & Houle, 1997, 1998). As observed with BA44, BA45 participates in a diversity of functions difficult to interpret with our current understanding of the brain (e.g., smelling of familiar odors) and probably reflects some inner speech during the performance of those tasks. BA45 participation in working memory (Rämä et al., 2001; Ranganath, Johnson, & D'Esposito, 2003) may also reflect the internal rehearsal of the information.

Brodmann's Area 8 (Part of Prefrontal Cortex; Lateral and Medial Supplementary Motor Area)

BA8 is usually regarded as the "frontal eye field." However, functional studies report that BA8 participates in a wide diversity of functions, including motor (Perry, Zatore, Petrides, et al., 1999), language (Fox et al., 2000), executive functions (Crozier, Sirigu, Lehéricy, et al., 1999; Kübler, Dixon, & Garavan, 2006), memory (Rämä et al., 2001), and attention (Cheng, Fujita, Kanno, et al., 1995). Indeed, few studies refer to its participation in eye movements (horizontal saccadic eye movements) (Anderson, Jenkins, Brooks, et al., 1994; Miki, Nakajima, Miyauchi, et al., 1996). It is very interesting to note the participation of the SMA in motor learning supported by several studies (Brunia, de Jong, van den Berg-Lenssen, & Paans, 2000; Inoue, Kawashima, Satoh, et al., 2000; Matsumara, Sadoto, Kochiyama, et al., 2004). Usually it is accepted that the SMA participates in initiating, maintaining, coordinating, and planning complex sequences of movements performed in a particular order. Stimulation of the left SMA has been related to arrest of speech and its damage to a particular type of language disorder referred as "aphasia of the SMA" (initial mutism lasting about 2–10 days; virtually total inability to initiate speech; nearly normal speech repetition; normal language understanding; and absence of echolalia). BA8 also participates in memory processes, particularly in verbal working memory (Rämä et al., 2001).

Brodmann's Areas 9 and 10 (Part of the Prefrontal Cortex, Middle Frontal Gyrus)

BAs 9/10 have a significant participation in memory, particularly memory encoding, memory retrieval, and working memory (Pochon, Levy, Fossati, et al., 2002; Raye, Johnson, Mitchell, et al., 2002; Zhang, Leung, & Johnson, 2003). BAs 9/10 also have other evident executive functions, such as "executive control of behavior" (Kübler et al., 2006), "inferential reasoning" (Knauff, Mulack, Kassubek, et al., 2002), and "decision making" (Rogers, Owen, Middleton, et al., 1999). Their participation in complex language processes may suggest the use of verbal strategies in executive processing; in these cases (e.g., syntactic processing, metaphor comprehension, generating sentences, etc.) (Brown, Martinez, & Parsons, 2006; Shibata et al., 2007; Wang, Zho, Zhang, et al., 2008), an extensive network is activated, involving diverse language related areas.

Brodmann's Area 46 (Anterior Middle Frontal Gyrus)

The participation of the left anterior middle frontal gyrus in language (e.g., verbal fluency (Abrahams et al., 2003) and phonological processing (Heim, Opitz, Müller, & Friederici, 2003) is shared by other left prefrontal convexital areas. According to current knowledge of language disturbances associated with brain pathology, other linguistic functions potentially related with BA46, such as verbal initiative and language pragmatics, have not been fully approached in fMRI studies.

Brodmann's Area 47 (Inferior Frontal Gyrus, Pars Orbitalis)

A significant amount of language-related functions have been associated with BA47, including semantic processing (De Carli et al., 2007), phonological processing (De Carli et al., 2007), semantic encoding (Li, Gong, Yang, et al., 2000), and selective attention to speech (Vorobyev, Alho, Medvedev, et al., 2004). In these cases, BA47 is simply one of the multiple steps in the brain language processing network. It could be further speculated that in these verbal related functions, the inferior frontal gyrus may play a more emotional/motivational function. Moreover, anatomically, BA47 is adjacent to BA45, an evident language brain area. BA47 also participates in some clearly emotionally related activities—e.g., adverse emotional inhibition (Berthoz, Armony, Blair, & Dolan, 2002) and in executive functions—e.g., deductive reasoning (Goel et al., 1998).

Brodmann's Area 11 (Gyrus Rectus)

No language functions have been explicitly related with BA11. From the clinical perspective, it is usually assumed that BA11 (base of the frontal pole) is related with something that could be termed "personality integrity." Personality changes observed in individuals with a traumatic brain injury are thought to result from damage of this orbital frontal area. It could be conjectured that BA11 participates in some individuals' "style of reacting" or "emotional idiosyncratic style."

Brodmann's Areas 24 and 32 (Anterior Cingulated Gyrus)

The cingulate gyrus is part of the limbic system and hence has a direct participation in emotional behavior. Anterior cingulate gyrus damage can be associated with mutism and akinesia. Contemporary fMRI studies support its involvement in language initiative (e.g., Nathaniel-James, Fletcher, & Frith, 1997).

Table 7-2 summarizes the participation of different frontal areas in language and communication, according to contemporary neuroimaging studies.

The Role of Broca's Area in Language and Cognition

In the past decade there has been a significant interest in reanalyzing the function of Broca's area (e.g., Grodzinky & Amunts, 2006; Hagoort, 2005; Thompson-Schill, 2005). From the traditional point of view, Broca's area corresponds to BA44, but several contemporary authors

Table 7-2 Participation of Different Frontal Areas in Language and Communication, According to Contemporary Neuroimaging Studies

Brodmann's Area	Participation in Language and Communication
Area 6	Left supplementary motor area: language initiation speech motor programming
Area 44 (and 45)	Praxis of speech and grammar
Area 8	Sequencing movements in a particular order
Areas 9 and 10	Complex language processes
Area 46	Verbal fluency, phonological processing
Area 47	Semantic and phonological processing; attention to speech
Area 11	No evident language function
Areas 24 and 32	Verbal initiative

also include BA45. In the traditional aphasia literature, it was assumed that damage in Broca's area was responsible for the clinical manifestations observed in Broca's aphasia. Only with the introduction of the computed tomography scan did it become evident that the damage restricted to Broca's area was not enough to produce the "classical" Broca's aphasia; extension to the insula, lower motor cortex, and subjacent subcortical and periventricular white matter is required (Alexander, Naeser, & Palumbo, 1990). "Broca's area aphasia" ("minor Broca's aphasia") is characterized by mildly nonfluent speech, relatively short sentences, and mild agrammatism; phonetic deviations and a few phonological paraphasias can be observed (Mohr, Pessin, Finkelstein, et al., 1978); some foreign accent can also be noticed (Ardila, Rosselli, & Ardila, 1988).

Simultaneously including both BA44 and BA45 in Broca's area is problematic. BA44 is a premotor dysgranular area, whereas BA45 has a granular layer IV and belongs to the heteromodal prefrontal lobe (granular cortex) (Mesulam, 2002). So, from a cytoarchitectonic point of view, BA44 and BA45 are quite different. BA44 is a premotor area, whereas BA45 corresponds to the prefrontal cortex. From the aphasia perspective, some authors have referred to different clinical manifestations associated with damage in BA44 (Broca-type aphasia) and BA45 (transcortical motor/dynamic aphasia) (e.g., Luria, 1976). Some authors have also pointed out that indeed Broca's area is a collective term that can be fractionated into different subareas (Lindenberg, Fangerau, & Seitz, 2007).

Hagoort (2005, 2006) refers to the "Broca's complex" as including BA44 (premotor), as well as BA45 and BA47 (prefrontal cortex) (Figure 7-3). He argues that the Broca's complex is not a language specific area and that it becomes active during some non-language activities, such as mental imagery of grasping movements (Decety, Perani, Jeannerod, et al., 1994). Functionally defined sub-regions could be distinguished in the Broca's complex: BA47 and BA45 are involved in semantic processing; BA44, BA45, and BA46 participate in syntactic processing; and BA44 is involved in phonological processing. Hagoort (2005) proposes that "the common denominator of the Broca's complex is its role in selection and unification operations by which individual pieces of lexical information are bound together into representational structures spanning multiword utterances" (p. 166). Its core function is, consequently, *binding the elements of the language.*

Thompson-Schill (2005) analyzed the different deficits observed in cases of damage in Broca's area: articulation, syntax, selection, and verbal working memory, suggesting that there may be more than a single function. The author proposes a framework for describing the deficits

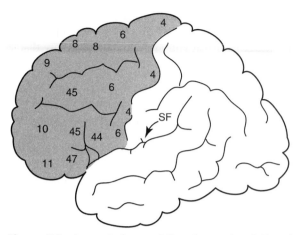

Figure 7-3 Anatomical map of Broca's complex. B45 and BA47 are involved in semantic processing; BA44, BA45 and BA46 participate in semantic processing; and BA44 and BA6 have a role in phonological processing. [Adapted from Hagoort, P. (2005). Broca's complex as the unification of space for language. In A. Cutler (Ed.), *Twenty-first century psycholinguistics: Four cornerstones* (p. 162). Mahwah, NJ: Lawrence Erlbaum Associates.]

observed in different patients. The proposed framework suggests that Broca's area may be involved in *selecting information among competing sources.* Fadiga, Craighero, and Roy (2006) speculate that the original role played by Broca's area relates to *generating/extracting action meanings;* that is, organizing/interpreting the sequence of individual meaningless movements. Ardila and Bernal (2007) conjectured that the central role of Broca's area was related to *sequencing motor/expressive elements.* Novick, Trueswell, and Thompson (2005) consider that the role of Broca's area is related with a general *cognitive control mechanism for the syntactic processing of sentences.*

Grodzinsky (2000, 2006) has presented an extensive analysis of the role of Broca's area. He proposed that most syntax is not located in Broca's area and its vicinity (operculum, insula, and subjacent white matter). This brain area does have a role in syntactic processing, but a highly specific one: *it is the neural home to receptive mechanisms involved in the computation of the relation between transformationally moved phrasal constituents and their extraction sites (syntactic movement).* He further assumes that Broca's area is also involved in the construction of higher parts of the syntactic tree in speech production. Interestingly, blood flow in Broca's area increases when subjects process complex syntax (Caplan, Alpert, Waters, & Olivieri, 2000). Syntax is indeed neurologically segregated, and its components are housed in several distinct cerebral locations far beyond the traditional ones (Broca's and Wernicke's regions). A new brain map for syntax would also include portions of the right cerebral hemisphere (Grodzinsky & Friederici, 2006).

In summary, regardless of the fact that expressive language disturbances have been associated for over a century with damage in the left inferior frontal gyrus (later known as "Broca's area"), currently there is incomplete agreement about its limits and its specific functions in language. Different proposals have been presented to explain language disturbances in so-called Broca's aphasia, including: binding the elements of the language (Hagoort, 2005); selecting information among competing sources (Thompson-Schill, 2005); generating/extracting action meanings (Fadiga et al., 2006); sequencing motor/expressive elements (Ardila & Bernal, 2007); acting as a cognitive control mechanism for the syntactic processing of sentences (Novick et al., 2005); constructing higher parts of the syntactic tree in speech production (Grodzinsky, 2000, 2006); and engaging in verbal working memory (Haverkort, 2005).

However, not only does Broca's area participate in linguistic processes, it also participates in nonlinguistic processes, such as memory—particularly working memory (Rämä et al., 2001; Ranganath et al., 2003; Sun, Zhang, Chen, et al., 2005), solving arithmetical tasks (Rickard, Romero, Basso, et al., 2000), music enjoyment (Koelsch, Fritz, Cramon, et al., 2006), and diverse motor tasks, such as observation of expressive gestures and motor acts (Lotze et al., 2006), motor imagery (Grezes & Decety, 2002), and understanding actions of other individuals (Fazio, Cantagallo, Craighero, et al., 2009). Departing from these observations, the existence of a mirror-neurons system in humans related with BA44 has been suggested (Rizzolatti & Craighero, 2004).

Transcortical (Extrasylvian) Motor Aphasia as a "Dysexecutive Aphasia"

Transcortical (extrasylvian) motor aphasia corresponds to Luria dynamic aphasia (Luria, 1976). It is characterized by nonfluent verbal output, a lack of verbal initiative, good comprehension, and good repetition of spoken language. Patients with this subtype of aphasia use as few words as possible, answer questions by reiterating many of the words and grammatical structures presented in the question (echolalia), and, on occasion, produce perseverative responses. Sentences tend to be started but not finished. Poor verbal fluency, impoverished narrative production, reduced use of complex and precise syntax, and poor inhibition of high-association responses have been described following left prefrontal damage (Kertesz, 1999). These patients perform speech series well once the series has been initiated. Recitation of nursery rhymes and naming the days of the week are often performed successfully if initiated by the examiner. Open-ended phrases are easily completed by these patients. Comprehension of spoken language is good, at least for conversational language. However, many patients have difficulty handling sequences of complex material, and some show defects in interpreting relational words. Interestingly, despite preserved language understanding, patients with this type of aphasia have difficulties following verbal commands.

The difficulty of these patients in initiating a response is complicated by significant apathy and behavioral withdrawal that is usually observed. These patients seem distant and not interested in engaging in social conversation. Luria (1980) proposed that in dynamic aphasia, the patient's behavior is not controlled by language, and the dissociation between language and overt behavior represents an executive control disorder impairing language at the pragmatic level. Some authors have supposed that in dynamic aphasia a selective impairment of verbal planning occurs (Costello & Warrington, 1989), particularly at the level of "macroplanning," that is, generating sequences of novel thoughts and ideas (Bormann, Wallesch, & Blanken, 2008). Alexander suggested that this type of aphasia could be more accurately defined as an executive function disorder rather than aphasia (2006). He proposed that the progression of clinical disorders from aphasia to discourse impairments can be interpreted as a sequence of procedural impairments from basic morphosyntax to elaborated grammar to narrative language, correlated with a progression of the focus of the damage from posterior frontal to polar, or lateral frontal to medial frontal, or both.

The ability of these aphasic patients to repeat utterances is unexpectedly good in dramatic contrast to their nonfluent spontaneous output. Although the patients often echo a word or phrase, they usually are not fully echolalic. The ability to name on confrontation is often limited. Three types of errors are found in confrontation naming: (1) Perseveration: the patient continues giving a past response for a new stimulus. (2) Fragmentation: the patient responds to a single feature of the stimulus, not to the whole stimulus. (3) Extravagant paraphasias: instead of the target name, the patient presents a free-association answer that becomes an extravagant deviation (Benson & Ardila, 1996).

Writing is almost always defective. Sentences are incomplete, and the patients must be continuously encouraged to continue writing. Complex aspects of writing, such as planning, narrative coherence, and maintained attention, are significantly disturbed ("dysexecutive agraphia," according to Ardila & Surloff, 2006).

Neurologic findings in this type of extrasylvian motor aphasia are variable. Hemiparesis is uncommon. Pathological reflexes involving the dominant limb are often present. Both conjugate deviation of the eyes and unilateral inattention have been recorded in the initial stages in some cases of dynamic aphasia. Damage is expected to involve BA45 (which is situated in front of Broca's area) and adjacent brain areas.

Extrasylvian (transcortical) motor aphasia can be interpreted as an executive function defect specifically affecting language use. The ability to actively and appropriately generate language appears impaired while the phonology, lexicon, semantics, and grammar are preserved. Extrasylvian (transcortical) motor aphasia could indeed be referred to as "dysexecutive aphasia" (Ardila, 2009).

Frontal Language Abilities and Metacognition

Disagreement persists around the potential unitary factor underlying executive functions. It can be suggested that "action representation" (i.e., internally representing movements) may constitute at least one basic metacognitive executive function factor. Several authors have argued that thought, reasoning, and other forms of complex cognition (metacognition) depend on an interiorization of actions. Vygotsky (1929, 1934/1962, 1934/1978), for instance, proposed that thought (and in general, complex cognitive processes) is associated with some inner speech. More recently, Lieberman (2002a, 2002b) suggested that language in particular and cognition in general arise from complex sequences of motor activities. Noteworthy, the frontal lobe, and particularly Broca's area, is involved in understanding actions of other individuals (Fazio et al., 2009).

Vygotsky's (1934/1962, 1934/1978) understanding of "higher mental functions" is roughly equivalent to "metacognitive executive functions." The central point in Vygotsky's (1934/1962) idea is that higher forms of cognition ("cognitive executive functions") depend on certain mediation (instruments), very specially, language. According to Vygotsky (1934/1962), the invention (or discovery) of these instruments will result in a new type of evolution (cultural evolution), not requiring any further biological changes. Thinking is interpreted as a covert motor activity ("inner speech").

Vygotsky (1929) assumes that thought and speech develop differently and independently having different genetic roots. Before 2 years of age, the development of thought and speech are separate. They converge and join at about the age of 2 years, and thought from this point ahead becomes language mediated (verbal thought). Language in consequence becomes the primary instrument for conceptualization and thinking. According to Vygotsky (1934/1962), speech develops first as external communicative/social speech, then egocentric speech, and finally inner speech.

Inner speech is for oneself while external, social speech is for others. Vygotsky considered that thought development is determined by language. School is intimately related with learning a new conceptual instrument: reading. Written language is an extension of oral language, and it represents the most elaborated form of language.

In brief, Vygotsky (1934/1962) argued that complex psychological processes (metacognitive executive functions) derive from language internalization. Thinking relies on the development of an instrument (language or any other), that represents a cultural product. Lieberman (2002a, 2002b) refers specifically to the origins of language. He postulates that neural circuits linking activity in anatomically segregated populations of neurons in subcortical structures and the neocortex throughout the human brain regulate complex behaviors such as walking, talking, and comprehending the meaning of sentences. The neural substrates that regulate motor control (the basal ganglia, cerebellum, and frontal cortex) in the common ancestor of apes and humans most likely were modified to enhance cognitive and linguistic ability. Lieberman (2002a, 2002b) suggests that motor activity is the departing point for cognition. Speech communication played a central role in this process. The neural bases of mankind's linguistic ability are complex, involving structures other than Broca's and Wernicke's areas. Many other cortical areas and subcortical structures form part of the neural circuits and are implicated in the lexicon, speech production and perception, and syntax. The subcortical basal ganglia support the cortical–striatal–cortical circuits that regulate speech production, complex syntax, and the acquisition of the motor and cognitive pattern generators that underlie speech production and syntax. They most likely are involved in learning the semantic referents and sound patterns that are instantiated as words in the brain's dictionary.

These two authors (Vygotsky and Lieberman), although using rather different approaches, have both postulated that the development of language and complex cognition are related with motor programming, sequencing, internalizing actions, and the like. Ardila (2009) argued that, historically, language developed in two different steps: initially as a lexical/semantic system, and more recently as a grammatical system. Grammar represents a sequencing of symbolic/linguistic elements (interiorization of actions), provides thinking strategies, and is related with the development of metacognitive executive functions.

The discovery of so-called "mirror neurons" represents a new element in understanding inner speech and action representation. A mirror neuron is a neuron which fires both when an animal performs an action and also when the animal observes the same action performed by another animal. In humans, brain activity consistent with mirror neurons has been found in the premotor cortex and the inferior parietal cortex (Rizzolatti & Craighero, 2004; Rizzolatti, Fadiga, Gallese, & Fogassi, 1996). These neurons (mirror neurons) appear to represent a system that matches observed events to similar, internally generated actions. As mentioned earlier, Broca's area participates in understanding actions of other individuals (Fazio et al., 2009).

Transcranial magnetic stimulation and positron emission tomography (PET) experiments suggest that a mirror system for gesture recognition also exists in humans and includes Broca's area (Rizzolatti & Arbib, 1998). The discovery of mirror neurons in Broca's area might have immense consequences for understanding the organization and evolution of mankind cognition (Arbib, 2006; Craighero, Metta, Sandini, & Fadiga, 2007). An obvious implication of mirror neurons is that they can participate in the internal representation of actions. PET studies have associated the neural correlates of inner language with activity of Broca's area (McGuire, Silbersweig, Murray, et al., 1996).

CONCLUSIONS

Despite the fact that the term "executive functions" was coined just a couple of decades ago, this concept has become a fundamental cornerstone in understanding human cognition. It has been observed that executive functions depend on extended dynamic networks including different brain areas, but the prefrontal cortex plays a major role in controlling and monitoring these areas. Noteworthy, "executive functions" is not a unitary concept, and the definition of executive functions includes two different dimensions: emotional/motivational (behavioral dimension), and metacognitive (cognitive dimension).

A diversity of communication disturbances can be observed in cases of frontal lobe pathology; some of them are more directly associated with social/emotional impairments in the use of language and are frequently found in cases of right frontal lobe pathology; others are more specifically related with the ability to use language as a cognitive instrument and are frequently observed in cases of left frontal lobe pathology. So-called transcortical (or extrasylvian)

motor aphasia could be interpreted as a defect in the executive control of language ("dysexecutive aphasia").

Contemporary neuroimaging studies have significantly advanced the understanding of the role of the frontal lobe in language. It has become evident that the prefrontal cortex has a monitoring role in language. Using neuroimaging techniques, it has been observed that the performance of a diversity of verbal tasks results in changes of the activation level in different prefrontal areas.

Traditionally, language production has been related with Broca's area; Broca's area corresponds to BA44, but several contemporary authors also include BA45. Regardless of the fact that it has been assumed that damage in Broca's area was responsible for the clinical manifestations observed in Broca's aphasia, contemporary studies have demonstrated that damaged restricted to this area only results in mildly nonfluent speech, relatively short sentences and mild agrammatism; phonetic deviations and a few phonological paraphasias can also be observed. The complete and classical Broca's aphasia requires significantly more extended lesions, including the opercular region, the precentral gyrus, the anterior insula, and the paraventricular and periventricular white matter.

The specific role of Broca's area has been polemic, and different suggestions have been presented, including binding the elements of language, selecting information among competing sources, generating/extracting action meanings, sequencing motor/expressive elements, acting as a cognitive control mechanism for the syntactic processing of sentences, constructing higher parts of the syntactic tree in speech production, and engaging in verbal working memory. However, Broca's area does not only participate in linguistic processes, but also in nonlinguistic processes such as observation of expressive gestures and motor acts, motor imagery, and understanding actions of other individuals. It has been suggested that the existence of a mirror-neurons system in humans is related with BA44.

Some authors have proposed that the development of metacognitive executive functions is related with motor programming, sequencing, and internalizing actions. Further, grammar represents a sequencing of symbolic/linguistic elements and is associated with the development of metacognitive executive functions.

ACKNOWLEDGMENT

My sincere gratitude to Melissa Marsal for her valuable help in editing this paper.

REFERENCES

Abrahams, S., Goldstein, L. H., Simmons, A., Brammer, M. J., Williams, S. C., Giampietro, V. P., et al. (2003). Functional magnetic resonance imaging of verbal fluency and confrontation naming using compressed image acquisition to permit overt responses. *Human Brain Mapping, 20*(1), 29–40.

Alexander, M. P. (2006). Impairments of procedures for implementing complex language are due to disruption of frontal attention processes. *Journal of the International Neuropsychological Society, 12*, 236–247.

Alexander, M. P., Benson, D. F., & Stuss, D. T. (1989). Frontal lobes and language. *Brain and Language, 37*, 656–691.

Alexander, M. P., Naeser, M. A., & Palumbo, C. (1990). Broca's area aphasia: Aphasia after lesions including the frontal operculum. *Neurology, 40*, 353–362.

Amunts, K., Weiss, P. H., Mohlberg, H., Pieperhoff, P., Eickhoff, S., Gurd, J. M., et al. (2004). Analysis of neural mechanisms underlying verbal fluency in cytoarchitectonically defined stereotaxic space—the roles of Brodmann areas 44 and 45. *Neuroimage, 22*(1), 42–56.

Anderson, S. W., & Tranel, D. (2002). Neuropsychological consequences of dysfunction in human dorsolateral prefrontal cortex. In J. Grafman (Ed.), *Handbook of Neuropsychology* (*Vol. 7*, 2nd ed., pp. 148–156). New York: Elsevier.

Anderson, T. J., Jenkins, I. H., Brooks, D. J., Hawken, M. B., Frackowiak, R. S., & Kennard, C. (1994). Cortical control of saccades and fixation in man: A PET study. *Brain, 117*, 1073–1084.

Anderson, V. (2001). Assessing executive functions in children: Biological, psychological, and developmental considerations. *Developmental Neurorehabilitation, 4*, 119–136.

Andres, P. (2003). Frontal cortex as the central executive of working memory: Time to revise our view. *Cortex, 39*(4–5), 871–895.

Andres, P., & Van der Linden, M. (2002). Are central executive functions working in patients with focal frontal lesions? *Neuropsychologia, 40*, 835–845.

Arbib, M. A. (2006). Aphasia, apraxia and the evolution of the language-ready brain. *Aphasiology, 20*, 1125–1155.

Ardila, A. (1984). Right prefrontal syndrome. In A. Ardila & F. Ostrosky-Sols (Eds.), *The right hemisphere: Neurology and neuropsychology* (pp. 171–193). London: Gordon and Breach Science Editors.

Ardila, A. (2004). A speech disorder associated with right Broca's homologous area pathology. *Acta Neuropsychologica, 2*, 45–52.

Ardila, A. (2008). On the evolutionary origins of executive functions. *Brain and Cognition, 68*(1), 92–99.

Ardila, A. (2009). Origins of the language: Correlation between brain evolution and language development. In S. M. Platek & T. K. Shackelford (Eds.), *Foundations of evolutionary cognitive neuroscience* (pp. 153–174). New York: Cambridge University Press.

Ardila, A. (2010). A proposed reinterpretation and reclassification of aphasic syndromes. *Aphasiology, 24* (3), 363–394.

Ardila, A., & Bernal, B. (2007). What can be localized in the brain? Towards a "factor" theory on brain organization of cognition. *International Journal of Neurosciences, 117*, 935–969.

Ardila, A., & Lopez, M. V. (1984). Transcortical motor aphasia: One or two aphasias? *Brain and Language, 22*, 350–353.

Ardila, A., Rosselli, M., & Ardila, O. (1988). Foreign accent: An aphasic epiphenomenon? *Aphasiology, 2*, 493–499.

Ardila, A. & Surloff, C. (2006). Dysexecutive agraphia: A major executive dysfunction sign. *International Journal of Neurosciences, 116*, 153–163.

Baddeley, A. (1986). *Working memory*. Oxford, UK: Oxford University Press.

Barbas, H. (2006). Organization of the principal pathways of prefrontal lateral, medial, and orbitofrontal cortices primates and implications for their collaborative interaction in executive functions. In J. Risberg & J. Grafman (Eds.), *The frontal lobes: Development, function and pathology* (pp. 21–68). Cambridge, MA: Cambridge University Press.

Barkley, R. A. (1997). *ADHD and the nature of self-control*. New York: Guilford Press.

Basho, S., Palmer, E. D., Rubio, M. A., Wulfeck, B., & Müller, R. A. (2007). Effects of generation mode in fMRI adaptations of semantic fluency: Paced production and overt speech. *Neuropsychologia, 45*(8), 1697–1706.

Benson, D. F., & Ardila, A. (1996). *Aphasia: A clinical perspective*. New York: Oxford University Press.

Benson, D. F., & Geschwind, N. (1971). Aphasia and related cortical disturbances. In A. B. Baker & L. H. Baker (Eds.), *Clinical neurology* (pp. 122–140). New York: Harper & Row.

Bernal, B., & Perdomo, J. (2007). *Brodmann's interactive atlas 1.1*. Retrieved from http://www.fmriconsulting.com/brodmann/

Berndt, R. S., & Caramazza, A. (1980). A redefinition of the syndrome of Broca's aphasia: Implications for a neuropsychological model of language. *Applied Psycholinguistics, 1*, 225–278.

Berthoz, S., Armony, J. L., Blair, R. J., & Dolan, R. J. (2002). An fMRI study of intentional and unintentional (embarrassing) violations of social norms. *Brain, 125*, 1696–1708.

Bhatnagar, S. C., Mandybur, G. T., Buckingham, H. W., & Andy, O. J. (2000). Language representation in the human brain: evidence from cortical mapping. *Brain and Language, 74*, 238–259.

Binder, J. R., Frost, J. A., Hammeke, T. A., Cox, R. W., Rao, S. M., & Prieto, T. (1997). Human brain language areas identified by functional magnetic resonance imaging. *Journal of Neuroscience, 17*(1), 353–362.

Bormann, T., Wallesch, C. W., & Blanken, G. (2008). Verbal planning in a case of 'Dynamic Aphasia': An impairment at the level of macroplanning. *Neurocase, 14*(5), 431–450.

Broca, P. (1861). Nouvelle observation d'aphémie produite par une lésion de la moitié postérieure des deuxième et troisième circonvolution frontales gauches. *Bulletin de la Société Anatomique, 36*, 398–407.

Brown, S., Martinez, M. J., & Parsons, L. M. (2006). Music and language side by side in the brain: A PET study of the generation of melodies and sentences. *The European Journal of Neuroscience, 23*(10), 2791–2803.

Brunia, C. H., de Jong, B. M., van den Berg-Lenssen, M. M., & Paans, A. M. (2000). Visual feedback about time estimation is related to a right hemisphere activation measured by PET. *Experimental Brain Research, 130*(3), 328–337.

Burton, M. W., Noll, D. C., & Small, S. L. (2001). The anatomy of auditory word processing: Individual variability. *Brain and Language, 77*(1), 119–131.

Calandra-Buonaura, G., Basso, G., Gorno-Tempini, M. L., Serafini, M., Pagnoni, G., & Baraldi, P., et al (2002). Human brain language processing areas identified by functional magnetic resonance imaging using a lexical decision task. *Functional Neurology, 17*(4), 183–191.

Caplan, D., Alpert, A., Waters, G., & Olivieri, A. (2000). Activation of Broca's area by syntactic processing under conditions of concurrent articulation. *Human Brain Mapping, 9*, 65–71.

Chayer, C., & Freedman, M. (2001). Frontal lobe functions. *Current Neurology and Neuroscience Reports, 1*, 547–552.

Cheng, K., Fujita, H., Kanno, I., Miura, S., & Tanaka, K. (1995). Human cortical regions activated by wide-field visual motion: An H2(15)O PET study. *Journal of Neurophysiology, 74*(1), 413–427.

Christoff, K., & Gabrieli, J. D. E. (2000). The frontopolar cortex and human cognition: Evidence for a rostrocaudal hierarchical organization within the human prefrontal cortex. *Psychobiology, 28*(2), 168–186.

Costello, A. L., & Warrington, E. K. (1989). Dynamic aphasia: The selective impairment of verbal planning. *Cortex, 25*, 103–114.

Craighero, L., Metta, G., Sandini, G., & Fadiga, L. (2007). The mirror-neurons system: Data and models. *Progress in Brain Research, 164*, 39–59.

Crozier, S., Sirigu, A., Lehéricy, S., van de Moortele, P. F., Pillon, B., Grafman J., et al. (1999). Distinct prefrontal activations in processing sequence at the sentence and script level: An fMRI study. *Neuropsychologia, 37*(13), 1469–1476.

Cummings, J. L. (1993). Frontal-subcortical circuits and human behavior. *Archives of Neurology, 50*, 873–880.

Damasio, A., & Anderson, S. W. (2003). The frontal lobes. In K. M. Heilman & E. Valenstein (Eds.), *Clinical Neuropsychology* (4th ed., pp. 404–446). New York: Oxford University Press.

Damasio, H., & Damasio, A. R. (1989). *Lesion analysis in neuropsychology*. New York: Oxford University Press.

Damasio, H., Grabowski, T., Frank, R., Galaburda, A. M., & Damasio, A. R. (1994). The return of Phineas Gage: Clues about the brain from the skull of a famous patient. *Science, 264*(5162), 1102–1105.

De Carli, D., Garreffa, G., Colonnese, C., Giulietti, G., Labruna, L., Briselli, E., et al. (2007). Identification of activated regions during a language task. *Magnetic Resonance Imaging, 25*(6), 933–938.

Decety, J., Perani, D., Jeannerod, M., Bettinard, V., Tadardy, B., Woods, R., et al. (1994). Mapping motor representations with positron emission tomography. *Nature, 371*, 600–602.

Delis, D. C., Kaplan, E., & Kramer, J. K. (2001). *Delis-Kaplan executive function system (D–KEFS)*. San Antonio: Harcourt Assessment, Inc.

Denckla, M. B. (1994). Measurement of executive function. In G. R. Lyon (Ed.), *Frames of reference for the assessment of learning disabilities: New views on measurement issues* (pp. 117–142). Baltimore, MD: Paul H. Brooks.

Denckla, M. B. (1996). A theory and model of executive function: A neuropsychological perspective. In G. R. Lyon & N. A. Krasnegor (Eds.), *Attention, memory, and executive function* (pp. 263–277). Baltimore, MD: Paul H. Brooks.

Dronkers, N. F. (1996). A new brain region for coordinating speech articulation. *Nature, 384*, 159–161.

Elliott, R. (2003). Executive functions and their disorders. *British Medical Bulletin, 65*, 49–59.

Eslinger, P. J., & Damasio, A. R. (1985). Severe disturbance of higher cognition after bilateral frontal ablation. *Neurology, 35*, 1731–1741.

Fadiga, L., Craighero, L., & Roy, A. (2006). Broca's region: A speech area? In Y. Grodzinky & K. Amunts (Eds.), *Broca's region* (pp. 137–152). New York: Oxford University Press.

Fazio, P., Cantagallo, A., Craighero, L., D'Ausilio, A., Roy, A. C., Pozzo, T., et al. (2009). Encoding of human action in Broca's area. *Brain, 132*(7), 1980–1988.

Feuchtwanger, E. (1923). *Die funktionen des Stirnhirns*. Berlin: Springer.

Filley, C. M., Young, D. A., Reardon, M. S., & Wilkening, G. N. (1999). Frontal lobe lesions and executive dysfunction in children. *Neuropsychiatry, Neuropsychology, and Behavioral Neurology, 12*, 156–160.

Fincham, J. M., Carter, C. S., van Veen, V., Stenger, V. A., & Anderson, J. R. (2002). Neural mechanisms of planning: A computational analysis using event-related fMRI. *Proceedings of the National Academy of Sciences of the United States of America, 99*(5), 3346–3351.

Foundas, A. L., Eure, K. F., Luevano, L. F., & Weinberger, D. R. (1998). MRI asymmetries of Broca's area: The pars triangularis and pars opercularis. *Brain and Language, 64*, 282–296.

Fox, P. T., Ingham, R. J., Ingham, J. C., Zamarripa, F., Xiong, J. H., & Lancaster, J. L. (2000). Brain correlates of stuttering and syllable production: A PET performance-correlation analysis. *Brain, 123*, 1985–2004.

Friedman, N. P., Miyake, A., Young, S. E., Defries, J. C., Corley, R. P., & Hewitt, J. K. (2008). Individual differences in executive functions are almost entirely genetic in origin. *Journal of Experimental Psychology: General, 137*(2), 201–225.

Fuster, J. M. (1989). *The prefrontal cortex* (2nd ed.). New York: Raven Press.

Fuster, J. M. (1997). *The prefrontal cortex: Anatomy, physiology, and neuropsychology of the frontal lobe* (3rd ed.). New York: Lippincott, Williams & Wilkins.

Fuster, J. M. (2001). The prefrontal cortex—an update: Time is of the essence. *Neuron, 30*, 319–333.

Fuster, J. M. (2002). Frontal lobe and cognitive development. *Journal of Neuropsychology, 31*, 373–385.

Fuster, J. M. (2008). *The prefrontal cortex* (4th ed.). Boston: Academic Press.

Godefroy, O., Cabaret, M., Petit-Chenal, V., Pruvo, J. P., & Rousseaux, M. (1999). Control functions of the frontal lobes: Modularity of the central-supervisory system? *Cortex, 35*(1), 1–20.

Goel, V., Gold, B., Kapur, S., & Houle, S. (1997). The seats of reason? An imaging study of deductive and inductive reasoning. *Neuroreport, 8*(5), 1305–1310.

Goel, V., Gold, B., Kapur, S., & Houle, S. (1998). Neuroanatomical correlates of human reasoning. *Journal of Cognitive Neuroscience, 10*(3), 293–302.

Goldberg, E. (2001). *The executive brain.* New York: Oxford University Press.

Goldman-Rakic, P. S., & Porrino, L. J. (1985). The primate mediodorsal (MD) nucleus and its projection to the frontal lobe. *The Journal of Comparative Neurology, 242,* 535–560.

Goodglass, H. (1993). *Understanding aphasia.* New York: Academic Press.

Grafman, J. (2006). Human prefrontal cortex: Processes and representations. In J. Risberg & J. Grafman (Eds.), *The frontal lobes: Development, function and pathology* (pp. 69–91). Cambridge, MA: Cambridge University Press.

Grezes, J., & Decety, J. (2002). Does visual perception of object afford action? Evidence from a neuroimaging study. *Neuropsychologia, 40,* 212–222.

Grodzinsky, Y. (2000). The neurology of syntax: Language use without Broca's area. *Behavioral and Brain Sciences, 23,* 1–21.

Grodzinsky, Y. (2006). The language faculty, Broca's region, and the mirror system. *Cortex, 42,* 464–468.

Grodzinsky, Y., & Amunts, K. (Eds.). (2006). *Broca's region.* New York: Oxford University Press.

Grodzinsky, Y., & Friederici, A. D. (2006). Neuroimaging of syntax and syntactic processing. *Current Opinions in Neurobiology, 16,* 240–246.

Hagoort, P. (2005). Broca's complex as the unification of space for language. In A. Cutler (Ed.), *Twenty-first century psycholinguistics: Four cornerstones* (pp. 157–172). Mahwah, NJ: Lawrence Erlbaum Associates.

Hagoort, P. (2006). On Broca, brain, and binding. In Y. Grodzinky & K. Amunts (Eds.), *Broca's region* (pp. 242–253). New York: Oxford University Press.

Harlow, J. M. (1868). Recovery from the passage of an iron bar through the head. *Massachusetts Medical Society Publications, 2,* 327–346.

Hausen, H. S., Lachmann, E. A., & Nagler, W. (1997). Cerebral diaschisis following cerebellar hemorrhage. *Archives of Physical Medicine and Rehabilitation, 78,* 546–549.

Haverkort, M. (2005). Linguistic representation and language use in aphasia. In A. Cutler (Ed.), *Twenty-first century psycholinguistics: Four cornerstones* (pp. 57–68). Mahwah, NJ: Lawrence Erlbaum Associates.

Heim, S., Eickhoff, S. B., & Amunts, K. (2008). Specialization in Broca's region for semantic, phonological, and syntactic fluency? *Neuroimage, 40*(3), 1362–1368.

Heim, S., Opitz, B., Müller, K., & Friederici, A. D. (2003). Phonological processing during language production: fMRI evidence for a shared production-comprehension network. *Cognitive Brain Research, 16*(2), 285–296.

Hillis, A. E., Work, M., Barker, P. B., Jacobs, M. A., Breese, E. L., & Maurer, K. (2004). Re-examining the brain regions crucial for orchestrating speech articulation. *Brain, 127,* 1479–1487.

Hobson, P., & Leeds, L. (2001). Executive functioning in older people. *Reviews in Clinical Gerontology, 11,* 361–372.

Inoue, K., Kawashima, R., Satoh, K., Kinomura, S., Sugiura, M., Goto, R., et al. (2000). A PET study of visuomotor learning under optical rotation. *Neuroimage, 11*(5 Pt. 1), 505–516.

Jacobs, R., Harvey, A. S., & Anderson, V. (2007). Executive function following focal frontal lobe lesions: Impact of timing of lesion on outcome. *Cortex, 43,* 792–805.

Jastrowitz, M. (1888). Beitrage zur Localization in Grosshirm and Uber deren prakitsche. Verwerthma. *Deutsche Medizinische Wochenschrift,14,* 81–83.

Kertesz, A. (1985). Aphasia. In J.A.M. Frederiks (Ed.), *Handbook of clinical neurology (Vol. 45): Clinical neuropsychology* (pp. 287–332). Amsterdam: Elsevier.

Kertesz, A. (1999). Language and the frontal lobe. In B. L. Miller & J. C. Cummings (Eds.), *The human frontal lobes: Functions and disorders* (pp. 261–277). New York: Guilford Press.

Kimberg, D., D'Esposito, M., & Farah, M. (1997). Cognitive functions in the prefrontal cortex—Working memory and executive control. *Current Directions in Psychological Science, 6,* 185–192.

Knauff, M., Mulack, T., Kassubek, J., Salih, H. R., & Greenlee, M. W. (2002). Spatial imagery in deductive reasoning: A functional MRI study. *Cognitive Brain Research, 13*(2), 203–212.

Koelsch, S., Fritz, T., V Cramon D. Y., Müller, K., & Friederici, A. D. (2006). Investigating emotion with music: An fMRI study. *Human Brain Mapping, 27*(3), 239–250.

Koziol, L. F., & Budding, D. E. (2009). *Subcortical structures and cognition.* New York: Springer.

Kübler, A., Dixon, V., & Garavan, H. (2006). Automaticity and reestablishment of executive control—An fMRI study. *Journal of Cognitive Neuroscience, 18*(8), 1331–1342.

Lafleche, G., & Albert, M. (1995). Executive function deficits in mild Alzheimer's disease. *Neuropsychology, 9,* 313–320.

Laiacona, M., De Santis, A., Barbarotto, R., Basso, A., Spagnoli, D., & Capitani, E. (1989). Neuropsychological follow-up of patients operated for aneurysms of anterior communicating artery. *Cortex, 25,* 261–273.

Lawrence, E. J., Shaw, P., Giampietro, V. P., Surguladze, S., Brammer, M. J., & David, A. S. (2006). The role of 'shared representations' in social perception and empathy: An fMRI study. *Neuroimage, 29*(4), 1173–1184.

Levin, H. S., Eisenberg, H. M. & Benton, A. L. (1991). *Frontal Lobe Function and Dysfunction.* New York: Oxford University Press.

Lezak, M. D. (1983). *Neuropsychological assessment* (2nd ed.). New York: Oxford University Press.

Li, P. C., Gong, H., Yang, J. J., Zeng, S. O., Luo, O. M., & Guan, L. C. (2000). Left prefrontal cortex activation during semantic encoding accessed with functional near infrared imaging. *Space Medicine & Medical Engineering, 13*(2), 79–83.

Lieberman, P. (2002a). *Human language and our reptilian brain.* Cambridge, MA: Harvard University Press.

Lieberman, P. (2002b). On the nature and evolution of the neural bases of human language. *Yearbook of Physical Anthropology, 45,* 36–62.

Lindenberg, R., Fangerau, H., & Seitz, R. J. (2007). "Broca's area" as a collective term? *Brain and Language, 102,* 22–29.

Lloyd, D. (2000). Virtual lesions and the not so-modular brain. *Journal of the International Neuropsychological Society, 6,* 627–635.

Lotze, M., Heymans, U., Birbaumer, N., Veit, R., Erb, M., Flor, H., et al. (2006). Differential cerebral activation during observation of expressive gestures and motor acts. *Neuropsychologia, 44*(10), 1787–1795.

Luria, A. R. (1969). Frontal lobe syndromes. In P. J. Vinken & G. W. Bruyn (Eds.), *Handbook of clinical neurology* (Vol. 2, pp. 725–757). Amsterdam: North Holland.

Luria, A. R. (1976). *Basic problems of neurolinguistics*. The Hague: Mouton.

Luria, A. R. (1980). *Higher cortical functions in man* (2nd ed.). New York: Basic.

Macmillan, M. (2000). Restoring Phineas Gage: A 150th retrospective. *Journal of the History of the Neurosciences, 9*(1), 42–62.

Macmillan, M. (2008). Phineas Gage – Unravelling the myth. *The Psychologist, 21*(9), 828–831.

Manthey, S., Schubotz, R. I., & von Cramon, D. Y. (2003). Premotor cortex in observing erroneous action: An fMRI study. *Cognitive Brain Research, 15*(3), 296–307.

Mantyla, T., Carelli, M. G., & Forman, H. (2007). Time monitoring and executive functioning in children and adults. *Journal of Experimental Child Psychology, 96*(1), 1–19.

Matsumura, M., Sadato, N., Kochiyama, T., Nakamura, S., Naito, E., Matsunami, K., et al. (2004). Role of the cerebellum in implicit motor skill learning: A PET study. *Brain Research Bulletin, 63*(6), 471–483.

McGuire, P. K., Silbersweig, D. A., Murray, R. M., David, A. S., Frackowiak, R. S. J., & Frith, C. D. (1996). Functional anatomy of inner speech and auditory verbal imagery. *Psychological Medicine, 26*, 38–39.

Mesulam, M. M. (1986). Frontal cortex and behavior. *Annals of Neurology, 19*, 320–325.

Mesulam, M. M. (2002). The human frontal lobes: Transcending the default mode through contingent encoding. In D. T. Stuss & R. T. Knight (Eds.), *Principles of frontal lobe function* (pp. 8–31). New York: Oxford.

Miki, A., Nakajima, T., Miyauchi, S., Takagi, M., & Abe, H. (1996). Functional magnetic resonance imaging of the frontal eye fields during saccadic eye movements. *Nippon Ganka Gakkai Zasshi, 100*(7), 541–545.

Miller, B. L., & Cummings, J. L. (1998). *The human frontal lobes: Functions and disorders*. New York: The Guilford Press.

Mitchell, R. L., & Phillips, L. H. (2007). The psychological, neurochemical and functional neuroanatomical mediators of the effects of positive and negative mood on executive functions. *Neuropsychologia, 45*(4), 617–629.

Miyake, A., Friedman, N., Emerson, M., Witzki, A., & Howerter, A. (2000). The unity and diversity of executive functions and their contributions to complex "frontal lobe" tasks: A latent variable analysis. *Cognitive Psychology, 41*, 49–100.

Mohr, J. P., Pessin, M. S., Finkelstein, S., Funkenstein, H. H., Duncan, G. W., & Davis, K. R. (1978). Broca's aphasia: Pathologic and clinical aspects. *Neurology, 28*, 311–324.

Morin, O., & Grèzes, J. (2008). What is "mirror" in the premotor cortex? A review. *Neurophysiologie Clinique, 38*(3), 189–195.

Nathaniel-James, D. A., Fletcher, P., & Frith, C. D. (1997). The functional anatomy of verbal initiation and suppression using the Hayling test. *Neuropsychologia, 35*,(4), 559–566.

Novick, J. M., Trueswell, J. C., & Thompson, S. L. (2005). Cognitive control and parsing: Reexamining the role of Broca's area in sentence comprehension. *Cognitive, Affective, & Behavioral Neuroscience, 5*, 263–281.

Novoa, O. P., & Ardila, A. (1987). Linguistic abilities in patients with prefrontal damage. *Brain and Language, 30*, 206–225.

Oppenheim, H. (1890). Zur Pathologie der Grosshirngeschwülste. *Archiv für Psychiatrie und Nervenkrankheiten, 21*, 560–587, 705–745.

Oppenheim, H. (1891). Zur Pathologie der Grosshirngeschwülste. *Archiv für Psychiatrie und Nervenkrankheiten, 22*, 27–72.

Osaka, N., Osaka, M., Mondo, H., Morishita, M., Fukuyama, H., & Shibasaki, H. (2004). The neural basis of executive function in working memory: An fMRI study based on individual differences. *NeuroImage, 21*, 623–631.

Pennington, B. F., & Ozonoff, S. (1996). Executive functions and developmental psychopathology. *Journal of Child Psychology and Psychiatry, 37*, 51–87.

Perecman, E. (Ed.). (1987). *The frontal lobes revisited*. New York: The IRBN Press.

Perry, D. W., Zatorre, R. J., Petrides, M., Alivisatos, B., Meyer, E., & Evans, A. C. (1999). Localization of cerebral activity during simple singing. *Neuroreport, 10*(18), 3979–3984.

Piguet, O., Grayson, G., Browe, A., Tate, H., Lye, T., Creasey, H., et al. (2002). Normal aging and executive functions in "old-old" community dwellers: Poor performance is not an inevitable outcome. *International Psychogeriatric Association, 14*, 139–159.

Platek, S. M., Keenan, J. P., Gallup, G. G., & Mohamed, F. B. (2004). Where am I? The neurological correlates of self and other. *Cognitive Brain Research, 19*, 114–122.

Pochon, J. B., Levy, R., Fossati, P., Lehericy, S., Poline, J. B., Pillon, B., et al. (2002). The neural system that bridges reward and cognition in humans: An fMRI study. *Proceedings of the National Academy of Sciences of the United States of America, 99*(8), 5669–5674.

Pribram, K. H., & Luria, A. R. (Eds). (1973). *Psychophysiology of the frontal lobes*. New York: Academic Press.

Rämä, P., Martinkauppi, S., Linnankoski, I., Koivisto, J., Aronen, H. J., & Carlson, S. (2001). Working memory of identification of emotional vocal expressions: An fMRI study. *Neuroimage, 13*(6, Pt. 1), 1090–1101.

Ranganath, C., Johnson, M. K., & D'Esposito, M. (2003). Prefrontal activity associated with working memory and episodic long-term memory. *Neuropsychologia, 41*(3), 378–389.

Rapp, A. M., Leube, D. T., Erb, M., Grodd, W., & Kircher, T. T. (2004). Neural correlates of metaphor processing. *Cognitive Brain Research, 20*(3), 395–402.

Raye, C. L., Johnson, M. K., Mitchell, K. J., Reeder, J. A., & Greene, E. J. (2002). Neuroimaging a single thought: Dorsolateral PFC activity associated with refreshing just-activated information. *Neuroimage, 15*(2), 447–453.

Rickard, T. C., Romero, S. G., Basso, G., Wharton, C., Flitman, S., & Grafman, J. (2000). The calculating brain: an fMRI study. *Neuropsychologia, 38*(3), 325–335.

Rizzolatti, G., & Arbib, M. A. (1998). Language within our grasp. *Trends in Neurosciences, 21*, 188–194.

Rizzolatti, G., & Craighero, L. (2004). The mirror neuron system. *Annual Review of Neuroscience, 27,* 169–192.

Rizzolatti, G., Fadiga, L., Gallese, V., & Fogassi, L. (1996). Premotor cortex and the recognition of motor actions. *Cognitive Brain Research, 3,* 131–141.

Roberts, A. C., Robbins, T. W., & Weiskrantz, I. (2002). *The prefrontal cortex: Executive and cognitive functions.* Oxford: Oxford University Press.

Rogers, R. D., Owen, A. M., Middleton, H. C., Williams, E. J., Pickard, J. D., Sahakian, B. J., et al. (1999). Choosing between small, likely rewards and large, unlikely rewards activates inferior and orbital prefrontal cortex. *The Journal of Neuroscience, 19*(20), 9029–9038.

Ross, E. D. (1981). The aprosodias: Functional-anatomical organization of the affective components of language in the right hemisphere. *Archives of Neurology, 140,* 695–710.

Salthouse, T. (1996). The processing-speed theory of adult age differences in cognition. *Psychological Review, 103,* 403–428.

Salthouse, T. (2005). Relations between cognitive abilities and measures of executive functioning. *Neuropsychology, 19,* 532–545.

Salthouse, T., Atkinson, T., & Berish, D. (2003). Executive functioning as a potential mediator of age-related cognitive decline in normal adults. *Journal of Experimental Psychology: General, 132,* 566–594.

Schiff, H. B., Alexander, M. P., Naeser, M. A., & Galaburda, A. M. (1983). Aphemia. Clinical-anatomic correlations. *Archives of Neurology, 40*(12), 720–727.

Schoenemann, P. T. (2006). Evolution of the size and functional areas of the human brain. *Annual Review of Anthropology, 35,* 379–406.

Schoenemann, P. T., Sheehan, M. J., Glotzer, L. D. (2005). Prefrontal white matter volume is disproportionately larger in humans than in other primates. *Nature Neuroscience, 8,* 242–252.

Schubotz, R. I., & von Cramon, D. Y. (2001). Functional organization of the lateral premotor cortex: fMRI reveals different regions activated by anticipation of object properties, location and speed. *Brain Research and Cognitive Brain Research, 11*(1), 97–112.

Semendeferi, K., Lu, A., Schenker, N., & Damasio, H. (2002). Humans and great apes share a large frontal cortex. *Nature Neuroscience, 5,* 272–276.

Shammi, P., & Stuss, D. T. (1999). Humour appreciation: A role of the right frontal lobe. *Brain, 122,* 657–666.

Shibata, M., Abe, J., Terao, A., & Miyamoto, T. (2007). Neural mechanisms involved in the comprehension of metaphoric and literal sentences: An fMRI study. *Brain Research, 1166,* 92–102.

Shuster, L. I., & Lemieux, S. K. (2005). An fMRI investigation of covertly and overtly produced mono- and multisyllabic words. *Brain and Language, 93*(1), 20–31.

Stout, J. C., Ready, R. E., Grace, J., Malloy, P. F. & Paulsen, J. S. (2003). Factor analysis of the frontal systems behavior scale (FrSBe). *Assessment, 10*(1), 79–85.

Stuss, D. T., & Alexander, M. P. (2000). Executive functions and the frontal lobe: A conceptual view. *Psychological Research, 63,* 289–298.

Stuss, D. T., & Alexander, M. P. (2007). Is there a dysexecutive syndrome? *Philosophical Transactions of the Royal Society, 362,* 901–915.

Stuss, D. T., & Benson, D. F. (1986). *The frontal lobes.* New York: Raven Press.

Stuss, D. T., Gallup, G. G., & Alexander, M. P. (2001). Frontal lobes and "theory of the mind." *Brain, 124,* 274–286.

Stuss, D. T., & Knight, R. T. (2002). *Principles of frontal lobe function.* New York: Oxford University Press.

Stuss, D. T., & Levine, B. (2002). Adult clinical neuropsychology: Lessons from studies of the frontal lobes. *Annual Review of Psychology, 53,* 401–433.

Sun, X., Zhang, X., Chen, X., Zhang, P., Bao, M., Zhang, D., et al. (2005). Age-dependent brain activation during forward and backward digit recall revealed by fMRI. *Neuroimage, 26*(1), 36–47.

Super, H., Spekreijse, H., & Lamme, V. A. (2001). A neural correlate of working memory in the monkey primary visual cortex. *Science, 293,* 120–124.

Thompson-Schill, S. L. (2005). Dissecting the language organ: A new look at the role of Broca's area in language processing. In A. Cutler (Ed.), *Twenty-first century psycholinguistics: Four cornerstones* (pp. 173–190). Mahwah, NJ: Lawrence Erlbaum Associates.

Trousseau, A. (1864). De L'aphasie, maladie décrite recémment sous le nom impropre d'aphemie. *Gaz Hop Civ Mil, 37,* 13–4, 25–6, 37–9, 49–50.

Vorobyev, V. A., Alho, K., Medvedev, S. V., Pakhomov, S. V., Roudas, M. S., Rutkovskaya, J. M., et al. (2004). Linguistic processing in visual and modality-nonspecific brain areas: PET recordings during selective attention. *Cognitive Brain Research, 20*(2), 309–322.

Vygotsky, L. S. (1929). The problem of the cultural development of the child II. *Journal of Genetic Psychology, 36,* 415–432.

Vygotsky, L. S. (1934/1962). *Thought and language.* Cambridge, MA: MIT Press.

Vygotsky, L. S. (1934/1978). *Mind in society.* Cambridge, MA: Harvard University Press.

Wang, S., Zhu, Z., Zhang, J. X., Wang, Z., Xiao, Z., Xiang, H., et al. (2008). Broca's area plays a role in syntactic processing during Chinese reading comprehension. *Neuropsychologia, 46*(5), 1371–1378.

Zhang, J. X., Leung, H. C., & Johnson, M. K. (2003). Frontal activations associated with accessing and evaluating information in working memory: An fMRI study. *Neuroimage, 20*(3), 1531–1539.

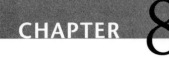

CHAPTER 8

Language and Communication Disorders Associated with Attentional Deficits

CHAPTER OUTLINE

Bruce Crosson and Matthew L. Cohen

LANGUAGE AND COMMUNICATION DISORDERS ASSOCIATED WITH ATTENTIONAL DEFICITS

Arousal, vigilance, intention, and attention are fundamental cognitive substrates that cannot be entirely separated from the cognitive processes they support. Together with working memory, they provide the scaffolding upon which language and other higher-level cognitive processes are carried out. Inevitably, brain damage and disease affect these substrates and thus interfere with higher cognitive processes that depend on them. This interference with cognitive processing can occur whether or not the cognitive process in question is directly affected by the brain damage. For example, when this underlying architecture of arousal, vigilance, intention, and attention is weakened, language operations become less efficient, and in severe cases, some language functions can become severely compromised. Hence, addressing the mechanisms of arousal, vigilance, intention, and attention can be important for understanding implications for communication, even in cases of relatively subtle deficits. To do

so, one must understand their anatomy and implications of their impairment for language and communication. Regarding intention and attention, understanding the implications of lateralization for these substrates is also important. In this chapter, we endeavor to first define arousal, vigilance, intention, and attention, and then to explore the impact of disorders of these processes on language and communication. Although addressing language and communication in this fashion is somewhat unconventional, there is much that can be learned by doing so. This is not only true for the clinician, but is particularly true for the researcher as well. The last couple of decades have yielded interesting findings in this regard, and hopefully, the next couple of decades will build on this foundation.

AROUSAL, VIGILANCE, INTENTION, AND ATTENTION MECHANISMS: THE BASICS

A basic understanding of intention and attention mechanisms will be necessary for understanding their impact on language and communication. Before beginning this discussion, an important distinction must be made. In much of the classical literature in cognitive psychology, attention and related processes are considered as hypothetical constructs and assigned certain properties. For example, attention is frequently considered to be a finite resource, portions of which can be allocated to some activity, much the same way that we might draw money from a bank account for one project or another. We do not believe that such metaphors are productive in understanding attention and related functions. Rather, we will consider attention and related functions to be processes arising from various activities that restrict the information we process or the actions we perform to a manageable level.

For example, consider having a conversation in a crowded room with many others talking around you. There may be three, or four, or even five conversations within earshot on which you might focus. What allows you to focus on the speech with the specific person to whom you are talking? That ability lies within the realm of *attention* (which we will define formally shortly). Put simply, we filter out the irrelevant sources of information (i.e., other conversations) using attention mechanisms and focus on the one source of information important to us. Why must we focus on a single source of information to the exclusion of others? The answer is that the brain system we use for language comprehension has a limited capacity in the amount of incoming linguistic information it can process at one time. These capacity limitations lie within the realm of working memory. Working memory can be defined as the ability to hold items in one's immediate grasp so that they can be used for other processes (e.g., comprehension of a communication). It is widely accepted that the number of items that can be held in working memory is limited. Attempts to quantify working memory capacity go at least as far back as the work of Miller (1956), but research has continued in this topic (Cowan, 2001). It is not our purpose to elaborate on working memory and its capacity. It suffices to note that limited capacity of processing resources constitutes a bottleneck in processing through which only a limited amount of information can pass. What concerns us here are the processes that keep a particular resource from being overwhelmed by more information than it can handle, which would lead to a deterioration in processing.

As a second example (on the output side), suppose you want to talk about your dog. You could choose a variety of words to describe your dog: "dog," "Lab," "Labrador," "Labrador retriever," "yellow Lab," "Gertrude" (real name), "Trudy" (nickname), "pet," etc. Which word(s) you choose will depend in part upon the context of the discussion and upon the shared knowledge of the listener, but in order to talk about your dog, you have to choose the word(s) to describe your dog each time you mention her. For the sake of efficiency, you do not say every word that might be used for your dog each time you mention her; you must select one. This selection is in the realm of *intention* (which will be defined formally later). The concept is that when we act, the action we choose will preclude other competing actions. Again, at the point of selection, there is a bottleneck at which time only one, or at least a very limited number of actions can be selected. The relevant issue here is not so much how we implement actions; rather, it is how we limit the selected actions to a level that can actually be performed to achieve our goals.

Now that we have discussed the assumption of limited capacity for processing incoming information or for executing actions, we can turn to more formal definitions of the components of attention. Posner and Boies (1971) broke attention down into three components: arousal, vigilance, and selective attention. Work reviewed by Heilman and colleagues (Heilman, Watson, & Valenstein, 2003), however, suggests that the selective attention component can be further divided into separate intention and attention processes. Arousal and vigilance are basic states supporting more complex forms of attention (Figure 8-1). Arousal refers to a physiological state underlying a general readiness to act or to receive and process incoming information. It can be contrasted with sleep or coma, states in which the organism is ready neither to act nor to receive and process incoming information. Arousal can be thought of as having degrees, and the greatest cognitive efficiency is assumed when one is neither hyperaroused nor hypoaroused. Since arousal supports vigilance, intention, and attention, these other forms of attention are affected when arousal is above or below optimal levels.

Vigilance refers to a state whereby attention is sustained over a fairly long period of time. It is necessary for tasks that require processing of incoming information and/or formulating actions over a long period of time. One example might be sustaining attention to road conditions, route considerations, and traffic when driving. Within the realm of language, vigilance would be needed to conduct a meeting or to hold a conversation. Arousal and vigilance are necessary for selective forms of intention and attention, which are discussed next.

We touched on intention and attention earlier. A good place to begin this elaboration regarding these two forms of attention is with the observation of the Russian neuroanatomist Vladimir Alekseyevich Betz that the brain is basically an elaboration of the spinal cord (Betz, 1874). That is, the anatomic organization of

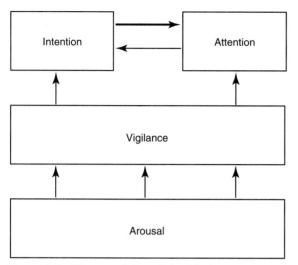

Figure 8-1 Diagram of the relationship between arousal, vigilance, intention, and attention. The diagram indicates that all other kinds of attention are dependent on an optimal level of arousal; thus, both hypoarousal and hyperarousal can cause problems downstream in attention systems. Most tasks require the ability to sustain intention and attention; for this reason, vigilance is also a necessary substrate for selecting actions or processing information. Intention and attention mechanisms also interact. Most frequently what we intend to do influences to what we attend, though external or internal stimuli also can capture attention and influence intention.

the spinal cord (motor functions in the anterior portion and sensory functions in the posterior portion) is recapitulated in the brain. Put another way, the anterior telencephalon (frontal lobes) is concerned with the planning and execution of action and the posterior telencephalon (temporal, parietal, and occipital lobes) is concerned with the sensation and perception of internal and external information. Although this idea is somewhat of an oversimplification, it is useful in conceptualizing brain organization (e.g., see Fuster, 2003).

Attention can be thought of as the ability to select for further processing one among many potential sources of sensory input. It is worth noting that this definition is essentially that of William James (1890). Thus, attention governs the processing of sensory information and the degree to which that information is processed. As such, it governs information processing in the posterior cortices. In the realm of language, attention would be important for listening to and processing a conversation with one person as opposed to listening and processing the surrounding conversations at a gathering of people. Another example might be that you are attending to the written information on

this page and processing it as opposed to looking at and processing the other stimuli that surround you.

Intention can be thought of as the action equivalent of attention, that is, the ability to select one among many potential actions for execution and to initiate that action. Hence, intention governs what actions are performed; therefore, intention mechanisms regulate a good deal of the information and action processing in anterior cortices. In the realm of language, if you were asked to name one kind of bird, you would have to select one to say among the dozens of kinds of birds you know. Another example would be choosing the best sentence structure to state an idea from among several potential structures. Intention also has been called "executive attention" by Fuster (2003), but the concept is essentially the same as that of intention.

To this point, we have discussed intention and attention as if they were entirely separate mechanisms. However, as we negotiate our surroundings in everyday life, intention and attention mechanisms influence each other. This interaction is represented in Figure 8-1 by the arrows between intention and attention mechanisms. Indeed, an important maxim is that what we intend to do determines to what we attend. For example, if I intend to pour a cup of coffee, I must attend to the location of the cup. From a communication standpoint, if I intend to carry on a conversation with you, I must attend to what you are saying. Nadeau and Crosson (1997) referred to this kind of attention as intentionally guided attention. It is represented by a somewhat larger arrow in Figure 8-1 because our intentions so commonly determine the items to which we attend. However, it is also true that attention can affect intention. For example, suppose you were at a baseball game and you notice that the ball has been hit into the stands right at you. Because of the impending danger, the ball will capture your attention, and you will take evasive action. As an example relevant to communication, imagine you are at a party talking to a friend and someone calls your name. The stimulus of someone calling your name will temporarily capture your attention and you will orient to that stimulus so that you can determine who is calling you and if any further action is necessary.

Before proceeding to a discussion of neural substrates, one further observation should be made regarding the nature of intention and attention mechanisms. To this point, our discussion about capacity limitations has revolved around the limited capacity within modality. For example, we noted that our processing of language is limited by the amount of information we can hold in our immediate attention (i.e., working memory). McNeil and his colleagues have studied the interface between attention and language, using dual task paradigms where either linguistic or nonlinguistic tasks compete with linguistic tasks (for a review, see Hula & McNeil, 2008). In general, the literature indicates that when linguistic and nonlinguistic tasks are performed almost simultaneously, they can interfere with each other, suggesting that they are competing for utilization of mechanisms common to both. For example, identifying a tone as high or low can interfere with picture naming. The usual interpretation is that the tasks are competing for utilization of attention (or intention) mechanisms or resources. Hence, simultaneous performance of tasks that require different kinds of processing may interfere with each other, for example, talking on a cell phone and driving a car. Finally, it is worth noting that Hula and McNeil (2008) attribute symptoms of aphasia to impairment in such attention mechanisms. We do not subscribe to this viewpoint, believing instead that impaired linguistic,

attention, and intention mechanisms contribute to the symptoms of various aphasia syndromes. Although further discussion of our differences in frameworks is beyond the scope of this chapter, it is worth reading Hula and McNeil's (2008) review for a different viewpoint.

NEURAL SUBSTRATES OF AROUSAL, VIGILANCE, INTENTION, AND ATTENTION

Since Moruzzi and Magoun (1949) demonstrated the role of the brainstem reticular formation, and particularly its midbrain component (Figure 8-2), in arousal, the midbrain reticular formation has been assumed to play a key role in arousal. However, since that time, it has been shown that arousal is affected by other structures as well, such as the thalamus (Figure 8-3).

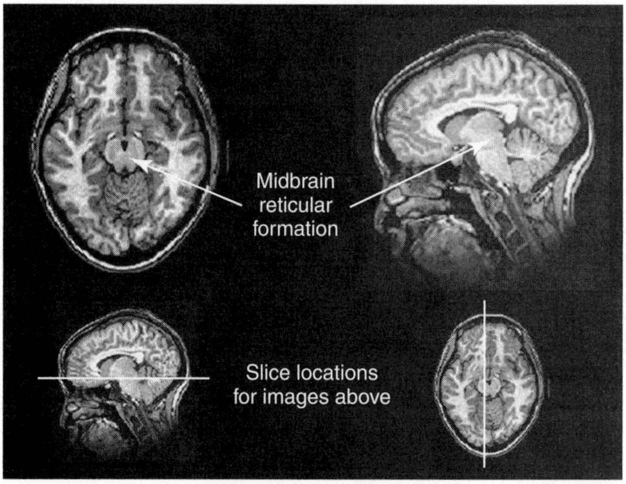

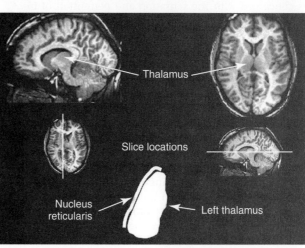

Figure 8-2 Midbrain reticular formation. These images show the approximate location of the midbrain reticular formation on an axial (*horizontal*) magnetic resonance image (*top left*) and on a sagittal (*vertical, front-to-back*) image (*top right*). The slice location for the axial slice is shown by the white horizontal line on the sagittal image (*bottom left*), and the slice location for the sagittal image is shown by the line on the axial image (*bottom right*).

Figure 8-3 Thalamus. The thalamus is shown on a sagittal magnetic resonance image (*top left*) and on an axial image (*top right*). Slice locations for each of these images are shown below the respective images. At the *bottom center* of the figure is a schematic representation of the relationship between the nucleus reticularis and the left thalamus in an axial orientation.

Sherman and Guillery (2006) reviewed the literature indicating that thalamic rhythms have a role in arousal. In the state of sleep, for example, thalamic relay cells reside in mode of rhythmic bursting, where fidelity of information transfer to the cortex is low. In the waking state, thalamic neurons are often in a single-spike, high fidelity mode of information transfer, where the output and input show good correspondence. The nucleus reticularis is a thin shell of neurons surrounding the lateral and anterior aspects of the thalamus in which corticothalamic and thalamocortical axons give off collaterals (Figure 8-3). The main inhibitory (GABAergic) target of cells in the nucleus reticularis are cells in the various thalamic nuclei. The firing mode of cells in the nucleus reticularis appears to affect the mode (burst versus single-spike) of thalamic relay nuclei. In turn, the midbrain reticular formation projects to the nucleus reticularis. Many of the profound effects of the midbrain reticular formation on arousal and, in turn, on intention and attention, are thought to be mediated by these connections at the thalamic level (Heilman et al., 2003). Finally, Heilman et al. (2003) have noted that specific cholinergic pathways involving the midbrain reticular formation may be involved in arousal.

The neurobiology of vigilance has not received as much attention in the literature as the neurobiology of arousal. However, it is clear that adequate arousal is necessary for vigilance. Hence, damage to or dysfunction in any of the arousal mechanisms mentioned earlier will lead to problems in vigilance. Indeed, subtle problems in arousal may be manifested as disturbances in vigilance. Further, sustaining intention or attention over time requires the vigilance to do so. As a result, it is likely that frontal mechanisms involved in intention (see later) are also involved in vigilance. Frontopontine fibers, for example, are known to reach the vicinity of

the pontine reticular formation (Parent, 1996), where they could affect the ascending reticular formation and modulate or help to sustain arousal (Figure 8-4).

The anatomy of intention (and attention) has been discussed by Heilman and colleagues (2003). As noted earlier, intention mechanisms regulate processing in the anterior cortices. Medial frontal cortices are known to be involved in the intention aspects of language, and damage to these cortices results in akinetic mutism (Barris & Schuman, 1953; Nielsen & Jacobs, 1951), a syndrome where language expression (and other activities) are initiated only with externally guided (exo-evoked) stimuli, such as very significant urging by an examiner or other person interacting with the patient. The supracallosal medial frontal cortex (Figure 8-5) can be divided into the anterior cingulate gyrus, the rostral cingulate zone, the supplementary motor area (SMA), and the pre–supplementary motor area (pre-SMA). Based on our research in word production, the portion of this cortex at the junction of pre-SMA and the rostral cingulate zone seems to be most important for word finding (Crosson, Sadek, Bobholz, et al., 1999; Crosson, Sadek, Maron, et al., 2001; Crosson, Benefield, Cato, et al., 2003).

The basal ganglia (Figure 8-6) are also involved in the intentional aspects of language, though their influence may be more subtle. These influences seem to be regulated by cortical-basal ganglia-cortical circuits (Figure 8-7) that are connected primarily, though not exclusively, to the frontal lobes (Alexander, DeLong, & Strick, 1986; Middleton & Strick, 2000). Crosson and colleagues (Crosson, Benjamin, & Levy, 2007) have adapted models of movement (Gerfen, 1992; Mink, 1996; Penney & Young, 1986) to explain empirical data regarding the participation of the basal ganglia in language (Copland, 2003; Copland, Chenery, & Murdoch, 2000b; Crosson et al., 2003). The essentials of the

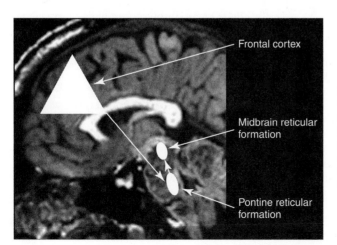

Figure 8-4 Frontal influence on midbrain reticular formation. A schematic representation of one pathway by which the frontal lobes might influence the midbrain reticular formation is overlaid onto a mid-sagittal magnetic resonance image. Essentially, descending fibers from frontal cortex synapse in the pontine reticular formation, which, in turn, sends ascending fibers to the midbrain reticular formation.

Figure 8-5 Divisions of medial frontal and medial posterior cortex relevant to language. A sagittal image of the medial wall of the cerebral hemisphere is shown (*upper left*). On an enlargement of the same image (*center*), the relevant frontal structures are: the anterior cingulate gyrus, the rostral cingulate zone, pre–supplementary motor area (SMA), and SMA. The medial motor cortex is plotted for reference. Relevant medial posterior structures are the posterior cingulate gyrus and the precuneus. A typical activity pattern for medial frontal cortex during category member generation is shown (*bottom right*). The vertical green line divides pre-SMA from SMA; both are active, but the activity also extends into the rostral cingulate zone. *BA 32*, Brodmann's area 32.

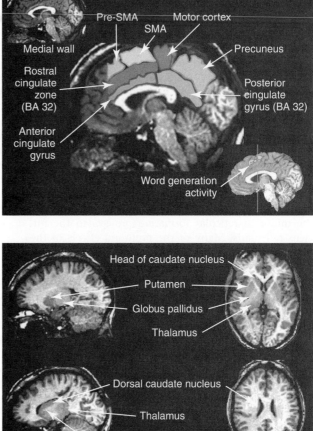

Figure 8-6 Basal ganglia. The location of the basal ganglia (caudate nucleus, putamen, and globus pallidus) and thalamus are shown in sagittal (*left*) and axial (*right*) magnetic resonance images. For sagittal images, the *bottom image* is medial to the *top image*. For axial images, the *bottom image* is superior to the *top image*.

model are that the basal ganglia enhance actions selected for execution (see Figure 8-7) and suppress alternative actions competing with the selected action (see Figure 8-7). In other words, the basal ganglia can be thought of as increasing the signal-to-noise ratio for a given output (i.e., behavior) (Kischka et al., 1996). Nambu and colleagues (Nambu, Tokuno, & Takada, 2002) have proposed that the basal ganglia also reset (clear) the system to allow switching from one action to another (see Figure 8-7).

The effects of basal ganglia damage or dysfunction on language are more subtle than those of medial frontal damage. It is well established now that basal ganglia damage alone does not cause aphasia (Hillis, Wityk, Barber, et al., 2002; Nadeau & Crosson, 1997). Thus, patients with Parkinson disease or basal ganglia lesions might demonstrate deficits in aphasia batteries only for the most difficult tasks, like naming low frequency items or word fluency (i.e., naming as many items as possible beginning

with a given letter or belonging to a given semantic category) (Copland, Chenery, & Murdoch, 2000a). However, the effects of Parkinson disease or basal ganglia lesion are seen on more complex language tasks, such as defining words or stating two concepts for an ambiguous sentence. The effects of medial frontal damage would be more pervasive than those of Parkinson disease or basal ganglia lesion because of the patient's inability to initiate their own responses after medial frontal damage.

A final distinction regarding intention should be made. That is the difference between endo-evoked and exo-evoked intention (Heilman et al., 2003). Endo-evoked intention refers to the selection and initiation of action (including cognitive actions) based on some internal motivation or state, while exo-evoked intention refers to behavior that is evoked by external stimulation. The akinesia (lack of or decreased movement) seen in patients with Parkinson disease can be thought

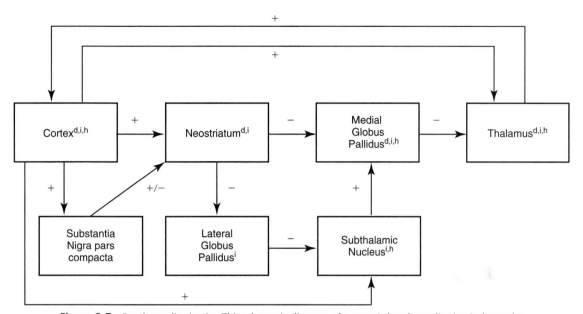

Figure 8-7 Basal ganglia circuits. This schematic diagram of a generic basal ganglia circuit shows the three subloops. These subloops are closed starting in an area of cortex and ending in the same area of cortex. The direct subloop includes cortex → neostriatum → medial globus pallidus → thalamus ←→ cortex (structures with a superscripted "d"). The indirect subloop includes cortex → neostriatum → lateral globus pallidus → subthalamic nucleus → medial globus pallidus → thalamus ←→ cortex (structures with a superscripted "i"). Structures in the hyperdirect subloop include cortex → subthalamic nucleus → medial globus pallidus → thalamus ←→ cortex (structures with a superscripted "h"). The "+" indicates the excitatory neurotransmitter glutamate, the "−" indicates the inhibitory neurotransmitter GABA, and the "±" indicates dopamine, which has a net facilitation effect on neostriatal neurons projecting into the direct subloop and a net suppression effect on neostriatal neurons projecting into the indirect subloop.

of as a disorder of endo-evoked intention; Parkinsonian patients have difficulty initiating behavior based on internal thoughts or motivations. However, if a strong external stimulus is applied (e.g., if someone were to shout "fire"), the difficulty initiating action (e.g., jumping up and moving away from danger) is mitigated.

As noted earlier, attention governs which sources of information are selected for further processing in the posterior cortices. The medial posterior cortices (posterior cingulate/precuneus region, Figure 8-5) and the parietal lobe play a large role in attention (Heilman et al., 2003). The effects of parietal lesions on attention often have hemispatial consequences on the side of space opposite of the lesion. It has been shown, for example, that patients with parietal lesions might perform language tasks better when stimuli are presented in their ipsilesional hemispace (Coslett, 1999). Thalamic nuclei also play a crucial role in attention (Sherman & Guillery, 2006). Essentially, this mechanism involves the firing modes in which thalamic neurons reside, as discussed earlier. There is a high fidelity mode of

information transfer from the periphery (single spike mode) for attended to items and a low fidelity mode of information transfer (burst mode) for unattended items. These authors have speculated that even cortico-cortical operations might be governed by similar mechanisms.

As noted earlier, intention and attention systems interact constantly during our everyday existence. Nadeau and Crosson (1997) called this relationship between the two systems intentionally guided attention, and they posited an anatomic mechanism (Figure 8-8).

Essentially, the frontal lobes are thought to influence thalamic nuclei through connections with the nucleus reticularis, surrounding the thalamus, which in turn regulates the state (single spike versus burst mode) of thalamic nuclei. Hence, this frontal-thalamic system intimately links intention and attention. The great irony about intention and attention is that intention governs much of what we attend to in our lives, but, as pointed out by Fuster (2003), intention is much less studied than attention.

Frontal Cortex

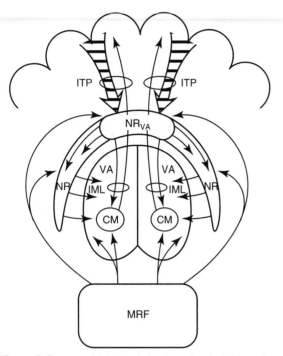

Figure 8-8 Frontal-inferior thalamic peduncle (ITP)–nucleus reticularis (NR) mechanism. This schematic diagram shows the frontal cortex projecting to the thalamus primarily through the ITP. The ITP pierces the NR through its ventral anterior component (NR_{VA}). The ITP gives of collaterals in the NR_{VA} which synapse on dendrites from neurons of more posterior segments of the NR. The neurons of the various NR segments send inhibitory projections into various thalamic nuclei affecting their state. These structures and connections are thought by Nadeau and Crosson (1997) to be the mechanism responsible for intentionally guided attention. This diagram also shows projections from the midbrain reticular formation (MRF) to the NR and to the centromedian nucleus of the thalamus (CM). *IML,* internal medullary lamina. [Reprinted from Brain and Language, Vol 58 (3), Stephen E. Nadeau and Bruce Crosson, Subcortical Aphasia, pp. 355–402, Copyright (1997), with permission from Elsevier.]

This form of attention (i.e., intentionally guided attention) may be compromised in aging. Cohen (manuscript in preparation) has recently demonstrated differences in the neural substrates of semantic fluency (saying as many items as one can in a category) between persons in their seventh and eighth decades of life and compared to younger counterparts in their third decade. There are three major differences between the older groups: First, during a semantic fluency task, persons in their eighth decade of life show much more extensive areas of increased neuronal activity in both hemispheres than persons in their seventh decade of life. Second, persons in their eighth decade demonstrate no areas of activity decrease during semantic fluency compared to a visual fixation baseline, whereas persons in their seventh decade maintain areas of decreased activity, though to a lesser degree than younger controls. Third, across subjects, activity levels in regions of activity become highly correlated in the eighth decade, while there are few positive correlations between regions active during the seventh decade. Put simply, persons in their eighth decade seem to lose their ability to selectively engage those areas needed for a task and to suppress those that are not needed; in other words, intentionally guided attention becomes compromised.

A final consideration in discussing intention and attention concerns laterality. This topic is covered in detail by Heilman et al. (2003). Regarding intention, the hand one uses to perform an activity (right versus left), the hemispace in which one performs an activity (right versus left), and the directionality of movement (rightward versus leftward) all are governed by the hemisphere opposite the intended arm, hemispace, or direction. Regarding attention, the side of body midline (right versus left), the side of head midline (right versus left), and the side of gaze midline (right versus left) can all be affected by the hemisphere opposite the side of body, head, or gaze midline to which attention is being paid. However, this simple schema is modulated by two other facets of brain organization: (1) In right-handed persons, left (dominant) hemisphere movement mechanisms often impact or control nondominant hemisphere mechanisms. (2) The right parietal lobe seems to be able to take both right and left space into account while the left hemisphere seems to be predominately designed to consider the right side of space.

EFFECTS OF AROUSAL, VIGILANCE, INTENTION, AND ATTENTION IMPAIRMENTS ON LANGUAGE AND COMMUNICATION

Because arousal, vigilance, intention, and attention are processes on which other forms of cognition are scaffolded, impairment of these mechanisms can impact language and communication. The effects are often subtle, but when the scaffolding collapses catastrophically, the effects can be dramatic. Below, the sampling of disorders of attention given earlier is expanded. Each attentional mechanism (arousal, vigilance, intention, attention) is addressed separately.

Impairments in Arousal

A good model for addressing the effects of arousal on communication is recovery from coma. Coma can be thought of as having gradations rather than as an all-or-nothing phenomenon. Indeed, Teasdale and Jennett (1974) developed the Glasgow Coma Scale (GCS) for grading coma severity. The GCS assesses verbal responses, along with eye opening and motor responses, to derive an index of how impaired a patient's consciousness is. This scale is now widely used as a means for describing levels of consciousness in acute traumatic brain injury.

In the deepest coma, a patient will not open his/her eyes or make any sound or movement. As arousal increases and consciousness returns, a patient who eventually may have no impairment or only subtle impairments in communication progresses through stages. Thus, as a patient emerges from a coma, he/she first may utter incomprehensible sounds, such as a grunt or a moan. Subsequently, he/she might progress from isolated, inappropriate words to confused and disoriented language. This latter condition can be referred to as a confusional state. Language and communication may be fairly complex and grammatically organized at this point, but often, it is not appropriate to the surroundings. For example, the patient may think they are at a different time and place. Communication also may be disinhibited, characterized by the patient making inappropriate personal or sexual remarks. Confusional states are not limited to patients recovering from coma; they also can exist in patients with frontal damage (e.g., frontal tumors), with herpes encephalitis, Wernicke-Korsakoff's syndrome, or other disorders (Bauer, Grande, & Valenstein, 2003; Damasio & Anderson, 2003). It is important to note that patients in confusional states frequently are not laying down permanent memories. Thus, these patients may not remember what they have said or what was said to them once such material has escaped their immediate attention.

Andersson, Norberg, and Hallberg (2002) assessed samples of communication in 51 cases of elderly patients with acute confusional state after orthopedic injury. Patients were described as speaking more or less continuously without addressing anyone in particular, changing unpredictably from one topic to another, asking questions without waiting for answers, and returning to the same topics multiple times. They were prone to misinterpreting communications and events, drawing from their own more remote history to explain circumstances around them. In another study of older patients with acute confusional state, Wallesch and Hundsalz (1994) found patients with acute confusional state made picture naming errors at a similar rate to

patients with Alzheimer disease. However, patients with confusional state were more likely to give unrelated responses than patients with dementia, suggesting that the nature of the naming impairment is different between the two kinds of disorders. Even so, the finding of significant naming errors in patients with acute confusional state indicates that arousal deficits can affect the basic language function of naming.

Impairments in Vigilance

Impairments in vigilance result in an inability to sustain concentration on a source of information or performance of a task over time. They are common in persons with attention deficit-hyperactivity disorders. Vigilance can also be compromised when we are fatigued. Impairments in vigilance are characterized by the affected person losing track of the task they are performing. In the realm of language and communication, a person with impaired vigilance might lose track of a subject about which they are talking or lose track of a verbal input from others in a conversation, thereby compromising their comprehension of other people's speech.

Impairments in Intention

As noted earlier, at its most basic level, intention involves the selection and execution of one action from many possible actions. Impairments of intention can be dramatic or quite subtle. Discussed briefly earlier, akinetic mutism is a dramatic example on the severe end of the spectrum and is characterized by a lack of initiation of spontaneous behavior, including language. Sometimes, repetition of words or short phrases can be coaxed from the patient with substantial urging. Two seminal case reports in the early 1950s (Barris & Schuman, 1953; Nielsen & Jacobs, 1951) described this syndrome with large medial frontal lesions. The clinical course of the syndrome after medial frontal lesion depends on the extent of the lesion, in particular, whether it is unilateral or bilateral. Unilateral lesions usually are followed by a good recovery, but in cases of bilateral lesion, some degree of the syndrome often persists (Damasio & Anderson, 2003). Although the usual cause of akinetic mutism is medial frontal damage, it also can occur with bilateral paramedian artery infarcts (e.g., Cavanna, Bertero, Cavanna, et al., 2009; van Domburg, ten Donkelaar, & Notermans, 1996). In these later cases, the symptoms also can persist for a long time.

Damage to or disease of the basal ganglia can cause more subtle intentional deficits vis-à-vis language. Nadeau and Crosson (1997) indicated that basal ganglia strokes should not cause aphasia if the cortex was not affected, and Hillis et al. (2002) provided strong empirical support for this conclusion in acute striato-capsular infarcts using magnetic resonance perfusion imaging. Hence, basic language functions remain intact in dominant hemisphere basal ganglia lesions as long as peri-Sylvian language cortices are not involved. Yet, David Copland, Helen Chenery, Tony Angwin, and their colleagues and students at the University of Queensland have explored this area. Copland et al. (2000a) showed that patients with chronic left basal ganglia lesions and patients with Parkinson disease did not have deficits on most subtests of aphasia batteries, with the exception of word fluency and naming pictures associated with low-frequency words. Yet, on more complex language tests, impairment was relatively pervasive. Examples of impairments include an inability to give both alternative meanings for semantically ambiguous sentences or to give precise definitions for words. This group has done extensive work to characterize these deficits. For example, Copland (Copland, 2003; Copland et al., 2000b) demonstrated changes in semantic priming, particularly when the intervals between primes and targets allowed for top-down cognitive processing to affect priming. Crosson et al. (2007) suggested that patients' deficits in these studies could be accounted for by an interruption of the enhancement of selected behaviors and/or suppression of competing behaviors, but it is clear that this explanation does not account for all of the semantic priming findings of the University of Queensland group (e.g., Angwin, Chenery, Copland, et al., 2004). Subsequent studies from this group have endeavored to define the parameters of suppression (inhibition) of language behaviors that are affected in Parkinson disease (e.g., Castner, Copland, Silburn, et al., 2007). The interested reader is referred to their extensive work.

A related area is difficulty in processing complex syntax, which has been demonstrated to be impaired in Parkinson disease. In recent years, evidence has mounted that these deficits are due to intentional and working memory deficits (e.g., Grossman, 1999; Lee, Grossman, Morris, et al., 2003; Novais-Santos, Gee, Shah, et al., 2007). In 1999, Grossman wrote, " . . . findings suggest that the sentence comprehension deficit in Parkinson disease is due in large part to limitations in the strategic distribution of cognitive resources such as selective attention that contribute to processing of complex material" (p. 387). The top-down influence on attention implicated in this statement would be an example of intentionally guided attention. This concept is consistent with differences in anterior cingulate activity between Parkinson disease and control participants during sentence processing (Grossman, Crino, Reivich, et al., 1992).

Another disorder of intention involves the inability to switch from one behavior to another. In its most severe form, this problem is referred to as perseveration. Patients who perseverate may (or may not) perform a behavior in an appropriate context initially, but the behavior is then repeated in contexts for which it is not appropriate. Frequently, patients with perseveration lose the ability to monitor their performance and have no idea that the perseverated behavior is inappropriate (Luria, 1973). A clinical example from the language domain might be demonstrated by patients who are being asked to define words. When asked to define the word *bed*, they might say, "a place to sleep," an appropriate definition. But, then the concept of sleep might find its way into other definitions for which it is not appropriate, for example when defining *flower* or *television*. Such inappropriate repetition can be manifested in conversation as well as in clinical testing.

A more subtle inability to switch between behaviors is the inability to multitask. Persons with this deficit have difficulty switching from one task to another without inordinately interrupting the tasks from which or to which they are switching. This form of attention is strongly related to but dissociable from divided attention, the attentional counterpart to this ability (discussed later). In the realm of language, a patient unable to multitask might be unable to switch between carrying on a conversation and performing some other behavior without interrupting the conversation at an inappropriate place.

A related problem is impairment in performing two behaviors simultaneously. Frequently, performing two behaviors simultaneously comes at a cost to one behavior. For example, neurologically normal participants who perform speeded, repetitive finger tapping while also performing a phonemic fluency task demonstrate a decrease in finger tapping speed (Bowers, Heilman, Satz, & Altman, 1978; Hellige & Longstreth, 1981; Simon & Sussman, 1987). It is possible that dual task performance can cause an inordinate cost for one of the behaviors when an impairment of intention exists. For example, De Monte, Geffen, May, et al. (2005) showed that in acute mild traumatic brain injury finger tapping while repeating words slows finger tapping more than for participants with orthopedic injuries. The expected extrapolation to daily behaviors would be that talking could abnormally interfere with the performance of other behaviors (or vice versa, depending on what task is prioritized).

Paradoxically, the reverse can also be true; the cost of dual task performance on one behavior can be diminished by an injury. This circumstance can reflect a change in the ability of one behavior to influence another. For example, Mennemeier and colleagues (1997) reported reduced right-hand finger tapping speed in a patient with a small lesion primarily occupying the centromedian/parafascicular complex of the left thalamus (i.e., the caudal portion of the thalamic intralaminar nuclei). When the patient performed finger tapping during a phonemic fluency task, her finger tapping speed increased and was at a level similar to that of neurologically normal controls during dual-task performance. The authors posited that the unusual facilitation of performance was related to disruption of projections from the centromedian/parafascicular complex to the basal ganglia. One way to think about this finding is that there is a loss of normal suppression of finger tapping behavior because of the loss of the influence of the basal ganglia on finger tapping.

Finally, some attention should be given to the lateralized aspects of intention. The effects of some lesions on upper extremity movements can be lateralized. Heilman et al. (2003) have explained these effects. In limb akinesia, patients have inordinate difficulty initiating movement and/or demonstrate movement abnormalities with the arm on the opposite side of the lesion that cannot be accounted for by impairment of the motor system nor by attention deficits (e.g., neglect). The slowing of right-hand tapping (i.e., during single-task performance) in Mennemeier and colleagues' (1997) case would be an example of a mild form of limb akinesia (i.e., hypokinesia). As noted earlier, the lesion was in the left thalamic intralaminar nuclei. In hemispatial akinesia, the patient has inordinate difficulty moving the hand and arm when they are in the hemispace opposite to the lesion. For example, Coslett, Schwartz, Goldberg, et al. (1993) evaluated a patient with left-hemisphere lesions whose left arm movements were much less abnormal on the side ipsilateral to the lesion as opposed to on the side contralateral to the lesion. Lesions were in the left anterior cingulate and left temporoparietal regions. In directional akinesia, performance is worse when movement is in the direction toward the side opposite to the lesion and better when the direction is away from the side opposite to the lesion. Heilman et al. (2003) gave the example of patients who cannot initiate gaze toward the side opposite their lesion. Although these deficits are most often seen after focal disturbances, such as stroke, there is evidence that they can also occur with degenerative processes (Cohen et al., 2010).

The implications of these lateralized forms of akinesia for language are not entirely clear. However, the fact that left-hemisphere lesions might affect movement of the non-paretic right hand (e.g., Mennemeier et al., 1997) or affect movement in the right hemispace (e.g., Coslett, Schwartz, Goldberg, et al., 1993) raises the possibility that damaged intention mechanisms could affect language. For example, the patient of Coslett et al. (1993) performed better on language tasks when attention was directed to the ipsilesional hemispace, but it is uncertain whether this is an effect of intention mechanisms or attention mechanisms since structures associated with both were damaged. However, evidence from Crosson and colleagues (Crosson et al., 2005, 2009; Crosson, Fabrizio, Singletary, et al., 2007; Richards et al., 2002) highlights the importance of intention for language.

Implications of Intention Mechanisms for Aphasia Treatment

These authors have engaged an intentional mechanism to assist in reorganizing language production to the previously nondominant frontal lobe. The conceptual rationale for this treatment was as follows: If a patient has a relatively severe, chronic aphasia, it indicates that the dominant hemisphere has not reorganized on its own to facilitate language. Indeed, a recent study by Parkinson, Raymer, Chang, et al. (2009) showed that in patients with chronic aphasias, patients with larger left frontal lesions showed better recovery of naming ability and more progress in a naming therapy than patients with smaller left frontal lesions. How can this counter-intuitive finding be explained? One possible explanation is that residual left frontal cortex, because of its previous association with language functions, tries to take over a function it cannot adequately perform, interfering with the ability of other areas to assume naming functions. Thus, right frontal mechanisms might be more capable of taking over this function than residual left frontal cortex, but it is hindered in doing so by left frontal activity. When such left frontal cortex is damaged by lesion, it cannot interfere with attempts of right frontal cortex to assume this function. Thus, in chronic aphasia, right frontal cortex may be a more likely place to which to reorganize at least some language production functions than residual left frontal cortex.

The question is, then, how can you engage right frontal mechanisms in a way that they assume a role in language production. We reasoned that if we engaged right frontal intention mechanisms, they would in turn activate right lateral frontal mechanisms capable of participating in language production. Hence, we employed an intentional manipulation, opening a box with the left hand in the left hemispace and pressing a button in a button array, to initiate a picture naming trial. Note the use of both left side of the body and left hemispace in which the action was performed to engage right-hemisphere intention mechanisms. Further, after errors, subjects performed a circular gesture with their left hand when repeating correct responses given by the therapist. Finally, the treatment was designed for patients with nonfluent aphasia, because this type of aphasia is more commonly associated with left frontal lesions than fluent aphasias. It should be noted that this rationale assumes some overlap between intention mechanisms for language and those for hand movement.

Initial findings were positive, demonstrating that nonfluent patients receiving this treatment improved (Richards et al., 2002). A follow-up study (Crosson et al., 2007) showed that patients relearned words faster with this intention treatment than with a control treatment with an attention manipulation. Finally, Crosson et al. (2009) showed that the treatment was successful in creating a rightward shift in frontal activity. Thus, preliminary studies of this treatment indicate that it is successful both in provoking a faster rate of relearning words and in shifting frontal activity rightward during word production in patients with nonfluent aphasia. Thus, findings suggest that this intention mechanism can be used to leverage therapeutic improvement in patients with nonfluent aphasia.

Impairments in Attention

As noted earlier, at its most basic level, attention can be conceptualized as selecting one from many sources of information for further processing. Like intention deficits, attention deficits can be obvious or rather subtle. At the more obvious end of the spectrum are patients for whom information decays so rapidly that they cannot select it for further processing. Martin and colleagues (Martin, Dell, Saffran, & Schwartz, 1994; Martin & Saffran, 1992; Martin, Saffran, & Dell, 1996) studied such a patient. When first studied, the patient's digit and word spans were less than a single item, and the patient was classified as having a Wernicke's aphasia. The authors could explain many of this patient's deficits and some aspects of his recovery using a model with very rapid decay of information at the input side. It can be argued that this is really a deficit in auditory-verbal short-term memory; indeed, Martin et al. did just that. However, as just pointed out, extremely rapid decay of information leaves it unavailable for further processing; so if one does not care to classify this problem as an attention deficit, then it is at least necessary to consider the impact of the deficit for attention. On the auditory-verbal processing side of the equation, if information is lost before it can be processed further, then comprehension will be compromised. Comprehension problems are a defining characteristic of

Wernicke's aphasia, the kind of language problem this patient demonstrated early in his recovery. It is not clear how much the rapid decay of information contributed to his comprehension deficit, per se, but Martin and colleagues did show that it may have contributed to the semantic errors the patient eventually made in repetition. The point here is that disrupting attention processes will affect comprehension as well as other processes.

More subtle deficits in attention certainly can affect communication as well. For example, an inability to select one source of information among multiple potential sources would lead one to be distracted by stimuli not relevant to the task at hand. An example relevant to communication is the inability to focus on one voice among many voices in a crowded room. In this circumstance, one could miss parts of conversations, which in turn could compromise comprehension. Indeed, this is a frequent complaint among persons who have experienced mild to moderate traumatic brain injury.

One important aspect of attention is the degree to which it is driven from top-down mechanisms, in other words, the degree to which it is driven by intention mechanisms. As previously stated, what we intend to do often determines the things to which we must attend. Indeed, the act of making a conscious decision to attend to a specific source of information is an act of intention. Thus, it is often difficult to separate an attention preference from the actions and decisions from which it flows, and persons with compromised intention mechanisms, often will have attention deficits as well, i.e., show an inability effectively to select one source of information for further processing when multiple sources are available.

It follows that more complex forms of attention are frequently intentionally driven. This observation can be applied to divided attention, when one must attend to multiple stimuli at the same time (attention system) in order to act on them (i.e., multitasking, involving intention processes). That is to say that attending to two sources of information is often the product of what we intend to do. Problems with divided attention may only be noticeable when attention demands are high. As applied to communication, for example, patients may be unable to perform other activities while talking without losing track of the thoughts driving speech. Likewise, switching attention (disengaging from one source, then engaging another source of information) is most often intentionally driven. Without this ability patients remain fixed on a source of information, such as a speaker, when they should have switched their attention to another source, such as second or third speakers.

There is evidence that these latter kinds of attention are impaired in patients with aphasia. For example, Murray, Holland, and Beeson (1997) showed that the performance of patients with aphasia deteriorated more than that of neurologically normal controls during either a distraction which they did not have to attend (requiring suppression of divided attention) or during dual-task performance (requiring divided attention). Deterioration in performance did not correlate with severity of aphasia, and it happened even with nonverbal distracters, suggesting that there is a separate attention deficit coexisting with the aphasia and not merely a byproduct of the aphasia. Clearly, this kind of problem can exacerbate problems with basic language functions in environments with distracters or when multitasking is required. From an experimental standpoint, studies such as that of Murray et al. (1997) involve the active performance of tasks (i.e., they engage intention as well as attention mechanisms). This presents an interesting interpretive challenge because when tasks engage both intention and attention mechanisms, it is hard to know if the change in performance is related to effects on intention mechanisms, to effects on attention mechanisms, or the interaction of the two. From the standpoint of rehabilitation, this is an important distinction because underlying mechanism of the deficit should dictate how the problem is approached. It should be pointed out that the literature on language or aphasia in dual processing tasks has recently been reviewed by Hula and McNeil (2008) and the reader is referred to this review for further information.

Spatial attention problems have implications for language and specifically for aphasia. Heilman et al. (2003) have noted that spatial attention can be divided by side of body midline, side of head midline, or side of gaze midline (all right versus left). In right parietal lesions, it is not uncommon for patients to fail to attend (i.e., neglect) stimuli on the left side of their body. This problem is less commonly seen for the right side of space with left parietal lesions, prompting speculation that the left hemisphere attends to the right side of space, while the right hemisphere attends to both sides of space. Although spatial neglect is less common on the right side of space after left-hemisphere lesion than vice versa, there is evidence that subtle spatial attention deficits on the right (contralesional) side are present in patients with aphasia. For example, Petry and colleagues (Petry, Crosson, Gonzalez Rothi, et al., 1994) gave patients with aphasia and neurologically normal controls a task in which they responded to a target presented to the left or right of gaze midline and participants responded as quickly as they could by pressing a computer

key. Prior to the appearance of the target, participants frequently were given a cue on the side of the target; less frequently, they were either cued to the side opposite that on which the target would appear or were not cued at all. Neurologically normal participants showed no leftward or rightward bias in their reaction times to the target on any of these kinds of trials. However, participants with aphasia showed slower reaction times to targets on the right side either when there was no cue or when they were first cued to the left, suggestive of subtle spatial attentional deficits.

Coslett (1999) showed the practical consequences of this kind of attention bias. For some patients with parietal lesions, performance on language tests improved when test stimuli were given in the ipsilesional as opposed to the contralesional hemispace. An important aspect of this finding is that it was true for patients with right as well as left parietal lesions. This finding was important because it indicated that language performance could be impacted by spatial attention deficits even when no aphasia was present (i.e., when the patient had a right parietal lesion). Thus, this result clearly showed that compromised spatial attention systems could affect language performance.

Although spatial neglect can negatively impact reading, a somewhat different and interesting interface between spatial neglect and language is neglect dyslexia (e.g., Ellis, Flude, & Young, 1987; Hillis & Caramazza, 1990). It usually involves the left side of words. Some patients with right-hemisphere lesions will misread two or more letters on the left side of a printed word and replace the target word with a real word with two or more letters on the right side of the replacement word that are the same as the letters of the target word. However, cases of left-hemisphere lesion have been reported in which the right side of words is misread while the left side is not (e.g., Crosson, 1999; Hillis & Caramazza, 1990). Neglect dyslexia differs from pure neglect in that patients seem to know that letters exist in the impaired hemispace, as they replace the target letters with other letters making a real word but one different from the target. In contrast, patients with simple neglect often appear to be unaware of the left side of a word or words on the left side of a page. Often, the internal representation of the misread word in neglect dyslexia seems to be disrupted, since spelling is disrupted as well as reading. However, in some cases, the problem appears to be at earlier stages of visual processing, since oral spelling is better than reading (e.g., Crosson, 1999; Ellis et al., 1987). Again, it seems that spatial attention can impact language with either left- or right-hemisphere lesion.

Implications of Attention Mechanisms for Aphasia Treatment

The ability to change performance by moving stimuli into the ipsilesional hemispace (Coslett, 1999) opens up the possibility of using this manipulation for therapeutic purposes to facilitate the relearning of words or other language processes. Indeed, Dotson, Singletary, Fuller, et al. (2008) presented stimuli 45 degrees into patients' ipsilesional hemispace in a picture-naming treatment for three patients with fluent aphasia and showed that two of the three patients improved with treatment. Fluent aphasia was chosen as the target for this treatment because of the association of fluent aphasias with posterior lesions in general and because attention mechanisms, as described earlier are associated with posterior, sensoriperceptual systems. The two patients who improved had a moderately severe anomia, while the patient who did not improve had a profound anomia, naming almost no pictures correctly during probes for any of the 8 baseline or 30 treatment sessions. Training had some degree of specificity for the items being trained. While these preliminary findings are promising, the nature of the A-B study design (baseline sessions followed by a treatment phase) limits our ability to definitively conclude that the attention manipulation was responsible for some or all of the treatment effect.

CONCLUSIONS

Attention processes can be divided into arousal, vigilance, intention, and attention proper. These processes form a foundation for all cognitive functions. Hence, impairments in any of these processes caused by brain lesion or disease can cause impairments in communication ranging from subtle to severe. Further, impairments in these mechanisms can exacerbate basic language deficits in aphasia, but it may also be possible to manipulate these mechanisms in the service of aphasia treatment. Although recent studies have made advances in understanding the interactions of attention processes with language, there is still much to learn. Understanding these interactions is important not only for descriptive or diagnostic reasons, but also because of the treatment implications. This chapter has attempted to provide a foundation by addressing attention impairments and their impact on communication. Assessment and therapeutic implications will be covered in Chapter 12. As research and conceptualization of this important area continues, it should improve our ability to address the variety of implications for communication and language.

ACKNOWLEDGMENTS

Work on this chapter was supported by a Department of Veterans Affairs Rehabilitation Research and Development Senior Research Career Scientist Award (Grant B6364L) and a National Institute on Deafness and Other Communication Disorders Award (Grant R01 DC007387) to the first author. No approval of the content of this chapter by the Department of Veterans Affairs is implied.

REFERENCES

Alexander, G. E., DeLong, M. R., & Strick, P. L. (1986). Parallel organization of functionally segregated circuits linking basal ganglia and cortex. *Annual Review of Neuroscience, 9*, 357–381.

Andersson, E. M., Norberg, A., & Hallberg, I. R. (2002). Acute confusional episodes in elderly orthopaedic patients: The patients' actions and speech. *International Journal of Nursing Studies, 39*(3), 303–317.

Angwin, A. J., Chenery, H. J., Copland, D. A., Arnott, W. L., Murdoch, B. E., & Silburn, P. A. (2004). Dopamine and semantic activation: An investigation of masked direct and indirect priming. *Journal of the International Neuropsychological Society, 10*(1), 15–25.

Barris, R. W., & Schuman, H. R. (1953). [Bilateral anterior cingulate gyrus lesions; syndrome of the anterior cingulate gyri.]. *Neurology, 3*(1), 44–52.

Bauer, R. M., Grande, L., & Valenstein, E. (2003). Amnesic disorders. In K. M. Heilman & E. Valenstein (Eds.), *Clinical neuropsychology* (4th ed., pp. 495–573). New York: Oxford University Press.

Betz, W. (1874). Anatomischer Nachweis zweier Gehirncentra. *Centralblad fur die Medizinische Wissenschaft, 12*, 578–580, 595–599.

Bowers, D., Heilman, K. M., Satz, P., & Altman, A. (1978). Simultaneous performance on verbal, nonverbal and motor tasks by right-handed adults. *Cortex, 14*(4), 540–556.

Castner, J. E., Copland, D. A., Silburn, P. A., Coyne, T. J., Sinclair, F., & Chenery, H. J. (2007). Lexical-semantic inhibitory mechanisms in Parkinson's disease as a function of subthalamic stimulation. *Neuropsychologia, 45*(14), 3167–3177.

Cavanna, A. E., Bertero, L., Cavanna, S., Servo, S., Strigaro, G., & Monaco, F. (2009). Persistent akinetic mutism after bilateral paramedian thalamic infarction. *Journal of Neuropsychiatry and Clinical Neurosciences, 21*(3), 351.

Cohen, M. L., Burtis, B., Williamson, J. B., Kwon, J. C., & Heilman, K. M. (2010). Action-intentional spatial bias in a patient with posterior cortical atrophy. *Neurocase, 16*(6), 529–534.

Copland, D. (2003). The basal ganglia and semantic engagement: Potential insights from semantic priming in individuals with subcortical vascular lesions, Parkinson's disease, and cortical lesions. *Journal of the International Neuropsychological Society, 9*(7), 1041–1052.

Copland, D. A., Chenery, H. J., & Murdoch, B. E. (2000a). Persistent deficits in complex language function following dominant nonthalamic subcortical lesions. *Journal of Medical Speech-Language Pathology, 8*, 1–14.

Copland, D. A., Chenery, H. J., & Murdoch, B. E. (2000b). Processing lexical ambiguities in word triplets: Evidence of lexical-semantic deficits following dominant nonthalamic subcortical lesions. *Neuropsychology, 14*(3), 379–390.

Coslett, H. B. (1999). Spatial influences on motor and language function. *Neuropsychologia, 37*(6), 695–706.

Coslett, H. B., Schwartz, M. F., Goldberg, G., Haas, D., & Perkins, J. (1993). Multi-modal hemispatial deficits after left hemisphere stroke. A disorder of attention? *Brain, 116*(Pt 3), 527–554.

Cowan, N. (2001). The magical number 4 in short-term memory: A reconsideration of mental storage capacity. *Behavioral and Brain Sciences, 24,* 87–185.

Crosson, B. (1999). Subcortical mechanisms in language: Lexical-semantic mechanisms and the thalamus. *Brain and Cognition, 40*(2), 414–438.

Crosson, B., Bacon Moore, A., McGregor, K. M., Chang, Y. L., Benjamin, M., Gopinath, K., et al. (2009). Regional changes in word-production laterality after a naming treatment designed to produce a rightward shift in frontal activity. *Brain and Language, 111,* 73–85.

Crosson, B., Benefield, H., Cato, M. A., Sadek, J. R., Moore, A. B., Wierenga, C. E., et al. (2003). Left and right basal ganglia and frontal activity during language generation: Contributions to lexical, semantic, and phonological processes. *Journal of the International Neuropsychological Society, 9*(7), 1061–1077.

Crosson, B., Benjamin, M., & Levy, I. F. (2007). Role of the basal ganglia in language and semantics: Supporting cast. In J. J. Hart & M. Kraut (Eds.), *Neural basis of semantic memory* (pp. 219–243). New York: Cambridge University Press.

Crosson, B., Fabrizio, K. S., Singletary, F., Cato, M. A., Wierenga, C. E., Parkinson, R. B., et al. (2007). Treatment of naming in nonfluent aphasia through manipulation of intention and attention: A phase 1 comparison of two novel treatments. *Journal of the International Neuropsychological Society, 13*(4), 582–594.

Crosson, B., Moore, A. B., Gopinath, K., White, K. D., Wierenga, C. E., Gaiefsky, M. E., et al. (2005). Role of the right and left hemispheres in recovery of function during treatment of intention in aphasia. *Journal of Cognitive Neuroscience, 17*(3), 392–406.

Crosson, B., Sadek, J. R., Bobholz, J. A., Gokcay, D., Mohr, C. M., Leonard, C. M., et al. (1999). Activity in the paracingulate and cingulate sulci during word generation: An fMRI study of functional anatomy. *Cerebral Cortex, 9*(4), 307–316.

Crosson, B., Sadek, J. R., Maron, L., Gokcay, D., Mohr, C. M., Auerbach, E. J., et al. (2001). Relative shift in activity from medial to lateral frontal cortex during internally versus externally guided word generation. *Journal of Cognitive Neuroscience, 13*(2), 272–283.

Damasio, A. R., & Anderson, S. W. (2003). The frontal lobes. In K. M. Heilman & E. Valenstein (Eds.), *Clinical neuropsychology* (4th ed., pp. 404–446). New York: Oxford University Press.

De Monte, V. E., Geffen, G. M., May, C. R., McFarland, K., Heath, P., & Neralic, M. (2005). The acute effects of mild traumatic brain injury on finger tapping with and without word repetition. *Journal of Clinical and Experimental Neuropsychology, 27*(2), 224–239.

Dotson, V. M., Singletary, R., Fuller, R., Koehler, S., Bacon Moore, A., Rothi, L. J. G., et al. (2008). Treatment of word-finding deficits in fluent aphasia through the manipulation of spatial attention: Preliminary findings. *Aphasiology, 22,* 103–113.

Ellis, A. W., Flude, B. M., & Young, A. W. (1987). "Neglect dyslexia" and the early visual processing of letters in words and nonwords. *Cognitive Neuropsychology, 4,* 439–464.

Fuster, J. (2003). *Cortex and mind: Unifying cognition.* New York: Oxford University Press.

Gerfen, C. R. (1992). The neostriatal mosaic: multiple levels of compartmental organization in the basal ganglia. *Annual Review of Neuroscience, 15,* 285–320.

Grossman, M. (1999). Sentence processing in Parkinson's disease. *Brain and Cognition, 40*(2), 387–413.

Grossman, M., Crino, P., Reivich, M., Stern, M. B., & Hurtig, H. I. (1992). Attention and sentence processing deficits in Parkinson's disease: The role of anterior cingulate cortex. *Cerebral Cortex, 2*(6), 513–525.

Heilman, K., Watson, R., & Valenstein, E. (2003). Neglect and related disorders. In K. Heilman & E. Valenstein (Eds.), *Clinical neuropsychology* (pp. 296–346). New York: Oxford University Press.

Hellige, J. B., & Longstreth, L. E. (1981). Effects of concurrent hemisphere-specific activity on unimanual tapping rate. *Neuropsychologia, 19*(3), 395–405.

Hillis, A. E., & Caramazza, A. (1990). The effects of attentional deficits on reading and spelling. In A. Caramazza (Ed.), *Cognitive neuropsychology and neurolinguistics: Advances in models of cognitive function and impairment* (pp. 211–275). Hillsdale, NJ: Lawrence Erlbaum and Associates.

Hillis, A. E., Wityk, R. J., Barker, P. B., Beauchamp, N. J., Gailloud, P., Murphy, K., et al. (2002). Subcortical aphasia and neglect in acute stroke: The role of cortical hypoperfusion. *Brain, 125*(Pt 5), 1094–1104.

Hula, W. D., & McNeil, M. R. (2008). Models of attention and dual-task performance as explanatory constructs in aphasia. *Seminars in Speech and Language, 29*(3), 169–187.

James, W. (1890). *Principles of psychology* (Vol. 2). New York: Holt.

Kischka, U., Kammer, T., Maier, S., Weisbrod, M., Thimm, M., & Spitzer, M. (1996). Dopaminergic modulation of semantic network activation. *Neuropsychologia, 34*(11), 1107–1113.

Lee, C., Grossman, M., Morris, J., Stern, M. B., & Hurtig, H. I. (2003). Attentional resource and processing speed limitations during sentence processing in Parkinson's disease. *Brain and Language, 85*(3), 347–356.

Luria, A. R. (1973). *The working brain: An introduction to neuropsychology* (B. Haigh, Trans.). New York: Basic Books.

Martin, N., Dell, G. S., Saffran, E. M., & Schwartz, M. F. (1994). Origins of paraphasias in deep dysphasia: Testing the consequences of a decay impairment to an interactive spreading activation model of lexical retrieval. *Brain and Language, 47*(4), 609–660.

Martin, N., & Saffran, E. M. (1992). A computational account of deep dysphasia: Evidence from a single case study. *Brain and Language, 43*(2), 240–274.

Martin, N., Saffran, E. M., & Dell, G. S. (1996). Recovery in deep dysphasia: Evidence for a relation between auditory—verbal STM capacity and lexical errors in repetition. *Brain and Language, 52*(1), 83–113.

Mennemeier, M., Crosson, B., Williamson, D. J., Nadeau, S. E., Fennell, E., Valenstein, E., et al. (1997). Tapping, talking and the thalamus: Possible influence of the intralaminar nuclei on basal ganglia function. *Neuropsychologia, 35*(2), 183–193.

Middleton, F. A., & Strick, P. L. (2000). Basal ganglia and cerebellar loops: Motor and cognitive circuits. *Brain Research Reviews, 31*(2–3), 236–250.

Miller, G. E. (1956). The magical number seven plus or minus two: Some limits on our capacity for processing information. *Psychological Review, 63*(2), 81–97.

Mink, J. W. (1996). The basal ganglia: Focused selection and inhibition of competing motor programs. *Progress in Neurobiology, 50*(4), 381–425.

Moruzzi, G., & Magoun, H. W. (1949). Brain stem reticular formation and activation of the EEG. *Electroencephalography and Clinical Neurophysiology, 1*(4), 455–473.

Murray, L. L., Holland, A. L., & Beeson, P. M. (1997). Auditory processing in individuals with mild aphasia: A study of resource allocation. *Journal of Speech, Language, and Hearing Research, 40*(4), 792–808.

Nadeau, S. E., & Crosson, B. (1997). Subcortical aphasia. *Brain and Language, 58*(3), 355–402; discussion 418–423.

Nambu, A., Tokuno, H., & Takada, M. (2002). Functional significance of the cortico-subthalamo-pallidal 'hyperdirect' pathway. *Neuroscience Research, 43*(2), 111–117.

Nielsen, J. M., & Jacobs, L. L. (1951). Bilateral lesions of the anterior cingulate gyri; report of case. *Bulletin of the Los Angeles Neurological Society, 16*(2), 231–234.

Novais-Santos, S., Gee, J., Shah, M., Troiani, V., Work, M., & Grossman, M. (2007). Resolving sentence ambiguity with planning and working memory resources: Evidence from fMRI. *Neuroimage, 37*(1), 361–378.

Parent, A. (1996). *Carpenter's human neuroanatomy* (9th ed.). Baltimore: Williams & Wilkins.

Parkinson, B. R., Raymer, A., Chang, Y. L., Fitzgerald, D. B., & Crosson, B. (2009). Lesion characteristics related to treatment improvement in object and action naming for patients with chronic aphasia. *Brain and Language, 110*(2), 61–70.

Penney, J. B., Jr., & Young, A. B. (1986). Striatal inhomogeneities and basal ganglia function. *Movement Disorders, 1*(1), 3–15.

Petry, M. C., Crosson, B., Gonzalez Rothi, L. J., Bauer, R. M., & Schauer, C. A. (1994). Selective attention and aphasia in adults: preliminary findings. *Neuropsychologia, 32*(11), 1397–1408.

Posner, M. I., & Boies, S. W. (1971). Components of attention. *Psychological Review, 78*, 391–408.

Richards, K., Moore, A., Singletary, F., Rothi, L., Clayton, M., & Crosson, B. (2002). *Two novel treatments utilizing intentional and attentional mechanisims in rehabilitation of nonfluent aphasia*. Paper presented at the Rehabilitation Research for the Twenty-First Century: The New Challenges, Washington, DC.

Sherman, S. M., & Guillery, R. W. (2006). *Exploring the thalamus and its role in cortical function* (2nd ed.). Cambridge, MA: MIT Press.

Simon, T. J., & Sussman, H. M. (1987). The dual task paradigm: speech dominance or manual dominance? *Neuropsychologia, 25*(3), 559–569.

Teasdale, G., & Jennett, B. (1974). Assessment of coma and impaired consciousness. A practical scale. *Lancet, 2*(7872), 81–84.

van Domburg, P. H., ten Donkelaar, H. J., & Notermans, S. L. (1996). Akinetic mutism with bithalamic infarction. Neurophysiological correlates. *Journal of the Neurological Sciences, 139*(1), 58–65.

Wallesch, C. W., & Hundsalz, A. (1994). Language function in delirium: A comparison of single word processing in acute confusional states and probable Alzheimer's disease. *Brain and Language, 46*(4), 592–606.

CHAPTER 9

Memory Disorders and Impaired Language and Communication

CHAPTER OUTLINE

Randi Martin and L. Robert Slevc

MEMORY DISORDERS AND IMPAIRED LANGUAGE AND COMMUNICATION

Understanding and producing language are complicated cognitive tasks that draw on several different memory systems. To link information from different parts of a sentence, some type of short-term memory (STM) or working memory (WM) system is needed. To understand word meanings and analyze the structure of a sentence, it is necessary to draw on long-term memory (LTM) representations for word meanings and the allowable grammatical sequences in the language. In order to make sense of discourse and draw appropriate inferences it is necessary to draw on memory of events and facts and episodic memory about when and where a conversation took place are needed. Damage to these STM and LTM systems thus impacts language processing, and the nature of these impacts can inform our understanding of language deficits. In this chapter, we will consider first the consequences for language

processing of damage to STM, or WM, and then the consequences of damage to LTM systems. Figure 9-1 provides a diagram of the various types of memory systems considered in this chapter.

Disorders of Short-Term Memory and Working Memory

As discussed in Chapter 5, current theorists distinguish between passive STM systems and a WM system (Engle, Tuholski, Laughlin, & Conway, 1999). For instance, a passive storage system is assumed to be involved in standard span tasks that involve repeating back a list of digits or words. A WM system, in contrast, is thought to reflect a capacity for both maintaining information and operating on that information—thus, encompassing both storage and processing (Daneman & Carpenter, 1980). More complex tasks, like reading span or operation span (Figure 9-2), have been used to tap WM capacity. In the reading span task, individuals read aloud sentences and attempt to remember the last word of each sentence, recalling these last words at the

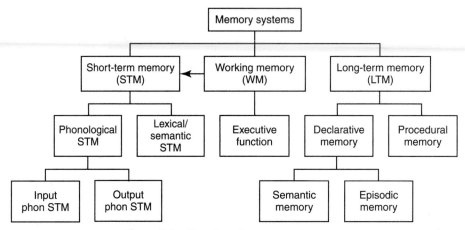

Figure 9-1   Overview of memory systems.

Reading span

<u>Set size</u> 3
Although the sun was warm, there was a strong BREEZE.
The cowboys herded the cattle through the mountain PASS.
All of the basketball players rode the bus to the nearby ARENA.

Recall: breeze, pass, arena

Operation span

<u>Set size</u> 4
$9-(5*1)= ?$ T
$(5*2)-4= ?$ F
$8-(3*2)= ?$ V
$(4*3)-6= ?$ A

Recall: T, F, V, A

Figure 9-2   Examples of reading span and operation span test materials.

end of a set of sentences (which might vary from 3 to 7 sentences in length). In the similar operation span task, individuals carry out an arithmetic problem on each trial and then are asked to remember a letter or word following the problem (Turner & Engle, 1989). Again, at the end of a series of arithmetic problems, they attempt to recall the series of letters. In both cases, information has to be maintained while other processing is being carried out.

Short-Term Memory Deficits

Phonological Versus Semantic Short-Term Memory Deficits

Aphasic patients are almost universally impaired on simple span tasks involving word list recall (Martin & Ayala, 2004). While neurally healthy adults may have a STM span of about 7 digits and 5 words, aphasic patients typically have spans of 1 to 3 items. A large body of research has examined the causes of these STM deficits and their consequences for aphasic patients' language comprehension and production. In some theoretical positions, the passive storage involved in word span tasks is assumed to be a buffer that maintains phonological representations (e.g., Baddeley, 1986). In other approaches that take a more language-based approach to STM, both phonological and semantic information are thought to support word list retention. R. Martin and colleagues (e.g., Martin, Shelton & Yaffee, 1994) and N. Martin and colleagues (e.g., Martin & Saffran, 1997) have provided patient data supporting the latter view. For instance, Martin et al. (1994) and Martin and He (2004) have shown that some patients show a deficit specifically in maintaining phonological information and others show a deficit specifically in maintaining semantic information. Those with a phonological STM deficit fail to show the standard effects of phonological variables on span performance (e.g., failing to show an effect of phonological similarity of the words in the list) but do show effects related to semantic variables (e.g., performing better with word lists than lists made up of nonwords such as "pem, dat, tur"). Patients with a semantic STM deficit show the reverse pattern, showing effects of phonological variables, but failing to show effects of semantic variables (for instance, performing at the same level on word and nonword lists). Two tasks that have been shown to discriminate the patients with semantic and phonological STM deficits are the category and rhyme probe tasks (Figure 9-3). In both tasks, patients hear a list of words followed by a probe word. In the category

• Rhyme probe (phonological retention)

Word 1	Word 2	Word 3	...	Probe	Response
disc	frog	sock	...	lock	(y)

• Category probe (semantic retention)

Word 1	Word 2	Word 3	...	Probe	Response
table	dog	sock	...	cat	(y)

Figure 9-3 Examples of category and rhyme probe trials.

probe task, subjects must judge if the probe word is in the same category as any of the list words. In the rhyme probe task, subjects judge whether the probe word rhymes with any of the list words. Patients with a phonological STM deficit perform better on the category than the rhyme probe task, whereas the patients with a semantic STM deficit perform better on the rhyme that the category probe task. (See also Barde, Schwartz, Chrysikou, & Thompson-Schill, 2010; Hoffman, Jefferies, Ehsan, et al., 2009; Wong & Law, 2008, for recent replications of these findings.) N. Martin and colleagues have presented other data showing different effects of semantic and phonological variables on recall of words which are correlated with patients' semantic and phonological processing

abilities. For instance, a composite measure of semantic processing is correlated with imageability effects on span, whereas a composite measure of phonological processing is correlated with frequency effects on span.

Based on these dissociations, Martin, Lesch, and Bartha (1999) presented a model of verbal STM that includes separate capacities for retaining semantic and phonological information (Figure 9-4). On the left hand side of Figure 9-4 are the types of knowledge representations that one has about words. On the right are buffers used to maintain these different types of representations. In addition to separate buffers for semantic and phonological information, as shown in Figure 9-4, separate capacities are assumed for maintaining input and output phonological representations. Input representations are those derived from the perception of speech. Output representations are those used in speech production. Martin et al. (1999) and others (e.g., Allport, 1984; Shallice & Butterworth, 1977) have presented evidence showing that patients can have poor retention of spoken words on the input side but show normal patterns of speech production (implying preserved output phonological retention), whereas other patients can show normal retention of phonological representations during speech perception but have difficulty in maintaining phonological information used in production.

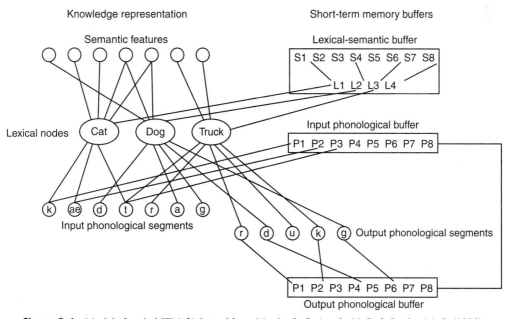

Figure 9-4 Model of verbal STM. [Adapted from Martin, R. C., Lesch, M. F., & Bartha, M. C. (1999): Independence of input and output phonology in word processing and short-term memory. *Journal of Memory & Language, 41,* 3–29.]

Effects of Short-Term Memory Deficits on Comprehension

A surprising finding coming out of studies carried out during the late 1980s and early 1990s was that a phonological STM deficit appeared to have few consequences for sentence comprehension, even for complex sentences with a large intervening distance between the words that needed to be linked together (e.g., Butterworth, Campbell, & Howard, 1986; Caplan & Waters, 1999; Martin et al., 1994; Martin & Romani, 1994). Martin and Romani (1994) and Martin and He (2004), however, reported that a semantic STM deficit (but not a phonological STM deficit) was related to deficits in comprehending certain sentence types. Specifically, in a task in which subjects had to indicate whether sentences were sensible or anomalous, the patients had difficulty making those judgments for sentences in which several adjectives came before a noun (e.g., "rusty old red wagon" versus "rusty old red swimsuit") or several nouns came before a verb (e.g., "glasses, vases, and mirrors cracked" versus "rugs, vases, and mirrors cracked"). They did much better when the adjectives followed the noun (e.g., "the wagon was old, red, and rusty") or the nouns followed the verb (e.g., "the movers cracked the mirrors, vases, and glasses"). These authors argued that in the "before" conditions, individuals had to maintain the meanings of the adjectives or nouns in an unintegrated fashion until the respective noun or verb was processed, thus overloading their restricted STM capacity. In contrast, in the "after" condition, each adjective could be integrated as a modifier of the noun as it was heard and each noun could be integrated as an object of the verb as it was heard. The assumption was that once these integrations had been made, the STM representation was no longer needed. Given the poor performance of the patients with semantic STM deficits and the good performance of the patient with a phonological STM deficit, these authors argued that the retention of semantic information, rather than phonological information, was critical for maintaining the words prior to integration.

Effects of Short-Term Memory Deficits on Production

A role for STM in comprehension may seem intuitively necessary, whereas a role in production may seem less obvious. However, in production, one does not typically retrieve one word and then utter it, retrieve the next word and utter it, and so on. Instead, speech is typically produced in fluent stretches, which implies some degree of advance planning of two or more words. This advance planning would presumably rely on STM resources to support the representations of several words prior to their articulation.

Martin and colleagues have reported evidence from aphasic patients suggesting that semantic STM capacity is critical for this advance planning in production. In one study, Martin and Freedman (2001) showed that patients with a semantic STM deficit had difficulty producing adjective-noun phrases (e.g., "long blonde hair"), tending to produce these utterances in piecemeal fashion (Figure 9-5). For example, for the target utterance of "small leaf", patient AB produced, "It's a leaf. It's small." These same patients did better when asked to produce the same information in a sentence frame (e.g., "The leaf is small"). A patient with a phonological STM deficit performed at a normal level for both utterance types. In a related study, Martin, Miller, and Vu (2004) showed that patients with a semantic STM deficit had difficulty producing sentences that began with a conjoined noun phrase (e.g., "the ball and the block moved") compared to sentences that began with a single noun (e.g., "the ball moved"). A patient with a phonological STM deficit showed a latency difference between the two sentence types that was well within the range of controls. Martin and colleagues concluded that speakers plan at a phrasal level, attempting to plan all of the lexical-semantic representations for a phrase prior to beginning phonological retrieval for that phrase. The normal performance for the patient with a phonological STM deficit in the two studies might be attributed to the fact that there is very limited planning at the phonological level (which was within the capacity of the patient) or to a dissociation between input and output phonological retention (Martin et al., 1999). That is, there may be separate capacities for maintaining phonological representations involved in speech perception and those involved in speech production (Shallice & Butterworth, 1977; Romani, 1992). The patient studied by Martin and colleagues may have had a deficit on the input side but not on the output side (Martin et al., 1999).

Effect of Short-Term Memory Deficits on Learning

Although a phonological STM deficit appears to have few consequences for sentence comprehension and production, it does have consequences for the learning of novel phonological forms (i.e., the learning of new words or names) (Baddeley, Papagno, & Vallar, 1988; Freedman & Martin, 2001). Freedman and Martin (2001) showed contrasting patterns of learning impairments

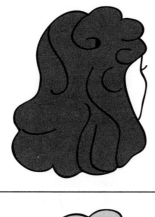

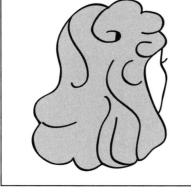

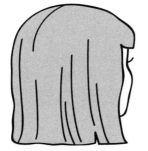

Figure 9-5 Pictorial for stimulus for eliciting "long blonde hair." Patients are asked to describe the boxed picture in a way that would distinguish it from the other pictures. [Adapted from Martin, R. C., & Freedman, M. L. (2001). Short-term retention of lexical-semantic representations: Implications for speech production. *Memory, 9,* 261–280.]

for patients with phonological and semantic STM deficits. Those with phonological STM deficits had greater difficulty learning foreign translations of English words than in learning new meanings for known words. Those with semantic STM deficits showed the reverse pattern, indicating that semantic STM was needed to transfer new semantic information to LTM. Thus, there was a code-specific relation between short-term retention and long-term learning.

Working Memory Deficits

Although STM and WM are different theoretical concepts, performance on the tests used to tap the two is usually correlated to a moderate degree for healthy subjects, presumably because WM performance relies to some extent on storage in passive storage systems (e.g., in a phonological STM buffer) and because STM tests rely on processing to some extent (e.g., whatever strategies subjects might use to help remember a list of words) (Engle et al., 1999). Since aphasic patients are so impaired at simple span tasks, they are typically very impaired at WM tasks as well if only because of the contribution of passive storage to WM measures. Consequently, one may look to other patient groups such as those with dementia of the Alzheimer type (DAT patients) or with Parkinson's disease, whose performance is better preserved on simple span tasks, to examine the effects of WM deficits on sentence processing.

Interpretive Versus Postinterpretive Aspects of Sentence Processing

Caplan and Waters and colleagues (see Caplan & Waters, 1999, for an overview) carried out several studies examining the role of WM in sentence comprehension. They demonstrated that both DAT and Parkinson disease patients had preserved phonological retention and rehearsal but had very reduced WM capacities as measured by tasks like the reading span task (e.g., a WM span of less than one in the case of the DAT patients). For both patient groups, they showed that the effect of syntactic complexity was no greater than for controls. However, both groups showed an exaggerated effect of the number of propositions in the sentence. (See examples of variations in syntactic complexity and number of propositions in Table 9-1.) Caplan and Waters (1999) explained these findings on the grounds that different WM resources support interpretive versus postinterpretive aspects of sentence processing. By interpretive processing, they refer to "the processes of recognizing words and appreciating their meanings and syntactic features; constructing syntactic and prosodic representations; and assigning thematic roles, focus, and other aspects of propositional and discourse-level semantics . . . " (p. 78). By postinterpretive processing, they refer to "remembering the content of a sentence, using the meaning of a sentence to plan action, reasoning on the basis of sentence meaning" and other related processes (p. 79). For interpretive aspects, they assume a dedicated WM system for language processing that is

Table 9-1	Sentence Materials Varying on Syntactic Complexity and Number of Propositions
Syntactically simple	The child spilled the juice that stained the rug.
Syntactically complex	The juice that the child spilled stained the rug.
One proposition	The magician performed the stunt and the joke.
Two propositions	The magician performed the stunt that included the joke.

From Caplan, D., Alpert, N., & Waters, G. (1998). Effects of syntactic structure and propositional number on patterns of regional cerebral blood flow. *Journal of Cognitive Neuroscience*, 10, 541–552.

not tapped by standard span tasks (either simple or complex). For postinterpretive processing, general WM resources are drawn upon. Thus, in order to accommodate their findings, they have to assume that variations in syntactic complexity affected interpretive processes whereas variations in number of propositions affected postinterpretive processes.

Working Memory and Executive Function

A number of studies in the literature on healthy individuals have demonstrated a relation between WM capacity and the ability to allocate attention to external stimuli and internal representations and to inhibit attention to interfering material. For instance, there is a negative correlation between WM capacity and the size of the standard Stroop effect (Kane & Engle, 2003), which reflects the degree of interference in naming the ink color of a written color word (e.g., saying "green" to the word "red" written in green ink). Attention allocation is thought to be one aspect of executive function (EF), which involves coordinating goal-directed behavior. A recent study by McCabe, Roediger, McDaniel, et al., (2010) found a very high correlation between factor scores for WM (derived from several measures of complex span) and EF (derived from several standard EF tasks such as the Wisconsin Card Sorting task).

These findings suggest that deficits in WM might be related to deficits in aspects of EF. Hamilton and Martin (2005, 2007) presented evidence that an aphasic patient (ML) who showed a semantic STM deficit had difficulty inhibiting verbal information, but not nonverbal information. For instance, he showed a verbal Stroop effect that was many standard deviations outside the normal range but showed an effect within normal range on a

spatial analogue to the Stroop effect. On a recognition probe task (that is, a task in which subjects decide if a probe word matches an item in a previous list), ML showed highly exaggerated interference effects if the probe matched an item in a previous list or was even phonologically or semantically related to a previous list item. Hamilton and Martin (2005) proposed that the patient had a specific difficulty in inhibiting irrelevant verbal representations. A study by Biegler, Crowther, and Martin (2008) showed that this patient and another with a semantic STM deficit had exaggerated difficulty in repeatedly naming items from the same semantic category. They suggested that this repeated naming from the same category led to an overactivation of all of the terms in the category. Difficulty in inhibiting the incorrect names led to increasingly longer naming latencies for same-category items relative to different category items. They hypothesized that the left inferior frontal gyrus (Figure 9-6), which was affected in these patients, is involved in verbal inhibition. A deficit in inhibition could cause difficulty in spontaneous speech, where one needs to inhibit what has already been talked about to produce the next words.

Recently, Barde et al. (2010) have offered another interpretation of the interference effects demonstrated by ML in the recognition probe task described earlier (Hamilton & Martin, 2007). They suggest that the effects can be accounted for by reactivation of the prior list item by the rhyming or semantically related probe word and a rapid loss of the semantic or phonological features of the probe that makes it difficult for the patient to verify whether the item matches the probe or not. They present data from 20 aphasic patients with varying degrees of semantic and phonological

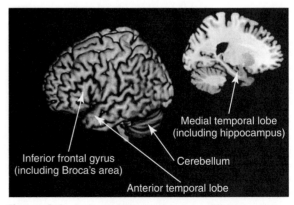

Figure 9-6 Brain structures related to different memory systems.

STM deficits. Consistent with their hypothesis, they show that the degree of phonological interference is accounted for by the degree of phonological STM deficit and the degree of semantic interference is accounted for by the degree of semantic STM deficit. It is unclear how their hypothesis can account for ML's difficulties on the Stroop task (or more recent data indicating an exaggerated picture-word interference effect; Biegler et al., 2008). However, it is possible that these are simply co-occurring deficits for ML and not causally related to the STM deficit. Only the investigation of a large number of patients on STM as well as single word tasks involving interference can address this issue.

Semantic Control

Recently, Hoffman, et al. (2009) proposed that EF deficits are the source of semantic impairments in aphasia (see further discussion later). That is, they argue that aphasic patients do not have a disruption of semantic knowledge per se but instead have a deficit in controlling access in a task-dependent fashion to appropriate aspects of semantic knowledge. These patients' lesions in left frontal and/or parietal regions are thought to underlie their semantic control deficit as these regions have been implicated in executive functioning (Collette, Hogge, Salmon, & van der Linden, 2006). This control deficit contrasts with a deficit in semantic knowledge representation, which is observed in semantic dementia (Box 9-1). They further argue that patients with a semantic STM deficit are those who have the most mild semantic control deficits. Patients with more severe semantic control deficits demonstrate obvious difficulties on processing single words such as in picture naming or picture-word matching. For patients with mild control deficits, their difficulties in semantic processing appear only when they have to process word lists rather than single words. However, semantic difficulties with single words can be observed for even the mildly affected patients if they are put under some kind of pressure (i.e., time pressure or having to select words from strongly interfering words).

Selection Deficits

As discussed earlier, a number of lines of evidence suggest that the left inferior frontal gyrus (LIFG; see Figure 9-6) is involved in inhibiting verbal representations. Thompson-Schill and colleagues have made a more general proposal, arguing that the LIFG is involved in selection, that is, in selecting target representations from competing ones (e.g., see Thompson-Schill, Bedny, & Goldberg, 2005, for an overview). This selection could be involved in choosing, for example, a synonym from a

---

Box 9-1

Conditions Associated with Semantic Memory Deficits

Semantic dementia, a subtype of **frontotemporal dementia,** is a neurodegenerative disease that leads to the loss of semantic memory and is associated with damage primarily in the temporal lobes (in contrast to other forms of frontotemporal dementia that involve greater degeneration in frontal regions).

Semantic aphasia refers to semantic deficits resulting from stroke, and typically involves lesions to inferior frontal and temporoparietal regions in the left hemisphere. Semantic aphasia can be best characterized as a deficit in accessing semantic memory rather than a deficit in semantic memory itself.

Herpes simplex virus encephalitis (HSVE) is a viral infection of the central nervous system that leads to inflammation of the brain, especially in the temporal lobes, and is often associated with deficits in episodic and semantic memory (as well as with a variety of other symptoms including hallucinations and personality changes).

Alzheimer disease is a degenerative disease leading to atrophy across a wide variety of brain regions. Alzheimer disease is primarily associated with deficits in episodic memory, but also leads to semantic memory deficits, especially for living things.

---

closely related word, judging the relatedness of word meanings on a particular dimension, or producing a name for a picture when several names might be appropriate. Thompson-Schill and Botvinick (2006) have suggested that this selection deficit arises from difficulty in biasing the cognitive system toward targeted information rather than in inhibiting nontarget information (see Botvinick, Braven, Barch, et al., 2001). This line of work has been extended to explain sentence comprehension deficits in patients with LIFG damage. In particular, Novick, Trueswell, and Thompson-Schill (2005) argued that the LIFG was part of a frontal system involved in detecting conflicting representations and in sentence processing initiated the reanalysis of a misinterpreted sentence. As Broca's area is part of the LIFG, they suggested that sentence processing deficits in patients with damage to Broca's area might be interpreted as due to a difficulty in reanalysis rather than to a syntactic deficit per se. Recently, Novick, Kan, Trueswell, and Thompson-Schill (2009) presented evidence that a patient with damage to the LIFG had great difficulty overcoming the tendency to interpret "on the mat" as the destination in the sentence "Put the frog on the mat in the box." In comparison, patients with frontal damage but without LIFG damage performed in a normal fashion. They further showed that the patient with LIFG was impaired a number of nonsentence tasks involving the resolution of conflict whereas the non-LIFG patients were not.

Summary of Short-Term Memory and Working Memory Deficits and Their Role in Language Processing

Reduced STM span, as often observed in aphasia, has few consequences for language comprehension and production if the span deficit reflects difficulty maintaining phonological information. In contrast, a deficit in maintaining semantic information causes difficulties for both comprehension and production. Phonological STM is important, however, for learning new phonological information; similarly, semantic STM is important for learning new semantic information. There is controversy whether semantic STM deficits reflect a rapid loss of semantic information or a deficit in various EFs (such as an inhibition deficit). Deficits in more complex WM appear to affect the ability to carry out what have been termed post-interpretive aspects of sentence processing rather than more on-line interpretive aspects (Caplan & Waters, 1999).

Semantic Memory Deficits

The preceding discussion has focused on STM systems and their role in retrieving, maintaining, and manipulating representations of meanings, facts, and general world knowledge drawn from LTM. These representations are a part of long-term *semantic memory*, referring to memory of meanings, concepts, and general world knowledge that are unrelated to specific experiences, and are thus a crucial part of language processing. Deficits in semantic memory can occur as a result of a variety of neurological conditions, including semantic dementia, stroke, herpes simplex virus encephalitis (HSVE), and Alzheimer disease (see Box 9-1), and can have drastic consequences for language.

Semantic Dementia

Semantic dementia is a subtype of frontotemporal dementia (and a further subtype of primary progressive aphasia) that results from atrophy of the anterior temporal lobes (see Figure 9-6) bilaterally, though often the atrophy is greater in the left hemisphere (Mummery, Patterson, Price, et al., 2000). Patients suffering from semantic dementia show a progressive loss of both productive and receptive vocabulary, stemming from a loss of semantic knowledge (Hodges & Patterson,

2007; Snowden, Goulding, & Neary, 1989; Warrington, 1975). Semantic dementia patients typically first lose knowledge of fine-grained features of concepts while retaining knowledge of more common or typical features. Thus words tend to be replaced with more general terms (e.g., "animal" instead of "camel") and less typical features are omitted when drawing (e.g., if asked to draw a camel, a semantic dementia patient would likely include a head, two ears, and four legs, but omit distinctive features such as the hump). This correspondence between word production and drawing suggests that the loss of semantic knowledge in semantic dementia is multimodal, as is further evidenced by a corresponding loss of knowledge of how to use objects in the later stages of the disease (Bier & Macoir, 2010; Hodges, Bozeat, Lambon Ralph, et al., 2000). Semantic dementia patients also typically develop symptoms of surface dyslexia, where irregularly spelled words (e.g., yacht) are read as if they were regular (Woollams, Lambon Ralph, Plaut, & Patterson, 2007) demonstrating the role of semantic memory in processing of exception words (i.e., words with irregular grapheme-to-phoneme correspondences).

Semantic dementia has been particularly influential because the deficit seems to be limited to semantic memory. Despite their severe semantic memory impairment, semantic dementia patients seem to have preserved syntactic processing, phonology, calculation ability, and drawing skills (at least in the earlier stages; Ash, Moore, Antani, et al., 2006; Hodges et al., 1999). Semantic dementia contrasts with progressive nonfluent aphasia, another form of frontotemporal dementia, which shows essentially the opposite pattern: impaired syntactic and phonological production in the context of spared semantic knowledge (Grossman, 2010). Importantly, patients with semantic dementia also appear to have relatively preserved episodic memory (i.e., memory for events, though the semantic memory deficits can make this difficult to demonstrate; Hodges & Patterson, 2007).

The amodal nature of the semantic memory deficit in semantic dementia suggests a relatively general role of the anterior temporal lobes in semantic memory. One recent proposal along these lines is that the anterior temporal lobes serve as a "hub" that integrates distributed modality-specific semantic information (Jefferies, Baker, Doran, & Lambon Ralph, 2007; Jefferies & Lambon Ralph, 2006; Lambon Ralph & Patterson, 2008; Patterson, Nestor, & Rogers, 2007; Rogers, Lambon Ralph, Garrard et al., 2004; see also Damasio, 1989). Some of the major motivations for this type of theory come from differences between patients with semantic dementia and stroke patients with semantic memory deficits.

Semantic Memory Deficits from Stroke

Although semantic memory deficits are not one of the typical symptoms of aphasia from stroke, they do sometimes arise from left-hemisphere stroke, leading to what is sometimes called *semantic aphasia*. As is true in semantic dementia, semantic aphasia is associated with semantic deficits on both verbal and nonverbal tasks. However, as mentioned earlier, these seemingly similar symptoms may have two distinct cognitive and neurological bases (e.g., Jefferies et al., 2007; Jefferies & Lambon Ralph, 2006; Patterson et al., 2007). One reason to assume different bases is that the neurological damage in semantic dementia and semantic aphasia are very different: while semantic dementia primarily affects the anterior temporal lobes, semantic aphasia generally involves left-hemisphere lesions to inferior frontal and/or temporoparietal regions (see Figure 9-6; in general, stroke very rarely leads to focal anterior temporal lesions simply as a function of the vascular system; Wise, 2003).

Behavioral evidence also indicates differences between the semantic memory deficits in semantic dementia and semantic aphasia. In particular, while anomia (difficulty finding words) is a ubiquitous symptom in both semantic aphasia and semantic dementia, anomia in semantic aphasia seems to reflect problems *finding* words whereas anomia in semantic dementia seems to reflect a lack of anything to find. One piece of evidence for this is that semantic aphasia patients benefit from phonemic cuing (i.e., when given the first sound of the target word) whereas semantic dementia patients show no such benefit. Also, semantic dementia patients show performance consistency across tasks (i.e., will be impaired both at producing the word "camel" and at drawing a camel) and are affected by item frequency/familiarity (as mentioned earlier). This suggests that the actual stored knowledge (e.g., of camels) is lost. In contrast, semantic aphasia patients tend to not show consistency across tasks that require different types of semantic knowledge and their performance is not affected by frequency. These patterns suggest that the semantic deficit in semantic aphasia is not a loss of the semantic memories per se but rather a deficit in *accessing* that intact knowledge (Jefferies et al., 2007; Jefferies & Lambon Ralph, 2006; Warrington & Shallice, 1979).

This differentiation between damage to an amodal semantic hub (in semantic dementia) and damage to semantic access mechanisms (in semantic aphasia), while appealing, has been challenged for a variety of reasons (see, e.g., Rapp & Caramazza, 1993). A more recent proposal is that semantic aphasia results not from a deficit in some (underspecified) access mechanism(s) but rather results from a deficit in the cognitive control processes that manage the retrieval of semantic memories (Jefferies & Lambon Ralph, 2006). By this account, semantic retrieval in semantic aphasia should not necessarily be variable over repeated testing (as is predicted by the original semantic access deficit account; Warrington & Shallice, 1979) but should vary as a function of the control demands of the task. There is evidence to support this claim (Jefferies et al., 2007; Jefferies & Lambon Ralph, 2006); however, it is as yet unclear if this semantic control mechanism is equivalent to some (or all) aspects of the EF systems involved in controlling and coordinating other complex tasks (Miyake, Friedman, Emerson, et al., 2000). Nevertheless, the distinction between storage and access/control seems to be a promising approach to our understanding of semantic memory deficits.

Semantic Memory Deficits from Herpes Simplex Virus Encephalitis and Alzheimer Disease

The most common memory deficits associated with HSVE are in long-term episodic memory rather than in semantic memory. However, some cases of HSVE are associated with semantic memory deficits, specifically cases that involve anterior temporal lobe damage (Kapur, Barker, Burrows, et al., 1994). Similarly, Alzheimer's disease is associated primarily with deficits in episodic memory, but semantic memory deficits emerge as well in later stages of the disease (Kramer et al., 2003). Semantic memory problems in HSVE and Alzheimer's disease often seem to be specific to living things, leaving preserved knowledge of man-made things and artifacts (e.g., Silveri, Daniele, Giustolisi, & Gainotti, 1991; Warrington & Shallice, 1984). This type of category-specific deficit has often been used to argue for separate neural representation of the memory of living and nonliving things (Caramazza & Shelton, 1998; see also, e.g., Barsalou, 1999). However, others have suggested that this dissociation might emerge in a unitary distributed semantic system based on other differences between living and nonliving things (e.g., Tyler, Moss, Durrant-Peatfield, & Levy, 2000). For example, living things may have more shared features and relatively fewer distinctive features than nonliving things, essentially making them more confusable (Noppeney et al., 2007).

Semantic Memory and Language: Conclusion

Semantic memory—as the mechanism underlying our knowledge of words and concepts—noncontroversially plays a critical role in language processing. The actual nature of semantic memory is somewhat more controversial. While there is broad agreement that semantic memory involves a wide distribution of brain regions

(Martin, 2007), debates over whether semantic memory is an entirely distributed network (e.g., Barsalou, 1999) or relies on an amodal semantic hub (e.g., Rogers et al., 2004) are ongoing. Understanding the role of the anterior temporal lobes is an important part of this debate, and neuropsychological deficits (especially semantic dementia) will likely continue to be a crucial piece of the puzzle (see Simmons & Martin, 2009).

Procedural Memory Deficits

Most work on the relationship between memory and language processing (both in normal populations and in language disorders) has focused on the role of explicit memory systems such as short-term and WM or long-term declarative memory (e.g., semantic memory). The role of nondeclarative systems like procedural memory have received less attention, presumably because there is less of an intuitive link between this system and the type of knowledge used in language. There are, however, good reasons to think that procedural memory plays an important role in language processing. This may seem more intuitive when thinking of language as a skill that is acquired via general learning mechanisms (e.g., Elman et al., 1997), in which case procedural memory is likely to be particularly important in domains where linguistic knowledge is learned implicitly, such as syntactic and morphological knowledge (e.g., Saffran, Aslin, & Newport, 1996).

The most explicit model of the role procedural memory plays in language processing is the *declarative/ procedural model* (Ullman, 2001, 2004, 2007; Ullman, Corkin, Coppola, et al., 1997), which relies on the well-established distinction between declarative and procedural memory. Declarative memory refers to conscious recall of information and events and is subserved by medial temporal and temporal-parietal regions, whereas procedural memory refers to nonconscious memory for how to do things and relies on frontal regions, the basal ganglia, and the cerebellum (Squire & Zola, 1996). With regard to language processing, the declarative/procedural model suggests that our knowledge of words (i.e., the mental lexicon) relies on declarative memory systems (including semantic memory), whereas our knowledge of linguistic rules (i.e., morphological and syntactic knowledge) relies on procedural memory systems.

Much of the research looking for dissociations between declarative- and procedurally-based aspects of language processing has investigated inflectional morphology, especially the distinction between regular and irregular verbs (e.g., Ullman et al., 1997). The basic idea is that tensed forms of regular verbs like *look* are conjugated via morphological rules (e.g., past tense employs an –*ed* suffixation rule, yielding *looked*) whereas

the tensed forms of irregular words like *go* (e.g., *went*) must be retrieved from the mental lexicon (Dell, 1986). A straightforward prediction of this model is that patients who have deficits in declarative memory and spared procedural memory—such as patients with semantic dementia, Alzheimer disease, and anterograde amnesia—should show deficits with irregular forms but preserved processing of regular morphology and syntax. In contrast, patients with deficits in procedural memory with (relatively) spared declarative memory should show the opposite pattern.

Evidence supporting this *procedural deficit hypothesis* (Ullman & Pierpont, 2005) is discussed later, focusing first on developmental and then on acquired (or adult-onset) deficits. It is important to note upfront that much of this evidence is subject to alternative explanations. For example, dissociations between the processing of regular and irregular morphology do not necessarily imply that regulars and irregulars rely on qualitatively different memory systems (or qualitatively different systems of other types, e.g., Pinker, 1994); these dissociations can also arise in single-system connectionist models under the assumption that irregular morphology relies more on semantic (and less on phonological) information than does regular morphology (Joanisse & Seidenberg, 1999). In general, these are controversial issues (even within the restricted domain of inflectional morphology) and are beyond the scope of this chapter. For the purposes of this section, we simply assume the dual-memory-system approach of the procedural/ declarative model (Ullman et al., 1997), while cautioning the reader that the conclusions given later might be quite different under competing models.

Developmental Deficits in Procedural Memory and Language

The idea that the "rule-based" aspects of language (in particular, syntactic and morphological processes) are acquired through implicit procedural mechanisms implies that children with procedural memory deficits should show corresponding difficulties in learning these rule-based aspects of language. Three general types of developmental disorders have been suggested to show linguistic deficits stemming from underlying deficits in procedural memory: specific language impairment, dyslexia and dysgraphia, and autism spectrum disorders (Box 9-2).

Procedural Memory and Specific Language Impairment

Specific language impairment (SLI) is a developmental language disorder that (as can be gathered from the name) is specific to language and not associated with

Box 9-2

Conditions Associated with Procedural Memory Deficits

Specific language impairment (SLI) is a developmental language disorder that does not result from brain injury or hearing loss and is not accompanied by other developmental disorders. SLI is associated particularly with syntactic and morphological problems in language and has been argued to reflect an underlying deficit in procedural memory.

Dyslexia and dysgraphia are developmental disorders in reading (dyslexia) and writing (dysgraphia) that may reflect underlying problems with phonological processing.

Autism spectrum disorders (ASD) are developmental disorders that typically involve social and linguistic impairments and repetitive behavior. ASD includes autism as well as Asperger syndrome, which involves less severe cognitive and linguistic deficits.

other conditions such as mental retardation, neurological injury, hearing impairment, or psychological trauma (Leonard, 1998). The extent to which SLI is a "pure" language deficit is controversial, and SLI seems to be a fairly heterogeneous diagnosis (van der Lely, 2005). Nevertheless, one of the hallmark symptoms of SLI is a deficit in morphological and syntactic aspects of language (Rice, Tomblin, Hoffman, et al., 2004), which are just the "rule-based" aspects predicted to be impaired given a deficit in procedural memory (Ullman & Pierpont, 2005).

Indeed, morphological deficits in SLI seem to affect regular more than irregular morphology and syntactic deficits in SLI seem to spare lexicalized aspects of syntax such as argument structure (see Ullman & Pierpont, 2005, for a review). These dissociations are relative: SLI is also associated with less severe deficits in irregular morphology, but Ullman and Pierpont (2005) point out that this could reflect compensatory use of declarative memory to store linguistic forms that would otherwise be generated by procedural rule-based processes. Additionally, because the declarative and procedural memory systems rely on different neural systems, the procedural deficit hypothesis predicts that individuals with SLI should show abnormalities in frontal regions, the basal ganglia, and other regions associated with procedural learning. Ullman and Pierpont (2005) summarize anatomical evidence to this end (e.g., Jernigan, Hesselink, Sowell, & Tallal, 1991); however, the neurobiology and neuroanatomy of SLI are not yet well

understood (Friederici, 2006) so such claims must be taken with caution.

An important prediction of the procedural deficit hypothesis is that SLI should also be associated with procedural learning/memory deficits (and spared declarative memory) in *nonlanguage* tasks. Ullman and Pierpont (2005) point out that problems with complex sequential motor skills (e.g., Owen & McKinlay, 1997) fit with a procedural learning deficit, and people with SLI are also impaired on some types of procedural learning tasks. One such task is the serial reaction-time (SRT) task, in which participants simply respond to the location of stimuli with a button press. These stimuli either occur in a specific sequence of locations or occur randomly; when stimuli occur in a specific sequence, people began to implicitly learn the sequence and respond faster (compared to when the location varies randomly). Tomblin, Mainela-Arnold, and Zhang (2007) found that while adolescents with SLI showed some procedural learning in this task (i.e., they were faster with sequenced stimuli), they improved more slowly than did typically developing participants and their rate of learning correlated with grammatical impairment but not with vocabulary size.

Kemény and Lukács (2009) looked at a different test of procedural learning called the Weather Prediction task (Knowlton, Squire, & Gluck, 1994). In this task, participants predict the weather (by choosing either *sunshine* or *rain*) after seeing cues that are differentially predictive (e.g., Cue 1 predicts sunshine in 77% of cases, Cue 3 in 42%, etc.) and are told if their prediction was right or wrong. Over time, predictions improve for typical participants as well as for amnesic patients, showing that the task does not rely on declarative memory (at least in the relatively early stages of the task; Knowlton et al., 1994). Children with SLI showed worse performance and less improvement than adults or age-matched typically developing children (Kemény & Lukács, 2009), providing further evidence for a deficit in nonlinguistic procedural learning in SLI.

Remember, however, that the critical point for the procedural deficit hypothesis (and the declarative/procedural model in general) is that procedural memory should be impaired *in the context of spared declarative memory*. Some recent work suggests that while children with SLI do well on nonverbal declarative memory tasks, they show impaired performance on verbal declarative memory tasks (Lum, Gelgic, & Conti-Ramsden, 2010). Thus SLI does not seem to be *uniquely* associated with a procedural memory deficit, but it is not yet clear if declarative memory deficits are of comparable severity as procedural memory deficits in SLI.

Overall, these data lend at least some support to the procedural deficit hypothesis of SLI. Of course, SLI is a complex and not-well-understood syndrome, and there are many other accounts with similarly equivocal support. For example, SLI has been argued to reflect a deficit in language-specific syntactic and morphological mechanisms (van der Lely, Rosen, & McClelland, 1998), a deficit in auditory processing (Tallal, Stark, & Mellits, 1985), a deficit in processing speed (Bishop, 1994), or a deficit in phonological WM (Montgomery, 1995). Some (or perhaps even all) of these deficits could reflect an underlying deficit in the systems underlying procedural memory (Ullman & Pierpont, 2005), or might simply reflect other variants of the relatively heterogeneous diagnosis of SLI.

Procedural Memory and Dyslexia/Dysgraphia

Developmental dyslexia and dysgraphia are disorders marked by difficulties in reading and writing, respectively, that are not due to deficits in vision, hearing, or education (American Psychiatric Association, 1994). As is true for SLI, the underlying cause of dyslexia and dysgraphia are controversial, due at least partially to their relative heterogeneity (Heim, Tschierse, Amunts, et al., 2008). Current influential accounts of dyslexia (and dysgraphia, though there is considerably less research) suggest an underlying phonological deficit (Ramus, 2004; Stanovich, 1988), or a general deficit in the magnocellular sensory processing stream (Livingstone, Rosen, Drislane, & Galaburda, 1991).

Interestingly, dyslexia has also often been associated with clumsiness and minor motor difficulties, which fits with the suggestion that dyslexic children have trouble making skills automatic (Nicolson & Fawcett, 1990), and with the related proposal that dyslexia and dysgraphia reflect an underlying deficit in the procedural learning and memory system (Nicolson & Fawcett, 2007; 2011; Ullman, 2004). Supporting this view, brain regions showing structural and functional abnormalities in dyslexia—including inferior frontal regions and the cerebellum (among other regions, see Démonet, Taylor, & Chaix, 2004, for a review)—correspond well with those underlying procedural memory.

However, behavioral evidence supporting a procedural deficit in dyslexia is mixed. Dyslexia has been associated with nonlinguistic problems in sequence learning (in SRT tasks, as described earlier) in both children (Vicari, Marotta, Menghini, et al., 2003) and adults (Stoodley, Harrison, & Stein, 2006). However, other work has not found deficits in SRT tasks or in artificial grammar learning tasks (Rüsseler, Gerth, & Münte, 2006). Thus the role of procedural memory in dyslexia is not yet entirely clear, but is receiving more

attention as evidenced, e.g., by a recent special issue of the Annals of the New York Academy of Sciences devoted entirely to "Learning, Skill Acquisition, Reading, and Dyslexia" (Eden & Flowers, 2008).

Procedural Memory and Autism Spectrum Disorders

A procedural memory deficit has also been proposed to play a role in autism spectrum disorder (ASD), a developmental disorder involving a wide range of social and communicative impairments (American Psychiatric Association, 1994). Although a wide variety of neurological abnormalities are associated with ASD (see, e.g., Courchesne, Redcay, Morgan, & Kennedy, 2005), some of these anatomical and functional abnormalities are in areas corresponding to the neurological substrates of procedural memory, such as the cerebellum and in the frontal lobe (Carper & Courchesne, 2000). And, as predicted by the procedural deficit hypothesis (Ullman et al., 1997), use of syntax and regular inflectional morphology is often impaired in ASD (at least among subtypes with language impairments; Tager-Flusberg, 2006), whereas declarative linguistic knowledge (e.g., vocabulary and irregular morphology) is relatively unimpaired (Ullman, 2004; Walenski, Tager-Flusberg, & Ullman, 2006).

Procedural learning in ASD has been investigated in nonlinguistic domains as well. Some evidence suggests that individuals with ASD show less procedural learning than do typically developing individuals in tasks such as the SRT task (Gordon & Stark, 2007; Mostofsky, Goldberg, Landa, & Denckla, 2000), whereas other studies find no such differences (Brown, Aczel, Jiménez, Kaufman, & Grant, 2010). A recent fMRI study investigated the fronto-temporal-parietal networks involved in procedural memory while learning an artificial grammar and found that individuals with ASD (unlike typically developing individuals) showed no facilitation from additional cues and no modulation of activity with learning (Scott-Van Zeeland, McNealy, Wang, et al., 2010). Thus, there seems to be important differences in the functioning of procedural memory in ASD; however, it remains to be seen how well these differences can account for ASD-related language deficits.

Acquired Deficits in Procedural Memory and Language

The declarative/procedural model suggests that procedural memory is involved not only in the acquisition of rule-based aspects of language, but also in the application of those rules, thus procedural memory deficits have also been implicated in acquired language deficits. In particular, a deficit in procedural memory has been claimed to underlie the linguistic deficits in some types of aphasia, Parkinson disease, and Huntington disease. Findings from these groups contrast interestingly with acquired deficits in declarative knowledge, such as Alzheimer disease, in which the opposite patterns (e.g., impairment on irregular more than regular morphology) are often observed (Ullman et al., 1997).

Procedural Memory and Aphasia

Ullman and colleagues (Ullman, 2004; Ullman et al., 2005, 1997) have suggested that fluent aphasia (aka receptive or posterior or Wernicke's aphasia) results from damage primarily to the declarative system and nonfluent, agrammatic aphasia (aka productive or anterior or Broca's aphasia) results from damage primarily to the procedural system. Indeed, there is evidence that agrammatic aphasic patients with left frontal lesions show more difficulty with regular than irregular past tense morphology, whereas fluent aphasic patients with left temporoparietal lesions show more difficulty with irregular than regular morphology (Ullman et al., 2005; see also Marslen-Wilson & Tyler, 1997; Miozzo & Gordon, 2005). However, agrammatic patients have also been reported who perform worse on irregular than regular morphology (e.g., de Diego Balaguer, Costa, Sebastián-Galles, et al., 2004) and agrammatic aphasia does not seem to be associated with deficits in nonlinguistic procedural memory such as performance on SRT tasks (Goschke, Friederici, Kotz, & van Kampen, 2001; Orrell, Eves, Masters, & Macmahon, 2007). Interestingly, agrammatic Broca's aphasics have been found to show deficits in procedural memory tasks that involve linguistic stimuli (phoneme sequences; Goschke et al., 2001), suggesting that some aspects of procedural learning for language may rely on domain-specific systems (Conway & Pisoni, 2008).

Procedural Memory and Other Acquired Language Deficits

Ullman (2004) proposes a number of other acquired syndromes in which language deficits can be thought of as arising from an underlying deficit in procedural memory, including Parkinson's and Huntington's disease. While linguistic deficits are not the hallmark symptoms of these syndromes, they involve disorders in areas important for procedural memory, particularly in the basal ganglia (Albin, Young, & Penney, 1989) and so the procedural deficit hypothesis predicts these patients should show abnormalities in syntax and irregular morphological processing. Indeed there is some evidence that Parkinson and Huntington disease patients show abnormal use of morphology (with Parkinson patients having trouble with regular morphology and

Huntington patients overusing regular morphological rules; Ullman et al., 1997), and these syndromes also involve deficits in procedural memory in SRT tasks (Knopman & Nissen, 1991; Siegert, Taylor, Weatherall, & Abernethy, 2006). However, other work has not found deficits in irregular morphology in these groups (Longworth, Keenan, Barker, et al., 2005) and neither Parkinson's nor Huntington's patients necessarily show deficits in other procedural memory tasks such as artificial grammar learning (Knowlton, Squire, Paulsen, et al., 1996; Witt, Nühsman, & Deuschl, 2002).

Procedural Memory and Language: Conclusion

As can be seen from the preceding discussion, the procedural deficit hypothesis (Ullman & Pierpont, 2005) is not without its problems. The idea that regular and irregular morphology are processed in independent memory systems (a claim on which the perceptual deficit hypothesis is predicated) is controversial (see, e.g., Kielar, Joanisse, & Hare, 2008; Pinker & Ullman, 2002) and many disorders of procedural memory do not unambiguously have corresponding deficits in rule-based aspects of language. [Yet another seemingly problematic counterexample comes from individuals with Williams syndrome, who appear to have deficits in procedural memory (Vicari, Bellucci, & Carlesimo, 2001) yet show impaired performance on irregular but not regular morphology (Clahsen & Almazan, 1998)—opposite the pattern predicted by the procedural deficit hypothesis.]

Nevertheless, the procedural deficit hypothesis is appealing as it is able to provide a unified account for a variety of language deficits—both developmental and acquired—within the context of the well-studied differentiation between declarative and procedural memory. Future versions of the perceptual deficit hypothesis may need to take different types of procedural memory into account (i.e., the common dissociations between perceptual learning on SRT tasks and artificial grammar tasks suggests at least some differentiation in perceptual memory systems) in order to capture the variety of memory-related language deficits.

Long-Term Episodic Memory Deficits

The procedural deficit hypothesis contrasts procedural memory systems with declarative memory, which includes both semantic and episodic memory. Deficits in semantic memory (e.g., as in semantic dementia, see earlier) clearly show the importance of semantic LTM for language processing. However it is less clear to what extent language processing depends on long-term episodic memory—that is, the memory system that allows us to remember past experiences (Tulving, 1972, 2002).

Deficits in episodic memory (Box 9-3) are associated with *anterograde amnesia* resulting from damage to the medial temporal lobes. Severely amnesic patients can have normal STM spans (Baddeley & Warrington, 1970), show preserved syntactic processing and memory (e.g., Ferreira, Bock, Wilson, & Cohen, 2008), and seem to have spared semantic memory. However, most amnesic patients are unable to learn new semantic information after the onset of amnesia, including new word meanings (Gabrieli, Cohen, & Corkin, 1988; Manns, Hopkins, & Squire, 2003) and often have preserved episodic memory for events occurring prior to the onset of amnesia (Wilson & Baddeley, 1988), which instead suggests impaired ability to create new long-term memories (be they semantic or episodic) within a single system of LTM (Squire, Stark, & Clark, 2004). Still, cases of developmental amnesia have been reported where episodic memory is severely disrupted despite relatively preserved semantic memory (Baddeley, Vargha-Khadem, & Mishkin, 2001; Vargha-Khadem, Gadian, Watkins, et al., 1997), fitting with the proposal that episodic memory deficits result from hippocampal damage, whereas semantic memory deficits involve damage to cortical regions (Mishkin, Suzuki, Gadian, & Vargha-Khadem, 1997).

This illustrates one problem with determining the role of long-term episodic memory deficits in language processing; namely that the existence of deficits specific to episodic (and not semantic) memory is somewhat controversial. Additionally, amnesia is generally assumed to not involve language problems (Milner, 2005), and even the rare individuals who show severely disrupted episodic memory in the context of preserved semantic memory seem to have normal language ability (Vargha-Khadem et al., 1997). Together, this suggests no crucial role for episodic memory in language learning or processing.

That said, the common view that language skills are preserved in amnesia has been questioned, based largely on evidence from the famous amnesic patient H.M. H.M.'s medial temporal lobes were resected as treatment for severe epilepsy, after which he was profoundly amnesic (Scoville & Milner, 1957). Although H.M.'s language abilities were originally reported to be normal (Milner, Corkin, & Teuber, 1968), later work suggested that H.M. had linguistic deficits that paralleled his memory problems. In particular, MacKay and colleagues have amassed a variety of evidence that H.M. had trouble detecting multiple meanings in ambiguous sentences (MacKay, Stewart, & Burke, 1998), showed syntactic processing deficits (MacKay, Burke, & Stewart, 1998; MacKay, James, Taylor, & Marian, 2007), and developed a deficit in the processing of low-frequency words (James & MacKay, 2001; MacKay & Hadley, 2009).

As mentioned earlier, these deficits may not reflect a deficit in *episodic* memory, but might instead reflect problems forming new *semantic* memories (e.g., H.M.'s language processing decrements could plausibly reflect a gradual deterioration of semantic knowledge). Additionally, there are reasons to be cautious of these findings: Other work has failed to find any evidence for language deficits in H.M. (Kensinger, Ullman, & Corkin, 2001; Skotko, Andrews, & Einstein, 2005; Skotko, Rubin, & Tupler, 2008) or has suggested that H.M.'s language deficits are idiosyncratic and unrelated to his temporal lobe lesions (Schmolck, Kensinger, Corkin, & Squire, 2002; Stefanacci, Buffalo, Schmolck, & Squire, 2000). One concern related to this second point is that H.M.'s surgery was performed to treat intractable epilepsy, and there is evidence that epilepsy is associated with abnormal language processing (particularly with word-finding difficulties; Mayeux, Brandt, Rosen, & Benson, 1980).

Episodic Long-Term Memory and Language: Conclusion

The relative lack of deficits specific to episodic LTM combined with the controversy over the existence of a separate system for episodic memory at all (Squire et al., 2004) leaves little evidence for a relationship between long-term episodic memory and language processing. It is, however, clear that H.M. and other amnesic patients have considerable trouble learning new semantic information (and, of course, impaired episodic memory presumably leaves one with fewer things to discuss).

CONCLUSIONS

Impairments in language and communication are typically considered linguistic deficits, however many of these linguistic problems arise as a function of problems in underlying memory systems. This should not

---

Box 9-3

A Condition Associated with Long-Term Memory Deficits

Anterograde amnesia refers to an inability to create new declarative memories, typically following traumatic brain injury or some types of drug use. Anterograde amnesia is associated with bilateral damage to the medial temporal lobes, including the hippocampi.

be surprising: language is a complicated system with many cognitive demands, and so relies heavily on most (perhaps even all) aspects of memory. Deficits in short-term and WM affect the ability to learn words, to plan phrases and sentences, and to comprehend complex propositions. Deficits in long-term semantic memory affect knowledge of words and access to semantic information. Deficits in procedural memory affect the use of structural processes (e.g., syntax and morphology) and deficits in episodic memory impact communicative content. Of course, many questions and issues remain, but the increasing amount of work investigating the role of memory systems in language holds promise not only for our understanding of these systems, but also for improved diagnosis and treatment of language and communicative disorders.

REFERENCES

Albin, R. L., Young, A. B., & Penney, J. B. (1989). The functional anatomy of basal ganglia disorders. *Trends in Neurosciences, 12*(10), 366–375.

Allport, D. A. (1984). Auditory verbal short-term memory and conduction aphasia. In H. Bouma & D. G. Bouwhuis (Eds.), *Attention and performance X: Control and language processes* (pp. 351–364). Hove, UK: Lawrence Erlbaum Associates Ltd.

American Psychiatric Association. (1994). *DSM-IV: Diagnostic and statistical manual of mental disorders* (4th ed.). Washington, DC: American Psychiatric Association.

Ash, S., Moore, P., Antani, S., McCawley, G., Work, M., & Grossman, M. (2006). Trying to tell a tale: Discourse impairments in progressive aphasia and frontotemporal dementia. *Neurology, 66*(9), 1405–1413.

Baddeley, A. D. (1986). *Working memory.* Oxford, UK: Clarendon Press.

Baddeley, A. D., Papagno, C., & Vallar, G. (1988). When long-term learning depends on short-term storage. *Journal of Memory and Language, 27*, 586–595.

Baddeley, A. D., Vargha-Khadem, F., & Mishkin, M. (2001). Preserved recognition in a case of developmental amnesia: Implications for the acquisition of semantic memory? *Journal of Cognitive Neuroscience, 13*(3), 357–369.

Baddeley, A. D., & Warrington, E. K. (1970). Amnesia and the distinction between long- and short-term memory. *Journal of Verbal Learning and Verbal Behavior, 9*, 176–189.

Barde, L. H. F., Schwartz, M. F., Chrysikou, E. G., Thompson-Schill, S. L. (2010). Reduced short-term memory span in aphasia and susceptibility to interference: Contribution of material-specific maintenance deficit. *Neuropsychologia, 48*, 909–920.

Barsalou, L. W. (1999). Perceptions of perceptual symbols. *Behavioral and Brain Sciences, 22*(4), 637–660.

Biegler, K. A., Crowther, J. E., & Martin, R. C. (2008). Consequences of an inhibition deficit for word production and comprehension. *Cognitive Neuropsychology, 25*, 493–527.

Bier, N., & Macoir, J. (2010). How to make a spaghetti sauce with a dozen small things I cannot name: A review of the impact of semantic-memory deficits on everyday actions. *Journal of Clinical and Experimental Neuropsychology, 32*(2), 201.

Bishop, D. V. M. (1994). Grammatical errors in specific language impairment: Competence or performance limitations? *Applied Psycholinguistics, 15*(4), 507–550.

Botvinick, M. M., Braver, T. S., Barch, D. M., & Carter, C. S., & Cohen, J. D. (2001). Conflict monitoring and cognitive control. *Psychological Review, 108*, 624–652.

Brown, J., Aczel, B., Jiménez, L., Kaufman, S. B., & Grant, K. P. (2010). Intact implicit learning in autism spectrum conditions. *The Quarterly Journal of Experimental Psychology, 63*, 1789–1812.

Butterworth, B., Campbell, R., & Howard, D. The uses of short-term memory: A case study. *Quarterly Journal of Experimental Psychology, 1986, 38*, 705–737.

Caplan, D., Alpert, N., & Waters, G. (1998). Effects of syntactic structure and propositional number on patterns of regional cerebral blood flow. *Journal of Cognitive Neuroscience, 10*, 541–552.

Caplan, D., & Waters, G. S. (1999). Verbal working memory and sentence comprehension. *Brain and Behavioral Sciences, 22*, 77–126.

Caramazza, A., & Shelton, J. R. (1998). Domain-specific knowledge systems in the brain: The animate-inanimate distinction. *Journal of Cognitive Neuroscience, 10*(1), 1–34.

Carper, R. A., & Courchesne, E. (2000). Inverse correlation between frontal lobe and cerebellum sizes in children with autism. *Brain, 123*(4), 836–844.

Clahsen, H., & Almazan, M. (1998). Syntax and morphology in Williams syndrome. *Cognition, 68*(3), 167–198.

Collette, F., Hogge, M., Salmon, E., & van der Linden, M. (2006). Exploration of the neural substrates of executive functioning by functional neuroimaging, *139*, 209–221.

Conway, C. M., & Pisoni, D. B. (2008). Neurocognitive basis of implicit learning of sequential structure and its relation to language processing. *Annals of the New York Academy of Sciences, 1145*, 113–131.

Courchesne, E., Redcay, E., Morgan, J. T., & Kennedy, D. P. (2005). Autism at the beginning: Microstructural and growth abnormalities underlying the cognitive and behavioral phenotype of autism. *Development and Psychopathology, 17*(3), 577–597.

Damasio, A. R. (1989). The Brain Binds Entities and Events by Multiregional Activation from Convergence Zones. *Neural Computation, 1*(1), 123–132.

Dell, G. S. (1986). A spreading-activation theory of retrieval in sentence production. *Psychological Review, 93*(3), 283–321.

Démonet, J., Taylor, M. J., & Chaix, Y. (2004). Developmental dyslexia. *The Lancet, 363*(9419), 1451–1460.

de Diego Balaguer, R., Costa, A., Sebastián-Galles, N., Juncadella, M., & Caramazza, A. (2004). Regular and irregular morphology and its relationship with agrammatism: Evidence from two Spanish-Catalan bilinguals. *Brain and Language, 91*(2), 212–222.

Eden, G. F., & Flowers, D. L. (2008). Introduction. *Annals of the New York Academy of Sciences, 1145*(1), ix-xii.

Elman, J. L., Bates, E. A., Johnson, M. H., Karmiloff-Smith, A., Parisi, D., & Plunkett, K. (1997). *Rethinking Innateness: A Connectionist Perspective on Development*. Cambridge, MA: MIT Press.

Engle, R. W., Tuholski, S. W., Laughlin, J. E., & Conway, A. R. (1999). Working memory, short-term memory, and general fluid intelligence: A latent-variable approach. *Journal of Experimental Psychology: General, 128*(3), 309–331.

Ferreira, V. S., Bock, K., Wilson, M. P., & Cohen, N. J. (2008). Memory for syntax despite amnesia. *Psychological Science, 19*(9), 940–946.

Freedman, M., & Martin, R. (2001). Dissociable components of short-term memory and their relation to long-term learning. *Cognitive Neuropsychology, 18*, 193–226.

Friederici, A. D. (2006). The neural basis of language development and its impairment. *Neuron, 52*(6), 941–952.

Gabrieli, J. D. E., Cohen, N. J., & Corkin, S. (1988). The impaired learning of semantic knowledge following bilateral medial temporal-lobe resection. *Brain and Cognition, 7*(2), 157–177.

Gordon, B., & Stark, S. (2007). Procedural learning of a visual sequence in individuals with Autism. *Focus on Autism and Other Developmental Disabilities, 22*(1), 14–22.

Goschke, T., Friederici, A. D., Kotz, S. A., & van Kampen, A. (2001). Procedural learning in Broca's aphasia: Dissociation between the implicit acquisition of spatio-motor and phoneme sequences. *Journal of Cognitive Neuroscience, 13*(3), 370–388.

Grossman, M. (2010). Primary progressive aphasia: clinicopathological correlations. *Nature Reviews Neurology, 6*(2), 88–97.

Hamilton, A. C., & Martin, R. C. (2005). Dissociations among tasks involving inhibition: A single case study. *Cognitive, Affective, & Behavioral Neuroscience, 5*, 1–13.

Hamilton, A., & Martin, R. C. (2007). Proactive interference in a semantic short-term memory deficit: Role of semantic and phonological relatedness. *Cortex, 43*, 112–123.

Heim, S., Tschierse, J., Amunts, K., Wilms, M., Vossel, S., Willmes, K., Grabowska, A., & Huber, W. (2008). Cognitive subtypes of dyslexia. *Acta Neurobiologiae Experimentalis, 68*(1), 73–82.

Hodges, J. R., & Patterson, K. (2007). Semantic dementia: a unique clinicopathological syndrome. *The Lancet Neurology, 6*(11), 1004–1014.

Hodges, J. R., Bozeat, S., Lambon Ralph, M. A., Patterson, K., & Spatt, J. (2000). The role of conceptual knowledge in object use Evidence from semantic dementia. *Brain, 123*(9), 1913–1925.

Hodges, J. R., Patterson, K., Ward, R., Garrard, P., Bak, T., Perry, R., & Gregory, C. (1999). The differentiation of semantic dementia and frontal lobe dementia (temporal and frontal variants of frontotemporal dementia) from early Alzheimer's disease: a comparative neuropsychological study. *Neuropsychology, 13*(1), 31–40.

Hoffman, P., Jefferies, E., Ehsan, S., Hopper, S., & Lambon Ralph, M. A. (2009). Selective short-term memory deficits arise from impaired domain general semantic control mechanisms. *Journal of Experimental Psychology: Learning, Memory and Cognition, 35*, 137–156.

James, L. E., & MacKay, D. G. (2001). H.M., word knowledge, and aging: support for a new theory of long-term retrograde amnesia. *Psychological Science, 12*(6), 485–492.

Jefferies, E., Baker, S. S., Doran, M., & Lambon Ralph, M. A. (2007). Refractory effects in stroke aphasia: A consequence of poor semantic control. *Neuropsychologia, 45*(5), 1065–1079.

Jefferies, E., & Lambon Ralph, M. A. (2006). Semantic impairment in stroke aphasia versus semantic dementia: a case-series comparison. *Brain, 129*(8), 2132–2147.

Jernigan, T. L., Hesselink, J. R., Sowell, E., & Tallal, P. (1991). Cerebral structure on magnetic resonance imaging in language- and learning-impaired children. *Archives of Neurology, 48*(5), 539–545.

Joanisse, M. F., & Seidenberg, M. S. (1999). Impairments in verb morphology after brain injury: A connectionist model. *Proceedings of the National Academy of Sciences of the United States of America, 96*(13), 7592–7597.

Kane, M. J., & Engle, R. W. (2003). Working memory capacity and the control of attention: The contributors of goal neglect, response competition, and task set to Stroop interference. *Journal of Experimental Psychology: General, 132*, 47–70.

Kapur, N., Barker, S., Burrows, E. H., Ellison, D., Brice, J., Illis, L. S., Scholey, K., et al. (1994). Herpes simplex encephalitis: long term magnetic resonance imaging and neuropsychological profile. *Journal of Neurology, Neurosurgery & Psychiatry, 57*(11), 1334–1342.

Kemény, F., & Lukács, A. (2009). Impaired procedural learning in language impairment: Results from probabilistic categorization. *Journal of Clinical and Experimental Neuropsychology*, 1–12.

Kensinger, E. A., Ullman, M. T., & Corkin, S. (2001). Bilateral medial temporal lobe damage does not affect lexical or grammatical processing: evidence from amnesic patient H.M. *Hippocampus, 11*(4), 347–360.

Kielar, A., Joanisse, M. F., & Hare, M. L. (2008). Priming English past tense verbs: Rules or statistics? *Journal of Memory and Language, 58*(2), 327–346.

Knopman, D., & Nissen, M. J. (1991). Procedural learning is impaired in Huntington's disease: evidence from the serial reaction time task. *Neuropsychologia, 29*(3), 245–254.

Knowlton, B. J., Squire, L. R., Paulsen, J. S., Swerdlow, N. R., & Swenson, M. (1996). Dissociations within nondeclarative memory in Huntington's disease. *Neuropsychology, 10*(4), 538–548.

Knowlton, B. J., Squire, L., & Gluck, M. A. (1994). Probabilistic classification learning in amnesia. *Learning & Memory, 1*(2), 106–120.

Kramer, J. H., Jurik, J., Sha, S. J., Rankin, K. P., Rosen, H. J., Johnson, J. K., & Miller, B. L. (2003). Distinctive neuropsychological patterns in frontotemporal dementia, semantic dementia, and Alzheimer disease. *Cognitive and Behavioral Neurology: Official Journal of the Society for Behavioral and Cognitive Neurology, 16*(4), 211–218.

Lambon Ralph, M. A., & Patterson, K. (2008). Generalization and differentiation in semantic memory: insights from semantic dementia. *Annals of the New York Academy of Sciences, 1124*, 61–76.

Leonard, L. B. (1998). *Children with specific language impairment*. Cambridge, MA: MIT Press.

Livingstone, M. S., Rosen, G. D., Drislane, F. W., & Galaburda, A. M. (1991). Physiological and anatomical evidence for a magnocellular defect in developmental dyslexia. *Proceedings of the National Academy of Sciences of the United States of America, 88*(18), 7943–7947.

Longworth, C. E., Keenan, S. E., Barker, R. A., Marslen-Wilson, W. D., & Tyler, L. K. (2005). The basal ganglia and rule-governed language use: evidence from vascular and degenerative conditions. *Brain, 128*(Pt 3), 584–596.

Lum, J. A. G., Gelgic, C., & Conti-Ramsden, G. (2010). Procedural and declarative memory in children with and without specific language impairment. *International Journal of Language & Communication Disorders, 45*(1), 96–107.

MacKay, D. G., & Hadley, C. (2009). Supra-normal age-linked retrograde amnesia: lessons from an older amnesic (H.M.). *Hippocampus, 19*(5), 424–445.

MacKay, D. G., Burke, D. M., & Stewart, R. (1998). H.M.'s language production deficits: Implications for relations between memory, semantic binding, and the hippocampal system. *Journal of Memory and Language, 38*(1), 28–69.

MacKay, D. G., James, L. E., Taylor, J. K., & Marian, D. E. (2007). Amnesic H.M. exhibits parallel deficits and sparing in language and memory: Systems versus binding theory accounts. *Language and Cognitive Processes, 22*(3), 377.

MacKay, D. G., Stewart, R., & Burke, D. M. (1998). H.M. revisited: relations between language comprehension, memory, and the hippocampal system. *Journal of Cognitive Neuroscience, 10*(3), 377–394.

Manns, J. R., Hopkins, R. O., & Squire, L. R. (2003). Semantic memory and the human hippocampus. *Neuron, 38*(1), 127–133.

Marslen-Wilson, W. D., & Tyler, L. K. (1997). Dissociating types of mental computation. *Nature, 387*(6633), 592–594.

Martin, A. (2007). The representation of object concepts in the brain. *Annual Review of Psychology, 58*(1), 25–45.

Martin, N., & Ayala, J. (2004). Measurements of auditory-verbal STM span in aphasia: Effects of items, task, and lexical impairment. *Brain and Language, 89*, 464–483.

Martin, N., & Saffran, E. M. (1997). Language and auditory-verbal short-term memory impairments: Evidence for common underlying processes. *Cognitive Neuropsychology, 14*, 641–682.

Martin, R. C., & Freedman, M. L. (2001). Short-term retention of lexical-semantic representations: Implications for speech production. *Memory, 9*, 261–280.

Martin, R. C., & He, T. (2004). Semantic short-term memory deficit and language processing: A replication, *Brain and Language, 89*, 76–82.

Martin, R. C., Lesch, M. F., & Bartha, M. C. (1999). Independence of input and output phonology in word processing and short-term memory. *Journal of Memory & Language, 31*, 2–39.

Martin, R. C., Miller, M., & Vu, H. (2004). Working memory and sentence production: Evidence for a phrasal scope of planning at a lexical-semantic level. *Cognitive Neuropsychology, 21*, 625–644.

Martin, R. C., & Romani, C. (1994). Verbal working memory and sentence comprehension: A multiple-components view. *Neuropsychology, 8*, 506–523.

Martin, R. C., Shelton, J., & Yaffee, L. (1994). Language processing and working memory: Neuropsychological evidence for separate phonological and semantic capacities. *Journal of Memory and Language, 33*, 83–111.

Mayeux, R., Brandt, J., Rosen, J., & Benson, D. (1980). Interictal memory and language impairment in temporal lobe epilepsy. *Neurology, 30*(2), 120–125.

McCabe, D. P., Roediger, H. L., McDaniel, M. A., Balota, D. A., Hambrick, D. Z. (2010). Relationship between working memory capacity and executive functioning: Evidence for a common executive attention construct. *Neuropsychology, 24*, 222–243.

Milner, B. (2005). The medial temporal-lobe amnesic syndrome. *Psychiatric Clinics of North America, 28*(3), 599–611.

Milner, B., Corkin, S., & Teuber, H. (1968). Further analysis of the hippocampal amnesic syndrome: 14-year follow-up study of H.M. *Neuropsychologia, 6*(3), 215–234.

Miozzo, M., & Gordon, P. (2005). Facts, events, and inflection: when language and memory dissociate. *Journal of Cognitive Neuroscience, 17*(7), 1074–1086.

Mishkin, M., Suzuki, W. A., Gadian, D. G., & Vargha-Khadem, F. (1997). Hierarchical organization of cognitive memory. *Philosophical Transactions of the Royal Society B: Biological Sciences, 352*(1360), 1461–1467.

Miyake, A., Friedman, N. P., Emerson, M. J., Witzki, A. H., Howerter, A., & Wager, T. D. (2000). The unity and diversity of executive functions and their contributions to complex "frontal lobe" tasks: a latent variable analysis. *Cognitive Psychology, 41*(1), 49–100.

Montgomery, J. W. (1995). Sentence comprehension in children with Specific Language Impairment: The role of phonological working memory. *Journal of Speech, Language and Hearing Research, 38*(1), 187–199.

Mostofsky, S. H., Goldberg, M. C., Landa, R. J., & Denckla, M. B. (2000). Evidence for a deficit in procedural learning in children and adolescents with autism: implications for cerebellar contribution. *Journal of the International Neuropsychological Society: JINS, 6*(7), 752–759.

Mummery, C., Patterson, K., Price, C., Ashburner, J., Frackowiak, R., & Hodges, J. R. (2000). A voxel-based morphometry study of semantic dementia: Relationship between temporal lobe atrophy and semantic memory. *Annals of Neurology, 47*(1), 36–45.

Nicolson, R. I., & Fawcett, A. J. (2011). Dyslexia, dysgraphia, procedural learning and the cerebellum. *Cortex, 47*, 117–127.

Nicolson, R. I., & Fawcett, A. J. (1990). Automaticity: A new framework for dyslexia research? *Cognition, 35*(2), 159–182.

Nicolson, R. I., & Fawcett, A. J. (2007). Procedural learning difficulties: reuniting the developmental disorders? *Trends in Neurosciences, 30*(4), 135–141.

Noppeney, U., Patterson, K., Tyler, L. K., Moss, H., Stamatakis, E. A., Bright, P., Mummery, C., et al. (2007). Temporal lobe lesions and semantic impairment: a comparison of herpes simplex virus encephalitis and semantic dementia. *Brain, 130*(4), 1138–1147.

Novick, J. M., Kan, I. P., Trueswell, J. C., Thompson-Schill, S. L. (2009). A case for conflict across multiple domains: Memory and language impairments following damage to ventrolateral prefrontal cortex. *Cognitive Neuropsychology, 26*, 527–567.

Novick, J. M., Trueswell, J. C., & Thompson-Schill, S. L. (2005). Cognitive control and parsing: Reexamining the role of Broca's area in sentence comprehension. *Cognitive, Affective, and Behavioral Neuroscience, 5,* 263–281.

Orrell, A. J., Eves, F. F., Masters, R. S. W., & Macmahon, K. M. M. (2007). Implicit sequence learning processes after unilateral stroke. *Neuropsychological Rehabilitation: An International Journal, 17*(3), 335–354.

Owen, S. E., & McKinlay, I. A. (1997). Motor difficulties in children with developmental disorders of speech and language. *Child: Care, Health and Development, 23*(4), 315–325.

Patterson, K., Nestor, P. J., & Rogers, T. T. (2007). Where do you know what you know? The representation of semantic knowledge in the human brain. *Nat Rev Neurosci, 8*(12), 976–987.

Pinker, S. (1994). *The language instinct.* New York: William Morrow and Company.

Pinker, S., & Ullman, M. T. (2002). The past and future of the past tense. *Trends in Cognitive Sciences, 6*(11), 456–463.

Ramus, F. (2004). Neurobiology of dyslexia: a reinterpretation of the data. *Trends in Neurosciences, 27*(12), 720–726.

Rapp, B., & Caramazza, A. (1993). On the distinction between deficits of access and deficits of storage: A question of theory. *Cognitive Neuropsychology, 10*(2), 113–141.

Rice, M. L., Tomblin, J. B., Hoffman, L., Richman, W. A., & Marquis, J. (2004). Grammatical tense deficits in children with SLI and nonspecific language impairment: Relationships with nonverbal IQ over time. *Journal of Speech, Language and Hearing Research, 47*(4), 816–834.

Rogers, T. T., Lambon Ralph, M. A., Garrard, P., Bozeat, S., McClelland, J. L., Hodges, J. R., & Patterson, K. (2004). Structure and deterioration of semantic memory: A neuropsychological and computational investigation. *Psychological Review, 111*(1), 205–235.

Romani, C. (1992). Are there distinct input and output buffers? Evidence from an aphasic patient with an impaired output buffer. *Language and Cognitive Processes, 7,* 131–162.

Rüsseler, J., Gerth, I., & Münte, T. F. (2006). Implicit learning is intact in adult developmental dyslexic readers: Evidence from the serial reaction time task and artificial grammar learning. *Journal of Clinical and Experimental Neuropsychology, 28*(5), 808.

Saffran, J. R., Aslin, R. N., & Newport, E. L. (1996). Statistical learning by 8-month-old infants. *Science, 274*(5294), 1926–1928.

Schmolck, H., Kensinger, E. A., Corkin, S., & Squire, L. R. (2002). Semantic knowledge in patient H.M. and other patients with bilateral medial and lateral temporal lobe lesions. *Hippocampus, 12*(4), 520–533.

Scott-Van Zeeland, A. A., McNealy, K., Wang, A. T., Sigman, M., Bookheimer, S. Y., & Dapretto, M. (2010). No neural evidence of statistical learning during exposure to artificial languages in children with autism spectrum disorders. *Biological Psychiatry, 68,* 345–351.

Scoville, W. B., & Milner, B. (1957). Loss of recent memory after bilateral hippocampal lesions. *Journal of Neurology, Neurosurgery, and Psychiatry, 20*(1), 11–21.

Shallice, T., & Butterworth, B. (1977). Short-term memory impairment and spontaneous speech. *Neuropsychologia, 15,* 729–735.

Siegert, R. J., Taylor, K. D., Weatherall, M., & Abernethy, D. A. (2006). Is implicit sequence learning impaired in Parkinson's disease? A meta-analysis. *Neuropsychology, 20*(4), 490–495.

Silveri, M., Daniele, A., Giustolisi, L., & Gainotti, G. (1991). Dissociation between knowledge of living and nonliving things in dementia of the Alzheimer type. *Neurology, 41*(4), 545–546.

Simmons, W. K., & Martin, A. (2009). The anterior temporal lobes and the functional architecture of semantic memory. *Journal of the International Neuropsychological Society, 15*(5), 645–649.

Skotko, B. G., Andrews, E., & Einstein, G. (2005). Language and the medial temporal lobe: Evidence from H.M.'s spontaneous discourse. *Journal of Memory and Language, 53*(3), 397–415.

Skotko, B. G., Rubin, D. C., & Tupler, L. A. (2008). H.M.'s personal crossword puzzles: understanding memory and language. *Memory, 16*(2), 89–96.

Snowden, J. S., Goulding, P. J., & Neary, D. (1989). Semantic dementia: A form of circumscribed cerebral atrophy. *Behavioural Neurology, 2*(3), 167–182.

Squire, L., Stark, C. E., & Clark, R. E. (2004). The medial temporal lobe. *Annual Review of Neuroscience, 27*(1), 279–306.

Squire, L., & Zola, S. (1996). Structure and function of declarative and nondeclarative memory systems. *Proceedings of the National Academy of Sciences of the United States of America, 93*(24), 13515–13522.

Stanovich, K. E. (1988). Explaining the differences between the dyslexic and the garden-variety poor reader: The phonological-core variable-difference model. *Journal of Learning Disabilities, 21*(10), 590–604.

Stefanacci, L., Buffalo, E. A., Schmolck, H., & Squire, L. R. (2000). Profound amnesia after damage to the medial temporal lobe: A neuroanatomical and neuropsychological profile of patient E. P. *The Journal of Neuroscience, 20*(18), 7024–7036.

Stoodley, C. J., Harrison, E. P., & Stein, J. F. (2006). Implicit motor learning deficits in dyslexic adults. *Neuropsychologia, 44*(5), 795–798.

Tager-Flusberg, H. (2006). Defining language phenotypes in autism. *Clinical Neuroscience Research, 6*(3–4), 219–224.

Tallal, P., Stark, R. E., & Mellits, D. (1985). The relationship between auditory temporal analysis and receptive language development: Evidence from studies of developmental language disorder. *Neuropsychologia, 23*(4), 527–534.

Thompson-Schill, S. L., Bedny, M., & Goldberg, R. F. (2005). The frontal lobes and the regulation of mental activity. *Current Opinion in Neurobiology, 15,* 219–224.

Thompson-Schill, S. L., & Botvinick, M. M. (2006). Resolving conflict: A response to Martin and Cheng (2006). *Psychonomic Bulletin & Review, 13,* 402–408.

Tomblin, J. B., Mainela-Arnold, E., & Zhang, X. (2007). Procedural learning in adolescents with and without Specific Language Impairment. *Language Learning and Development, 3*(4), 269.

Tulving, E. (1972). Episodic and semantic memory. In E. Tulving & W. Donaldson (Eds.), *Organization and memory*. New York: Academic Press.

Tulving, E. (2002). Episodic memory: From mind to brain. *Annual Review of Psychology, 53*(1), 1–25.

Turner, M. L. & Engle, R. W. (1989). Is working memory capacity task dependent? *Journal of Memory and Language, 28*, 127–154.

Tyler, L. K., Moss, H. E., Durrant-Peatfield, M. R., & Levy, J. P. (2000). Conceptual structure and the structure of concepts: A distributed account of category-specific deficits. *Brain and Language, 75*(2), 195–231.

Ullman, M. T. (2001). A neurocognitive perspective on language: The declarative/procedural model. *Nature Reviews Neuroscience, 2*(10), 717–726.

Ullman, M. T. (2004). Contributions of memory circuits to language: The declarative/procedural model. *Cognition, 92*(1–2), 231–270.

Ullman, M. T., Pancheva, R., Love, T., Yee, E., Swinney, D., & Hickok, G. (2005). Neural correlates of lexicon and grammar: evidence from the production, reading, and judgment of inflection in aphasia. *Brain and Language, 93*(2), 185–238.

Ullman, M. T., & Pierpont, E. I. (2005). Specific language impairment is not specific to language: The procedural deficit hypothesis. *Cortex, 41*(3), 399–433.

Ullman, M. T. (2007). The biocognition of the mental lexicon. In *The Oxford handbook of psycholinguistics* (pp. 267–286). Oxford, UK: Oxford University Press.

Ullman, M. T., Corkin, S., Coppola, M., Hickok, G., Growdon, J. H., Koroshetz, W. J., & Pinker, S. (1997). A neural dissociation within language: Evidence that the mental dictionary is part of declarative memory, and that grammatical rules are processed by the procedural system. *Journal of Cognitive Neuroscience, 9*(2), 266–276.

van der Lely, H. K. J. (2005). Domain-specific cognitive systems: insight from Grammatical-SLI. *Trends in Cognitive Sciences, 9*(2), 53–59.

van der Lely, H. K., Rosen, S., & McClelland, A. (1998). Evidence for a grammar-specific deficit in children. *Current Biology, 8*(23), 1253–1258.

Vargha-Khadem, F., Gadian, D. G., Watkins, K. E., Connelly, A., Van Paesschen, W., & Mishkin, M. (1997). Differential effects of early hippocampal pathology on episodic and semantic memory. *Science, 277*(5324), 376–380.

Vicari, S., Bellucci, S., & Carlesimo, G. A. (2001). Procedural learning deficit in children with Williams syndrome. *Neuropsychologia, 39*(7), 665–677.

Vicari, S., Marotta, L., Menghini, D., Molinari, M., & Petrosini, L. (2003). Implicit learning deficit in children with developmental dyslexia. *Neuropsychologia, 41*(1), 108–114.

Walenski, M., Tager-Flusberg, H., & Ullman, M. T. (2006). Language in autism. In *Understanding autism: From basic neuroscience to treatment.* (pp. 175–203). Boca Raton, FL: Taylor and Francis Books.

Warrington, E. K. (1975). The selective impairment of semantic memory. *Quarterly Journal of Experimental Psychology, 27*(4), 635–657.

Warrington, E. K., & Shallice, T. (1979). Semantic access dyslexia. *Brain, 102*, 43–63.

Warrington, E. K., & Shallice, T. (1984). Category specific semantic impairments. *Brain, 107*(3), 829–853.

Wilson, B., & Baddeley, A. D. (1988). Semantic, episodic, and autobiographical memory in a postmeningitic amnesic patient. *Brain and Cognition, 8*(1), 31–46.

Wise, R. J. S. (2003). Language systems in normal and aphasic human subjects: functional imaging studies and inferences from animal studies. *British Medical Bulletin, 65*(1), 95–119.

Witt, K., Nühsman, A., & Deuschl, G. (2002). Intact artificial grammar learning in patients with cerebellar degeneration and advanced Parkinson's disease. *Neuropsychologia, 40*(9), 1534–1540.

Woollams, A. M., Lambon Ralph, M. A., Plaut, D. C., & Patterson, K. (2007). SD-squared: on the association between semantic dementia and surface dyslexia. *Psychological Review, 114*(2), 316–339.

Wong, W., & Law, S.-P. (2008). The relationship between semantic short-term memory and serial recall of known and unknown words and nonwords: Data from two Chinese individuals with aphasia. *Journal of Experimental Psychology: Learning, Memory, and Cognition, 34*, 900–917.

Language Processing Disorders

Tracy Love and Kathleen Brumm

INTRODUCTION

In normal conversation, we tend to take the remarkable processes of language comprehension and production for granted. We are seemingly able to carry on conversations rapidly and effortlessly, expressing ourselves to others and understanding what others convey to us. Yet, comprehension and production are exceedingly complex, using a multitude of processes that occur during normal language processing and spanning multiple language levels from basic phonological processing, lexical access, syntactic analysis, and discourse level processing, among others.

Often, we are unaware of how complex and specialized language processes must be until we or someone we know experiences neural trauma. Scientists first began to learn about these processes and the architecture of the language system by examining language disorders in individuals who have survived some type of neural injury. Those early explorations led to broad behavioral descriptions of the general components of language (production, comprehension) and, more recently, of the levels of processing involved in each of these components.

The goal of this chapter is to examine the nature and time-course of language processing in individuals who have survived brain damage. We discuss acquired language disorders and their potential underpinnings from a processing perspective. Our discussion is based upon an examination of the psychological evidence for disordered sentence-level[1] language processing in acquired language disorders. Alongside this evidence, we examine specific neural regions that, when damaged, lead to aberrant language processing.

Several principles guide the work of this chapter. The first is that to understand the nature of language processing, one must first understand the various methods that have been used by researchers in the field. We discuss those methods and consider their advantages and limitations for the study of language processing.

The second principle of this chapter is that the brain can use a variety of techniques or approaches to process language. These include automatic processes, problem solving, specialized strategies, meta-linguistic reflection, and others. We examine how language processing can go awry at any of a number of stages, from an initial or automatic operation to the arrival of final understanding. As this is a large area to cover (speech perception through discourse, with all that comes between), we limit our focus to the lexical (word) and sentence structure building portions of auditory language processing, which are particularly germane to the disorders found in the aphasias.

Finally, our third principle is that evidence from language disorders arising from localized, acquired neural trauma (specifically stroke) can help illuminate the functional roles of brain regions that are (critically) involved in language processing (Box 10-1).

---

[1]As discussed in Chapter 6, the sentence is often considered the basic unit of analysis in language processing, and as discussed throughout this chapter, it is at the sentence level where language processing disorders are frequently observed (although difficulties can certainly span all levels, including in discourse).

We then present the categories (types) of language disorders subsequent to stroke and discuss empirical evidence that addresses the relationship between brain and language. We also briefly discuss more subtle impairments of language that can occur following damage to the side of the brain that does not typically dominate language (in most individuals, the right hemisphere).

What is to be gained by such explorations? By understanding the different levels of language processing and the neural and cognitive architectures underlying them, we hope to learn how and when they interact in the unimpaired listener. Such investigations aid us in understanding how language processing is disrupted once brain damage occurs, and may aid in refining neurologically informed models of language processing. A comprehensive and accurate model of the language process could lead to the development of specialized treatment protocols for individuals with language disorders (see Chapter 14).

A Historical Perspective

A brief historical review of early research into language processing disorders will help to illustrate how contemporary research in the field has emerged. Prior to the 1800s, there were numerous reports of language disturbances in individuals who had sustained some type of brain injury. However, there was little attempt to correlate particular disorders with specific injuries. Much of what we now know about how the brain processes language first arose during the mid to late 1800s in published case and group study reports of individuals who had acquired language impairments subsequent to a stroke. This language disorder

---

Box 10-1

Focal Versus Diffuse Neural Trauma and Language Disorders

ACQUIRED LANGUAGE DISORDERS

Acquired language disorders refers to language deficits that results from neural trauma (stroke, traumatic brain injury) or neurological disease (e.g., Alzheimer, Parkinson, schizophrenia), all of which result in some degree of language impairment.

STROKE

A disruption in blood supply can result in relatively focal death of brain cells. This can occur from a blockage (ischemic stroke) or from a bleed (hemorrhagic stroke). Most aphasia research has been conducted with stroke survivors because of the ability to link aberrant behavior to a certain area of compromised brain. Here, one can investigate the deficits present after the stroke and assume the other regions of the brain, not affected by the blockage or bleed, are still structurally and somewhat functionally intact.

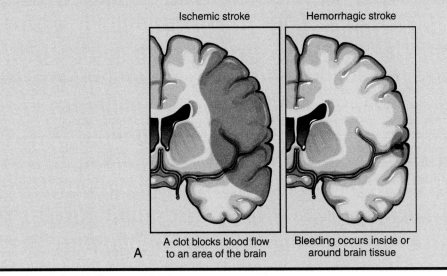

Ischemic stroke | Hemorrhagic stroke

A   A clot blocks blood flow to an area of the brain | Bleeding occurs inside or around brain tissue

From Nucleus Medical Media www.nucleusinc.com

Continued

Box 10-1

Focal Versus Diffuse Neural Trauma and Language Disorders—cont'd

TRAUMATIC BRAIN INJURY (TBI)

This is the most common form of brain damage in individuals under 40 years of age. TBIs are classified as either "open" or "closed" head injuries, with the former resulting from a penetrating trauma (e.g., gunshot wound) and the latter from accidents (e.g., car crash) where the brain ricochets inside the skull.

Mechanism of Closed Head Injury

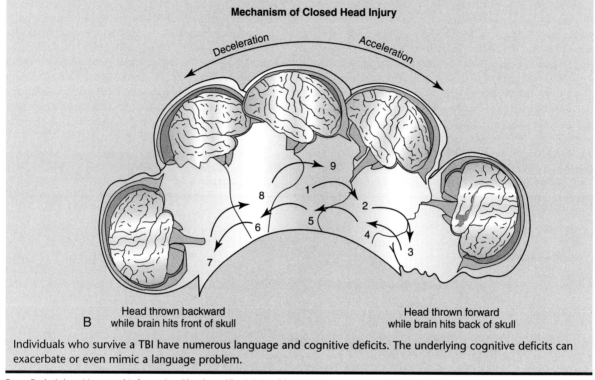

Deceleration

Acceleration

B   Head thrown backward
while brain hits front of skull

Head thrown forward
while brain hits back of skull

Individuals who survive a TBI have numerous language and cognitive deficits. The underlying cognitive deficits can exacerbate or even mimic a language problem.

From Brain Injury News and Information Blog http://braininjury.blogs.com

---

is now referred to as *aphasia* and is characterized by an impaired ability to produce and/or comprehend language in the spoken, signed or written modalities (see Appendix 10-1 for a more detailed timeline of the field).

Aphasia arises secondary to neural trauma (typically stroke) and impedes the proper functioning of brain regions that support language. In most individuals, this involves damage to the left hemisphere of the brain. Aphasia is not the result of deficits in sensory, intellect, or with psychiatric functioning.[2] It

is also not due to muscle weakness or a general cognitive disorder, though there are those who suggest that cognitive processes such as attention and memory are compromised in aphasia, as well as language (see Chapters 8 and 9).

The study of aphasia through history, which can be traced to as early as the Egyptian era (3000 to 2500 BC), has been an interesting, albeit winding road. Often influenced, and usually limited by, erroneous contemporary beliefs ranging from the functional roles of human organs to explanations of human behavior, it is not surprising that we find contradictory hypotheses. Aristotle (c. 360 BC) linked the localization of mental function to the heart, although centuries earlier, ancient Egyptians had already associated language expression with head injuries (Edwin Smith Surgical Papyrus, see Breasted, 1930; Garcia-Albea, 1999). Still

---

[2]Historically, this was not always the case. In the late 1800s, there was a movement in which intelligence, sensory function, and psychiatric function were argued to be implicated in aphasia. (Goldstein, 1924-original citation; Head, 1926; Jackson, 1878; Marie, 1906; Trousseau, 1865), see Appendix 10-1.

others focused on the relationship between language deficits and intelligence or general cognitive function (see Appendix 10-1).

In 1861 French neurologist Dr. Paul Broca provided perhaps the most well-known initial description of a language impairment subsequent to focal brain damage (Broca, 1861). In a now famous case, Broca described a patient who had lost the ability to produce speech, with the exception of a single word ("tan"), yet demonstrated spared comprehension. Upon the patient's death and subsequent autopsy, Broca discovered damage to the left inferior frontal region of this patient's brain (Figure 10-1, BA 44-45), and he therefore attributed speech output abilities to this circumscribed neural region. In this way, "Broca's aphasia" came to be known as primarily a speech production disorder following damage to left inferior frontal regions of the brain.

Ten years later, German neurologist Dr. Karl Wernicke was also investigating the relationship between localized brain damage and language impairments (Wernicke, 1874). He noted that language deficits could occur following damage to parts of the brain other than the left inferior frontal region, and that symptoms differed depending on the brain regions involved. Specifically, Wernicke posited a link between the left superior temporal gyrus and language comprehension (see Figure 10-1), after observing that patients with damage to this region demonstrated comprehension impairments. From this, "Wernicke's aphasia" was

characterized as a disorder of language comprehension following damage to the left superior temporal gyrus. It was the work of Broca and Wernicke that spurred early investigations of brain injury and its effect on language (among other behaviors).

Two important observations should be noted regarding "aphasia" research during this time.[3] First, scientists were operating under the assumption that particular language functions (e.g., production, auditory comprehension) were controlled by specific neural regions, and thus assumed that damage to that region resulted in a specific language deficit. While this characterization of brain–behavior relationships is intuitively appealing, later in this chapter we will discuss how a good deal of research has since shown this line of thought to be inadequate. Language is much more complex than a simple "input–output" system.

During the early era of aphasia research, the field of aphasiology was *descriptive*—language disorders were characterized based on direct observable behaviors (i.e., the patient's overt symptoms). However, several years after Broca and Wernicke described patterns of language impairment in their patients, the Wernicke-Lichtheim model was introduced (Lichtheim, 1885), which marked the first attempt to *predict* patterns of aphasia following stroke. This model, shown in Box 10-2, anticipated aphasia subtypes, or *groups*, based on symptoms and site of neural trauma. Symptoms were cast in terms of language activities, like speaking and listening; "lesions" (injury) within the core areas and the connections between them were used to predict patterns of language impairment in aphasia. For example, damage to the motor center would yield a Broca's type of aphasia, while a lesion to the auditory center would yield a Wernicke's type of aphasia. A lesion to the auditory-motor pathway would yield a disconnection syndrome, such as conduction aphasia, characterized by the inability to repeat what is heard. Hence, this model ushered in an era of aphasiology that could be characterized as "connectionism.[4]" During this era, connectionism assumed that higher mental

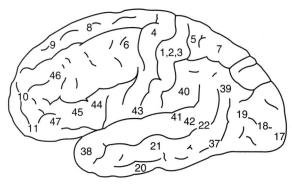

Figure 10-1 Left hemisphere of brain with Brodmann area labels overlaid. German neurologist Korbinian Brodmann (1909) provided a roadmap for the organization of the human brain by painstakingly mapping 52 cortical regions. Each area, now known as *Brodmann areas* (BA), is a region of the cerebral cortex that is defined based on its cytoarchitecture, or organization of cells. Historically, regions which have been implicated in language processing are BA 44, 45, and 22, although a number of neural regions have now been demonstrated to contribute to language performance.

[3]The term "aphasia" is quoted because during the 1800s, the literature is filled with writings strongly debating the appropriate term to use to describe these disorders; see Appendix 10-1.

[4]Note that connectionism in the late 1870s refers to something different than the way connectionism is used today. Today, the term "connectionism," (also known as parallel distributed processing) refers to the use of artificial neural networks, computers, to model cognition (Feldman & Ballard, 1982).

Box 10-2

Adaptation of the Wernicke-Lechtheim Model of Language Disturbance in Aphasia

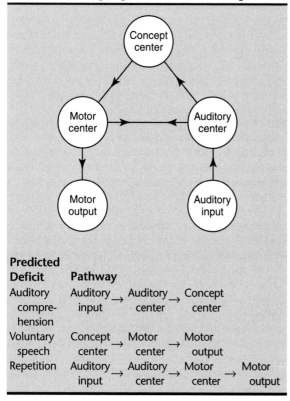

Predicted Deficit	Pathway		
Auditory comprehension	Auditory input →	Auditory center →	Concept center
Voluntary speech	Concept center →	Motor center →	Motor output
Repetition	Auditory input →	Auditory center →	Motor center → Motor output

functions were dependent on the connections between different centers in the cortex (Ahlsén, 2006). A more modern proponent of connectionism, Norman Geschwind, advanced the theory that disconnections between neural regions could lead to language disturbances (Geschwind, 1965). Connectionism remained an important concept in aphasiology for many years (and variants of this work remain active topics of research).

The contemporary era of aphasia research (and the focus of this chapter) was ushered in by Caramazza and Zurif (1976) and others, who examined the dissociation between different levels of language processing deficits in aphasia (see Accounts of Language Deficits in Aphasia later in this chapter). Indeed, current research aims to uncover the processing deficits in aphasia that may account for observable language deficits. Before we discuss this process-oriented research, we first introduce and briefly describe the

major types/syndromes of aphasia, to set the stage for a discussion of processing differences between these syndromes.

TYPES OF APHASIA

In this section we present some of the major classifications (or subtypes) of aphasia. Note here that we are describing the prototype of each of the main subtypes of aphasia. "Pure" cases of any given type of aphasia are seldom observed.

Broca's aphasia is typically characterized by halting, *nonfluent speech*. Grammatical function words (such as "is," "and," "the") and inflections (for tense, agreement, number, gender), are often omitted in language production (spoken or written), with mainly root content words being produced. Someone with Broca's aphasia may say "boy girl fall" to mean "The boy and the girl are falling" (Figure 10-2, *A*, *B*). Language production is therefore described as telegraphic or agrammatic ("without grammar"). In the 1970s, it was discovered that this agrammatic component of Broca's aphasia also extends to *comprehension*. The failure to detect comprehension deficits in Broca's patients was likely due to the fact that comprehension of single words and simple sentences (mostly) appears relatively intact. We now know that language impairment in Broca's aphasics extends to comprehension of more complex sentence constructions such as noncanonical structures (i.e., passives and object-relatives, see Chapter 6). This impairment for noncanonical sentences was investigated by Caramazza and Zurif (1976), who noted that Broca's patients demonstrated poor comprehension for sentences containing reversible noun phrases (e.g., "The boy was chased by the girl," where either of the nouns *boy* or *girl* can perform the action *chase*). This was in stark contrast to the group's ability to understand noncanonical sentences that did not contain reversible constituents (e.g., in "The ice cream was eaten by the boy," only the animate noun *boy* can perform the action *eat*, thus reducing the likelihood that patients would believe ice cream to be the subject of the sentence). This finding of Broca's patients' difficulty in understanding noncanonical sentence structures led to the term "overarching agrammatism," which refers to the fact that the grammatical constituents of language are not employed in either the production or comprehension of sentences (this will be discussed in more detail shortly). In addition to agrammatism, repetition abilities may also be impaired in this group (Table 10-1).

Broca's aphasia, and a subtype known as *agrammatic aphasia*, commonly occur following damage to the left

Speech sample from a patient with Broca's Aphasia
(Patient was shown a picture book of Cinderella and asked to retell the story).

Experimenter: Tell me the story.

Patient: Happy. B- all- ballerina. I can't say it. Uh, name.

Experimenter: That's OK. Just keep going.

Patient: Sisters two. Mother evil. Mop- ing. Dress. Bird and, uh, mouse. One, two, three. Uh, angels? Fairy! Crying and uh, uh, mother uh, mother lock- ed it.

Experimenter: Oh.

Patient: Yeah! Mommy, mommy, mommy! And uh, horse and dog. Wands. Uh, uh, muck lock lop moppins [muffins]. And uh, mouse and birds or?

Experimenter: I don't know.

Patient: Oh well. Uh, bored. Curl. Pretty. And, uh, twelve. Shoe. Uh, run- ning. Yeah. And uh, sisters. Um, shoe? One. Shoe? Right there? Bigger. Uh, and uh, that's right.

Experimenter: Hmm?

Patient: That's right (motions putting on a shoe).

Experimenter: Fits right.

Patient: Yeah. And affer [ever] and ever.

Experimenter: Great job.

A

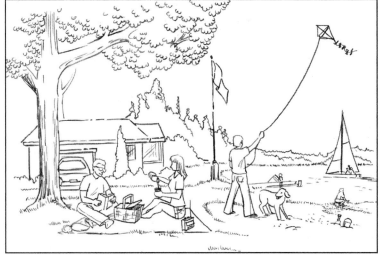

Figure 10-2 A, Speech sample from an individual with Broca's aphasia, retelling the Cinderella story. **B,** Same individual's written description from the Western Aphasia Battery. [**A** is Courtesy of the Cognitive Neuroscience Laboratory, SDSU. **B** is from Kertesz, A. (1982). Western Aphasia Battery. New York: Grune and Stratton.]

She a girl.
Man a book.
Chicken a sand.
Dog
Radio off.
Sande - feel.
B   a girl dride.

Table 10-1   Types of Aphasia and Associated Symptomotology

Aphasia Types	Production	Comprehension	Repetition	Naming
Nonfluent				
Broca's	Halting, agrammatic	Impaired for noncanonical syntax	Poor	Poor
Transcortical motor	Halting, agrammatic	Impaired for noncanonical syntax	Intact	Poor
Global	Severely impaired	Severely impaired	Poor	Poor
Fluent				
Anomia	Fluent, with word-finding problems, circumlocutions	Intact	Intact	Moderate-poor
Wernicke's	Fluent, facile, paraphasias	Poor	Poor	Poor
Transcortical sensory	Fluent, facile, paraphasias	Poor	Intact	Poor
Conduction	Fluent, facile	Intact	Poor	Intact

inferior frontal regions (Figure 10-3).[5] However, there have been reports of individuals with Broca's-like behaviors who have sustained damage to other, subcortical, regions (Alexander, Naeser, & Palumbo, 1987; Fridriksson, Bonilha, & Rorden, 2007), and inconsistencies of this sort make it difficult to precisely characterize brain–behavior relationships.

Similar to Broca's aphasia, patients with ***transcortical motor aphasia*** are *nonfluent* and may produce telegraphic or agrammatic speech. However, these individuals, unlike those with Broca's aphasia, typically demonstrate intact repetition. Brain injury with this group tends to be in areas surrounding Broca's area, in the anterior superior frontal lobe.

In contrast to the halting, agrammatic speech observed in Broca's or transcortical motor aphasics, a patient with **Wernicke's aphasia** has facile language production and speech that contains grammatical structure. In this type of fluent aphasia, the "preserved" speech fluency originally led researchers to regard Wernicke's aphasia solely as an impairment of comprehension. Research has since shown, however, that language production in this syndrome is also impaired and typically contains many instances of paraphasias, as exemplified in Table 10-2.

Paraphasias in Wernicke's aphasia may include *jargon* or *neologistic paraphasias* (among others), which are utterances that sound like words of the speaker's language, but are in fact not real words. For instance, a patient with Wernicke's aphasia may produce a neologism like "glick," which is not a true word but conforms to phonological rules of the language (Figure 10-4).

Neologisms are suggestive of either impaired word finding or semantic processing in Wernicke's aphasia. As illustrated in Figure 10-3, damage to the posterior temporal regions is most often implicated in this type of aphasia.

Similar to Wernicke's aphasia, ***transcortical sensory aphasia*** consists of empty or jargon-filled speech. People with this rare type of aphasia cannot comprehend what others say to them. Unlike Wernicke's aphasia, however, these individuals can repeat words or sentences. Lesions to areas of the brain near Wernicke's area often lead to this type of fluent aphasia.

Conduction aphasia was originally described by Wernicke. It is classically defined as a disorder of impaired repetition of auditory material. More recent research has indicated that word-finding is impaired in the disorder, and that individuals with conduction aphasia often produce phonemic paraphasias in ongoing speech (Baldo, 2008; Fridriksson, 2010). Injury to the supramarginal gyrus (see Figure 10-1, BA 40) and arcuate fasciculus is commonly associated with conduction aphasia (see Figure 10-3).

Global aphasia is the most severe of the aphasia types, in which both language comprehension and production are profoundly impacted, rendering the individual severely impaired. Brain lesions typically span across the frontal and temporal lobes. By contrast, ***anomic aphasia***, or "Anomia," is perhaps the mildest form of the disorder and is characterized by problems recalling words or names.[5] Individuals with this impairment frequently use circumlocutions (speaking in a roundabout way) to express words that they cannot recall or produce. Persons with anomic aphasia may not show other obvious signs of impairment and may in fact produce relatively fluent speech. Comprehension may be mildly impacted in this group with repetition most often intact.

---

[5]Anomia is a prominent feature of many aphasia syndromes.

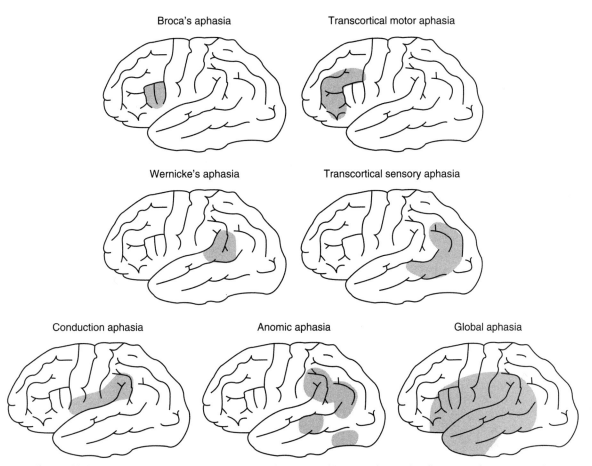

Figure 10-3   An illustration of typical sites of neural injury resulting in aphasia. This illustration demonstrates the typical 1:1 lesions associated with these syndromes. It is important to not confuse the correlation of structure with that of function. There is considerable variability in lesion sites with respect to damage to cortical and subcortical tissue.

Table 10-2   Examples of Paraphasias

Paraphasia Type	Description	Example
Phonemic (Literal)	Substitution of one phoneme for another within a single word	/pun/ for /spun/ /tevilision/ for /television/
Neologistic (Jargon, Gibberish)	Substitution of word sounds phonetically and semantically unrelated to the target words	/glick/ for /pencil/
Semantic (Verbal)	Substitution of one word for another, but not always semantically related	/flew/ for /soared/

Lesion localization in this group is the least reliable of all the aphasias. Most often, there is injury affecting temporal and parietal regions (Fridriksson, 2010).

Some words of caution: In any discussion of language disorders resulting from neural trauma, it is important to bear in mind that diagnoses and classifications (type and severity of aphasia) are based primarily on a patient's symptomology, thus being descriptive in nature. The descriptive nature of this process, relying on overt responses during assessment, can result in overgeneralizing a patient's ability or inability. This can cause difficulty in the interpretation of patient performance on language assessments as any one assessment may not capture the *entirety* of a language disorder. As an example, consider a

Speech sample from a patient with Wernicke's aphasia
(Patient was shown a picture book of Cinderella and asked to retell the story.)

Experimenter: Are you ready? OK let's hear it.

Patient: First I started with a s- little, small it was the lady's little which wa- was thing that I wanted before I could remember, but I can't do it now. This uh- I look carefully about what he he looked around but he couldn't really try it about there. At the same time, all these things, at least one, two, three people. Which were clever to the people. This, this and she supposed to do that. I don't know, but anyway, they say thinking.

And I just couldn't with him carrying from absolutely doing this. While I'm doing absolutely nothing, uh, that I made, made, made him and I was pushing this stuff, all this stuff was going. And all this was going anyway. So I look at that point and, um, at those points, I had put the, you know, the one, two, three of the people were doing this and putting everything through it, which I did.

And, um, at that time, um, I clevered what how much that little thing she went right here. Which is fine. I did as much as I could. At the same time, at the beginning, she started to look at the um, girl who is looking for all this stuff that was going through while he was there and I watched and watched that stuff that was going and through I looked at the mice doing that.

It was very good and so on and the first thing I saw them do was this lovely small little thing for of and I said ooh!

First, I could feel the other girls were playing there and I was trying as much as I could to do that I never as much as I could and that's probably tried.

A

Figure 10-4 **A,** Speech sample from an individual with Wernicke's aphasia, retelling the Cinderella story. **B,** An individual with Wernicke's aphasia's written description of The Cookie Theft picture. [**A** is Courtesy of the Cognitive Neuroscience Laboratory, SDSU. **B** from Goodglass, H., & Kaplan, E. (1972). *Boston diagnostic aphasia examination*. Philadelphia: Lea & Febiger.]

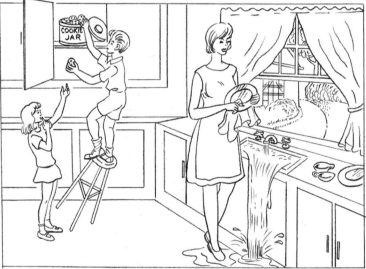

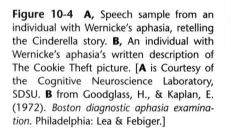

Cookies are ~~tef~~ four looking for the boy and little girl. The will ~~tet~~ ~~turd~~ hit the button of the ~~to~~ boy. Mother is not finding much to help the ~~fo~~ ~~ear~~ ~~dag~~ day of the sink and dishes. Water in the floor is a ~~twisted~~ ~~bad~~ water on the floor and miking all over the shoes. Miss ~~maug~~

B is a muss.

situation in which a researcher or clinician wishes to measure a patient's auditory language comprehension abilities and uses a task known as sentence-picture matching. Individuals are presented with a sentence and two (or more) pictures and are asked to choose the picture that matches the sentence. A patient with an underlying sentence comprehension deficit may be able to use a strategy rather than his/her linguistic knowledge to correctly perform the task, and thus this task may underestimate the full magnitude of a patient's language comprehension deficit. As an illustration, recall the earlier discussions of overarching agrammatism; prior to Caramazza and Zurif's work on sentence comprehension in reversible sentence constructions, it was thought that Broca's patients maintained intact language comprehension, thus resulting in claims that these individuals had a primary production problem with intact comprehension. We now know that these claims were inaccurate and that many comprehension assessment results were based on the ability of Broca's patients to use world knowledge to figure out the meaning of certain sentences (e.g., ice cream cannot eat boys).

Another note of caution: research on the neural underpinnings of language is still in its infancy. A great deal of research has shown that although a particular area of the brain may be implicated in a specific language function (either through patient studies or in functional neuroimaging experiments), one cannot assume that a particular brain region is *solely* responsible for the process under investigation (i.e., that a particular language function *lives* in a specific brain region). A damaged brain region that is implicated in language processing may have only been an important part of a *network* of different brain regions that were critical to that particular level of processing. Likewise, if experiments demonstrate a link between normal operation of a specific language process and a region of the brain, this does not mean that this area exclusively serves that process, to the exclusion of other cognitive processes. Thus, localization of function is not as simple as assuming a direct 1:1 relationship between specific brain damage patterns and subsequent language impairment.

We now turn to a discussion of language processing in aphasia and begin with a discussion of the different techniques used to measure behavior.

Language Processing in Aphasia

Methodologies Used to Study Language Processing

The Study of Language Processing via Off-line Methodologies

Until the 1970s, it was standard practice to use one methodological approach to examine language ability in patients with language disorders. Typically, this approach took the form of an untimed meta-linguistic task. Such a task measures language processing *after* the event of interest (e.g., after an entire sentence has been heard). These types of tasks are considered "off-line" measures and reflect what listeners ultimately understand a sentence to mean. They allow individuals to consciously reflect on the problem and use all the resources available to them at the time to determine the final meaning of a sentence. Examples from aphasia research include sentence-picture matching, grammaticality judgment, and paraphrasing (e.g., Caramazza & Zurif, 1976; Friedmann, 2006; Linebarger, Schwartz, & Saffran, 1983) (see Chapter 6, Box 6-2, for additional discussion).

While off-line methodologies are informative in providing information as to how individuals ultimately understand or interpret language, these tasks do not allow for an examination of the moment-by-moment operations of sentence processing as they are occurring in real-time. In an off-line task, if an individual demonstrates poor sentence comprehension performance, it is unclear *why* the individual could not accurately perform the task. For instance, consider a sentence-picture matching task in which an individual with Broca's aphasia demonstrates poor performance with noncanonical sentences. A number of factors could contribute to this end result: the individual might have an underlying lexical deficit (knowledge of word meanings); an underlying structure building deficit (inability to link the incoming words to build structural relationships among them); or an inability to retain the sentence and match it to the pictures (working memory deficit). Thus, while informative, off-line methodologies alone do not allow for precise characterization of the underlying processes that contribute to language impairments. Additionally, the task demands of off-line methodologies may draw the participant's attention to the linguistic material under investigation, and in doing so alter the nature of the comprehension process. From this point on, we limit our discussion of off-line tasks and focus primarily on evidence garnered from on-line experiments.

The Study of Language Processing via On-line Methodologies

To understand the complete details of the comprehension process, language scientists require methods that can capture the moment-by-moment unfolding of comprehension. "On-line" tasks do just this, and allow researchers to observe language processing both while it is occurring and without conscious reflection on the part of the participant. With on-line experimental techniques and the right kinds of experimental designs, researchers can examine the individual stages or components of language processing, and in populations with language disorders, investigate which of these stages may be impaired. In keeping with the goals of this chapter, we briefly summarize on-line methodologies that have been (and are currently) used to study auditory sentence comprehension in Table 10-3 (see also Chapter 6, Box 6-1).

Taken together, these on-line methodologies can provide complementary evidence regarding the nature of language processing. These methods have been critical in the development of accounts of language deficits in aphasia.

Accounts of Language Deficits in Aphasia

In this section we discuss different accounts that have been proposed to describe the observable language deficits in aphasia. We focus on evidence from Broca's aphasia, as the majority of work has examined deficits in patients aphasics of this type. We conclude with a brief summary of sentence processing research in Wernicke's aphasia.

Representation and Processing

Theoretical accounts of sentence processing deficits in Broca's patients generally fall in to two categories: representational or processing theories. Representational accounts attribute deficits to the inability to construct particular syntactic representations. Processing deficit accounts suggest that aphasic patients maintain implicit linguistic knowledge of a language, but are unable to effectively make use of this knowledge. Representational

accounts will be discussed first, followed by processing accounts.

Representational Accounts of Broca's Aphasia Deficits

Within this theoretical framework of aphasiology, researchers make use of linguistic theory to account for patterns of deficits that are exhibited by patients with aphasia. These accounts sometimes claim that patients with aphasia are unable to mentally represent certain linguistic elements during language processing, or alternatively, suggest that linguistic theory is necessary to describe the deficit patterns in production or comprehension.

Production. In the realm of production, the *Tree Pruning Hypothesis* is a predominant linguistically-motivated theory of production deficits in Broca's aphasia. Within this framework, production deficits are ascribed to impairment among Broca's patients in the ability to represent elements of a linguistic tree. Consider (1) and (2) (from Friedmann, 2006):

1. Today the boy <u>walks.</u>
2. Yesterday the boys <u>walked.</u>

Here, the verb *walk* is inflected for tense (e.g., present or past), and must also agree with the person, gender or number of the subject (e.g., *the boy/boys*). Now consider Figure 10-5, which represents a linguistic tree structure for such a phrase, and note that Agreement (Agr) and Tense (T) are represented by separate nodes (see Chapter 6 for a discussion of tree structure representations; example from Friedmann, 2006; Pollock, 1989; additional reference from Grodzinsky, 2000a). Here, the

Table **10-3**	Methodologies Commonly Used in the Study of Language Processing in Aphasia		
Methodology	**Elements of Language Processing Studied**	**Strengths**	**Limitations**
Event-related potentials	• Various levels of language processing: phonological, lexical-semantic, syntactic, discourse-level	• Good temporal resolution • No secondary task required • Not limited to single data point per stimulus	• Only indicates the *signatures* of language processing, not the processes themselves • Concern about participant attention if no secondary task used
Eye-tracking	• Lexical integration • Syntactic processing • Discourse-level processing	• Good temporal resolution • No secondary task required • Not limited to single data point per stimulus	• Only indicates the signatures of language processing, not the processes themselves • Concern about participant attention if no secondary task used • Possible use of strategy, may alter comprehension processes
Cross-modal priming	• Lexical access • Syntactic processing	• Indicates precisely which elements of the sentence are processed ("activated") at point of interest	• Only one data point per stimulus item • Dual-task demand may be difficult for some patients

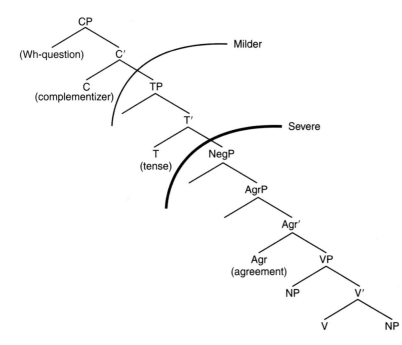

Figure 10-5 An illustration of the linguistic tree (see Chapter 6) proposed by the Tree Pruning Hypothesis of production deficits in Broca's aphasia. [From Friedmann, N. (2006). Generalizations on variations in comprehension and production: A further source of variation and a possible account. *Brain and Language, 96,* 151–153.]

important element to note is that Tense is represented at a higher node than Agreement. Interestingly, a good number of cross-linguistic studies (many in which tense and agreement are more richly inflected than in English), have demonstrated that individuals with Broca's aphasia show dissociation in the production of Agreement and Tense. For example, given the following prompt in (3), participants should produce a verb that is inflected for tense and must agree with the subject (past tense, third-person feminine singular, e.g., "jumped"; from Friedmann & Grodzinsky, 1997):

3. The girl wanted to jump, so she stood on the diving board and _____.

Participants with aphasia tend to be impaired in their production of *tense* but not in *agreement*, both for these types of sentence prompts and in elicited speech. At first glance this dissociation is surprising, since both of these elements are inflected on the verb and relate information about the nature of the action that is occurring. However, the Tree Pruning Hypothesis contends that individuals with Broca's aphasia have an impairment in representation and/or use of the higher nodes on the syntactic tree, which include the node for Tense. Meanwhile, the node for Agreement is intact, and Broca's patients can thus use this linguistic element during production.

Comprehension. As mentioned earlier, Broca's aphasia was originally thought to be a production deficit. Caramazza and Zurif's (1976) demonstrated that Broca's patients not only had deficits in speech production, but

also in comprehension. Prior to that study, off-line sentence–picture matching studies presented nonreversible sentences (such as (4)) to patients, in which the nouns in the sentence represent both inanimate (ice cream) and animate (man) constituents (Linebarger et al., 1983).

4. The ice cream was eaten by the man.

Real world knowledge allows for the supposition that the only noun in the sentence which can perform the *eating* action is the *man*, which is the animate noun. Hence, individuals with Broca's aphasia correctly choose *man* as the subject of the sentence.

Caramazza and Zurif presented reversible sentences such as (5):

5. The boy was chased by the girl.

Note that although both (4) and (5) make use of passive sentence constructions, in which the recipient of the action precedes the verb, there are semantic differences between them. In (4), a listener can use meta-cognitive knowledge to determine that the man must perform the action in this sentence. However, the participants in (5) ("boy" and "girl") are semantically reversible. That is, either the boy or the girl can perform the action, so there are no semantic cues that a listener can use to interpret the meaning of this sentence. When individuals with Broca's aphasia were presented with semantically reversible sentences like (5), they demonstrated chance performance (statistically equivalent to guessing) on a sentence-picture matching task.

Based on the results of this study, Caramazza and Zurif introduced the term "overarching agrammatism" to describe the deficits in Broca's aphasia. The authors argued that Broca's patients were not only unable to *produce* fluent, grammatical sentences, but that syntactic abilities were globally impaired in this population, thus also affecting sentence *comprehension*. This combination of deficits across production and comprehension modalities gave rise to the notion of a central syntactic impairment in Broca's patients that affected receptive and expressive language in similar way (Berndt & Caramazza, 1980; Caramazza & Zurif, 1976).

Caramazza and Zurif's study helped to usher in the contemporary era of aphasia research, in which aphasic deficits are considered within a linguistically based framework. A slightly later study by Bradley, Garrett, and Zurif (1980) hypothesized that Broca's aphasics had lost the ability to understand and mentally represent closed class words; that is, the small function words of a language, such as "the, by, in, and."

Caplan and Futter (1986) proposed the *linearity hypothesis*, which claimed that Broca's patients evince difficulty in sentence comprehension because they lack the syntactic information needed to properly assign thematic roles (see Chapter 6 for details on thematic role assignment). As a result (and since they arguably only can label incoming lexical items), other cognitive strategies are required for comprehension. Caplan and Futter suggested that Broca's patients assign thematic roles via a linear sequence of nouns and verbs instead of building a hierarchical structure; that is, the first noun phrase (NP) is always considered the agent of the action described by the verb, and the second NP, the patient or theme of the action.

The Trace Deletion Hypothesis (TDH, also known as 'movement theory')

Grodzinsky (1986, 1995, 2000b, 2006) and Hickok, Conseco-Gonzalez, Zurif, and Grimshaw (1992) argued against the linearity hypothesis by claiming that patients can construct a normal, albeit incomplete, syntactic representation. These researchers have argued that the problem in comprehension arises from a deletion of a syntactic component (trace). This theory stems from observations that Broca's patients only exhibit comprehension difficulties noncanonical constructions, those constructions which contain the displacement or movement of a constituent from the underlying representation to a position earlier in the sentence. This movement purportedly leaves an empty category (or trace) which allows for the linking between that original position and the moved constituent, and ultimately the assignment of thematic roles (see Chapter 6 for

a discussion of the properties of traces). Unimpaired individuals are able to successfully comprehend sentences like (6) and (7) by automatically linking the moved element (*boy*) to the position from which it was displaced (the trace, immediately after the verb), thus allowing those two elements to "co-refer" (Frazier & d'Arcais, 1989; Garnsey, Tanenhaus, & Chapman, 1989; Hickok et al., 1992; McElree & Griffith, 1998; Nicol, 1988; Sussman & Sedivy, 2003; Tanenhaus & Trueswell, 1995; Traxler & Pickering, 1996; and many others).

6. Alyssa saw the boy$_i$ who the dancer kissed ____ $_i$ on the cheek.
7. The boy$_i$ was kissed ____ $_i$ by the dancer.

Persons with Broca's, or agrammatic aphasia, are unable to comprehend these sentences correctly, according to this account, because traces are deleted from the linguistic representation, resulting in the inability to properly assign a thematic role to the moved constituent. Both the first noun, *Alyssa* and the second noun, *the boy* in (6) are assigned the thematic role of Agent, but by different mechanisms. The first noun assignment is the result of a cognitive (nonlinguistic) linear strategy simply because it appears first, the second noun (*the boy*) is assigned agent status by the verb *kissed*, a proper structural assignment. Given that there are now two agents in the structural representation, the person with Broca's aphasia guesses as to "who did what to whom," resulting in random performance on, for example, sentence-picture matching tasks.

Processing-Based Accounts of Broca's Aphasia Deficits

The studies discussed earlier, which argue for a representational basis of deficits in Broca's aphasia, were certainly crucial for the advancement of the field. However, off-line tasks were primarily used, which disallowed any examination into the multiple levels of processing that occur during moment-by-moment sentence comprehension. More recent work has suggested a processing deficit that may underlie the inability to understand sentences containing traces, particularly for individuals with Broca's aphasia; we turn to this work later in the chapter.

Production. There has been a relative dearth of on-line studies of production deficits in aphasia. This is most likely due to the potential confounds of collecting time-sensitive productions from patients who may experience comorbidity of speech disorders (e.g., apraxia, dysarthria) alongside their aphasia. While on-line production studies in healthy individuals typically measure either reaction times or error patterns during production of target sequences, these measures would be inappropriate with aphasic individuals. It would be impossible to know whether differences in reaction times between conditions were due to processing differences between those conditions or rather due to speech-motor planning deficits. Error patterns are also not a good measure of production in aphasia, as again, it would be difficult to ascertain whether the errors were due to issues with on-line processing during production, or with motor planning or execution. We now briefly describe a model of speech production and discuss how it may contribute to an understanding of aphasic processing for language production.

One account of on-line production deficits in Broca's aphasia attributes agrammatic errors to timing problems during the synchronization of production processes (Kolk, 1995). Based on computational modeling, this account claims that sentence production occurs as a series of processing stages. Briefly summarized, lexical access occurs, followed by the insertion of lexical items into syntactic "slots" in order for production to occur. Kolk asserts that in individuals with Broca's aphasia, lexical access proceeds normally, but the root form of the words cannot be inserted properly into their syntactic slots. This inability is not due to a competency deficit because aphasic individuals can properly establish a sentence's syntactic framework, but is instead due to a processing deficit in that they are slower to insert appropriate lexical items into their slots.

In addition, Kolk adds that this syntactic slot filling is generally slower for complex sentence structures than for simple sentence constructions in unimpaired speakers. If so, slower slot filling in Broca's aphasia would disproportionately affect production of complex sentences over simpler ones. Kolk further contends that agrammatic speech is a form of message simplification, resulting from these timing problems. He argues that the production systems of patients are always overburdened and that their capacity to produce well-formed sentences is overwhelmed. Thus, he claims, aphasic speakers will simplify messages greatly to compensate for this limited capacity. Kolk's hypothesis may account for the telegraphic speech that is a hallmark of Broca's aphasia, as well as for the observation that patients typically fail in their production of noncanonical (more complex) syntactic constructions.

Comprehension. Unlike accounts that describe deficits in linguistic representational terms, processing-based accounts argue that core knowledge is intact but a person with aphasia cannot make use of that knowledge to support language function. There have been a number of processing theories put forth over the past four or five decades. We discuss some of the main accounts later.

The Mapping Hypothesis. The mapping hypothesis (Saffran, Schwartz, & Marin, 1980, Schwartz, Saffran, & Marin, 1980) attributes comprehension deficits in agrammatic patients to a deficit in mapping semantic roles onto sentence constituents (see Chapter 6 for a discussion of semantic/thematic roles). This theory asserts that the comprehension deficits found in Broca's patients are the result of an impairment in the final interpretative stage of processing. In a series of studies, Saffran and colleagues demonstrated that Broca's patients were able to identify grammaticality and plausibility violations in aurally presented sentences via judgment tasks. It was argued that Broca's patients do not have difficulty with complex syntax, but instead cannot map a verb's thematic roles (e.g., agent, theme) onto sentence constituents (i.e., they cannot map meaning to sentence structure) (Marshall, 1995). A main argument against this approach has to do with the reliance on off-line tasks to infer intact syntactic parsing. Swinney and Zurif (1995) argued that in order to appropriately evaluate syntactic parsing, one must distinguish syntactic and semantic systems via tasks sensitive to automatic processing levels.

On-line Evidence for Processing-Based Account in Aphasia. Recall our earlier discussion of the types of sentences that typically pose a comprehension challenge for individuals with Broca's aphasia; that is, noncanonical sentence constructions that involve displacement or movement of an argument. Example (6), repeated here for ease of reading, is an instance of such a sentence (here, an object-relative).

6. Alyssa saw the boy$_i$ who the dancer kissed $_{i(t)}$ ___ on the cheek.

Traces have been shown to have real time processing consequences (Swinney & Fodor, 1989). Lexical priming research with unimpaired individuals demonstrates a specific pattern of activation in these constructions: initial activation of the meaning of the displaced constituent (the object of this sentence, boy) and *re*activation at the offset of the verb *kissed*, its base-generated position before it is displaced (Hickok et al., 1992; Love, 2007; Love, Swinney, Walenski, & Zurif, 2008; Love & Swinney, 1996; Nicol, Fodor, & Swinney, 1994; Nicol & Swinney, 1989; Swinney & Osterhout, 1990; Tanenhaus, Boland, Garnsey, & Carlson, 1989). By contrast, Broca's patients do not show reactivation of the object at the offset of the verb (in real time) (Love et al., 2008; Swinney, Zurif, Prather, & Love, 1996; Zurif, Swinney, Prather, et al., 1993). This work has led to hypotheses that aim to account for on-line sentence processing in this population, and we highlight some of the predominant theories here.

Lexical Hypothesis. In attempting to understand the underpinnings of aberrant patterns of co-reference linking during sentence processing in Broca's aphasia (and off-line sentence comprehension impairments), some theories have focused on possible lexical retrieval impairments. The rationale for this argument is that a sentence structure cannot be built properly without the appropriate building blocks of a sentence (words). Thus a lexical deficit will lead to a breakdown in comprehension. Some studies have implicated ineffective or degraded lexical retrieval of function (e.g., closed class) words (e.g., Bradley et al., 1980; Friederici, 1983; Haarmann & Kolk, 1991), while others have implicated poor lexical access of content (e.g., open class) words (e.g., Utman, Blumstein, & Sullivan, 2001; Milberg, Blumstein, & Dworetzky, 1987; Love et al., 2008; Prather, Zurif, Love, & Brownell, 1997; Swinney et al., 1989; Zurif, Swinney, Prather, & Love, 1994; Zurif, Swinney, & Garrett, 1990).

The *lexical slow rise hypothesis* argues that the underlying nature of language deficits in Broca's population results from a slowed lexical access system (also termed "lexical activation"). Similar to the model proposed by Kolk in the production arena, this slow rise of lexical activation may result in lexical information "feeding" into syntactic processes too slowly, leading to breakdowns of automatic fast-acting structure-building, which eventually leads to the particular syntactic deficits seen in Broca's aphasia (e.g., Love et al., 2008). Indeed, recent evidence from on-line studies using cross-modal lexical priming (CMLP, see Table 10-3; see also Chapter 6) provides support for the lexical slow rise hypothesis. Participants in Love et al. (2008) heard sentences such as (8), while probe words were presented at one of a possible 5 time points during the sentence (each probe position indicated by *) :

8. The audience liked the wrestler$_i$ *1 that the *2parish priest condemned_____$_i$ *3 for *4 foul *5 language.

Here, the goal was to determine when healthy individuals and those with Broca's aphasia would access the direct object of the verb *condemned* ("*wrestler*"), both when it was first encountered at its displaced position, and again at its base-generated position after the verb. As expected from previous work, unimpaired participants showed access for the direct object at both its structurally licensed positions in the sentence, that is, at the offset of the object itself (*1) and at the offset of the verb (*3). By contrast, participants with Broca's aphasia did *not* show evidence of activation of the object at either of these test points. However, lexical activation among Broca's patients was observed, albeit at probe positions further downstream (*2, *4). Specifically, Broca's patients showed access of the object

300 msec after the word's offset and 500ms after the offset of the verb. This demonstrated intact comprehension of lexical access and structure building, yet only at delayed (later) time points. In other words, the pattern of activation for this NP during sentence comprehension was present, but temporally delayed in Broca's aphasia. Love et al. (2008) provided evidence that slowed lexical access/activation in Broca's aphasia might be an underlying cause of sentence comprehension deficits in this population.

Evidence from electrophysiological studies (ERP, see Table 10-1) might also support the assertion that on-line lexical processing is slowed in aphasia. Swaab, Brown, and Hagoort (1997) showed a delayed ERP component that is related to lexical/semantic processing (N400) in Broca's aphasia. The authors contended that this delay could be attributed to slowed lexical-semantic integration processes (see also Hagoort, Brown, & Swaab, 1996; Swaab, Brown, & Hagoort, 1998). In addition, recent eye-tracking evidence has provided support for the theory that lexical slowing in Broca's aphasia might underlie sentence comprehension difficulties (e.g., Dickey & Thompson, 2009; Thompson & Choy, 2009).

Syntax Hypothesis. In contrast to processing accounts that claim that lexical impairments underlie sentence comprehension deficits in Broca's aphasia, another body of theories claims that the source of impairment in this population lies within the syntactic system itself. According to these theories, termed "weak syntax" or "slow syntax," lexical access is purported to proceed normally, but the processes by which these lexical items are *combined* into syntactic structures is slowed (see Avrutin, 2006; Burkhardt, Avrutin, Piñango, & Ruigendijk, 2008; Piñango, 2000).

Piñango, Burkhardt, and colleagues argue for a *slow syntax* hypothesis whereby the nature of Broca's comprehension deficit is driven by a delay in the parser to combine syntactic categories during syntactic structure formation. Specifically, it is argued that there is a breakdown in the sequencing of syntactic linking (a fast acting process which ensures that arguments are syntactically linked) and the semantic linking of thematic roles (a later occurring process which linearly assigns an agent thematic role to the first occurring noun phrase). Because thematic role assignment is argued to depend on a fully formed syntactic structure (especially in the case of noncanonical constructions), delayed input from the syntactic system results in the availability of two competing interpretations, one from the intrusion of extrasyntactic information and the other from a protracted syntactic analysis. In a cross-modal lexical decision task, subjects were presented with sentences like:

9. The kid loved the *cheese*$_j$ which $_{j/i}$ the brand new mi*[1]crowave *melted* ___t$_i$ ye*[2]sterday *[3]afternoon while the entire family was watching TV.

Three probe positions were tested, a baseline position (400 msec before the verb, *1), 100 msec after the offset of the verb (*2, where thematic assignment occurs due to structural linking of the object and the trace) and a point 650 msec from the offset of the verb (*3).[6] Unimpaired subjects showed the previously reported finding of activation of the object (*cheese)* only at the offset of the verb (*melted*, *2). Broca's patients on the other hand showed activation of the object only at the latter, downstream probe position (*3).[7] These results are in line with those reported by Love et al. (2008, described earlier). Critically, however, one cannot rule out a lexical level deficit in this study as activation for the object itself (*cheese)* was not tested at the first instance of occurrence.

Additionally, some ERP experiments lend support to the theory that syntactic processing or structure building is aberrant in Broca's aphasia. Friederici et al. (1998) presented participants with aphasia with sentences that included semantic (10) or syntactic (11) violations.

10. The cloud was buried.
11. The friend was in the visited.

The authors reported that a Broca's patient failed to show a commonly found electrophysiological component (ELAN) to syntactic violations, but did show a later occurring component for syntactic reanalysis (P600). This patient also demonstrated an intact semantic component (N400), a finding contrary to Swaab et al. (1997) (see also Friederici, von Cramon, & Kotz, 1999). The researchers contended that the results indicate intact semantic, but disrupted syntactic processing in this individual. These results agree with theories of abnormal syntactic processing in Broca's aphasia, although some caution may be applied, as they represent findings from a single patient.

Cognitive Theories. Along with theories of disrupted lexical or syntactic processing in Broca's aphasia, some researchers have attributed sentence processing deficits to impairment of one or more cognitive abilities,

which may not be specific to language operations. A good deal of work in this area has examined short-term or working memory systems in Broca's aphasia, with an eye toward uncovering how resource allocation deficits may underlie comprehension impairment for complex sentences (Caplan & Waters, 1999; Caplan, Waters, DeDe, et al., 2007; see Chapters 9 and 13 in the text).

This work, collectively referred to as "resource allocation deficit theories" by some researchers, refers to a cognitive deficit that affects an entire set of cognitive operations, not just linguistic ones. The hypothesis within these theories is that individuals with Broca's aphasia can successfully comprehend and process simple, canonical sentences with the cognitive resources that are available to them. However, when sentences become more complex, the limited cognitive systems within which language processing occurs is taxed to the point of breakdown, and comprehension fails.

Sentence-Level Processing in Wernicke's Aphasia

While the majority of sentence processing work in aphasia has focused on deficits and patterns of processing in Broca's aphasia, several intriguing studies have examined the nature of on-line processing in Wernicke's aphasia as well. Such studies show that on-line processing deficits are not uniform across aphasia types (Swinney & Zurif, 1995; Zurif et al., 1993). Although individuals with Broca's aphasia show on-line processing deficits for sentences containing syntactic dependencies, research has indicated that individuals with Wernicke's aphasia are fully able to compute syntactic dependencies in real-time and to link constituents in a sentence during comprehension of complex sentences (e.g., Swinney & Zurif, 1995). However, as mentioned in the discussion of aphasia types, language comprehension (as measured via off-line indices) is impaired in Wernicke's aphasia, which leads one to question how on-line sentence processing proceeds in this population.

In Wernicke's aphasia, word-finding or semantic problems are theorized to be disordered and are thought to contribute to comprehension problems in this population. One of the few studies to examine on-line sentence processing in Wernicke's aphasia suggests a semantic-level deficit in this population (Shapiro et al., 1993). The authors investigated on-line *verb-argument structure* processing in Wernicke's aphasia. In short, verb argument structure concerns how many arguments are required to accompany a verb in order to satisfy that verb's thematic structure (see Chapter 6). The verb "hit" requires two (and only two) arguments: an "agent"

---

[6]The timing information for the three probe positions was provided in Burkhardt et al. (2008), but the exact visual positions of the probe points for this example sentence were not provided in the article. The markings of the three probe positions in the example sentence were inserted by the authors to assist the reader.

[7]We note that Broca's patients were not tested at the verb offset (*2) as it is argued that published reports had shown that Broca's patients do not evince activation at verb offset.

who performs the action and a "theme" who receives the action. Argument structure is considered to be relevant to the conceptual semantics of verbs. It is well known from work with unimpaired individuals that verb argument structure impacts on-line sentence processing load; specifically, verbs with more complex argument structures take longer to process than verbs with fewer arguments (Shapiro et al., 1987; Shapiro, Zurif, & Grimshaw, 1989). This increase in processing load is thought to reflect exhaustive activation of a verb's argument structure; thus, verbs with more complex argument structure will lead to greater processing load than verbs with less complex argument structures.

Results from Shapiro and colleagues' investigations of aphasia (e.g., Shapiro & Levine, 1990; Shapiro, Gordon, Hack, & Killackey, 1993) indicated abnormal on-line verb argument structure processing among individuals with Wernicke's aphasia, which is in contrast to the normal sensitivity of argument structure evinced by Broca's patients and unimpaired participants. Importantly, the insensitivity to argument structure in Wernicke's patients was observed irrespective of the syntactic complexity of the sentence in which the verbs were embedded. The authors contend that these findings signify a semantic processing deficit in Wernicke's aphasia, but one that requires a linguistic description.

The results from Shapiro and colleagues are supported by Friederici et al. (1999) in their ERP study of syntactic and semantic on-line processing. The authors report that their Wernicke's patient showed an expected ELAN response and a delayed P600 response to syntactically anomalous sentences, yet in this same patient, no N400 was observed when the patient heard semantic violations in sentences. This study therefore provides additional support for the theory that real-time syntactic processing remains intact in Wernicke's aphasia, while semantic processing is disrupted.

Shapiro and Friederici's studies, taken together with findings from on-line studies of syntactic processing in Broca's and Wernicke's aphasia (e.g., Love et al., 2008; Swinney & Zurif, 1995), suggest a dissociation in real-time sentence processing deficits. Whereas individuals with Broca's aphasia demonstrate on-line processing deficits in response to syntactic complexity, individuals with Wernicke's aphasia demonstrate real-time verb argument structure processing deficits. Note that these are not the only processing factors that underlie each aphasic type and associated pattern of behavior. Rather, the studies discussed here provide compelling evidence for distinct real-time processing impairments in these two groups during isolable stages of sentence comprehension.

Right Hemisphere Damage and Language Processing

The overwhelming majority of research that has considered the brain-behavior relationships underlying natural language processing has focused on the role of the left hemisphere and its subregions. This work has attempted to determine how different neuroanatomical regions cooperate to allow both language production and comprehension. This focus of this work has largely been driven by the lesion literature, in which damage to the left hemisphere has been shown to produce overt behavioral deficits in language, whereas damage to the right hemisphere seemingly produces cognitive deficits (such as attention deficits), which were considered to be nonlanguage specific. More recently, however, the role of the right hemisphere (RH) for efficient communication has been recognized. The finding that RH damage could influence language performance grew out of studies that used right hemisphere–damaged (RHD) patients as control subjects for aphasia studies. Many studies discovered that while RH patients performed better than aphasics in some tasks, they were not at the same level of performance as unimpaired control subjects (Gardner, 1994). More recent research has expanded these initial observations and now it is widely accepted that patients with RHD have a variety of language processing difficulties (see Tompkins, 2008, for an excellent review).

In the past few decades, researchers have embraced the role of prosody, nonliteral (figurative) interpretation, pragmatics, discourse comprehension, humor/sarcasm and inference, among others, as integral properties of language. The existing evidence has often demonstrated these language properties to be deficient in persons who have sustained unilateral damage to the right, but not the left, hemisphere. Thus, discovering the role of the RH's contribution to language can now be seen as central to any complete account of language comprehension and production. This section will discuss some of these language disturbances and the accounts which attempt to explain RHD comprehension deficits.

Overview of the Role of the RH in Language Processing

The overall view of the role of the RH in language processing has led to a view of the role of the RH as being centered on the development and maintenance of "alternative" or "secondary" interpretations during language comprehension (see e.g., Brownell, Potter, & Michelow, 1984; Brownell & Joanette, 1993; Burgess & Simpson, 1988; Chiarello, 1988; Faust, 2006; Joanette & Goulet, 1988; Tompkins, 1995). These characteristics of the right and left hemisphere have been described by

Beeman (1998) as consisting of an LH that can choose contextually relevant meanings ("fine coding") and the RH that activates and maintains more distantly related meanings ("coarse coding").

Coarse coding is argued to provide input that may be important for updating and revising interpretations during comprehension (Beeman, 1998; Faust, Barak, & Chiarello, 2006). Course coding has also been linked to one's ability to derive figurative meanings and draw inferences (Beeman, 1993, Beeman, Friedman, Grafman, et al., 1994). RHD patients have difficulties in all these areas and this has led some researchers to argue that RHD comprehension deficits reflect a coarse coding deficit (Beeman, 1993; Brownell, 2000; but see Klepousniotou & Baum, 2005, and Tompkins, Baumgaertner, & Lehman, 2000, for contrasting results).

Being able to understand communication requires the listener to go beyond the specifics of what was said and integrate all levels of information, thus allowing for the understanding of nonliteral language, which is said to be one-third of all communication. RHD individuals do not appear to appreciate the abstract meaning of figurative (nonliteral) language (Kempler, 1999). Work with RHD patients has shown a pervasive literalness in their interpretation of idiomatic and metaphorical expressions such as "He has a heavy heart" (e.g., Winner & Gardner, 1977).[8] Interestingly, left hemisphere-damaged (hereafter, LHD) aphasic subjects who exhibit gross "linguistic" deficits are not drawn to the incorrect (literal) interpretation of these items. Brownell et al. (1984) presented patients with word triads (such as "loving-hateful-warm") and asked them to choose the two words that were most closely related. RHD patients responded along denotative lines ("loving-hateful"). This was in contrast to LHD aphasics, who typically responded with connotative answers ("loving-warm") and unimpaired controls, who responded about equally with both types of relationships. Thus, a double disassociation was demonstrated between these two groups, such that the RHD subjects tend to prefer the more literal (denotative) groupings, whereas the LHD subjects choose the figurative (connotative) groupings (Brownell et al., 1984). This deficit in RHD processing of figurative words has been linked to the

inability of these patients to maintain alternative interpretations of lexical items.

Taking these results one step further, Tompkins (1990), in one of the few temporally "on-line" tasks of RH processing, has demonstrated that RHD patients possess an intact <u>un</u>conscious representation of metaphors, one that is not available during "off-line" testing procedures. In this seminal work, an auditory list priming paradigm[9] was used whereby participants (RHD, LHD and unimpaired controls) were asked to make lexical decisions to a list of successive auditorily presented word and nonword strings. In some instances the word preceding a target item (*open* for example) was related to the literal (*closed*) meaning of the target. In other cases the preceding word was related to the metaphorical (*honest*) meaning. All three populations studied (RHD, LHD, and unimpaired controls) showed similar patterns of priming for target words when either a metaphorical or literal item preceded them (see Chapter 6 for a more detailed discussion on priming). In showing that RHD patients showed facilitation for the metaphorical meaning of words, the authors concluded that RHD patients' access to metaphorical meaning is intact, but that RHD results in the inability to consciously interpret language was proposed (see also Tompkins et al., 1992).

The inability of RHD patients to understand multiple, sometimes competing, interpretations has been argued to cause this group to be overly literal in situations requiring access to alternate interpretations to assist in the understanding of sarcasm, inferences, humor and so forth (see for example, Brownell, Bihrle, & Michelow, 1986; Kaplan, Brownell, Jacobs, & Gardner, 1990; Weylman, Brownell, Roman, & Gardner, 1989; Winner, Brownell, Happe, et al., 1998). For example, Molloy, Brownell, and Gardner (1990) showed that RHD patients are impaired in their ability to use new information to reinterpret an utterance, in this case, the punch-line of a joke. The authors argue that when listening to a joke, the listener makes assumptions about where the story is going. When they hear the punch-line, they are forced to reinterpret their understanding during comprehension, since the meaning of the jokes goes against initial assumptions.

Similar deficits in pragmatics and discourse can be seen in a RHD patient's difficulty in identifying the main idea or "theme" during comprehension. Brownell et al. (1986) described RHD patients as being

---

[8]The overwhelming majority of research with RHD patients has relied on off-line metalinguistic tasks. However, research with less cognitively demanding on-line implicit measures have demonstrated intact abilities that are not evident in off-line tasks (see Tompkins & Baumgaertner, 1998; and Tompkins & Lehman, 1998, for a summary).

[9]In a list priming paradigm, words are presented in a continual fashion to reduce the use of strategies, expectancies, on the part of the subjects. See Prather et al. (1997) for a detailed description of the list priming paradigm.

able to process single sentences but unable to combine information across sentences (see also Hough, 1990). They provided subjects with two sentence vignettes for which half the time, the second sentence did not fit with the first (e.g., Sally brought a pen with her to meet the movie star. The article would include famous people's opinions about nuclear power). The latter sentence should provoke the listener to revise his/her initial interpretation. The RHD patients showed a failure to re-interpret, making them less able to infer the main theme.

We now turn our discussion to studies that looked at whether RHD patients can use sentence context to aid in the activation and selection of the appropriate meaning of ambiguous words. Similar to how idioms and metaphors can be argued to have multiple meaning representations, lexical ambiguities are single words in our lexicon which may have multiple meanings ("bug" can mean "insect" or "spy device"). Studies of lexical ambiguity processing in healthy individuals have indicated that *all* meanings of a lexical ambiguity are activated immediately upon hearing it (e.g., Swinney, Onifer, Prather, & Hirshkowitz, 1979). This immediate exhaustive activation for meanings of a lexical ambiguity occurs regardless of sentence context that might bias towards one meaning of the ambiguity. It is only shortly thereafter that the comprehender uses context to "select" the correct interpretation of a lexical item.[10] If it is the case that RHD individuals cannot maintain multiple meanings of an item, RHD patients should not show the availability of less frequent meanings at later points in sentence processing even if the context of the sentence is biased towards that less frequent meaning.

Grindrod and Baum (2003) used a cross-modal priming study with unimpaired individuals and RHD patients to investigate on-line access patterns for sentence-final lexical ambiguities. These ambiguities were embedded in sentence which biased towards one of two meanings of the lexical item (see (12) and (13) next). Among sentence-final ambiguities that have equally frequent meanings, one predicts that context will be used to select the appropriate meaning of the lexical ambiguity.

12. After writing a long message, he looked at the CARD (First meaning bias)
13. Although trying not to cheat, he looked at the CARD (Second meaning bias)

In (12), only activation of the greeting card meaning should be evident, whereas in (13), only the second meaning should be accessed. In their study, the authors found that the unimpaired group showed this pattern. However, RHD patients never evinced activation for the second meaning, leading the authors to conclude that this group was insensitive to context effects.

These results may help to explain why individuals with right hemisphere damage face discourse challenges; patients are unable to access multiple possible meanings of a linguistic constituent. This group's over-reliance on literal interpretations for nonliteral language, such as jokes, metaphors, and indirect request may also be a result of such a deficit. Individuals with right hemisphere damage may have only one interpretation available, thus not allowing them to "choose" between two possible interpretations for a given utterance. These individuals may then only be able to rely on the most common construal of the linguistic information.

CONCLUSIONS

Much of the literature described in this chapter also suggests that there are areas of the brain that are related to particular levels of language ability. Specifically, the anterior regions of the left hemisphere (those typically damaged in Broca's aphasia) seem to play a critical role in the fast-acting process of parsing. This includes accessing the meanings of words and building sentence structure. The posterior regions (those involved in Wernicke's aphasia) seem to be involved in the interpretation of the constructed constituents.

Individuals with Broca's aphasia demonstrate aberrant access to lexical items during auditory sentence processing and show delayed structure building, which result in specific comprehension deficits. In contrast, Wernicke's patients demonstrate intact parsing with hyperactivation of lexical items. It has been argued (e.g., Milberg, Blumstein, & Dworetzky, 1987) that these patients rely on intact frontal areas to perform syntactic structure building but are unable to integrate the semantics of the constituent components to interpret sentence meaning. Research in neuroimaging has played a large role in exploring how Broca's and Wernicke's brain regions interact and work together (or compensate) for particular deficits. Readers who are interested in this area are encouraged to consult Crosson, McGregor, Gopinath, et al. (2007). And finally, individuals with RHD evince deficits in the integration of lexical-semantic information, information that is critical for the interpretation of figurative language, jokes, indirect requests, and so forth.

---

[10]This pattern is found and predicted ONLY when the ambiguous words are presented within an on-going sentence, not at the end of the sentence. In the latter case, end of sentence wrap up effects (see Chapter 6) encourage top down influences resulting in context driven access (see Balogh, Zurif, Prather, et al., 1998, for a review).

Throughout this chapter, we have demonstrated that a language disorder can manifest in a variety of ways, and also that language processing research can provide insight into which levels of the language system have become impaired in patients with aphasia (and right hemisphere damage). We have noted that evidence from language processing research, especially on-line investigations, may help to clarify the types of language deficits that we see in our patients with aphasia. Importantly, we remind the reader that language processing deficits are not homogeneous across aphasia types (or RHD syndromes), and we feel that future language processing research may help clinicians and researchers to further distinguish between aphasia types and patterns of deficits. Importantly, given the intricacy of the language processing system, current research has only begun to unveil important patterns of language processing in individuals with language impairment. As we continue to examine linguistic processing in patient populations, discoveries in this field will help both scientists and clinicians to better characterize and understand aphasia, which will not only lead to a better understanding of the language architecture in general, but will also contribute to the development of specified treatments to ameliorate processing deficits in these patients.

REFERENCES

Ahlsèn, E. (2006). *Introduction to Neurolinguistics*. Amsterdam: John Benjamins.

Alexander, M. P., Naeser, M. A., & Palumbo, C. l. (1987). Correlations of subcortical CT lesion sites and Aphasia profiles. *Brain, 110*, 961–991.

Avrutin, S. (2006). Weak ayntax. In Y. Grodzinsky & K. Amunts (Eds.), *Broca's region*. New York: Oxford University Press.

Baldo, J. (2008). It's either a cook or a baker: Patients with conduction aphasia get the gist but lose the trace. *Brain and Language, 105*, 134–140.

Balogh, J., Zurif, E., Prather, P., Swinney, D., & Finkel, L. (1998). Gap-filling and end-of-sentence effects in real-time language processing: Implications for modeling sentence comprehension in aphasia. *Brain and Language, 61*, 169–182.

Beeman, M. (1993). Semantic processing in the right hemisphere may contribute to drawing inferences from discourse. *Brain and Language, 44*, 80–120.

Beeman, M. (1998). Coarse semantic coding and discourse comprehension In M. Beeman & C. Chiarello (Eds.), *Perspectives from cognitive neuroscience* (pp. 255–284). Mahwah: Lawrence Erlbaum.

Beeman, M., & Chiarello, C. (Eds.). (1998). *Right hemisphere language comprehension: Perspectives from cognitive neuroscience*. Hillsdale, NJ: Lawrence Erlbaum.

Beeman, M., Friedman, R., Grafman, J., Perez, E., Diamond, S., & Beadle Lindsay, M. (1994). Summation priming and coarse semantic coding in the right hemisphere. *Journal of Cognitive Neuroscience, 6*, 26–45.

Berndt, R. S., & Caramazza, A. (1980). A redefinition of the syndrome of Broca's aphasia: Implications for a neuropsychological model of language. *Applied Psycholinguistics, 1*, 225–278.

Bradley, D. C., Garrett, M. F., & Zurif, E. B. (1980). Syntactic deficits in Broca's aphasia. In D. Caplan (Ed.), *Biological studies of mental processes* (pp. 269–286). Cambridge, MA: MIT Press.

Breasted, J. (1930). The Edwin Smith Surgical Papyrus. *University of Chicago Press.*

Broca, P. (1861). Perte de la Parole, Ramollissement Chronique et Destruction Partielle du Lobe Antérieur Gauche du Cerveau. *Bulletin de la Société Anthropologique, 2*, 235–238.

Brodmann, K. (Ed.). (1909). *Vergleichende Lokalisationslehre der Grosshirnrinde in ihren Prinzipien dargestellt auf Grund des Zeelenbaues*. Leipzig: Barth.

Brownell, H., & Stringfellow, A. (1999). Making requests: Illustrations of how right-hemisphere brain damage can affect discourse production. *Brain & Language, 68*, 442–465.

Brownell, H. H. (2000). Right hemisphere contributions to understanding lexical connotation and metaphor. In Y. Grodzinsky, L. Shapiro & D. Swinney (Eds.), *Language and the brain: Representation and processing* (pp. 185–201). San Diego: Academic Press.

Brownell, H. H., Bihrle, A. H., & Michelow, D. (1986). Basic and subordinate level naming by agrammatic and fluent aphasic patients. *Brain and Language, 28*, 42–52.

Brownell, H. H., & Joanette, Y. (Eds.). (1993). *Narrative discourse in neurologically impaired and normal aging adults*. San Diego: Singular Publishing Group.

Brownell, H. H., Potter, H. H., & Michelow, D. (1984). Sensitivity to lexical denotation and connotation in brain-damaged patients: A double dissociation? *Brain and Language, 22*, 253–265.

Burgess, C., & Simpson, G. B. (1988). Cerebral hemispheric mechanisms in the retrieval of ambiguous word meanings. *Brain and Language, 33*, 86–103.

Burkhardt, P., Avrutin, S., Piñango, M. M., & Ruigendijk, E. (2008). Slower-than-normal syntactic processing in agrammatic Broca's aphasia: Evidence from Dutch. *Journal of Neurolinguistics, 21*, 120–137.

Caplan, D., & Futter, C. (1986). Assignment of thematic roles to nouns in sentence comprehension by an agrammatic patient. *Brain and Language, 27*, 117–134.

Caplan, D., Waters, G., DeDe, G., Michaud, J., & Reddy, A. (2007). A study of syntactic processing in aphasia: Behavioral (psycholinguistic) aspects. *Brain and Language, 101*, 103–150.

Caplan, D., & Waters, G. S. (1999). Verbal working memory and sentence comprehension. *Behavioral and Brain Sciences, 22*, 77–126.

Caramazza, A., & Zurif, E. (1976). Dissociation of algorithmic and heuristic processes in language comprehension: Evidence from aphasia. *Brain and Language, 3*, 572–582.

Chiarello, C. (1988). Lateralization of lexical processes in the normal brain: A review of visual half-field research. In H. A. Whitaker (Ed.), *Contemporary reviews in neuropsychology*. New York: Springer-Verlag.

Crosson, B., McGregor, K., Gopinath, K. S., Conway, T. W., Benjamin, M., Chang, Y.-L., et al. (2007). Functional MRI of language in aphasia: A review of the literature and the methodological challenges. *Neuropsychological Review, 17*, 157–177.

Dickey, M. W., & Thompson, C. (2009). Automatic processing of wh- and NP-movement in agrammatic aphasia. *Brain and Language, 99*, 63–64.

Faust, M., Barak, O., & Chiarello, C. (2006). The effects of multiple script priming on word recognition by the two cerebral hemispheres: Implications for discourse processing. *Brain and Language, 99*, 247–257.

Feldman, J., & Ballard, D. (1982). Connectionist models and their properties. *Cognitive Science, 6*, 205–254.

Frazier, L., & d'Arcais, G. B. F. (1989). Filler driven parsing: A study of gap filling in Dutch. *Journal of Memory and Language, 28*, 331–344.

Fridriksson, J. (2010). Impaired speech repetition and left parietal lobe damage. *The Journal of Neuroscience, 30*, 11057–11061.

Fridriksson, J., Bonilha, L., & Rorden, C. (2007). Severe Broca's aphasia without Broca's area damage. *Behavioral Neurology, 18*, 237.

Friederici, A. D. (1983). Aphasics' perception of words in sentential context: Some real–time processing evidence. *Neuropsychologica, 21*, 351–358.

Friederici, A. D., Hahne, A., & von Cramon, D. Y. (1998). First-pass versus second-pass parsing processes in a Wernicke's and a Broca's aphasic: Electrophysiological evidence for a double dissociation. *Brain and Language, 62*, 311–341.

Friederici, A. D., von Cramon, D. Y., & Kotz, S. A. (1999). Language related brain potentials in patients with cortical and subcortical left hemisphere lesions. *Brain, 122*, 1033–1047.

Friedmann, N. (2006). Generalizations on variations in comprehension and production: A further source of variation and a possible account. *Brain and Language, 96*, 151–153.

Friedmann, N., & Grodzinsky, Y. (1997). Tense and agreement in agrammatic production: Pruning the syntactic tree. *Brain and Language, 56*, 397–425.

García-Albea, E. (1999). Neurology in the medical papyruses of the pharaohs. *Revista de neurologia, 28*, 430–433.

Gardner, H. (1994). The stories of the Right Hemisphere. In W. Spaulding (Ed.), *Integrative views of motivation, cognition, and emotion*. Lincoln: University of Nebraska Press.

Garnsey, S. M., Tanenhaus, M. K., & Chapman, R. M. (1989). Evoked potentials and the study of sentence comprehension. *Journal of Psycholinguistic Research, 18*, 51–60.

Geschwind, N. (1965). Disconnexion syndromes in animals and man: Part II. *Brain, 88*, 585.

Goldstein, K. (1924). Uber Farbenamnesie. *Psychologische Forschung, 6*, 127.

Goodglass, H., & Kaplan, E. (1972). *Boston diagnostic aphasia examination*. Philadelphia: Lea & Febiger.

Grindrod, C. M., & Baum, S. R. (2003). Sensitivity to local sentence context information in lexical ambiguity resolution: Evidence from left- and right-hemisphere-damaged individuals. *Brain & Language, 85*, 503–523.

Grodzinsky, Y. (1986). Language deficits and the theory of syntax. *Brain and Language, 27*, 135–159.

Grodzinsky, Y. (1995). A restrictive theory of agrammatic comprehension. *Brain and Language, 50*, 27–51.

Grodzinsky, Y. (2000a). The neurology of syntax: Language use without Broca's area. *Behavioral and Brain Sciences, 23*, 1–71.

Grodzinsky, Y. (2000b). OverArching Agrammatism. In Y. Grodzinsky, L. Shapiro & D. Swinney (Eds.), *Language and the brain: Representation and processing—Studies presented to Edgar Zurif on his 60th birthday* (pp. 73–86). San Diego: Academic Press.

Grodzinsky, Y. (2006). A blueprint for a brain map of syntax. In Y. Grodzinsky & K. Amunts (Eds.), *Broca's region*. New York: Oxford University Press.

Haarmann, H., & Kolk, H. (1991). Syntactic priming in Broca's aphasics: Evidence for slow activation. *Aphasiology, 5*, 247–263.

Hagoort, P., Brown, C. M., & Swaab, T. Y. (1996). Lexical-semantic event-related potential effects in patients with left hemisphere lesions and aphasia, and patients with right hemisphere lesions without aphasia. *Brain, 119*, 627–649.

Head, H. (1926). *Aphasia and kindred disorders of speech* (Vol. 2, pp. 375). London: Cambridge University Press.

Hickok, G., Conseco-Gonzalez, E., Zurif, E. B., & Grimshaw, J. (1992). Modularity in locating Wh-gaps. *Journal of Psycholinguistic Research, 21*, 545–561.

Hough, M. (1990). Narrative comprehension in adults with right and left hemisphere brain-damage: Theme organization. *Brain and Language, 38*, 253–277.

Jackson, H. (1878). London Hospital: Remarks on non-protrusion of the tongue in some cases of aphasia. *The Lancet, 111*, 716–717.

Joanette, Y., & Goulet, P. (1988). Word-naming in right-brain-damaged subjects. In C. Chiarello (Ed.), *Right hemisphere contributions to lexical semantics* (pp. 1–18). Berlin: Springer-Verlag.

Kaplan, J., Brownell, H., Jacobs, J., & Gardner, H. (1990). The effects of right hemisphere damage on the pragmatic interpretation of conversational remarks. *Brain and Language, 38*, 315–333.

Kempler, D. (1999). Idiom comprehension in children and adults with unilateral brain damage. *Developmental Neuropsychology, 15*, 327–349.

Kertesz, A. (1982). *Western Aphasia Battery*. New York: Grune and Stratton.

Klepousniotou, E., & Baum, S. (2005). Processing homonymy and polysemy: Effects of sentential context and time-course following unilateral brain damage. *Brain and Language, 95*, 365–382.

Kolk, H. H. (1995). A time-based approach to agrammatic production. *Brain and Language, 50*, 282–303.

Lichtheim, L. (1885). On aphasia. *Brain, 7*, 433.

Linebarger, M. C., Schwartz, M. F., & Saffran, E. M. (1983). Sensitivity to grammatical structure in so-called agrammatic aphasics. *Cognition, 13*, 361–392.

Love, T. (2007). The Processing of non-canonically ordered constituents in long distance dependencies by pre-school children: A real-time investigation. *Journal of Psycholinguistic Research, 36,* 191–206.

Love, T., & Swinney, D. (1996). Coreference processing and levels of analysis in object-relative constructions: Demonstration of antecedent reactivation with the cross-modal priming paradigm. *Journal of Psycholinguistic Research, 25,* 5–24.

Love, T., Swinney, D., Walenski, M., & Zurif, E. (2008). How left inferior frontal cortex participates in syntactic processing: Evidence from aphasia. *Brain and Language, 107,* 203–219.

Marie, P. (1906). Revision de la question de l'aphasie: La troisime circonvolution frontale gauche ne joue aucun role special dans la fonction du langage. *Semaine Medicale, 26,* 241.

Marshall, J. (1995). The mapping hypothesis and aphasia therapy. *Aphasiology, 9,* 517.

McElree, B., & Griffith, T. (1995). Syntactic and thematic processing in sentence comprehension: Evidence for a temporal dissociation. *Journal of Experimental Psychology: Learning, Memory, & Cognition, 21,* 134–157.

Milberg, W., Blumstein, S. E., & Dworetzky, B. (1987). Processing of lexical ambiguities in aphasia. *Brain and Language, 31,* 138–150.

Molloy, R., Brownell, H., & Gardner, H. (1990). Discourse comprehension by right hemisphere stroke patients: Deficits of prediction and revision. In Y. Joanette & H. Brownell (Eds.), *Discourse ability and brain damage: Theoretical and empirical perspectives* (pp. 113–130). New York: Springer-Verlag.

Nicol, J., Fodor, J. D., & Swinney, D. (1994). Using cross-modal lexical decision tasks to investigate sentence processing. *Journal of Experimental Psychology: Learning, Memory, & Cognition, 20,* 1229–1238.

Nicol, J., & Swinney, D. (1989). The role of structure in coreference assignment during sentence comprehension. *Journal of Psycholinguistic Research, 18,* 5–19.

Nicol, J. L. (1988). *Coreference processing during sentence comprehension.* Cambridge, MA: Massachusetts Institute of Technology.

Piñango, M. M. (2000). Canonicity in Broca's sentence comprehension: The case of psychological verbs. In Y. Grodzinsky, L. P. Shapiro & D. Swinney (Eds.), *Language and the brain: Representation and processing* (pp. 327–350). San Diego, CA: Academic Press.

Pollock, J.-Y. (1989). Verb movement, universal grammar, and the structure of IP. *Linguistic Inquiry, 20,* 365–424.

Prather, P. A., Zurif, E., Love, T., & Brownell, H. (1997). Speed of lexical activation in nonfluent Broca's aphasia and fluent Wernicke's aphasia. *Brain and Language, 59,* 391–411.

Saffran, E. M., Schwartz, M. F., & Marin, O. S. M. (1980). The word order problem in agrammatism: Production. *Brain and Language, 10,* 263–280.

Schneiderman, E., & Saddy, J. D. (1988). A linguistic deficit resulting from right-hemisphere damage. *Brain and Language, 34,* 38–53.

Schwartz, M., Saffran, E., & Marin, O. S. M. (1980). The word order problem in agrammatism I: Comprehension. *Brain and Language, 10,* 249–262.

Shapiro, L. P., Gordon, B., Hack, N., & Killackey, J. (1993). Verb argument structure processing in complex sentences in Broca's and Wernicke's aphasia. *Brain and Language, 45,* 423–447.

Shapiro, L. P., & Levine, B. A. (1990). Verb processing during sentence comprehension in aphasia. *Brain and Language, 38,* 21–47.

Shapiro, L. P., Zurif, E., & Grimshaw, J. (1987). Sentence processing and the mental representation of verbs. *Cognition, 27,* 219–246.

Shapiro, L. P., Zurif, E. B., & Grimshaw, J. (1989). Verb processing during sentence comprehension: Contextual impenetrability. *Journal of Psycholinguistic Research, 18*(2), 223–243.

Sussman, R. S., & Sedivy, J. (2003). The time-course of processing syntactic dependencies: Evidence from eye movements. *Language and Cognitive Processes, 18,* 143–163.

Swaab, T., Brown, C., & Hagoort, P. (1997). Spoken sentence comprehension in aphasia: Event-related potential evidence for a lexical integration deficit. *Journal of Cognitive Neuroscience, 9,* 39–66.

Swaab, T. Y., Brown, C., & Hagoort, P. (1998). Understanding ambiguous words in sentence contexts: Electrophysiological evidence for delayed contextual selection in Broca's aphasia. *Neuropsychologia, 36,* 737–761.

Swinney, D., & Fodor, J. D. (1989). Introduction to special issue on sentence processing. *Journal of Psycholinguistic Research, 18,* 1–3.

Swinney, D., Onifer, W., Prather, P., & Hirshkowitz, M. (1979). Semantic facilitation across sensory modalities in the processing of individual words and sentences. *Memory and Cognition, 7,* 159–165.

Swinney, D., & Osterhout, L. (1990). Inference generation during auditory language comprehension. In A. C. Graesser & G. H. Bower (Eds.), *Inference and text comprehension: The psychology of learning and motivation* (Vol. 25). San Diego: Academic Press.

Swinney, D., & Zurif, E. (1995). Syntactic processing in aphasia. *Brain and Language, 50,* 225–239.

Swinney, D., Zurif, E., Prather, P., & Love, T. (1996). Neurological distribution of processing operations underlying language comprehension. *Journal of Cognitive Neuroscience, 8,* 174–184.

Swinney, D., Zurif, E. B., & Nicol, J. (1989). The effects of focal brain damage on sentence processing: An examination of the neurological organization of a mental module. *Journal of Cognitive Neuroscience, 1,* 25–37.

Tanenhaus, M., Boland, J., Garnsey, S., & Carlson, G. (1989). Lexical structure in parsing long-distance dependencies. *Journal of Psycholinguistic Research, 18,* 37–50.

Tanenhaus, M. K., & Trueswell, J. C. (1995). Sentence comprehension. In J. Miller & P. Eimas (Eds.), *Handbook of perception and cognition.* (pp. 217–262). San Diego: Academic Press.

Thompson, C., & Choy, J. J. (2009). Pronominal resolution and gap filling in agrammatic aphasia: Evidence from eye movements. *Journal of Psycholingustic Research, 38,* 255–283.

Tompkins, C. (1990). Knowledge and strategies for processing lexical metaphor after right or left hemisphere brain damage. *Journal of Speech and Hearing Research, 33,* 307–316.

Tompkins, C. (1995). *Right hemisphere communication disorders*. San Diego: Singular Publishing.

Tompkins, C. (2008). Theoretical considerations for understanding "understanding" by adults with right hemisphere brain damage. *Perspectives on Neurophysiology and Neurogenic Speech and Language Disorders, 18*, 45–54.

Tompkins, C., & Baumgaertner, A. (1998). Clinical value of online measures for adults with right hemisphere brain damage. *American Journal of Speech-Language Pathology, 7*, 68–74.

Tompkins, C., Baumgaertner, A., & Lehman, M. (2000). Mechanisms of discourse comprehension impairment after right hemisphere brain damage. *Journal of Speech, Language, and Hearing Research 43*, 62–78.

Tompkins, C., Boada, R., & McGarry, K. (1992). The access and processing of familiar idioms by brain-damaged and normally aging adults. *Journal of Speech and Hearing Research, 35*, 626–637.

Tompkins, C., & Lehman, M. (1998). Interpreting intended meanings after right hemisphere brain damage: An analysis of evidence, potential accounts, and clinical implications. *Topics in Stroke Rehabilitation, 5*, 29–47.

Traxler, M., & Pickering, M. J. (1996). Plausibility and the processing of unbounded dependencies: An eye-tracking study. *Journal of Memory and Language, 34*, 454–475.

Trousseau, A. (1865). Phlegmasia alba dolens. *Clinique Medicale de l'Hotel-Dieu de Paris, 3*, 654–712.

Utman, J. A., Blumstein, S. E., & Sullivan, K. (2001). Mapping from sound to meaning: Reduced lexical activation in Broca's aphasics. *Brain and Language, 79*, 444–472.

Wernicke, C. (1874). *Der aphasiche Symptomenkomplex*. Breslau: Cohn und Weigert.

Weylman, S. T., Brownell, H. H., Roman, M., & Gardner, H. (1989). Appreciation of indirect requests by left- and right-brain-damaged patients: The effects of verbal context and conventionality of wording. *Brain and Language, 36*, 580–591.

Winner, E., Brownell, H., Happe, F., Blum, A., & Pincus, D. (1998). Distinguishing lies from jokes: theory of mind deficits and discourse interpretation in right hemisphere brain-damaged patients. *Brain and Language, 62*, 89–106.

Winner, E., & Gardner, H. (1977). The comprehension of metaphor in brain-damaged patients. *Brain, 100*, 717–729.

Zurif, E., Swinney, D., & Garrett, M. (1990). *Lexical processing and syntactic comprehension in aphasia* (3rd ed.). Hillsdale, NJ: Erlbaum.

Zurif, E., Swinney, D., Prather, P., & Love, T. (1994). Functional localization in the brain with respect to syntactic processing. *Journal of Psycholinguistic Research, 23*, 487–497.

Zurif, E., Swinney, D., Prather, P., Solomon, J., & Bushell, C. (1993). An on-line analysis of syntactic processing in Broca's and Wernicke's aphasia. *Brain and Language, 45*, 448–464.

Early Reports of Language Disorders

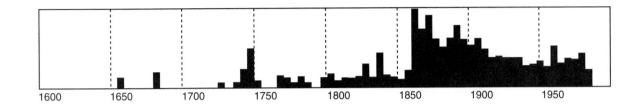

EGYPTIANS

- Edwin Smith Surgical Papyrus (c. 2500 BC), refers to "speechlessness" after head injury (Case 22)

GREEKS

- Homer: two types of speechlessness: Aphasia (loss of speech due to emotion; Aphonos (voiceless/soundless)
- Hippocrates (400 BC): APHONOS (loss of speech/voice) due to stroke
- Aristotle: the faculty of speech is located in the heart, not the head

ROMANS

- Valerius Maximus (around 30 AD) described a "very learned man from Athens" whose head was hit by a stone and who consequently suffered from a loss of his "memories for letters".
- Galen (103-200 AD) was the first one to localize thinking, perceiving and movement in the brain. First description of alexia, first hints of the separation of speech disturbance and paralysis (c. 30 AD)

15TH AND 16TH CENTURIES (RENAISSANCE PERIOD)

- Antonio Guainerio (1440s)—memory deficits result in language production problems
- Paracelsus (1500s)—linked head injuries to speech disturbances—paralysis sometimes occurs
- Nicolo Massa (late 1500s)—traumatic aphasia, or anarthrias (loss of the ability to produce speech)

17TH AND 18TH CENTURIES

- 1683, Peter Rommel: reports a case of "rare aphonia." A case of nonfluent conversational speech with spared "automatic" speech (e.g., the Lord's Prayer).
- 1745, Olaf Dalin: Preserved ability to sing despite severe nonfluent aphasia
- 1762, Giovanni Morgagni—presented cases of speechlessness in patients who have right side paralysis (hemiplegia)
- 1770, Johann Gesner (Die Spracharnnesie, The language amnesia): First clear description of fluent-type aphasias, which he called "speech amnesia." Deficits were not due to intellectual decline or loss of general memory, but to a specific impairment in verbal memory.

19TH AND 20TH CENTURIES

- 1801, Franz Fall—first to describe behavior links to specific areas (organs) in the brain, birth of phrenology
- 1825, Jean-Baptiste Bouillaud—first to describe the concept of inner speech (linking ideas to words) and that of articulation. Argued that there are different neural mechanisms involved in these processes
- 1825/1843, Jacques Lordat—introduced the term "alalia," a complete inability to speak, and made the distinction between verbal amnesia (loss of memory for words) and verbal asynergy (loss of the ability to pronounce words with the clear knowledge of what is desired to be said and no evidence of paralysis of the tongue)
- 1836, Marc Dax—language was seated in the left anterior frontal lobe

225

- 1861/1866, Paul Broca: "*Aphemia*, disorder in the faculty of language"—intelligence, hearing, comprehension, and thought are all intact. Linked to an area in the brain circumscribed to the left inferior frontal region.
- 1864, Armand Trousseau: "*Aphasia*, not aphemia"—intelligence, memory and attention almost always affected
- 1874, Karl Wernicke—fluent language disorder related to the left posterior part of the superior temporal gyrus
- 1877, Lichtheim & Kussmaul—generated models/theories linking lesions in areas of language centers (or connections between them)
- 1882, John Hughlings Jackson—aphasia is a cognitive disorder, is the inability to provide information (in speech or gesture)
- 1906, Pierre Marie—aphasia is an intellectual impairment; there was no one area of the brain that played a role in the function of language
- 1913, Arnold Pick— a psychological approach to the study of aphasia. Attempted to model agrammatism
- 1926, Henry Head—aphasia is a disorder in the symbolic formulation and expression. There is no center for speech, writing or reading. First to develop an assessment battery with both verbal and nonverbal tasks
- 1948, Kurt Goldstein—Gestalt approach to aphasia—aphasia is the inability to differentiate figure and background which results in an inability to abstract
- 1956, Roman Jakobson—used linguistic terminology to define motor and sensory aphasia
- 1950s/1960s, Luria, Geschwind, Goodglass—development of more refined aphasia classification systems and links to brain regions. Further interest in levels of language errors (phonemic—Blumstein, 1973; word—Geschwind, 1972; sentence—Zurif and Caramazzo, 1972, 1976).

REFERENCES AND SUGGESTED READINGS

Benton, A. L., & Joynt, R. J. (1960). Early descriptions of aphasia, from 400 B.C. til 1800. *Archives of Neurology, 3*, 205–222.

Brown, J., & Chobor, K. (1992). Phrenological studies of aphasia before Broca: Broca's aphasia or Gall's aphasia? *Brain and Language, 43*, 475–486.

Buckingham, H. (2006). A pre-history of the problem of Broca's aphasia. *Aphasiology, 20*, 792–810.

Code, C. H., & Tesak, J. (2007). *Milestones in the history of aphasia.* London: Psychology Press.

Eling, P. (1994). *Reader in the history of aphasia: From Franz Fall to Norman Geschwind.* Amsterdam: John Benjamins. An edited volume of the mentioned period.

Finger, S. (2000). *Minds behind the Brain. A History of the Pioneers and their Discoveries.* Oxford/New York: Oxford University Press.

Henderson, V. (1990). Alalia, aphemia and aphasia, *Archives of Neurology, 47*, 85–88.

Prins, R. S., & Bastiaanse, R (2006). Early history of aphasia. From 1700 B.C. till 1861. *Aphasiology, 20*, 761–792.

CHAPTER 11

Communication Following Executive Dysfunction

CHAPTER OUTLINE

Michael Cannizzaro and Carl Coelho

Symbolically based communication is susceptible to disruption secondary to acquired central nervous system dysfunction. Impairments of linguistic processing, as in aphasia, are often attributed to damage of the cortical and sub-cortical structures of the perisylvian language zone in the left cerebral hemisphere. However, when communication is disrupted due to alterations in cognitive functions not attributable to aphasia, cognitive-communication disorders result.

The American Speech-Language and Hearing Association (2005) defines cognitive-communication disorders as follows:

> Cognitive-communication disorders encompass difficulty with any aspect of communication that is affected by disruption of cognition. Communication may be verbal or nonverbal and includes listening, speaking, gesturing, reading, and writing in all domains of language (phonologic, morphologic, syntactic, semantic, and pragmatic). Cognition includes cognitive processes and systems (e.g., attention, perception, memory, organization, executive function). Areas of function affected by cognitive impairments include behavioral self-regulation, social interaction, activities of daily living, learning and academic performance, and vocational performance. (Association, 2005)

Cognitive impairments related to executive function/dysfunction (EF) and failures in cognitive control can negatively impact communication performance by affecting organization, output, efficiency, precision, abstraction, social referencing, appropriateness, and verbal learning abilities (Ylvisaker, Szekeres, & Feeney, 2001; 2008). Such cognitive-communication deficits are often associated with pathophysiology of the prefrontal cortex (PFC) and can be observable in the presence of relatively intact language skills (Coelho, 2007; Decker & Cannizzaro, 2007). For example, communicative impairments in persons who have sustained traumatic brain injuries (TBIs) are frequently attributed to damage of the PFC and subsequent EF dysfunction. Communication deficits following TBI are often apparent during complex communication tasks such as in the various forms of discourse (e.g., procedural, narrative, and conversational discourse) as opposed to disruptions at the word or sentence levels. Executive function abilities are necessary where successive information units (e.g., sentences or utterances) are combined to create meaningful discourse communication (Biddle, McCabe, & Bliss, 1996; Cannizzaro, Coelho, & Youse, 2002; Chapman, McKinnon, Levin, et al., 2001; Coelho, Ylvisaker, & Turkstra, 2005; Snow, Douglas, & Ponsford, 1998; Tucker & Hanlon, 1998). In this manner content, organization, appropriateness, and efficiency all become important features in the comprehension or production of a purposeful discourse message.

DEGENERATIVE DISORDERS AND COGNITIVE-COMMUNICATION IMPAIRMENT

Although TBI is one of the most common etiologies associated with PFC dysfunction, any disruption of the structure or function of the PFC or related cortical/subcortical neural circuitry may affect cognition, leading to EF deficits and subsequent cognitive-communication disorders. The prefrontal cortex is highly interconnected with the rest of the brain underscoring how damage in many cortical and subcortical areas can lead to dysfunction of the PFC and deficits in EF (Figure 11-1). For example, illnesses that lead to dementia such Huntington's disease (HD), Parkinson's disease (PD), Alzheimer's disease (AD), and frontotemporal lobar degeneration and its variants (e.g., frontotemporal dementia [FTD], primary progressive aphasia [PPA], and semantic dementia [SD]) can specifically impair prefrontal neural circuitry leading to impairments in cognition and communication (Miller & Cummings, 2007). Psychiatric disorders such as schizophrenia, major depression, bipolar disorder, and possibly obsessive-compulsive disorder can also have significant impact on EF related to dysfunction of the PFC with potential impacts related to communication and cognition (Miller & Cummings, 2007).

Difficulties with complex communication have been well documented with a number of non-aphasic disorders (e.g., AD, FTD, SD), primarily associated with the progressive deterioration of memory and EF skills in older adults (Ash, Moore, Antani, et al., 2006; Blair, Marczinski, Davis-Faroque, & Kertesz, 2007; Dijkstra, Bourgeois, Allen, & Burgio, 2004; Laine, Laakso, Vuorinen, & Rinne, 1998; Peelle & Grossman, 2008). As diseases such as AD, PPA, and FTD progress, there are measureable declines in basic language comprehension and production abilities, which can be documented via standardized aphasia batteries. These decrements in linguistic skills show different rates of decline (faster deterioration in PPA and FTD and slower deterioration in AD) but eventually reach similar overlapping profiles in disrupted language performance (Blair et al., 2007). In AD, deterioration of utterance level and inter-sentence cohesion may precede an inevitable decline in more complex discourse abilities such as maintaining thematic relevance and global measures of discourse cohesion (Dijkstra et al., 2004). Discourse assessments provide a sensitive measure of the cognitive-communicative decline in dementia, as persons with mild AD and mild cognitive impairment can demonstrate significant difficulties processing gist level in information in discourse (Chapman, Zientz, Weiner, et al., 2002). Although these changes in communication can appear subtle, the burden of dialogue can shift and differentially impact their communication partners (Dijkstra et al., 2004; Ripich, Vertes, Whitehouse, et al., 1991). However, certain disorders, such as the various manifestations of FTD, are

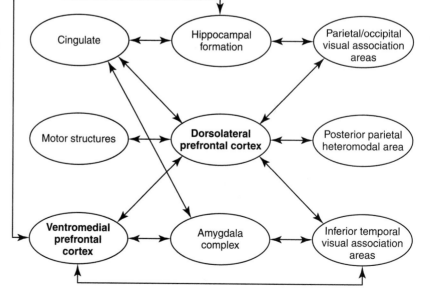

Figure 11-1 A summary of connectivity between the prefrontal cortex and other brain regions. The ventromedial and dorsolateral exhibit reciprocal connectivity with different posterior brain regions, with ventromedial prefrontal regions being associated with emotional processing areas (e.g., amygdala) and dorsolateral prefrontal regions associated with non-emotional sensory and motor areas (e.g., basal ganglia and parietal areas). [Adapted from Wood JN and Grafman J (2003). Human prefrontal cortex: Processing and representational perspectives. *Nat Rev Neurosci*, 4: 139–147.]

known to have a greater relative impact on EF performance and can manifest in more pronounced changes in cognitive-communication disruptions.

Frontotemporal dementia is a degenerative neurocognitive disorder characterized by alterations in behavior and communication skills with relatively less pronounced deficits in memory processes (Ash et al., 2006; Blair et al., 2007; Peelle & Grossman, 2008). In general, decreased communication fluency, as well as word and sentence level linguistic difficulties, are known to exist in most manifestations of FTD and are associated with atrophic changes in the left inferior frontal gyrus, the left insula, and portions of the left superior temporal gyrus (Ash et al., 2006; Ash, Moore, Vesely, et al., 2009; Blair et al., 2007). However, a specific variant with exacerbated impairment with social functioning and EF difficulties can present without aphasic symptoms, and exemplifies how deteriorations in EF can impact cognitive-communication (Ash et al., 2006; Peelle & Grossman, 2008). Ash and colleagues (2006) have documented specific organizational deficits in this group, with a failure to connect ideas in discourse at both a local (sentence to sentence) and global (theme or gist) levels, throughout relatively simple narrative discourse productions. This pattern of the disintegration of discourse components is related to cortical atrophy in the right prefrontal and temporal lobes, thought to be the anatomical correlate of the disorder (Ash et al., 2006; Peelle & Grossman, 2008). Additionally, poorly integrated discourse may be the most prominent change in communication ability in FTD with social executive impairments and these deficits are significantly correlated to clinically oriented behavioral measures of EF (Ash et al., 2006; Peelle & Grossman, 2008). Similar findings of poorly integrated discourse components measured on local and global levels have also been seen in patients with corticobasal degeneration (CB) (Gross, Ash, McMillan, et al., 2010). Persons with CB experience deficits related to cortical and subcortical changes that manifest in frontal and parietal symptoms, including social and EF deficits as well as motor planning difficulties (Gross et al., 2010).

Sub-cortical neurodegenerative disorders such as Parkinson's disease and Huntington's disease also provide evidence of measurable declines in cognitive-communication skills related to EF difficulties (Litvan, Frattali, & Duffy, 2005; Murray, 2000; Saldert, Fors, Stroberg, & Hartelius, 2010). Even during the early stages of HD, the comprehension of complex discourse can be impaired similar to persons who are in later stages of the disease progression (Murray & Stout, 1999; Saldert et al., 2010). Persons with HD generally demonstrate the ability to process main ideas during discourse comprehension but can be particularly challenged by detailed information and implied information, as well as the interpretation of figurative language (Chenery, Copland, & Murdoch, 2002; Murray & Stout, 1999). Additionally, persons with HD demonstrate large variations in a number of higher-level discourse comprehension skills such as the interpretation of metaphor and ambiguity in discourse (Saldert et al., 2010). Discourse production can also be compromised in PD and HD, leading to reduced output and decreased syntactic abilities, with shorter and less complex sentence constructions in discourse. Significantly less informative discourse has also been noted with an overall reduction of informational content and proportionally fewer informative utterances in simple discourse tasks produced by persons with HD (Murray, 2000).

But these phenomena are not strictly related to progressive disorders associated with aging and known neuropsychiatric pathology. College students who, by self-report, demonstrate characteristics of impulsive aggressive outbursts also show impairments of complex language function related to measureable EF deficits (Villemarette-Pittman, Stanford, & Greve, 2003). These appreciable differences in cognitive-communication skills indicate that planning of complex verbal output and organization of spoken communication were significantly difficult when compared to the communication of their peers. These behaviors were related to poor integration of information, the inclusion of inaccurate information, and awkward sequencing of information. These cognitive-communication challenges were significant even in the presence of intact basic language and other cognitive skills (Villemarette-Pittman et al., 2003).

LOCALIZED BRAIN DAMAGE, APHASIA, AND EXECUTIVE FUNCTION

Strokes and cerebrovascular disease in general can result in focal deficits such as hemiplegia/paresis and aphasia but also commonly result in cognitive deficits (Lesniak, Bak, Czepiel, et al., 2008; Zinn, Bosworth, Hoenig, & Swartzwelder, 2007). In a study of 200 consecutive admissions to a stroke unit, patients assessed with a broad cognitive battery (e.g., orientation, attention, gnosis, memory, praxis, visuospatial abilities, language, and EF) and re-assessed at 1 year after onset demonstrated that cognitive deficits were persistent in 72 percent of this population (Lesniak et al., 2008). Although the most common deficits noted were in the areas of attention and short-term memory, the presence of impaired EF in the second week after stroke emerged as the only predictor of functional recovery after 1 year (Lesniak et al., 2008). Similarly, Zinn and colleagues studied EF abilities in individuals with acute stroke and found that nearly 50 percent of their participants demonstrated impairments on measures of EF, and that such patients are at risk for failure to benefit fully from rehabilitation during the acute period and for several months following (Zinn et al., 2007).

Due to the common co-occurrence of aphasia and EF deficits following stroke, it is important to understand the unique and combinatorial impact on communication these deficits could have. Prescott and colleagues presented the Tower of Hanoi, a measure of complex problem solving, to individuals with aphasia and found that 30 percent of the group could not complete the task and those who did required significantly more time and moves to accomplish the task (Prescott, Gruber, Olsen, & Fuller, 1987). Glosser and Goodglass (1990) administered an EF battery to 22 individuals with left hemisphere brain damage and aphasia, to 19 with right hemisphere brain damage, and to 49 healthy controls. Results indicated that those individuals with left frontal lesions were significantly more impaired in EF than those with posterior or mixed lesions of the left hemisphere.

The relationship between cognitive abilities and specific communication treatment protocols has also been investigated. Individuals with aphasia who perform more poorly on assessments of non-verbal cognitive skills and measures of EF take longer to achieve performance criteria for context-based treatments (e.g., using compensatory communication strategies) and EF measures predicted communication performance at 6 months post treatment. Thus performance on the EF measures may be related to overall outcome, appropriateness of certain treatment types, and prescribed amount of treatment (Hinckley, Carr, & Patterson, 2001). This has also been demonstrated in investigations of cognitive flexibility with regard to the acquisition and use of varied symbols (i.e., alternate modes) for functional communication tasks. Persons with aphasia demonstrate the means to express concepts in an alternate mode; however, they can be persistent (i.e., preservative) in their attempts to use the verbal modality, albeit unsuccessfully. This suggests that cognitive flexibility, a component of EF, might be required for successfully using alternative modes communication (Purdy, Duffy, & Coelho, 1994). These relationships between EF and language also impact functional communication, defined as "the ability to receive or to convey a message, regardless of the mode, to communicate effectively and independently in a given natural environment" (Fridriksson, Nettles, Davis, et al., 2006,

p. 402). Correlations between functional communication abilities and EF are reported to be significant, suggesting that for individuals with aphasia, communicative success is related to or dependent on the integrity of EF skills as well as linguistic competency (Fridriksson et al., 2006).

The ultimate goal of aphasia therapy is to improve an individual's ability to communicate within real world contexts (i.e., in unpredictable settings with fluctuating conditions and demands). Successful everyday communication requires goal-oriented behavior and flexible problem solving, which characterize EF (Helm-Estabrooks, 2002). Additionally, second to language, EF was the aspect of cognition that was most vulnerable to the effects of brain damage associated with aphasia (Helm-Estabrooks, 2002). Therefore, it is not possible to predict a person's communicative success in everyday contexts on the basis of nonlinguistic cognitive skills or language performance alone. Thus, the implications of EF impairments for the management of individuals with aphasia must also been considered.

Overall, it is apparent that there is a complex relationship between nonlinguistic cognitive abilities, including EF, and language performance in persons with aphasia. These changes in cognitive abilities are prevalent in persons with aphasia and should be assessed separately. In particular, EF may play an important role in determining the success of various language and communication interventions and functional communication outcomes in persons with aphasia. Finally, for some individuals with aphasia, treatment of various aspects of cognition such as impaired EF may be an important consideration in conjunction with traditional linguistic-based and communication-based interventions.

KNOWLEDGE STRUCTURE, EXECUTIVE FUNCTION, AND DISCOURSE

In the most general sense, cognitive control and EF are manifest in the ability to perform in adaptive and responsive ways to novel or complex situations, and are necessary for appropriate cognition, emotional regulation, and social abilities such as communication (Lezak, Howieson, & Loring, 2004). Abstracting EF to fundamental elements reveals behaviors that are goal-directed, are achieved through the coordination of thought and action, are necessary for processing information, and are required for acting in a purposeful and appropriate manner (Grafman, 2006a; Miller & Wallis, 2009; Wood & Grafman, 2003). Communication can be seen as behavior (or as a particular set of behaviors) that is goal-directed for the purpose of exchanging information. Communication requires cognitive control for coordinating and organizing information (e.g., decoding many levels of input, linguistic ability, situational knowledge, pragmatic factors, performance, self-monitoring, etc.) via knowledge frameworks.

A number of theoretical explanations have been proposed to account for the information processing and knowledge representation utilized by the PFC, which enable us to engage in non-routine, complex activities and perform complicated tasks, including discourse (Gilbert & Burgess, 2008; Wood & Grafman, 2003; Wood, Knutson, & Grafman, 2005). This includes non-routinized, socially appropriate communication behaviors. Examples of such everyday behaviors include relating a story of a past event for the entertainment of others, explaining the steps necessary to complete a task, creating a message to persuade the opinion of others, and so on. Current models of EF involve top-down driven processes (organization, pragmatics, content selection, behavioral efficiency) that interact with more automatic cognitive processes (e.g., attention, speech motor control, linguistic processing) in response to specific task demands to attain relevant goals (Gilbert & Burgess, 2008). For example, your goal in reading this chapter (i.e., discourse

processing) might be to gain general knowledge about the relationship between EF disorders and their impact on communication. Similarly, your goal may also include short-term gains in extracting the necessary knowledge to pass an exam/course, or, more long-term, to improve your knowledge base in working with persons with cognitive-communication disorders. Either way, how you read the words will not change and is related to over-learned processes of word and text level decoding and semantic and syntactic processing for reading comprehension. However, when the reading objective presents itself (e.g., a conscious goal like preparation for an upcoming exam), you employ EF abilities related specifically to achieving the objective. The process for attending to or extracting particular themes of information for storage or memorization will be driven by your particular objectives. You may deploy a specific strategy such as outlining information, extracting key words, writing out definitions in your own words, or delineating general themes and sub-themes.

It has been suggested that the PFC is responsible for information consolidation (e.g., discourse processing) through the activation of unique stores of knowledge called structured event complexes (SECs) (Figure 11-2)

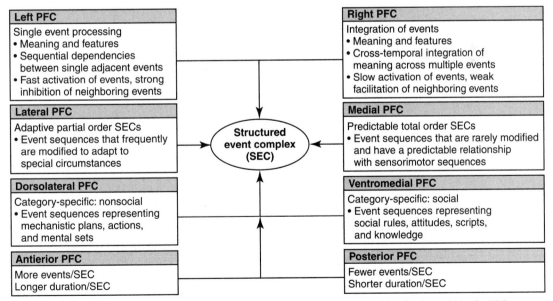

Figure 11-2 The representational forms of the SEC and their proposed localization within the PFC. Multiple subcomponents and their respective cortical areas can contribute to the formation or utilization of the SEC. For example, the telling of a well-known story with a predictable organizational format might rely heavily on both the right PFC and left PFC, especially in the medial aspects. Adapting the story (e.g., for children) could also rely on the ventromedial PFC to make it socially appropriate for a particular setting or group while contributions from the dorsolateral PFC could enhance mental states for that particular audience. [Adapted from Wood JN and Grafman J (2003). Human prefrontal cortex: Processing and representational perspectives. *Nat Rev Neurosci*, 4: 139–147.]

(Grafman, 1995; Grafman & Litvan, 1999; Partiot, Grafman, Sadato, et al., 1996; Sirigu, Cohen, Zalla, et al., 1998; Sirigu, Zalla, Pillon, et al., 1995; Wood & Grafman, 2003; Wood et al., 2005). These SECs are believed to be goal oriented, sequentially structured, thematic, and rule governed. Structured event complex information is thought to be stored as cognitive frameworks that are used to guide information processing and are encoded and retrieved as complete episodes (described below) and stored in the PFC (Wood & Grafman, 2003).

Structured event complex knowledge is used to encode and retrieve hierarchical sequences related to everyday life activities that are activated during information processing (Grafman, 2006a; 2006b; Krueger, Moll, Zahn, et al., 2007; Wood & Grafman, 2003; Wood et al., 2005). Examples of everyday events sequences are commonly occurring behaviors and can include anything from the routine and mundane (e.g., verbalizing the steps necessary for making the morning coffee) to novel cognitively challenging behaviors (e.g., writing out the information necessary to plan a dinner party for 100 guests), to the transcendent (e.g., discussing career goals and maintaining progress toward these goals over a 30-year span). This knowledge may include sequences such as activating previously learned information necessary for planning, organization, sub-goal routines, acting on plans, analysis of performance, and updating plans based on success of the SEC (Grafman, 2006b; Hewitt, Evans, & Dritschel, 2006). In this sense, goal-directed communication activities (e.g., relating personal information in the form of a narrative, comprehending the thoughts and feelings of others during a conversation) could be conceptualized as rule-governed frameworks for information processing that are employed to guide the comprehension and production of discourse communication. These frameworks are learned through repeated exposures to communicative situations that follow general patterns (i.e., organizational structure) and may include a number of important contextual factors (e.g., pragmatic rules, time constraints, etc.). For example, discourse in the form of fictional narratives are often comprised of a goal-directed episode made up of story grammar components that are considered to be one type of SEC (e.g., comprehension, production, memory encoding, event recall) (Grafman & Krueger, 2008; Rumelhart, 1975; Stein & Glenn, 1979; Krueger et al.; Wood et al., 2005). Because of the rich content, predictable organizational structure, and linguistic processing demands involved in discourse tasks, the analysis of discourse has become an important means for understanding cognitive-communication disorders.

Analysis of Discourse

The clinical examination of discourse has become a useful tool for studying communication skills in healthy children and adults, as well as in persons with acquired impairments subsequent to traumatic brain injury, stroke, and dementia (Arkin & Mahendra, 2001; Ash et al., 2006; Brookshire, Chapman, Song, & Levin, 2000; Coelho, 2007; Lehman Blake, 2006; Mar, 2004; McCabe & Bliss, 2006; Stemmer, 1999). Natural communication requires language processing beyond individual words or isolated sentences with the integration of smaller units of language into a coherent exchange of information (Gordon, 1993). Discourse encompasses a number of identifiable sub-genres (e.g., conversation, debate, picture description, story narrative, etc.), each with unique structure that defines and shapes the message components and their associations (Coelho et al., 2005; Fayol & Lemaire, 1993). The comprehension and production of discourse message represents complex behavior, which includes linguistic interpretation, organizational structure, and pragmatic rules. Since many levels of knowledge are necessary to construct a discourse, a number of methods of analysis have been devised to investigate these naturalistic communication acts (e.g., analysis of content, syntactic structure, cohesion, narrative structure, pragmatic behavior, etc.) (Table 11-1) (Cherney, Shadden, & Coelho, 1998; Mar, 2004).

The process of integrating information across successive utterances or sentences involves, among other things, updating contextual information with new information, monitoring for message coherence (e.g., personal knowledge, situational pragmatics, relationship between message components), and interpreting discourse as a unified whole (Ferstl & von Cramon, 2002; Ferstl, Neumann, Bogler, & von Cramon, 2008). The cognitive processes necessary for decoding semantics and syntax are employed as additional units of processed information that are combined, structured, and integrated until a complete message can be appreciated.

Recent investigations have implicated the PFC, and particularly the medial prefrontal cortex to contain stored knowledge (e.g., structured event complexes) that are experience guided, rule governed and somewhat predictable like a simple story (Krueger et al., 2007; Wood et al., 2005; Zacks & Tversky, 2009). Additionally, data from a recent study suggests that discourse information, presented in a simplistic and archetypical organizational pattern, reduces processing load to the point where comprehension becomes predictable and automatic (Cannizzaro, Dumas, Prelock, & Newhouse, 2010). In essence, SEC knowledge is a type of pattern abstraction of prior experience (e.g., exposure to stories

Table **11-1** Levels of Discourse and Analyses

LEVELS OF DISCOURSE INVESTIGATION	EXAMPLES OF ANALYSES
Word Level	Informational content
	Information efficiency/lexical productivity (e.g., words per minute)
	Reference & pronoun use
	Word-finding behavior
Sentence Level	Syntax structure/syntactic complexity
	Cohesion (intra- and inter-sentence)
Discourse Level/ Global Level	Story structure
	Topic maintenance
	Turn-taking behaviors
	Local coherence
	Global coherence
	Pragmatic ratings
	Impression ratings (e.g., effectiveness and efficiency)

Data from Mar, R. A. (2004). The neuropsychology of narrative: Story comprehension, story production and their interrelation. *Neuropsychologia, 42,* 1414–1434; and Cherney, L. R. Shadden, B. B., & Coelho, C. A. (1998). *Analyzing discourse in communicatively impaired adults* (pp. 1–8). Gaithersburg, MD: Aspen.

leads to a mental model or story schema); it is reasonable to assume that this prior experience with simplistic discourse patterns provides a base of experience that facilitates discourse processing (Maguire, Frith, & Morris, 1999; Cannizzaro et al., 2010; Krueger et al., 2007).

The accurate production and comprehension of a narrative requires a complex interaction of linguistic, cognitive, and pragmatic abilities that are sensitive to the particular deficits seen in such individuals demonstrating cognitive-communication impairments secondary to EF related communication impairments. In the sections that follow, narrative discourse analysis procedures are briefly described, findings from studies of populations with prefrontal cortex damage summarized, and samples of analyzed discourse narratives are presented that illustrate some characteristic deficits.

Discourse Analysis Procedures

The discourse analysis procedure commonly begins with the elicitation of a spoken narrative, minimally five sentences in length. Several narrative genres may be sampled, such as procedural (explaining how to make a sandwich), descriptive (describing a memorable vacation), or story narratives (generating an original story or retelling a previously presented story). These narratives types are referred to as monologic as opposed

to conversational discourse. The discourse samples are typically recorded, ideally videorecorded, and transcribed verbatim. The transcripts are then distributed into more basic units for analysis such as T-units, which are more reliably identified than sentences (Hughes, McGillivray, & Schmidek, 1997). A T-unit consists of an independent clause plus any dependent clauses associated with it (Hunt, 1970). Depending on the type of narrative elicited, numerous analyses may be performed, including within and across sentences or across an entire story text.

Sentence-Level Analyses

Examples of sentence-level analyses include measures of an individual's verbal output or productivity such as total number of T-units per narrative or words per T-unit. Complexity of sentence-level grammar might be measured by number of subordinate clauses per T-unit (Coelho, 2002).

Cohesion

An example of an across-sentence analysis is cohesion. Sentences are linked within a text by various types of meaning relations referred to as cohesive ties (Halliday & Hasan, 1976). The kinds of ties vary, depending on the communicative function of the text. An individual's frequency of use of various categories of cohesive ties is referred to as cohesive style and may vary depending on the discourse type (i.e., procedural, descriptive, stories, etc.) (Liles, Coelho, Duffy, & Zalagens, 1989). Analysis of cohesion may involve the frequency of occurrence of, for example, Halliday and Hasan's cohesive categories: Reference, Lexical, Conjunctive, Ellipsis, and Substitution (see Liles et al., 1989, or Mentis & Prutting, 1987, for operational definitions of these categories). Another index of cohesion is to examine cohesive adequacy. Each occurrence of a cohesive tie may also be judged as to its adequacy. A tie is judged "complete" if the information referred to by the cohesive marker is easily found and identified without ambiguity, or as "incomplete" or "erroneous" if the listener is guided to ambiguous information elsewhere in the text. The number of complete or error ties may be tallied as a percentage of the total number of ties in each story.

Coherence

Coherence ratings reveal how well an individual maintains and conveys the overall theme of a narrative. Each T-unit within a story is rated in terms of both local and global coherence (see Glosser & Deser, 1990; Van Leer & Turkstra, 1999). Global coherence refers to the relationship of the meaning or content of an utterance to the general topic of the story. Local coherence pertains to the relationship of the meaning or content of an utterance to that of the preceding utterance. Once the coherence has been rated for a story, two means are calculated, one for global coherence and a second for local coherence.

Story Grammar

Story grammar knowledge refers to the supposed regularities in the internal structure of stories that guide an individual's comprehension and production of the logical relationships (i.e., causal and temporal) between people and events. Episodes are the central unit in most models of story grammar (e.g., Frederiksen, Bracewell, Breuleux, & Renaud, 1990; Johnson & Mandler, 1980; Rumelhart, 1975; Thorndyke, 1977). The episode components are defined as statements about declared goals, attempts at solutions, and the consequences of the attempts. These components are referred to as Initiating Event, Attempt, and Direct Consequence (Stein & Glenn, 1979). The creation of episodes is evidence of story grammar knowledge and because it is cognitive in nature it is reasonable to believe that it may be disrupted by brain damage. Analysis of story grammar consists of looking at the number of complete episodes. An episode is judged as complete if it contains all three, logically related components: (a) an initiating event that prompts a character to formulate a goal-directed behavioral sequence; (b) an action or an attempt at achieving the goal; and (c) a direct consequence marking attainment or non-attainment of the goal. An additional measure is the proportion of T-units within the episode structure, in other words how much of the narrative is framed within episodes.

In considering the role of the PFC in language processing, story grammar, in particular, stands out as deserving of analysis since it may be considered a type of SEC. As discussed in the section on discourse analysis, story grammar refers to the purported regularities in the internal structure of narratives that guide an individual's comprehension and production of the logical relationships between people and events (i.e., temporal and causal). Components of episodes involve information units about stated goals, attempts at solutions, and the consequences of these attempts. Because the associations among components of an episode are considered logical and not bound by specific content, episode organization is described as cognitive in nature and potentially disrupted by damage to the PFC.

Completeness

For completeness, an inventory of key components (events and characters) for a given story can be created based on normative sampling (Le, Coelho, Mozeiko, &

Grafman, 2011). When key components are pooled across participants, these actions and events define distinct components of the story. In the examples given below, components were identified based on such a normative group. Components that were mentioned by 80% or more of the normative group were considered to be critical to the story and a total of five elements met the criterion for inclusion. Analysis on this level yields a completeness score, which is the total number of critical components included in each participant's story retelling compared to number of elements that are considered to be critical.

Narrative Discourse Samples

In this section narrative samples elicited from individuals with traumatic brain injury are presented and results of the discourse analyses summarized. All of the samples were drawn from a large database of Vietnam War veterans. The individuals with brain injuries survived severe penetrating head wounds and were 30-years post–onset of injury when the narrative samples were elicited. The story narratives of three individuals with damage exclusively to the prefrontal cortex, who also demonstrated moderately depressed scores on objective measures of executive functioning, appear below. These narratives are representative of the impairments seen following damage to the prefrontal cortex. Narratives of non–brain-injured Vietnam veterans are also presented for comparison purposes.

The narrative samples analyzed were all story narratives and were elicited in a story retelling format. Each participant was shown a 16-frame picture story, "Old McDonald Had an Apartment House" (Barrett, 1998), without a soundtrack on a computer screen. The story depicts the farmer Old McDonald's adjustment to urban living, including his attempts to grow vegetation indoors, which leads to conflict with his fellow tenants and the apartment owner. After viewing the story each participant was instructed to "Tell me that story you just watched." Each story was recorded and then transcribed verbatim and segmented into T-units. In the examples that follow, all story narratives are analyzed at multiple levels and the findings summarized.

Transcript NI 1: Non-injured Adult Male

1. Mr. McDonald and his wife had this apartment building which had several ten- [you know uh] tenants
2. and as time went by he turned it into a vegetable farm
3. had vegetables here there each and everywhere
4. [uh] then later on he brought in some animals
5. and his world [like] turned into old McDonald's farm instead of old McDonald's apartment house

6. [um] he had vegetables and animals [all over] all over the floor
7. [uh] eventually the people tenants started moving out because of all the vegetables and the animals
8. and eventually [uh] old McDonald and his wife [uh] lost the apartment building it looked like according to the pictures
9. [and] but the landlord or who he [owned owed] owed the house to or the apartments to found him a diced vegetable stand to sell his produce and stuff out of
10. and all his [uh] tenants became his customers

Summary for Transcript NI 1

In this story narrative, and the others that follow, the text has been segmented into T-units (spoken equivalent of a sentence-like structure), which are numbered. Certain words designated as revisions (e.g., "owned owed" in T-unit 9), repetitions (e.g., "all over" in T-unit 6), or fillers (e.g., "uh," "um," "you know uh") are bracketed and not considered in the overall analysis. In certain instances a high proportion of such utterances may be of interest and indicative of planning difficulty. Transcript 1 is a relatively efficient retelling of the picture story presented. Length is not excessive (10 T-units, 147 words) and grammatical complexity (subordinate clauses/T-unit = .20) is adequate (Table 11-2). Cohesive adequacy and coherence (local and global) are also

good. In other words, this individual was able to successfully link units of meaning across sentences (e.g., appropriate use of pronouns) and to maintain and convey the overall gist of the story from beginning to end. This non-injured participant generated a total of three episodes integrating all five of the critical components, which yielded a well-organized and complete retelling of the story.

Transcript NI 2: Non-injured Adult Male

1. this [um] McDonald, he lived in a apartment house
2. and [uh] his wife started to plant
3. and he decided he wanted to [uh] build a garden
4. and [uh,] so he planted [uh] vegetables and everything
5. and [he uh the the people uh uh uh] the other tenants [uh] weren't too thrilled about it
6. and [uh] fairly soon he had vegetables growing in the hallway and the tub, [uh], cows in the house and everything
7. [the uh,] all the tenants [uh] got mad and moved out
8. [and uh] he moved [uh] some more cows into the house and everything
9. he got so overwhelmed with [uh] produce in the house that [uh] I think the owner [uh] was furious about it

Table **11-2** Summary of Scores for Discourse Measures of the Five Transcripts of a Story Retelling Task for Five Participants (Two Non-injured Adult Males—NI 1 and 2, and Three Adult Males with Brain Injury—BI 1, 2, 3)

DISCOURSE MEASURES	NI 1	NI 2	BI 1	BI 2	BI 4
T-units	10	12	8	11	13
Words	147	179	162	144	125
Edited words	118	137	96	131	105
Subordinate clauses	2	3	1	2	0
Subordinate clauses/T-unit	.20	.25	.13	.18	0
Cohesive adequacy (complete ties/total ties)	.76	.70	.33	.48	.74
Local coherence	4.60	3.82	3.71	3.40	4.5
Global coherence	4.90	4.75	4.13	4.30	4.85
Story grammar (total episodes)	3	4	1	4	2
Proportion of T-units in episode structure	.90	.75	.25	1.00	.38
Completeness	5	5	2	4	5

Note. **T-Units** = total T-units in story narrative, **Words** = total number of words in story narrative, **Edited words** = total number of words minus revisions, repetitions and fillers, **Subordinate clauses** = total subordinate clauses in narrative, **Subordinate clauses/T-unit** = number subordinate clauses in story narrative divided by number of T-units, **Cohesive adequacy** = total number of complete ties divided by total number of cohesive ties, **Local and Global coherence** = mean ratings for story narrative, **Story grammar** = total number of episodes in narrative story, **Proportion of T-units in episode structure** = number of T-units within episodes divided by the total number of T-units in the narrative, **Completeness** = number of critical components mentioned in story narrative from a maximum of 5.

10. and [he uh,] I mean he [he he] was mad about it
11. [and uh] but he decided [to uh] since there was so much and the farmer was so good at producing [uh uh uh] vegetables and such that he [uh he] opened a [um] vegetable store for him
12. and they made a proposition to [uh] go into business together. [Boom.]

Summary for Transcript NI 2

This narrative, also generated by a non-injured participant, represents a good retelling of the story. Although it is seemingly less efficient, as indicated by a smaller proportion of T-units within episode structure, the narrator included all five of the critical content components, resulting in a complete story (see Table 11-2). This retelling is comparable to Transcript 1 in length and grammatical complexity as well as cohesive adequacy. The somewhat lower local coherence score did not detract from the overall gist of the story as indicated by the relatively high score for global coherence. Transcripts 1 and 2 illustrate some of the variability that is seen in "normal" speakers.

Transcript BI 1: Adult Male with Bilateral Lesion of Prefrontal Cortices (Ventromedial)

1. Well the first thing we've seen them together with the broom [and then uh the second thing I think it was uh I think it was I dunno {unintelligible, trails off}]
2. the third picture they were had a tomato plant and something like that
3. and the fourth picture [they had a,] he was growin [cabbage and uh] cabbage and all that stuff [and uh]
4. and [uh] third [he had] he had carrots growing [out of out of the] up in the roof on that thing [uh]
5. and [he uh] he [uh] had a bunch of [cows come into the house while they uh] cows in the house
6. [and and uh he uh] and one time when a cow was sittin on the stool [and and uh] and th the people was] the man was thinking of opening up [a] a [fruit,] fruit stand
7. and he was goin' {unintelligible} them in
8. and then he had the fruit stand opened up and everything [he he was] [and [uh] the next picture was [uh] that's about all I'll tell you]

Summary for Transcript BI 1

This transcript is characterized by numerous problems reflected in the scores of several different analyses (see Table 11-2). Story length is comparable to that of the stories produced by the two non-injured adults, although grammatical complexity is somewhat reduced. Cohesive adequacy is poor and problems begin immediately in T-unit 1 when the participant introduces the term

"them" followed by "they" in T-unit 2, and "he" in T-units 3, 4, and 5 without identifying who the pronouns refer to. The overall story is lacking in content, as reflected in the completeness score in which only two critical components are identified. This individual also only generated one episode; consequently only 25 percent of the T-units produced were within episodic structure. The resulting narrative is difficult to follow and would provide little meaningful information regarding the gist of the story to a naïve listener or reader.

This story was the worst of the three examples presented and was produced by an individual who had the lowest executive function scores and bilateral PFC lesions. Consistent with the reported consequences of PFC damage (Kaczmerek, 1984; Royall, Lauderbach, Cummings, et al., 2002), this individual produced fewer complex sentences and had difficulty developing the narrative in terms of a logical and temporally appropriate sequence, which are abilities associated with executive functions.

Transcript BI 2: Adult Male with Bilateral Lesion of Prefrontal Cortices

1. Old McDonald [umm] started a farm in his apartment first of all and started growing demolishing everything
2. then they started to fix it up
3. and Mrs. McDonald started to plant in the house
4. in the mean time Old McDonald had [umm] started to plant outside
5. then everybody come over and got mad at him because they had all these [uh] plants outside
6. and so they started growing 'em inside
7. and then the cattle cows decided they wanted to come inside.
8. so they come inside and ate all the vegetables in the living room all the carrots. (pause)
9. and then the manager of the apartment (pause) [ummm] got mad at him
10. but [uh] he had a kind heart and bought them their own [ah] vegetable place where they could sell their vegetables and grow 'em
11. and so [uh] the story [ha] has a happy ending

Summary for Transcript BI 2

This story retelling is distinguished from those of the non-injured participants by lower scores for cohesive adequacy and local coherence (see Table 11-2). By contrast, this participant generated four episodes and no T-units outside of episode structure. In addition this individual produced four of the five critical content components, which with the high story grammar scores resulted in a reasonable retelling of the story.

Although this individual also presents with bilateral PFC damage, his executive function scores are higher and his story narrative better than the story produced by participant BI 1. The primary limitations to the story involve a reduction of grammatical complexity and minor difficulty with local coherence. Overall story organization was good and completeness fair, which is consistent with his executive function scores.

Transcript BI 3: Adult Male with Lesion in Right Prefrontal Cortex

1. alright McDonald had an apartment house
2. and he grew vegetables
3. tried to raise cows [and he had vegetables.]
4. his wife had [a] a tomato plant on the kitchen table
5. wasn't doing too good
6. and then finally it started growing
7. and he was outside chopping wood
8. then he started growing vegetables [in the hou-] in the apartment house
9. and people were really getting upset about couple carrots coming through the floors
10. and he had mushrooms in the closet and cabbages on the floor
11. and the supervisor came by and saw what he was doing
12. and [I guess] he kicked him out
13. so he took all his vegetables [and] to a stand, and store whatever and sold 'em

Summary for Transcript BI 3

The final story narrative, produced by an individual with damage to the right PFC, is characterized by reduced grammatical complexity and poor story grammar with a good completeness score (see Table 11-2). It appeared that the individual producing this story narrative had difficulty integrating semantic units at the sentence and text levels. These findings are inconsistent with those reported for anterior right-sided brain damage in that he had no difficulty identifying critical story elements (Wapner, Hamby, & Gardner, 1981) as indicated by his completeness score of five. In spite of his good completeness score, his story grammar was relatively poor. This finding was consistent with his lower executive function scores. The resulting story narrative was complete but disorganized and grammatically simple.

SUMMARY AND DISCUSSION

These transcripts of story retelling and subsequent application of discourse analyses serve as examples of how damage to the PFC can manifest as cognitive communication impairments. Overall the number of words

and T-units included by the participants with brain injuries is generally comparable to non-injured participants, representing intact word-level linguistic ability. There are some apparent difficulties with grammatical complexity in all the discourse samples from the participants with brain injuries; however, this does not have an appreciable impact on the readability of the transcripts at the sentence level. The discourse samples lose their communicative impact due to the lack of clarity, completeness, and structure represented in the transcripts. The participants with brain injuries fail to incorporate clear reference (poor cohesion) for story characters introduced; do not include essential elements in their retellings (incomplete), leaving out events and character information; and fail to incorporate a logical sequential structure to organize information across the entire discourse sample (poor story grammar organization). In this representative sample, the discourse skills and cognitive communication challenges are generally consistent with poor performance on EF measures. Additionally, these difficulties in performance highlight the potential mismatch between relatively intact word and sentence level abilities in the face of marked cognitive communication impairments.

Discourse tasks are inherently demanding and have been described as the juncture where language and cognitive skills work in concert to create an efficient and effective message (Ylvisaker et al., 2008). Discourse analyses provide evidence of disrupted EF abilities and subsequent communication impairments in populations with damage or dysfunction of the PFC. Structured event complex knowledge, the type of information processing frameworks thought to be represented in the PFC, are at risk of disruption in populations with impaired prefrontal cortical functioning, at least in the case of linguistically-based story narratives (Cannizzaro et al., 2010).

These patterns of communication impairment have a number of implications for clinical practice. First, while it is well known that persons who have suffered a TBI often demonstrate changes in discourse ability measurable via story grammar analysis, little is known regarding effectiveness of treatment of these communication deficits (Cannizzaro et al., 2002; Coelho, 2002; 2007; Coelho et al., 2005; Ylvisaker et al., 2001). However, reducing the processing load during discourse communication, through the use of commonly occurring organizational patterns, may lead to improved comprehension and production abilities. Disrupted discourse and communication abilities following TBI are often characterized as being more debilitating than the physical consequences of the injury, reduce the quality of interpersonal relationships, and are thought of as a barrier to independent and productive employment (Coelho et al., 2005;

2007; McCabe and Bliss, 2006; Snow et al., 1998; Ylvisaker et al., 2001; 2007). Modification of discourse by using predictable and meaningful interaction frameworks may lead to improvements in communication between persons with TBI and their communication partners (McCabe & Bliss, 2006; Togher, McDonald, Code, & Grant, 2004). Narratives are a communication medium through which we learn, are able to relate our lives to others, and help us to remember events in context. A better understanding of the cognitive and neural architecture related to the function of these knowledge structures in communication may have implications for the thoughtful implementation of organizational structures for teaching narratives to children, improving cognitive performance in students and adults with and without brain damage, or assessing and treating the communication abilities of persons following neurological insult (Coyne, Baldwin, Cole, et al., 2009; Ferstl, Rinck, & von Cramon, 2005; Hewitt et al., 2006; Ylvisaker, 2003).

REFERENCES

Arkin, S., & Mahendra, N. (2001). Discourse analysis of Alzheimer's patients before and after intervention: Methodology and outcomes. *Aphasiology, 15,* 533–569.

Ash, S., Moore, P., Antani, S., McCawley, G., Work, M., & Grossman, M. (2006). Trying to tell a tale: Discourse impairments in progressive aphasia and frontotemporal dementia. *Neurology, 66,* 1405–1413.

Ash, S., Moore, P., Vesely, L., Gunawardena, D., McMillan, C., Anderson, C., et al. (2009). Non-fluent speech in frontotemporal lobar degeneration. *Journal of Neurolinguistics, 22*(4), 370–383.

Association AS-L-H (2005). *Roles of speech-language pathologists in the identification, diagnosis, and treatment of individuals with cognitive communication disorders: Position statement Secondary Titl.*: American Speech-Language Hearing Association.

Barrett, J. (1998). Old McDonald had an apartment house. New York: Atheneum Publishers.

Biddle, K. R., McCabe, A., & Bliss, L. S. (1996). Narrative skills following traumatic brain injury in children and adults. *Journal of Communication Disorders, 29,* 447–469.

Blair, M., Marczinski, C. A., Davis-Faroque, N., & Kertesz, A. (2007). A longitudinal study of language decline in Alzheimer's disease and frontotemporal dementia. *Journal of the International Neuropsychological Society, 13*(02), 237–245.

Brookshire, B. L., Chapman, S. B., Song, J., & Levin, H. S. (2000). Cognitive and linguistic correlates of children's discourse after closed head injury: A three-year follow-up. *Journal of the International Neuropsychological Society, 6,* 741–751.

Cannizzaro, M. S., Coelho, C. A., & Youse, K. (2002). Treatment of discourse deficits following TBI. *Perspectives on Neurophysiology and Neurogenic Speech and Language Disorders, 12,* 14–19.

Cannizzaro, M. S., Dumas, J., Prelock, P. P., & Newhouse, P. (2010). *What's the story with the prefrontal cortex; how story schema influences narrative discourse processing.* Poster session presented at the Cognitive Neuroscience Society, Montreal, QC Canada.

Chapman, S. B., McKinnon, L., Levin, H. S., Song, J., Meier, M. C., & Chiu, S. (2001). Longitudinal outcome of verbal discourse in children with traumatic brain injury: Three-year follow-up. *Journal of Head Trauma Rehabilitation, 16,* 441.

Chapman, S. B., Zientz, J., Weiner, M., Rosenberg, R., Frawley, W., & Burns, M. H. (2002). Discourse changes in early Alzheimer disease, mild cognitive impairment, and normal aging. *Alzheimer Disease & Associated Disorders 16*(3)(July/September), 177–186.

Cherney, L. R., Shadden, B. B., & Coelho, C. A. (1998). *Analyzing discourse in communicatively impaired adults* (pp. 1–8). Gaithersburg, MD: Aspen.

Chenery, H. J., Copland, D. A., & Murdoch, B. E. (2002). Complex language functions and subcortical mechanisms: Evidence from Huntington's disease and patients with non-thalamic subcortical lesions.

Coelho, C. (2007). Management of discourse deficits following traumatic brain injury: Progress, caveats, and needs. *Semin Speech Lang,* 122–135.

Coelho, C. A. (2002). Story narratives of adults with closed head injury and non-brain-injured adults: Influence of socioeconomic status, elicitation task, and executive functioning. *Journal of Speech, Language, and Hearing Research, 45,* 1232–1248.

Coelho, C. A., Ylvisaker, M., & Turkstra, L. S. (2005). Nonstandardized assessment approaches for individuals with traumatic brain injuries. *Semin Speech Lang, 26,* 223–241.

Coyne, J. T., Baldwin, C., Cole, A., Sibley, C., & Roberts, D. M. (2009). Applying real time physiologic measures of cognitive load to improve training. In D. Schmorrow, I. Estabrooke, & M. Grootjen (Eds.), *Foundations of Augmented Cognition. Neuroergonomics and Operational Neuroscience* (pp. 469–478). Springer Berlin/Heidelberg.

Decker J., & Cannizzaro, M. S. (2007). *The effectiveness of narrative discourse treatment in persons with chronic traumatic brain injury. Title.* Poster session presented at the Annual Convention of the American Speech-Language Hearing Association, Boston, MA.

Dijkstra, K., Bourgeois, M. S., Allen, R. S., & Burgio, L. D. (2004). Conversational coherence: Discourse analysis of older adults with and without dementia. *Journal of Neurolinguistics, 17*(4), 263–283.

Fayol, M., & Lemaire, P. (1993). Levels of approach to discourse. In Joanette H. H. B. Y. (Ed.), *Narrative discourse in neurologically impaired and normally aging adults.* San Diego, CA Singular Publishing Group, pp. 3–21.

Ferstl, E. C., Neumann, J., Bogler, C., & von Cramon, D. Y. (2008). The extended language network: A meta-analysis of neuroimaging studies on text comprehension. *Human brain mapping, 29.*

Ferstl, E. C., Rinck, M., & von Cramon, D. Y. (2005). Emotional and temporal aspects of situation model processing during text comprehension: An event-related fMRI study. *Journal of Congitive Neuroscience, 17,* 724–739.

Ferstl, E. C., & von Cramon, D. Y. (2002). What does the frontomedian cortex contribute to language processing: Coherence or theory of mind? *Neuroimage, 17,* 1599–1612.

Frederiksen, C. H., Bracewell, R. J., Breuleux, A., & Renaud, A. (1990). The cognitive representation and processing of discourse: Function and dysfunction. In Y. Joanette & H. H. Brownell (Eds.), *Discourse ability and brain damage: Theoretical and empirical perspectives* (pp. 69–112). New York: Springer-Verlag.

Fridriksson, J., Nettles, C., Davis, M., Morrow, L., & Montgomery, A. (2006). Functional communication and executive function in aphasia. *Clinical Linguistics and Phonetics, 20,* 401–410.

Gilbert, S. J., & Burgess, P. W. (2008). Executive function. *Current Biology, 18,* R110–R114.

Glosser, G., & Deser, T. (1990). Patterns of discourse production among neurological patients with fluent language disorders. *Brain and Language, 40,* 67–88.

Glosser, G., & Goodglass, H. (1990). Disorders in executive functions among aphasiac and brain damaged patients. *Journal of Clinical and Experimental Neuropsychology, 12,* 485–501.

Gordon, P. C. (1993). Computational and psychological models of discourse. In H. H. Brownell & Y. Joanette (Eds.), *Narrative discourse in neurologically impaired and normal aging adults* (pp. 23–46). San Diego, CA: Singular Publishing Group.

Grafman, J. (1995). Similarities and distinctions among current models of prefrontal cortical functions. In K. J. H. & F. B. J. Grafman (Eds.), *Structure and functions of the human prefrontal cortex* (pp. 337–368). New York: New York Academy of Sciences.

Grafman, J. (2006a). Human prefrontal cortex: Processes and representations. *The frontal lobes development, function and pathology, 69–91.*

Grafman, J. (2006b). Planning and the brain. *The Human Frontal Lobes: Functions and Disorders, 249.*

Grafman, J., & Krueger, F. (2008). The prefrontal cortex stores structured event complexes that are the representational basis for cognitively derived actions. In *Oxford Handbook of Human Action: Mechanisms of Human Action* (p. 197). New York, NY: Oxford University Press.

Grafman, J., & Litvan, I. (1999). Importance of deficits in executive functions. (statistical data included). *The Lancet, 354,* 1921.

Grant, D. A., & Berg, E. A. (1993). *Wisconsin Card Sorting Test.* Tampa, FL: Psychological Assessment Resources.

Gross, R. G., Ash, S., McMillan, C. T., Gunawardena, D., Powers, C., Libon, D. J., et al. (2010). Impaired Information Integration Contributes to Communication Difficulty in Corticobasal Syndrome. *Cognitive and Behavioral Neurology, 23*(1), 1–7. doi:10.1097/WNN.1090b1013e3181c1095e1092f1098.

Halliday, M. A. K., & Hasan, R. (1976). *Cohesion in English.* London: Longman Group Limited.

Helm-Estabrooks, N. (2002). Cognition and aphasia: A discussion and a study. *Journal of Communication Disorders, 35,* 171–186.

Hewitt J., Evans, J. J., & Dritschel, B. (2006). Theory driven rehabilitation of executive functioning: Improving planning skills in people with traumatic brain injury through the use of an autobiographical episodic memory cueing procedure. *Neuropsychologia, 44,* 1468–1474.

Hinckley, J. J., Carr, T. H., & Patterson, J. P. (2001). *Relationships between cognitive abilities, treatment time and treatment type in aphasia.* Paper presented at the Clinical Aphasiology Conference, Santa Fe, NM, June.

Hughes, D., McGillivray, L., & Schmidek, M. (1997). *Guide to narrative language.* Eau Claire, WI: Thinking Publications.

Hunt, K. (1970). Syntactic maturity in school children and adults. *Monographs of the Society for Research in Child Development, 35* (Serial No. 134).

Johnson, N. S., & Mandler, J. M. (1980). A tale of two structures: Underlying and surface forms in stories. *Poetics, 9,* 51–86.

Kaczmarek, B. (1984). Neurolinguistic analysis of verbal utterances in patients with focal lesions of frontal lobes. *Brain and Language, 21,* 52–58.

Krueger, F., Moll, J., Zahn, R., Heinecke, A., & Grafman, J. (2007). Event frequency modulates the processing of daily life activities in human medial prefrontal cortex. *Cereb. Cortex, 17,* 2346–2353.

Laine, M., Laakso, M., Vuorinen, E., & Rinne, J. (1998). Coherence and informativeness of discourse in two dementia types. *Journal of Neurolinguistics, 11*(1–2), 79–87.

Le, K., Coelho, C., Mozeiko, J., & Grafman, J. (2011). Measuring goodness of story narratives. *Journal of Speech, Language, and Hearing Research, 54,* 118–126.

Lesniak, M., Bak, T., Czepiel, W., Seniow, J., & Czlonkowska, A. (2008). Frequency and prognostic value of cognitive disorders in stroke patients. *Dementia and Geriatric Cognitive Disorders, 26,* 356–363.

Lehman Blake, M. (2006). Clinical relevance of discourse characteristics after right hemisphere brain damage. *American Journal of Speech-Language Pathology, 15,* 255–267.

Lezak, M. D., Howieson, D. B., & Loring, D. W. (2004). Executive functions and motor performance. In *Neuropsychological assessment, 4th ed* (pp. 611–646). New York: Oxford University Press.

Liles, B. Z., Coelho, C. A., Duffy, R. J., & Zalagens, M. R. (1989). Effects of elicitation procedures on the narratives of normal and closed head-injured adults. *Journal of Speech and Hearing Disorders, 54,* 356–366.

Litvan, I., Frattali, C., & Duffy, J. R. (2005). Characterizing and Assessing Speech and Language Disturbances. In I. Litvan (Ed.), *Atypical Parkinsonian Disorders* (pp. 255–276). Totowa, NJ: Humana Press.

Maguire, E. A., Frith, C. D., & Morris, R. G. M. (1999). The functional neuroanatomy of comprehension and memory: The importance of prior knowledge. *Brain, 122,* 1839–1850.

Mar, R. A. (2004). The neuropsychology of narrative: Story comprehension, story production and their interrelation. *Neuropsychologia, 42,* 1414–1434.

McCabe, A., & Bliss, L. S. (2006). Struggling to make sense: Patterns of impairment in adult narrative discourse. *Imagination, Cognition and Personality, 25,* 321–336.

Mentis, M., & Prutting, C. A. (1987). Cohesion in the discourse of normal and head-injured adults. *Journal of Speech and Hearing Research, 30,* 583–595.

Miller, B., & Cummings, J. (2007). *The human frontal lobes.* New York, NY: Guilford Press.

Miller, E., & Wallis, J. (2009). Executive function and higher-order cognition: Definition and neural substrates. *Encyclopedia of Neuroscience, 4*, 99–104.

Murray, L. L. (2000). Spoken language production in Huntington's and Parkinson's Diseases. *J Speech Lang Hear Res, 43*(6), 1350–1366.

Murray, L. L., & Stout, J. C. (1999). Discourse comprehension in Huntington's and Parkinson's Diseases. *Am J Speech Lang Pathol, 8*(2), 137–148.

Partiot, A., Grafman, J., Sadato, N., Flitman, S., & Wild, K. (1996). Brain activation during script event processing. *Neuroreport, 7*, 761–766.

Peelle, J. E., & Grossman, M. (2008). Language processing in frontotemporal dementia: A brief review. *Language and Linguistics Compass, 2*(1), 18–35.

Prescott, T., Gruber, J., Olson, M., & Fuller, K. (1987). Hanoi revisited. *Clinical Aphasiology, 17*, 249–258.

Purdy, M. H., Duffy, R. J., & Coelho, C. A. (1994). An investigation of the communicative use of trained symbols in aphasic adults following multimodality training. *Clinical Aphasiology, 22*, 345–356.

Ripich, D. N., Vertes, D., Whitehouse, P., Fulton, S., & Ekelman, B. (1991). Turn-taking and speech act patterns in the discourse of senile dementia of the Alzheimer's type patients. *Brain and Language, 40*(3), 330–343.

Royall, D. R., Lauderbach, E. C., Cummings, J. L., Reeve, A., Rummans, T. A., Kaufer, D. I., et al. (2002). Executive control function: A review of its promise and challenges for clinical research [Report from Committee on Research of the American Neuropsychiatric Association]. *Journal of Neuropsychiatry and Clinical Neurosciences, 14*, 377–405.

Rumelhart, D. E. (1975). Notes on a schema for stories. In *Representation and understanding: Studies in cognitive science* (pp. 211–236). New York: Academic Press.

Saldert, C., Fors, A., Stroberg, S., & Hartelius, L. (2010). Comprehension of complex discourse in different stages of Huntington's disease. *International Journal of Language & Communication Disorders, 45*, 656–669.

Sirigu, A., Cohen, L., Zalla, T., Pradat-Diehl, P., Van Eeckhout, P., & Grafman, J. (1998). Distinct frontal regions for processing sentence syntax and story grammar. *Cortex, 34*, 771–778.

Sirigu, A., Zalla, T., Pillon, B., Grafman, J., Dubois, B., & Agid, Y. (1995). Planning and script analysis following prefrontal lobe lesionsa. *Annals of the New York Academy of Sciences, 769*, 277–288.

Snow, P., Douglas, J., & Ponsford, J. (1998). Conversational discourse abilities following severe traumatic brain injury: A follow up study. *Brain Injury, 12*, 911–935.

Stein, N. L., & Glenn, C. G. (1979). An analysis of story comprehension in elementary school children. In Freedle R. O. (Ed.), *New directions in discourse processing* (pp. 53–120). Norwood, NJ: Ablex.

Stemmer, B. (1999). Discourse studies in neurologically impaired populations: A quest for action. *Brain and Language, 402*–418.

Thorndyke, P. W. (1977). Cognitive structures in comprehension and memory of narrative discourse. *Cognitive Psychology, 9*, 77–110.

Togher, L., McDonald, S., Code, C., & Grant, S. (2004). Training communication partners of people with traumatic brain injury: A randomized controlled trial. *Aphasiology, 18*, 313–335.

Tucker, F. M., & Hanlon, R. E. (1998). Effects of mild traumatic brain injury on narrative discourse production. *Brain Injury, 12*, 783–792.

Van Leer, E., & Turkstra, L. (1999). The effect of elicitation task on discourse coherence and cohesion in adolescents with brain injury. *Journal of Communication Disorders, 32*, 327–349.

Wapner, W., Hamby, S., & Gardner, H. (1981). The role of the right hemisphere in the apprehension of complex linguistic materials. *Brain and Language, 14*, 15–33.

Villemarette-Pittman, N. R., Stanford, M. S., & Greve, K. W. (2003). Language and executive function in self-reported impulsive aggression. *Personality and Individual Differences, 34*(8), 1533–1544.

Wood, J. N., & Grafman, J. (2003). Human prefrontal cortex: Processing and representational perspectives. *Nature Reviews Neuroscience, 4*, 139–147.

Wood, J. N., Knutson, K. M., & Grafman, J. (2005). Psychological structure and neural correlates of event knowledge. *Cerebral Cortex, 15*, 1155–1161.

Ylvisaker, M. (2003). Context-sensitive cognitive rehabilitation: Theory and practice. *Brain Impairment, 4*, 1–16.

Ylvisaker, M., Szekeres, S., & Feeney, T. (2001). Communication disorders associated with traumatic brain injury. In Chapey, R. (Ed.), *Language intervention strategies in aphasia and related neurogenic communication disorders, 4th ed* (pp. 745–807). Philadelphia: Lippincott, Williams & Wilkins.

Ylvisaker, M., Szekeres, S., & Feeney, T. (2008). Communication disorders associated with traumatic brain injury. In Chapey, R. (Ed.), *Language intervention strategies in aphasia and related neurogenic communication disorders* (pp. 879–962), *5th ed.* Philladelphia: Lippincott, Williams & Wilkins.

Zacks, J., & Tversky, B. (2009). Event structure in perception and conception. *Psychological Bulletin, 127*, 3–21.

Zinn, S., Bosworth, H. B., Hoenig, H. M., & Swartzwelder, H. S. (2007). Executive function deficits in acute stroke. *Archives of Physical Medicine and Rehabilitation, 88*, 173–180.

CHAPTER 12

Management of Acquired Language Disorders Associated with Attentional Impairment

CHAPTER OUTLINE

Richard K. Peach

Attention deficits in communicatively-disordered populations are well documented (Blake, Duffy, Myers, & Tompkins, 2002; Erickson, Goldinger, & LaPointe, 1996; Fillingham, Sage, & Lambon Ralph, 2006; Murray, 1999; Myers & Blake, 2008; Peach, Rubin, & Newhoff, 1994) and are frequently described as a contributing factor to the language impairments that are observed in these groups. That is, some of the language problems of communicatively-impaired individuals are thought to be due, at least in part, to a reduction in attentional abilities that are needed to (a) focus a listener on incoming verbal information while excluding competing or distracting information, (b) maintain a continuous record of conversation and context to support the interpretation of new information, and (c) construct coherent verbal outputs from among a number of contending alternatives (Crosson, 2000; Chapter 8, this text). For example, attentional impairments have been associated with problems in listening and reading comprehension following aphasia (Coelho, 2005; Murray, 2002; Murray, Keeton, & Karcher, 2006; Sinotte & Coelho, 2007), with the conversational problems observed in individuals with Alzheimer disease (Alberoni, Baddeley, Della Sala, et al., 1992), right-hemisphere damage (Myers & Blake, 2008) and traumatic brain injury (Stierwalt & Murray, 2002; Ylvisaker, Szekeres, & Feeney, 2008), and in the lexical and discourse deficits found in the language production of individuals with aphasia (Hula & McNeil, 2008, Murray, Holland, & Beeson, 1998), Alzheimer's disease (Kempler, Andersen, & Henderson, 1995; Neils, Roeltgen, & Greer, 1995), right-hemisphere damage (Myers & Blake, 2008), and traumatic brain injury (Ylvisaker et al., 2008).

It is not surprising, then, that some recent approaches to the rehabilitation of such language disorders have

241

emphasized the amelioration of a variety of attention deficits, including those concerned with selecting, sustaining, dividing, and alternating attention to both external and internal information. In such an approach, attention is typically conceived as a general pool of resources that are exogenous to but nonetheless critical for a variety of communicative behaviors. Treatments that stimulate and improve attentional processing might then be assumed to yield similar improvements in communication behaviors that depend on attention. Unfortunately, this has not been the case. While improvements in the specific skills necessary to perform a variety of tasks have been reported following attentional treatments, evidence for generalization of these improvements to related behaviors has been lacking (Park & Ingles, 2001; Sohlberg, Avery, Kennedy, et al., 2003).

These observations have led some to suggest that, in order for attentional treatments to be effective with regard to behaviors such as language, these treatments should be performed within the language domain and under conditions that compete for attentional resources (Fischler, 2000; Hula & McNeil, 2008). The premise underlying this position is that attentional processing is apt to improve only when such endogenous resources are deployed in the service of specific language tasks that requires control over and coordination of multiple processes, such as semantic, syntactic, and phonologic. Inasmuch as previous treatment studies have not necessarily focused on attention for specific cognitive tasks like language under conditions that challenge patients' attentional control, this may be one reason for the poor generalization of improved attention to untreated behaviors such as language.

Such an approach is consistent with the perspective that language is not simply an object of attention but rather is, in itself, an attention-focusing mechanism (Langacker, 2008). According to Crosson (2000), intention (the preparation to use language) "affects attention because the intention to perform a particular activity determines the particular internal and external sources of information to which we attend" (p. 375). For example, lexical selection (for both open- and closed-class words) engages central attentional mechanisms (Ayora, Jannsen, Dell'Acqua, & Alario, 2009; Hula & McNeil, 2008) while grammaticalized elements (conjunctions, prepositions, bound morphemes, etc.) direct the listener's attention to important aspects of sentences that convey the specific meanings intended by speakers or writers (Taube-Schiff & Segalowitz, 2005). In discourse, anaphoric constructions (i.e., those that use a noun or pronoun to refer to an entity that was previously mentioned) require that attention be directed to an antecedent occurring in an earlier sentence (Myachykov &

Posner, 2005). It might be expected then that problems in adequately "windowing" attention (directing the distribution of attention over a referent scene in a specific pattern) (Talmy, 2003) for these and other language tasks can produce the types of communication disturbances identified above.

In this chapter, the assessment and rehabilitation of attention deficits in cognitive-communication disorders are discussed using a language processing perspective. Emphasis is placed on the treatment of attentional problems as they unfold during specific linguistic tasks. Improvements in allocation of attentional resources during language processing should then produce improvements in communication functioning. Although there is scant evidence to suggest that language-based attention treatment will result in more favorable outcomes than those that have been reported in previous attention treatment programs, such a theoretically-motivated approach provides optimism for achieving improved communication outcomes that have heretofore been lacking.

ATTENTION DEFICITS IN POPULATIONS WITH ACQUIRED LANGUAGE DISORDERS

Attention deficits are among the most widely reported cognitive problems following brain damage and contribute to the acquired language disorders seen in these patients. A brief overview of the attention and language problems associated with various neuropathologies is provided here (see also Chapter 3 and Box 12-1).

Stroke

In a sample of consecutive patients with a wide range of ages and lengths of hospitalization and an even distribution of left and right hemisphere stroke, Hyndman, Pickering, and Ashburn (2008) found high levels of attention deficits at the time these patients were discharged to the community. Fifty-one percent of the patients demonstrated divided attention deficits while approximately 37 percent of the patients demonstrated sustained and auditory and visual selective attention deficits. While some improvements could be detected at 6 and 12 months after discharge, there was no clear recovery of attentional abilities in these patients.

Knopman, Roberts, Geda, et al. (2009) investigated the relationship between cognitive impairment and stroke in a population-based sample of elderly individuals with mild cognitive impairment (MCI) and no evidence of dementia. MCI was classified as either amnestic if there was evidence for memory impairment or nonamnestic if there was no memory impairment. Participants

Box 12-1

Functional Equivalency of Attention Deficits?

The language problems of brain-damaged individuals due to attentional deficits may be summarized as follows. Poorer confrontation naming, oral word reading, and auditory word recognition are observed when stimuli are presented in the contralesional hemispace to patients with parietal lobe lesions in either hemisphere. Problems with basic language tasks such as semantic judgment, lexical decision, word retrieval, and sentence production arise when they are performed under complex conditions that divide and compete for attention. Pragmatic disorders, including misinterpretation of conversations, irrelevant or inappropriate statements, and failure to appreciate non-literal meanings in discourse emerge when brain-damaged individuals fail to (a) detect, sustain, or disengage from important contextual cues, spatial locations, or stimulus categories; or (b) maintain or suppress alternate interpretations of a discourse that are necessary for its correct understanding. Sentence and discourse production may suffer when attention allocated to the contents of working memory is insufficient to allow full activation and/or elaboration of the plans for organizing linguistic outputs.

Although discussions of the impact of attentional deficits on language functioning have traditionally been organized according to the specific neuropathologies underlying those impairments (i.e., stroke to one hemisphere or the other, dementing processes, traumatic brain injury), it should not be surprising that attentional deficits arise following most types of brain damage. Inasmuch as the neural network that underlies attention is distributed with bilateral cortical and subcortical contributions (Filley, 2002; Knudsen, 2007; Mesulam, 1990, 1998), attentional deficits should be expected from most any type of brain damage. While it may appear that the attentional impairments identified above have been assigned unique status based upon their underlying neuropathologies, all of the language deficits associated with these clinical groups can be associated with four processes that are fundamental to attention: working memory (including spatial working memory), top-down sensitivity control, competitive selection, and automatic bottom-up filtering for salient stimuli (Knudsen, 2007) (see Figure 12-1). According to Knudsen, working memory is a highly dynamic form of memory that operates over seconds and temporarily stores information for detailed analysis. Competitive selection is the process that determines which information gains access to working memory. Top-down sensitivity control regulates the relative signal strengths of the different information channels that compete for access to working memory while salience filters automatically enhance responses to infrequent or biologically-important stimuli.

Despite the dissimilarity of the clinical populations that have been studied, it may be that the attentional impairments that are observed among these patients are functionally equivalent (Ylvisaker, Hanks, & Johnson-Green, 2003). When viewed through this lens, the lack of differences in attentional impairments demonstrated by patients with brain damage in contrasting regions of the same (Murray et al., 1997) or different cerebral hemispheres (Arvedson & McNeil, 1987; Coslett, 1999; Murray, 2000) should not be unexpected. And in the absence of evidence establishing that the attentional impairments on similar language tasks within and across different clinical populations are qualitatively different, the approaches taken to rehabilitation of communication problems secondary to attention deficits have continued to rely on treatments that address the fundamental processes described in patients with a variety of underlying neuropathologies (Coelho, 2005; Crosson, 2008, Crosson, Fabrizio, Singletary, et al., 2007; Dotson, Singletary, Fuller, et al., 2008; Helm-Estabrooks, Connor, & Albert, 2000; Murray, Keeton, & Karcher, 2006; Peck, Moore, & Crosson, 2004; Sinotte & Coelho, 2007; Youse & Coelho, 2009).

underwent nursing, neurological and neuropsychological evaluations to assign a clinical diagnosis. Stroke history was then obtained from the study participants and verified by medical records and the findings obtained in the neurological evaluation. Logistical regression analyses demonstrated a higher risk of MCI in study participants with a history of stroke. With regard to MCI subtype, the association of stroke was greater for nonamnestic versus amnestic MCI. A history of stroke was also found to be associated with lower functioning in

each of the cognitive domains that were tested except for memory. The association was found to be strongest for attention and executive functioning.

Arvedson and McNeil (1987) compared accuracy and oral response times from left-hemisphere damaged aphasic (LH), right-hemisphere nonaphasic (RH), and non-brain-damaged (NBD) individuals for two focused attention tasks (semantic judgment and lexical decision) under binaural listening conditions. For semantic judgment, the LH group was less accurate and had

Figure 12-1 Functional components of attention. Information about the world is transduced by the nervous system and is processed by salience filters that respond differentially to infrequent or important stimuli (bottom-up). Neural representations in various hierarchies encode information about the world, movements, memories, the animal's emotional state, etc. A competitive process selects the representation with the highest signal strength for entry into the circuitry that underlies working memory. Working memory can direct top-down bias signals that modulate the sensitivity of representations that are being processed in working memory. The selection process can also direct top-down bias signals that reflect the result of the competitive selection. Working memory and competitive selection direct eye movements and other orienting behaviors that modify the effects of the world on the animal's nervous system. Corollary discharges associated with gaze control modulate sensitivity control. Voluntary attention involves working memory, top-down sensitivity control, and competitive selection operating as a recurrent loop. [From Knudsen, E. L. (2007). Fundamental components of attention. *Annual Review of Neuroscience, 30,* 57–78.]

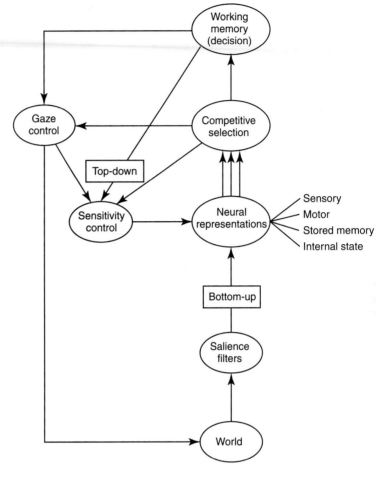

significantly longer response times than the NBD group. The RH group did not differ from either of the other two groups with regard to accuracy or response time. For lexical decision, both brain-damaged groups performed more poorly than the NBD group although there were no group differences for overall response times. Arvedson and McNeil (1987) concluded that the performance deficits observed in both groups were consistent with problems in attention and resource allocation.

Coslett (1999) investigated verbal processing following left and right hemisphere strokes as a function of the side of space to which subjects directed their attention. The study was motivated by reports of improved performance in stroke patients on a variety of sensory and motor tasks when stimuli were presented in the ipsilesional versus the contralateral hemispace. Unlike previous studies, however, this study sought to assess

(in addition to other goals) the degree to which hemispatial influences affect language processing, a behavior that doesn't appear to have a critical dependence on spatial representations. Because of the documented role of the parietal lobes in spatial functioning, Coslett predicted that patients with parietal lobe lesions would perform best when stimuli were presented in the ipsilesional space.

Subjects with left and right ischemic infarctions of parietal, non-parietal, and subcortical regions were assessed on three language tasks: confrontation naming, oral word reading, and auditory word recognition. Stimuli were presented to either the left or right side of body midline. The results demonstrated that the majority of subjects with parietal lobe lesions, whether of the left or right hemisphere, performed significantly worse when responding to language stimuli presented in the contralesional as compared to the ipsilesional hemispace. No other subjects demonstrated this pattern. Coslett interpreted the data in terms of a spatial registration hypothesis that suggests that all perceived stimuli are coded (i.e., marked) by the individual according to their location in space. Such marking binds a token specifying the location of stimuli to sensory and motor coordinate systems relevant to the position of focal attention. Binding is assumed to depend upon spatial attention, a limited capacity resource that activates the corresponding token and, once highlighted, bestows a processing advantage on the object or action linked to that token. When listening to a speaker, lexical retrieval and semantic search are linked to a token specifying the location of the person on the spatial map, which thus facilitates language processing. This account suggests that individuals with disrupted spatial processing will perform less well on verbal tasks when they require linkages to a location mediated by the impaired spatial system. Coslett suggests that this is one reason for the facilitation of language processing observed in individuals with acquired language disorders when they are gazing directly at a speaker.

Further support for the spatial registration hypothesis might be found in a study by Ansaldo, Arguin, and Lecours (2004). In their longitudinal investigation of recovery from Wernicke aphasia in a patient with a left parietotemporal stroke, they demonstrated that improved lexical semantic processing, as assessed by a lexical decision task, was correlated with presentation in the left visual but not right visual hemispace. An interaction between the grammatical class and the imageability of the lexical stimuli presented to the left visual hemispace suggested that the right hemisphere contributions to the observed recovery were linguistic. But correlations between the patient's global (nonlateralized) lexical and attentional performance, as assessed by the Nonverbal Stroop Test, suggested that recovery was mediated by attentional factors as well. While the authors conclude that the findings associated with presentations to the left visual hemispace likely represented premorbid language abilities of the right hemisphere, the observed language facilitation may just as well have been associated with the lexical highlighting that resulted with presentations in the ipsilesional hemispace.

Murray (2000) evaluated the influence of attentional deficits resulting from left-hemisphere (aphasic) and right-hemisphere brain damage (RBD) on word retrieval following stroke. Subjects completed phrases that were either highly (responses are drawn from a limited or closed set of choices) or minimally (responses are from open set with many plausible choices) constrained under a series of conditions with increasing attentional demands. In the single-task condition, subjects completed the phrases or discriminated tones (high versus low) in isolation (i.e., without distraction). In the focal attention condition, phrase and tone stimuli were presented simultaneously but the subjects completed one task only (phrase completion or tone discrimination). In the divided attention condition, subjects heard the phrase and tone stimuli simultaneously, discriminated the tones, and then completed the phrases. For both LH and RH groups, word retrieval accuracy was influenced by attentional demands. Neither group performed differently from a non-brain-damaged group in the single-task condition. However, in the focused and divided attention conditions, non-brain-damaged subjects performed significantly better than LH and RH subjects. Murray interpreted the lack of differences in the word retrieval abilities of the two brain-damaged groups as evidence that the deficits were not of purely linguistic origin. Instead, the results provide support for a negative interaction between attention and language processing in both aphasic and RBD subjects.

Aphasia

Murray, Holland, and Beeson (1997) found evidence for attention and resource allocation deficits on auditory-linguistic listening tasks in stroke patients with mild aphasia. Patients with frontal versus posterior lesions were compared to normal listeners on semantic judgment and lexical decision tasks during three listening conditions: isolation, focused attention, and divided attention. In the isolation condition, subjects performed either task without distraction; in the focused attention condition, subjects listened to competing primary and secondary stimuli but completed the primary listening task only. In two divided attention conditions, subjects again listened to competing primary and secondary stimuli but were required to complete both tasks. The type of distraction in the secondary task was either verbal (semantic judgment and lexical decision competing with each other) or nonverbal (semantic judgment or lexical decision competing with a tone discrimination task).

While aphasic and control subjects performed comparably during isolation conditions, both aphasic groups performed less accurately and more slowly than the normal group during the focused and divided attention conditions. The performance differences between the groups increased as the complexity of the listening conditions increased. Greater dual-task interference was observed in aphasic and normal subjects when the secondary task was verbal versus nonverbal. Murray et al. (1997) concluded that (a) the differences between aphasic and normal subjects on auditory-linguistic tasks are more quantitative than qualitative and support the concept of attention allocation inefficiency as an explanatory construct for aphasic performance; (b) the underlying cause of these inefficiencies is damage to a diffusely-represented attentional network that involves both frontal and posterior components; and (c) the greatest decrements in aphasic performance should be expected when linguistic processing demands competition for verbal attentional resources.

Murray, Holland, and Beeson (1998) found that these attentional impairments also negatively influence the spoken language production of individuals with mild aphasia. In this study, the morphosyntactic, lexical, and pragmatic characteristics of picture descriptions produced by normal and aphasic speakers were assessed under conditions imposing increasing demands on attention allocation (isolation, focused attention, and divided attention). The distracter in this study was the tone discrimination task. When compared to normal speakers, aphasic subjects produced significantly fewer well-formed utterances and significantly more simple versus complex sentences in the divided attention condition. They also produced significantly fewer words, more word-finding errors, and fewer correct information units (Nicholas & Brookshire, 1993) as attentional demands increased. The number of unsuccessful utterances (failure to communicate accurate and novel information or failure to follow directions) also increased significantly in the divided attention conditions when compared to isolation or the focused attention condition.

Right-Hemisphere Brain Damage

In a retrospective chart review of a large inpatient rehabilitation unit, Blake and colleagues (2002) found relationships between attentional and other cognitive deficits and the presence of acquired pragmatic disorders associated with hypo-responsiveness, hyper-responsiveness, and interpersonal interactions. In addition, basic deficits in expressive and receptive language functions were found in approximately one quarter of their patient sample. Myers and Blake (2008) suggest that attentional deficits impair RBD patients' ability to (a) appreciate visual and verbal cues within the context of communication, (b) shift attention during conversations, and (c) sustain attention to the communication environment and filter distractions. They also suggest that attentional deficits place more demands on cognitive resources, especially as interactions become more complex. These contribute to difficulties in forming and maintaining inferences about

the meaning of verbal communications. As a result, RBD patients often miss the overall theme, or central point, of narratives.

According to Myers and Blake (2008), communicative interactions increase in complexity when they require participants to form elaborative inferences. Elaborative inferences require an individual to attend to and make predictions about the emotions or motives of a conversational partner and therefore go to the implied rather than literal meaning of a communication. Doing so requires integration of multiple cues or selecting from several possible interpretations. Selective attention deficits may interfere with the ability to filter extraneous information and recognize important contextual cues that may manifest as seemingly irrelevant interpretations of, and responses to, the communication environment (e.g., attending to and/or describing isolated details of an integrated scene, failing to appreciate jokes or indirect requests, or producing inappropriate statements based on faulty inferences during discourse).

These problems appear to arise in discourse when revision of an initial inference is required for correct interpretation. Two different theories of faulty lexical-processing have been described to account for these deficits. One suggests that RHD patients activate diffuse semantic fields in response to lexical inputs that include distant and unusual semantic features; the fields are shaped by context and modulated by attention and time course. These large semantic fields provide course interpretations of words that are frequently ambiguous but important for understanding natural language (Jung-Beeman, 2005; Tompkins, Fassbinder, Scharp, & Meigh, 2008). It has been suggested that the problems RHD patients have with comprehending inferences may stem from difficulty sustaining distant activations that are needed to correctly interpret non-literal interpretations of a discourse (Tompkins, Scharp, Meigh, & Fassbinder, 2008).

A second theory suggests that RHD patients maintain initial interpretations even when the context indicates that they are inappropriate (Tompkins, Baumgaertner, Lehman, and Fassbinder, 2000). That is, RBD patients appear to activate both initial and revised inferences, but have difficulty suppressing an irrelevant or incompatible interpretation once it has been activated. Deficient suppression therefore might be understood as an impairment of inhibition (as conceived in models of selective attention) resulting from the demands suppression places on attentional resources (Tompkins et al., 2000; Tompkins, Blake, Baumgaertner, & Fassbinder, 2002). More recent evidence has confirmed that RBD patients generate and generally maintain inferences similarly to non-brain-damaged individuals (Blake, 2009) although these inferences did not concern ambiguities as in previous work.

Alzheimer Disease

Attentional impairments following Alzheimer disease (AD) are now well known (Belleville, Chertkow, & Gauthier, 2007; Foldi, Lobosco, & Schaefer, 2002; Levinoff, Saumier, & Chertkow, 2005). In their review of attentional functions in AD, Parasuraman and Haxby (1993) suggest that attentional deficits may appear coincidentally with the memory deficits that arise in the earliest stages of the disease. While selective attention may be spared in some patients, disengagement of attention, attentional switching between spatial locations and stimulus categories, divided attention for auditory, visual, and motor tasks, and sustained attention in conditions requiring effortful processing have been found to be impaired in even mildly affected individuals.

While the potential for attention deficits to disrupt language is recognized (Foldi et al., 2002), few studies have investigated this relationship directly. Alberoni et al. (1992) found that patients with AD have difficulty following even simple conversations and that this problem becomes amplified when the conversation involves multiple participants and/or they move from one location to another. They attributed this impairment to divided attention deficits that make it difficult for these patients to shift and refocus attention as well as track and remember the individual contributions and locations of each participant to a conversation. Deficits in attentional control (i.e., the focusing on and recall of important information) may also contribute to these conversational difficulties (Castel, Balota, & McCabe, 2009).

Kempler, Andersen, and Henderson (1995) assessed naming in patients with AD and found highly variable performance that was associated with attentional performance. Participants who consistently erred on the same items over two occasions were thought to demonstrate a deficit in lexical semantic representations while those who inconsistently erred on stimulus items were thought to demonstrate deficits in lexical access. The less consistent participants were significantly more impaired on tasks assessing attention. Patient severity (disease, anomia) could not account for the results. The authors concluded that impaired attention, along with deficits in lexical knowledge, contribute to anomia in AD.

Neils, Roeltgen, and Greer (1995) investigated the spelling abilities of people with mild AD. Participants completed tests of direct and delayed word copying, spelling to dictation for regular, irregular, and nonwords, and written picture description. They also completed tests of sustained attention (letter cancellation), visual attention (visual search), and language ability (Boston Naming Test). The percentages of phonemically implausible (PI) spelling errors for the AD participants as well as for a group of matched normal participants were calculated for the real words in the test battery. AD participants were found to produce more PI spelling errors than their normal counterparts. The two visual attention tests were found to be better predictors of these errors than the language test.

Participants with mild AD also produced more errors for delayed versus direct copying and for longer versus shorter dictated words. When considering all the errors produced by these participants (phonemically plausible and implausible), the results suggested that their spelling errors are due to breakdowns in linguistic (plausible errors) and post-linguistic (implausible errors) processes. The evidence from the attentional tests, as well as the patterns obtained for copying and words of varying lengths, suggested that the post-linguistic processing breakdown is at the level of the graphemic buffer.

The typical pattern of cognitive decline in AD is generally thought to be one of early episodic memory loss followed by combinations of attention-executive, language, and visuospatial impairment, although there is growing evidence of atypical focal cortical presentations of AD (Alladi, Xuereb, Bak, et al., 2007). Recently, Davidson, Irizarry, Bray, et al. (2009) analyzed the scores obtained from administration of the Mini-Mental Status Examination and the Mattis Dementia Rating Scale-2 to a large group of patients with mild/moderate AD to explore the existence of cognitive subgroups within this sample. Four subgroups were identified: a mild group and a severe group with fairly uniform impairment across cognitive domains that were distinguished by the severity of their impairments; a memory group with impairment of memory and orientation and relative sparing of attention, construction, and language; and an attention/construction group with impairments in attention and construction and relative sparing of memory and orientation. The attention/construction group was also characterized by language impairment at levels that were similar to those observed in the severe group. Separate groups with prominent deficits in language and visuospatial construction were not identified.

From these studies, it can be suggested that not all patients with AD will have language impairments.

However, for those who do, particularly those with mild AD, attentional deficits appear to be a causative factor, along with linguistic breakdowns, for the language problems of these individuals.

Traumatic Brain Injury

Impairments to language (Coelho, 2007; Hagen, 1984; Levin, 1981; Sarno, Buonaguro, & Levita, 1986) and attention (Stierwalt & Murray, 2002; Willmott, Ponsford, Hocking, & Schonberger, 2009) are reported frequently following traumatic brain injury (TBI). In a study of 25 participants with severe closed head injuries, impairments in lexical-semantic and sentential semantic skills, verbal fluency, complex auditory comprehension, and attentional operations were found to comprise a set of "cardinal" cognitive-linguistic deficits following TBI (Hinchliffe, Murdoch, Chenery, et al., 1998). The co-occurrence of these deficits suggests that the problems these individuals have with language may be a result of difficulties in allocating attentional resources effectively for linguistic cognitive operations (Peach, 1992). That is, TBI, even in mild cases, may affect how much and how rapidly linguistic information can be processed (Whelan, Murdoch, & Bellamy, 2007).

The profile of language deficits following TBI is generally referred to as confused or disorganized, which suggests that the disorder is due, at least in part, to problems in verbal planning (Alexander, 2002). Recent work has demonstrated that TBI patients have difficulty planning sentences in isolation (Ellis & Peach, 2009) and in discourse (Deschaine & Peach, 2008). Deficient planning for sentences in discourse have been found to be related to difficulties allocating attention for complex tasks (as indexed by the Trail Making Test, Part B) and suggest that the problem may be part of a more global planning impairment resulting from executive dysfunction. Such difficulties might be thought to result from impairment to the supervisory attentional system, a voluntary, top-down component of the executive system that facilitates the activation of mental schemas that are needed to interpret inputs and determine subsequent actions (Shallice, 1982). Sentential and discourse impairments therefore might be seen as a failure of executive control over cognitive and linguistic organizing processes (Ylvisaker, Szekeres, & Feeney, 2008).

Patients who suffer TBI often have difficulties participating in conversations; these difficulties can be linked to their attentional impairments (Coelho, 2007; Stierwalt & Murray, 2002). They tend to demonstrate problems with maintaining or extending the topic of discussion, using reference, and integrating relevant information because of poor sustained or selective attention. Their communication may be incoherent due to difficulty attending to and maintaining a plan for discourse as well as the listener's perspective. They also produce socially inappropriate output because of a failure to attend to social cues.

SPECIFICITY OF ATTENTION INTERVENTIONS FOR LANGUAGE DISORDERS

The outcomes associated with attentional treatments for acquired language disorders have been weak (Rohling, Faust, Beverly, & Demakis, 2009) and are most likely due to the generalized or non-specific approach that these studies have taken with regard to attention intervention. For example, Helm-Estabrooks, Connor, and Albert (2000) used nonlinguistic tasks to treat sustained, selective, and alternating attention. Researchers at the University of Florida treat spatial attention by increasing their patients' orientation to left hemi-space during picture naming so as to exploit right-hemisphere attention mechanisms (Crosson et al., 2007; Dotson et al., 2008; Peck et al., 2004). Still others (Coelho, 2005; Murray et al., 2006, Sinotte & Coelho, 2007; Youse & Coelho, 2009) have treated focused, alternating, selective, and divided attention using a variety of linguistic stimuli (numbers, letters, words) and tasks that are included in Attention Process Training II (Sohlberg, Johnson, Paule, Raskin, & Mateer, 2001), a program to treat attention impairments in patients with mild cognitive impairments. While all of these approaches assume that improved language will result from increased attention to linguistic stimuli, none of them are motivated by an analysis of the ways that specific linguistic processes recruit select attentional operations in the service of language.

The need for specificity in attention treatment has been addressed previously. Sturm, Willmes, Orgass, and Hartje (1997) demonstrated that specific attention functions improve in patients with localized vascular lesions only when specific training is received for that function. In this study, computer based programs were used to train the intensity (alertness, vigilance) and selectivity (selective and divided attention) aspects of attention. Even when patients demonstrated deficits in both domains of intensity or selection, improvements were only noted for the single domain that received training. This was particularly evident for the intensity aspects of attention. Specific attention training for alertness has also been found to contribute to reorganization of the right-hemisphere functional network known to subserve the alertness domain in normal subjects. Similar reorganization was not observed for right-hemisphere brain-damaged patients who received non-specific (memory) training for alertness (Sturm, Longoini, Weis, et al., 2004).

Park and colleagues (Park, Proulx, & Towers, 1999; Park & Ingles, 2001; Park & Barbuto, 2005) find no evidence to support approaches that incorporate direct training of distinct attentional components (e.g., sustained, selective, divided, and alternating attention). They have found, however, that attention treatments that focus on learning or relearning of specific skills that are important to desired outcomes or behaviors that have functional significance resulted in significant improvement.

An interesting outcome, for the purposes of this chapter, regarding the need for specificity in attention training was reported by Curran, Hussain, and Park (2001, as cited in Park & Barbuto, 2005). In their study, patients with mild cognitive impairment following stroke learned novel naturalistic actions (goal-directed activities that require the production of several actions in a particular order that cannot be learned prior to instruction, e.g., preparing an unfamiliar recipe) more effectively when the trainer verbally described the action while demonstrating it than when no verbal description accompanied the demonstration. The authors hypothesized that the verbal descriptions facilitated learning of the actions by enabling the patients to develop a more accurate conceptual representation of the novel actions. However, in more severely impaired patients, the additional information may actually impair performance because of the demands integrating verbal and visuo-spatial information place on patients with more limited cognitive resources (Green, Rich, & Park, 2003; Park & Barbuto, 2005).

It may also be, however, that the verbal descriptions directed the patients' attention to the relevant environmental information and, in this way, focused attention to facilitate the development of mental representations for these actions. Such a view is consistent with normal interactions between attention and language. With more severe impairments and limited resources, processing deficits for complex language arise and restrict the patients' ability to focus attention in a meaningful way, thus resulting in poor performance on the training tasks.

These observations support the conclusion that treatment for language disorders due to attentional impairments is better served by addressing the underlying attentional deficits within the context of specific linguistic operations. That most previous treatment studies for language disorders associated with attentional impairments have not done so offers an explanation for the weak outcomes that have been observed. Of course, to address attentional deficits through language treatment requires an appreciation of some of the ways

that language operates as an attention director. This is addressed in the next section.

LANGUAGE AND ATTENTION

Accounts of sentence processing that argue for modularity—that is, autonomy of lexical access and syntactic analysis—are not uncommon (e.g., Frazier & Fodor, 1978; Fodor & Frazier, 1980; Swinney, 1979). These accounts consider sentence processing to be an isolated process independent of the conversational and real-world contexts in which such sentences occur. An alternative approach suggests that the processor *attends* to the referents that are being described (Altmann, 1996). That is, sentence processing focuses attention on the relevant aspects of the real-world context. Language processing therefore cannot be separated from the real-world context onto which the language must be mapped.

Such fundamental relationships between language and attention can be expressed in the related concepts of grounding and windowing. Grounding refers to a speaker's use of linguistic elements to direct a hearer's attention to a particular meaning within a discourse (Langacker, 2008; Taube-Schiff & Segalowitz, 2005). Windowing refers to the way in which languages use explicit mention to place a coherent referent situation into the foreground of attention; omission of any mention of other portions of the situation places that information into the background of attention (Talmy, 2003).

Grounding

The meanings of specific utterances sharing similar lexical items can be quite diverse semantically depending upon which "thing" is identified or which process is described with respect to time and reality. Interpretations are based on the speaker-hearer interaction in the current discourse context.

Grounding elements are used to bridge such gaps. A grounding element specifies the status of the thing profiled by a nominal or the process profiled by a finite clause (broadly, nouns and verbs) with regard to the ground (the speech event, the participants—speaker and hearer, their interaction, and the immediate circumstances, e.g., the time and place of speaking).

> Through nominal grounding (e.g., the, this, that, some, a, each, every, no, any), the speaker directs the hearer's attention to the intended discourse referent, which may or may not correspond to an actual individual. Clausal grounding (e.g., -s, -ed, may, should, will) situates the profiled relationship with respect to the speaker's current conception of reality. (Langacker, 2008, p. 259)

Grounding establishes a connection between the interlocutors and the content evoked by a nominal or finite clause even while the ground remains covert. For example, the demonstrative *this* indicates that the nominal it points to is close to the speaker but it does not refer to the speaker explicitly. At the same time, grounding reflects an asymmetry between the conceptualizers and what is conceptualized.

For conceptions evoked as meanings of linguistic expressions, the speaker and the hearer are the primary conceptualizers whose interactions in producing and understanding an utterance form the ground. Individually and together, the speaker and hearer function as the *subject* of conception and figure, at least minimally, in the meaning of every utterance (Figure 12-2). An important aspect of the subject's activity is the focusing of attention. Within the full scope of awareness for the content of an utterance, the subject attends to a certain region (Langacker's "onstage" region) and further singles out some onstage linguistic or grammaticized element as the focus of attention. This is the *object* of conception, which can be either a thing or a relationship. As the focused object of conception, it is interpreted most clearly with respect to the context and the listener (see Figure 12-2).

Taube-Schiff and Segalowitz (2005) provided evidence that such grammaticized elements require a listener to refocus attention when such attention-directing words are encountered in natural language. In their study, participants demonstrated greater demands for attentional control (operationalized as shift costs in an alternating runs experimental design) when judging spatial (above-below) or temporal (past-present) function words embedded in phrases. Greater shift costs were also observed in a grammatically dissimilar condition (participants required to shift between spatial and temporal function words) versus a grammatically similar condition (participants required to shift between spatial words describing a vertical dimension, i.e., above-below, or a proximal condition, i.e., near-far). The authors concluded that "language itself acts as an attention-focusing mechanism, shaping the creation of a mental construction by the recipient that corresponds to the sender's meaning" (p. 516).

Coventry, Lynott, Cangelosi, and colleagues (2010) examined how such spatial language (e.g., *the bottle is over the glass*) directs attention to a visual scene. Two views have been offered as to how this might occur. In the first, spatial language directs the hearer's attention to a reference object in the array being described and then specifies how attention should be switched to the object to be located. A second view takes into account how objects are experienced and used in the world. So, according to the first view, the sentence above would activate a minimal representation of a bottle oriented in the standard position higher than a glass. In the second view, the sentence would activate knowledge that includes the placement of the objects according to the way objects typically interact. Following two experiments designed to discriminate how spatial language drives visual attention, Coventry and colleagues concluded that spatial language comprehension is associated with a situational representation of how objects usually function. Spatial language therefore is thought to summon a range of perceptual simulations (i.e., dynamic routines) of the typical interactions among objects, including motion processing where attention is directed to objects not mentioned in the heard sentence (see **path windowing** below).

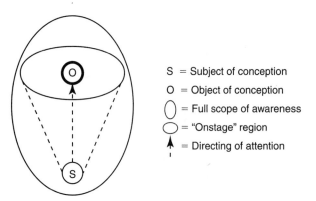

S = Subject of conception
O = Object of conception
◯ = Full scope of awareness
⬭ = "Onstage" region
⬆ = Directing of attention

Figure 12-2   The subject and object of conception must not be confused with subject and object as specifically grammatical notions. The speaker and the hearer are the principal subjects of conception, even when implicit, whereas grammatical subjects and objects are overt nominal expressions that generally refer to other entities. From Langacker, R. L. (2008). *Cognitive grammar: A basic introduction.* New York: Oxford University Press.

Windowing

Language can be used to direct one's attention over a referent scene in a certain pattern, with the greatest attention being placed in one or more windows of a scene. Such referent situations are referred to as event frames, sets of conceptual elements and interrelationships that are evoked together. Those elements or interrelationships that are conceived as the central identifying core of a particular event are said to be windowed (foregrounded) while those that are conceived as peripheral or incidental are said to be gapped (backgrounded).

Talmy (2003) describes several types of event frames and the types of windowing that operate on these events (Table 12-1). The first is a **path event frame,** which gives rise to **path windowing.** A path event frame refers to the entirety of a path of motion. There are three categories of paths: open, closed, and fictive. *Open paths* concern the paths that are described by objects that are physically in motion during a period of time and have beginning and ending points that are in different locations in space. For example, the sentence in (1) illustrates an open path event with maximal windowing over the whole of the conceived path while (1a) presents examples of gapping over one portion of the path and (1b) shows windowing over a single portion of the path.

(1) (a) Maximal windowing: The crate that was in the aircraft's cargo bay fell out of the plane through the air into the ocean.
   (b) Medial gapping: The crate that was in the aircraft's cargo bay fell out of the plane into the ocean.
   (c) Initial gapping: The crate that was in the aircraft's cargo bay fell through the air into the ocean.

(d) Final gapping: The crate that was in the aircraft's cargo bay fell out of the plane through the air.
(e) Initial windowing: The crate that was in the aircraft's cargo bay fell out of the plane.
(f) Medial windowing: The crate that was in the aircraft's cargo bay fell through the air.
(g) Final windowing: The crate that was in the aircraft's cargo bay fell into the ocean.

Closed paths are similar to open paths except the beginning and ending points coincide at the same location in space and essentially form a circuit. An example is provided in (2). Within a specified context, the whole event can be evoked by any of the widowing alternatives.

(2) [I need the milk.]
   (a) Full windowing: Go get it out of the refrigerator and bring it here.
   (b) Medial windowing: Get it out of the refrigerator.
   (c) Final windowing: Bring it here.
   (d) Final gapping: Go get it out of the refrigerator.
   (e) Initial gapping: Get it out of the refrigerator and bring it here.
   (f) Medial gapping: Go bring it here.

Table 12-1 Event Frames and Associated Types of Windowing*

EVENT FRAME	DEFINITION	TYPE OF WINDOWING
Path	Entirety of a path in motion	Path windowing
(a) Open	(a) objects are physically in motion during a period of time, have beginning and ending points in different locations in space	
(b) Closed	(b) beginning and ending points of path at same location in space and form a circuit	
(c) Fictive	(c) attribute figurative motion to static objects in space	
Causal chain	Sequence of linked events or sub-events where causality is associated with boundaries between each sub-event and linked successor	Causal-chain windowing
Cycle	Used to direct strongest attention to particular phase of iterating cycle; overall event is sequential but may have no clear beginning, middle, or end	Phase windowing
Participant interaction	Situational complex consisting of two parts: (1) a primary circumstance and (2) some individual interacting with that circumstance on two or more occasions; heightened attention placed on one or the other of the interactions fixes point for locating temporal perspective	Participant interaction windowing
Interrelationship	Conceptual complex comprised of parts that are not autonomous in themselves but intrinsically relative with respect to each other, i.e., the presence of one such part necessarily entails the presence of the other parts	Interrelationship windowing
(a) Motion	(a) Figure and ground cover both motion and location where figure is a moving or conceptually movable entity and ground is a stationary entity within a scene	Figure-ground windowing
(b) Factuality	(b) Displays property of supporting factuality windowing for placement of two alternatives within a single frame; constitute **comparison frame**	Factuality windowing

*See Text for Examples of Sentences Displaying Each Event Frame.
Adapted from Talmy, L. (2003). The windowing of attention in language. In *Toward a cognitive semantics volume I: Concept structuring systems* (pp. 258–309). Cambridge, MA: The MIT Press.

Fictive motion sentences attribute figurative motion to static objects in space. In fictive motion sentences, a motion verb is applied to a subject that is not literally capable of physical movement (e.g., the path swings along the cliff, the tattoo runs along his spine) (Ramscar, Matlock, & Boroditsky, 2009; Ramscar, Matlock, & Dye, 2009). According to Talmy (2003), a spatial configuration that is otherwise conceived as static can be alternatively conceptualized as being sequentialized and include a path of fictive motion. One such *fictive path* is the trajectory of a person's focus of attention shifting over a conceived scene. When a sentence can direct the hearer's attention along such a path, it is amenable to the same types of windowing patterns as is possible with paths involving physical motion. One example would be sentences such as those in (3) containing the "across from" construction in which the focus of attention is directed along a path that traverses two reference points.

(3) (a) Maximal windowing:
       My bike is across the street from the bakery.
       Patti sat across the table from Kevin.
    (b) Medial gapping:
       My bike is across from the bakery.
       Patti sat across from Kevin.
    (c) Initial gapping:
       My bike is across the street.
       Patti sat across the table.

A **causal-chain event** consists of a sequence of linked event or subevents where causality is associated with the boundaries between each subevent and its linked successor (Talmy, 2003). Causal-chain events exhibit **causal-chain windowing** of attention. A characteristic of these constructions is gapping of the entire medial portion of the sequence as in (4).

(4) I broke the window.
    (a) Full windowing: I threw the rock that I picked up and broke the window.
    (b) Full windowing: I broke the window by hitting it with a rock.

Talmy (2003) suggests that the medial gapping of causal sequences reflects a cognitive structuring in which a particular state or event and its occurrence are conceptualized together in the foreground of attention while little or no attention is given to the intervening mediating stages.

Sentences containing a **cycle event frame** use **phase windowing** to direct one's strongest attention to a particular phase of an iterating cycle. The overall event is sequential but may have no clear beginning, middle, or end. In the case where the overall event is a motion event and one cycle constitutes a closed path of the type described above, these labels become departure phase, away phase, and return phase while a base phase (the state of locatedness) is labeled as the home phase. The sentences in (5) demonstrate alternative options for windowing attention on these phases.

(5) (a) Departure phase windowing:
       The pen kept falling off the table.
    (b) Return phase windowing:
       I kept putting the pen back on the table.
    (c) Departure phase plus return phase windowing:
       The pen kept falling off the table and I kept putting it back.

According to Talmy (2003), "the language affords the speaker alternatives of attentional windowing on essentially the same event frame with the addressee feasibly able to infer the different gapped portions of each alternative so as to reconstruct back to the same single event frame" (p. 281). The sentence in (5c) also induces a conceptual running together of the departure and return phases (conceptual splicing) with backgrounding of the home (the pen lying on the table) and away phases (the pen lying on the floor).

Cycle event frames can also support referentially nonequivalent phase windowings (i.e., where a phase window is created by an external coincident event rather than by the same single referent described thus far). The sentences in (6) illustrate this coincidence for the three phases of this cycle. For (6c), the return phase refers to Smith returning the location to which he had gone.

(6) When I phoned,
    (a) Smith was always just about to step out of his office. [departure phase]
    (b) Smith was always just stepping out of his office. [away phase]
    (c) Smith had always just stepped out of his office [return phase]

The **participant-interaction event frame** refers to a situational complex consisting of two parts: a) a primary circumstance and b) some individual interacting with that circumstance on two or more occasions. **Participant-interaction windowing** places heightened attention on one or the other of these interactions so that that interaction becomes the addressee's point for locating his/her temporal perspective (Talmy, 2003). This type of event frame is similar to the preceding types in that it includes a sequence of phenomena differing through time and that differing windows of attention differ with respect to their temporal placement. The sentences in (7) illustrate this type of event frame and can be interpreted as referring to a single situational complex.

(7) (a) John met a woman at the party last week. Her name was Linda.
    (b) John met a woman at the party last week. Her name is Linda.

In this event, the primary circumstance is that of a woman having the name Linda. According to Talmy (2003), the first interaction in (a) is John's encounter with Linda. The second interaction in (b) is the speaker's consideration of the woman's name at the moment of speaking. The tense differences in the second sentences of (7a) and (7b) place the attentional windows over one or the other of these interactions. In (7a), the use of the past tense marker does not apply to the main referent of the sentence (the woman named Linda), but rather, to the time of the first participant interaction (John's encounter with the woman). The use of the present tense in (7b) indicates the adoption of the temporal perspective of the second interaction, i.e., the present moment. The participant-interaction event frame therefore evokes the entirety of a situation while establishing selective attention for only subportions of that event frame.

An **interrelationship event frame** is a conceptual complex that is contained or comprised of parts that are not autonomous in themselves but intrinsically relative with respect to each other; that is, the presence of one such part necessarily entails the presence of the other parts. Talmy (2003) notes that **interrelationship windowing** is permitted over one part or another of such a complex while mention of the remaining part is omitted but still understood. Two types of interrelationship event frames are described: a figure-ground interrelationship and a factual-counterfactual interrelationship.

In the figure-ground interrelationship, the figure and ground are parts of a motion event (covering both motion and location) where the figure is a moving or conceptually movable entity within the scene and the ground is a stationary reference entity within the scene. Each is characterized with respect to the other. This **motion event frame** is conceptually irreducible (i.e., no part can exist without the rest) but can be partitioned into components that support differential **figure-ground windowing** of attention. To illustrate, Talmy refers to a scene where paint is peeling off a wall; the paint is understood to function as the figure relative to the wall as ground. Two counterpart constructions that gap reference to the figure and then the ground are provided in (8).

(8) (a) The paint is peeling (from the wall).
    (b) The wall is peeling (of its paint).

Given the original scene, (8a) refers to the windowing of the figure (plus the activity) and gapping of the ground while (8b) windows the ground (plus the activity) while gapping the figure.

The factual-counterfactual interrelationship is expressed by constructions that present a referent as being the case or, alternatively, not being the case. In pairs of such constructions, they are positive-negative counterparts of each other but make the same overall statement. A speaker can choose either one of the constructions, but in so doing, selects whether greater attention should be given to something that was or was not the case. Since each member of these pairs entails the other, Talmy refers to this type of interrelationship event frame as a **factuality event frame** and the heightened attention given to one or the other of these referent types as **factuality windowing.**

Factuality event frames also display the property of supporting factuality windowing for not just one of the alternatives, but for placement of both alternatives within a single frame. So, while main attention is directed toward one of the alternatives, the other is present in a backgrounded way to act as a basis for comparison. For Talmy (2003), an event frame that evokes larger-frame conceptualizations such as these can be further said to constitute a **comparison frame.** The following constructions evoke comparison frames for the occurrence or nonoccurrence of some referent.

(9) (a) I didn't go to John's party last night.
    (b) I went to the movies last night because they were playing my favorite film.
    (c) Sue may have gone to John's party last night.
    (d) Did Sue go to John's party last night?
    (e) I would have gone to John's party last night if I had had the time.

In (9a), the corresponding unrealized positive event is evoked (i.e., *I went to John's party last night*). In (9b), the inclusion of a *because*-clause evokes the unrealized negative counterpart by including a reason or cause without which the event would not have occurred. Placing the referent at some point along a continuum of certainty, as in (9c), also evokes consideration of events at the opposite end of the scale. The interrogative form in (9d) has at its main semantic point the occurrence or nonoccurrence of the referent. And (9e) uses an overtly counterfactual event to evoke its factual complement—that is, *going to the party*.

Similarly, certain lexical items also incorporate within their meaning notions of realization and nonrealization. Talmy (2003) offers the following examples.

(10) (a) I missed the target.
     (b) I regret that I lent him money.
     (c) I succeeded in opening the window.

In (10a), the verb *missed* seems to also evoke the occurrence of the projectile hitting the target. The verb *regret* in (10b) evokes the desired nonoccurrence of that event. And in (10c), the use of the verb *succeed* set up a comparison frame by suggesting the possibility of the event's nonoccurrence, a comparison that would be lacking without its use, as in *I opened the window.*

Finally, multiple instances of windowing can occur simultaneously with respect to several concurrent event frames. The sentences in (11) demonstrate successively greater instances of windowing.

(11) (a) Simple path event with medial gapping
The ball rolled off the lawn back onto the lawn.
(b) Simple path event with initial and medial gapping
The ball rolled back onto the court.
(c) Interrelationship event frame: motion event frame with figure windowing and ground gapping
The ball rolled back.
(d) Causal-chain with gapped motion event
I rolled the ball back.
(e) Cycle-event frame with return phase windowing
I kept rolling the ball back.
(f) Factuality event frame with comparison event windowing consideration of counterfactual and gapping consideration of factual
If I hadn't kept rolling the ball back, there would have been no game.

To summarize, cognition segments various phenomena into coherent conceptual packets called event frames and has the further ability to direct greatest attention to particular portions of the event frame while placing the remainder in the background of attention. The creation of a linguistic window over portions of a conceptual complex links the attentional system with the corresponding parts of the cognitive system processing that complex. Talmy (2003) refers to this process as "the windowing of attention" when language includes explicit linguistic material for the portions to be foregrounded (windowed) and the exclusion of any linguistic material for the portions to be backgrounded (gapped). In this way, the language system can direct the limited cognitive resources of the attentional system to the information that the user establishes as the most relevant based on larger concerns or goals.

Word and Sentence Processing

Recent evidence has suggested that word production draws upon central attentional resources. Ferreira and Pashler (2002) used dual-task methods (psychological refractory period paradigm) to investigate whether the word production stages of lemma selection, phonological form selection, and/or phoneme selection are subject to a processing bottleneck like that which has been identified in attention research. Picture naming tasks in a sentence context that manipulated cloze

constraints, lexical frequency, and conceptually- and phonologically-related distractor words were performed concurrently with a tone discrimination task to determine if any of these stages of word production share central processing resources between the two tasks. The results were expected to provide evidence for whether language processing shares resources with other processing mechanisms or generally operates with dedicated (modular), language-specific mechanisms (see above).

Ferreira and Pashler found that some aspects of word production that are seemingly automatic, such as lemma selection and phonological word-form selection, are subject to a central bottleneck (require privileged use of resources) while other aspects, such as phoneme selection, operate independently of a central bottleneck (Figure 12-3). That is, performance on the tone discrimination task slowed as a function of close constraint, lexical frequency, and the conceptual relatedness of the distractor words (manipulations that were expected to influence lemma and phonological form selection) in the picture naming task while tone discrimination latencies were not influenced by manipulations of the phonological relatedness of the distractor words (which were expected to influence phoneme selection). The authors concluded therefore that word production shares central attention resources with other nonlinguistic tasks.

Ayora, Janssen, Dell'Acqua, and Alario (2009) used similar dual-task methods to that of Ferreira and Pashler (2002) to investigate whether the retrieval of open-class words (i.e., nouns, verbs, adjectives, adverbs) differs from that of closed-class words (e.g., determiners, pronouns, prepositions, conjunctions) in terms of the attentional resources that are required. The study was motivated by theories that suggest that the two classes of words are retrieved differently during language production. That is, open-class words are selected on the basis of semantic information while closed-class words are represented abstractly and automatically during the construction of the syntactic frame. Participants named pictures with determiner noun phrases composed of a closed-class word (a determiner) and an open-class word (a noun) while concurrently discriminating the pitch of auditory tones. Noun retrieval was manipulated by the lexical frequency of the target items. The ease of determiner retrieval was controlled with a congruency manipulation (congruent versus incongruent) for French possessive and demonstrative determiners that uses grammatical gender-determiner form associations.

Increased lexical frequency resulted in shorter picture-naming and tone discrimination latencies. Noun phrases

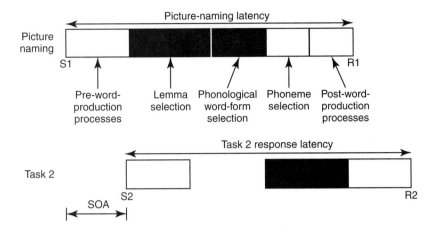

Figure 12-3 Schematic of the stages of word production in terms of their sensitivity to a central processing bottleneck. Filled rectangles represent processes in each task that are subject to a central processing bottleneck and therefore cannot occur simultaneously. S1, R1, S2, and R2 designate stimuli and responses for Task 1 and Task 2. SOA = stimulus onset asynchrony. [From Ferreira, V. S., & Pashler, H. (2002). Central bottleneck influences on the processing stages of word production. *Journal of Experimental Psychology: Learning, Memory, and Cognition, 28*(6), 1187–1199.]

with incongruent determiners resulted in longer latencies in both the picture naming task and in the tone discrimination task. Ayora and colleagues concluded that domain-general central processing mechanisms are required for noun production as well as the correct determiner form. The findings suggested that determiner form retrieval cannot rely on automatic, language-dedicated mechanisms for closed-class word retrieval.

Sentence processing requires not only comprehension of content words and their syntactically-derived relationships but also analysis of the context in which the sentence appears. The relationship between a sentence and its context is indicated by its focus structure where focus represents the new information that is unrecoverable from the preceding discourse (Cutler & Fodor, 1979). Speakers use devices like accent or topicalization (placing of a topic at the beginning of a sentence) to direct listeners' attention to the focus of the sentence. In the following example provided by Cutler and Fodor, the word *blue* has been topicalized:

(12) Blue, the hat was, that the man on the corner was wearing.

Cutler and Fodor (1979) suggest that particular attention is directed to the processing of focused words when a sentence is being understood (p. 56). Acoustic and linguistic cues therefore direct the listener's attention to the semantic focus of the sentence during comprehension.

Another linguistic cue employed to direct attention to an entity previously mentioned in an oral or written text is the use of a pronoun or noun phrase (anaphora resolution) (Myachykov & Posner, 2005). For example, when the antecedent is the subject of the first clause of a complex sentence, then an anaphoric pronoun will assume the position of subject in the second clause. It is also the case that the first mentioned entity in a sentence has a greater chance of being referred to subsequently by a pronoun.

The choice of anaphoric expression also depends on the distance separating the anaphora from its antecedent. A general rule is the larger the textual distance, the more likely that a noun phrase will be used to refer to the antecedent; the shorter the distance, the more likely that a pronoun will be used (Myachykov & Posner, 2005). When a new entity is introduced, an indefinite noun or proper name is often used. When an anaphoric pronoun is used, the cognitive search for the antecedent is likely to be short-ranged, confined to a few preceding clauses, and highly automatic. However, the use of a definite noun requires a longer-ranged, less automatized and attentionally-demanding search for the antecedent. Greater attention is required, therefore, to resolve referential ambiguity raised by the use of anaphora when a longer distance occurs between a referent and its antecedent (Myachykov & Posner, 2005).

External cues may also direct attention and in so doing influence the choice of syntactic subject during sentence production. It has been shown that for both static and dynamic events, the assignment of syntactic subject varies depending on a visual cue (Tomlin, 1997, and Forrest, 1996, as cited in Myachykov & Posner, 2005). So, when subjects are asked to describe a stimulus in which attention is cued to one or the other sides of a stimulus array (e.g., a heart and a star), the choice of syntactic subject will vary according to the cue (i.e., *the heart is to the left of the star* versus *the star is to the right of the heart*). Similarly, when subjects are asked to describe an unfolding event (e.g., the eating of a dark fish by a light fish), the choice of syntactic subject is also determined by the cue (i.e., *the dark fish was eaten by the light fish* versus *the light fish ate the dark fish*).

In summary, it has been shown that language acts as an attention director to facilitate activation of the intended meanings conveyed by words, sentences, and discourse. The conception intended by a speaker is grounded by the use of specific grammaticized lexical elements to focus attention on a particular meaning in a particular context. Listeners refocus their attention during language as new lexical elements are encountered. In the special case of spatial elements, the listener's attention is not only directed to particular objects in a visual scene, but also to the functional relationships between them.

Speakers further direct listeners' attention by using language to window (highlight) specific portions of a referent scene, such as an event. Such windowing is performed over a number of different types of events and highlights the central identifying core of the event that the speaker deems most relevant. Linguistic cues such as topicalization and the choice of anaphoric expression are used to direct listeners' attention to the focus of sentences, that is, new and antecedent information.

Finally, certain aspects of word production draw upon central attentional resources. Specifically, lemma and phonological form selection are subject to a processing bottleneck that suggests that these phases of word processing are resource intensive. This appears to be the case for both open- and closed-class words.

From the preceding review, it has been shown that language processing is dependent upon adequate attentional functioning in the service of language. When applying these observations to individuals with acquired language disorders and attentional impairments, it may be inferred that the language disruption may represent: (a) a failure of an impaired language mechanism to sufficiently direct attention to critical linguistic constituents necessary for the processing of meaning, (b) a failure of language processing secondary to inadequate recruitment of attentional resources that are essential for the interpretation of linguistic cues, (c) a failure of language processing due to reduced capacity or allocation of attentional resources that support language processing, or (d) some combination of all of the above. Whichever may be the underlying cause for the observed language deficits, it appears that, in all instances, the focus of the intervention for improved language functioning should be on the use of attention-directing language tasks. In the following sections, such a management approach is presented.

ASSESSMENT OF ATTENTION IN PATIENTS WITH ACQUIRED LANGUAGE DISORDERS

Standardized Testing

Generally, current clinical practice regarding assessment of attentional impairments in patients with acquired language disorders consists of determining the extent to which a variety of attentional domains are impaired without recourse to their direct influence on language functioning. Assessments may be performed in unstructured (interview, observational) or structured (scales, standardized testing) contexts to provide evidence as to whether and how these impairments interfere with daily activities and social communication (Murray, 2002; van Zomeran & Spikman, 2005).

van Zomeran and Spikman categorize attentional impairments following brain damage into those of control and those of speed or processing capacity. This scheme aligns with Knudsen's (2007) fundamental attentional processes of working memory and competitive selection (see above); the executive and perceptual factors underlying attentional assessment measures identified by Moosbrugger, Goldhammer, and Schweizer (2006); and the two major areas of attentional assessment, deployment and encoding, described by Mapou and Mateer (1996). Measures that assess attentional control include those that test focused, sustained, divided, and higher-order (executive) attention while those that assess speed test speed of information processing. Most measures of attention however are multifaceted and cannot be fit easily into these distinct components. Many are considered measures of working memory (Strauss, Sherman, & Spreen, 2006). Because attention cannot be captured in a single definition, it can be argued that it cannot be assessed with a single test. According to van Zomeren & Brouwer (1992), there may be no *tests* of attention, only assessments of behavior with special interest for the attentional components that underlie it.

With these caveats in mind, Table 12-2 provides a representative, but by no means exhaustive, listing of attention tests organized by whether they primarily assess attentional control or speed of information processing. Assessment scales, therefore, have been excluded from this listing. While some tests overlap both categories, the table provides the primary attentional components that are targeted by each tool. It should be noted that impaired attentional processing is not always a global problem and may impair one input or output modality more than others (Lezak, Howieson, & Loring, 2004).

Table 12-2 Standardized Tests for Assessing Attention

TEST	ATTENTIONAL PROCESS(ES)	REFERENCE
Attentional Control		
Digit Span Forward	Attention Span	
Letter Cancellation Test	Hemi-attention, focused attention	Lezak et al., 2004
Behavioural Inattention Test	Hemi-attention, focused attention	Wilson et al., 1987
d2 Test of Attention	Hemi-attention, focused attention	Brickencamp & Zillmer, 1998
Continuous Performance Tests (Conners, Vigil)	Focused attention, sustained attention	Conners, 2004
Continuous Performance Test of Attention	Focused attention, sustained attention	Cicerone, 1997
Stroop Tests	Focused attention, sustained attention	Strauss et al., 2006
Brief Test of Attention	Divided attention	Schretlen, 1997
Trail Making Tests (Trail Making Test; Oral Trail Making Test; Color Trails Test)	Divided attention	Strauss et al., 2006
Test for Attentional Performance	Divided attention, sustained attention	Zimmermann & Fimm, 1995
Sustained Attention for Response Task	Sustained attention	Robertson et al., 1997; Manly & Robertson, 2005
Test of Everyday Attention	Visual and auditory selective attention, sustained attention, attentional switching, divided/sustained attention	Robertson et al., 1994
Digit Span Backwards	Working memory	Lezak et al., 2004
Listening and Reading Span Tasks	Working memory	Caspari et al., 1998; Daneman & Carpenter, 1980; Tompkins et al., 1994
N-Back Task	Working memory	Callicott et al., 1999
Controlled Oral Word Association Test	Executive attention	Strauss et al., 2006
Tower of London	Executive attention	Shallice, 1982
Wisconsin Card Sorting Test	Executive attention	Heaton et al., 1993
Behavioural Assessment of Dysexecutive Syndrome	Executive attention	Wilson et al., 1996
Processing Speed		
Computerized Test of Information Processing	Speed of information processing	Tombaugh & Rees, 2008
Paced Auditory Serial Attention Test (PASAT)	Sustained, divided attention, concentration, working memory, speed of information processing	Gronwall, 1977
Digit Symbol-Coding	Focused attention, speed of information processing	Wechsler, 1997
Symbol Digit Modalities Test	Focused attention, speed of information processing	Smith, 1991

Some have argued that, because many of these tests use linguistic stimuli to assess attention, the results obtained from the use of these tests in patients with acquired language disorders may be confounded and therefore invalid (see e.g., Murray, 2002). On the other hand, it has also been recognized recently that any test of the influence of attentional impairments on language processing must utilize linguistic stimuli in order to provide appropriate insight regarding the influences of one on the other (McNeil, Hula, & Sung, 2011). As McNeil and colleagues state, the problem with the latter approach is that the language deficits cannot be unambiguously attributed to attentional impairments because of the demands on linguistic processing in language-disordered individuals (p. 566). They suggest that the Stroop Test and Stroop-like tasks offer a possible remedy for this problem.

The Stroop task produces a response interference effect between automatic and controlled processes that provides a key role in understanding attention by tapping supervisory control (MacLeod, 1992; van Zomeren & Brouwer, 1992). The task involves rapidly naming the color of the ink for a printed color word in a congruent condition, where the color of the ink matches the printed word (e.g., the word "blue" printed in blue ink), and in an incongruent condition, where the color of the ink does not match the printed word (e.g., the word "yellow" printed in blue ink). The interference effect is manifested as increased difficulty (increased reaction times, more errors) for naming words in the incongruent condition when compared to a neutral condition (naming a color patch or reading a color word in black ink). Response facilitation (shorter reaction times, fewer errors) is observed in the congruent condition relative to the neutral condition. The interference effect is attributed to the requirement to inhibit the automatic activation of the word in favor of the controlled processing necessary to name the color (but note the results of Ferreira and Pashler, 2002, and Ayora et al., 2009, discussed above regarding arguments concerning automatic activation of open- and closed-class lexical items).

McNeil and colleagues (2011) reviewed the few studies that have used Stroop tasks to investigate attentional impairments in individuals with aphasia and found contradictory results with regard to the presence of an interference effect. In one study (Cohen, Meier, & Schulze, 1983, as cited in McNeil et al., 2011), patients with two different types of aphasia showed significantly less interference to incongruent linguistic stimuli than was observed in a control group, suggesting the patients with aphasia either did not have automatic access to word meanings or that they had superior inhibitory processes for the color word. In another study (Wiener, Conor, & Obler, 2004, as cited in McNeil et al., 2011), a small group of patients with Wernicke aphasia showed a larger interference effect than was observed in a control group, which was interpreted as evidence for deficit of inhibition for lexical/semantic language processing. Because patients with aphasia demonstrated low error rates in these studies, McNeil et al. concluded that Stroop tasks may provide an appropriate method for evaluating attention-related facilitation, inhibition, and goal-maintenance in persons with aphasia. To this end, McNeil, Kim, Lim, and colleagues (2010) investigated the effects of several color word congruent and incongruent Stroop tasks in persons with aphasia and normal adults in the context of a reading comprehension test (the Computerized Revised Token Test-R-Stroop [CRTT-R-wf-Stroop]). Both groups showed vigilance and interference effects on RT ratios reflecting costs in sustained attention, interference/suppression effects and attentional switching. Both groups showed a facilitation effect on the CRTT-R-wf score. Unlike the NA, the PWA showed no attentional effects for the number of correct responses on the color adjectives.

Dual-Tasks

In the description of language impairments associated with attentional impairments provided above, it was shown that the source of such impairments is generally not one of elementary (i.e., perceptual) attentional processing, but rather one related to more central processes having to do with the graded allocation of processing resources. Dual-task assessment provides an index of the interference that occurs during language processing when listeners/speakers must control and coordinate allocation of attentional resources for semantic, syntactic, and phonologic processes. For this reason, dual-task assessment would be the preferred approach for measuring the influence of impairments to attentional control during language processing. Table 12-3 provides an overview of some of the dual-task methods that have been employed to assess attentional mechanisms in patients with acquired language disorders (Box 12-2).

The majority of dual-task methods require laboratory instrumentation and therefore have not found their way into the general clinical assessment procedures for patients with acquired language disorders (McNeil et al., 2011). Two approaches from Table 12-3, however, appear to have the potential for clinical use because of either their reliance on typical clinical methods or their potential for being adapted to clinical use. LaPointe and Erickson (1991) used an auditory vigilance/card sorting dual-task. An audio-taped list of monosyllabic words with a randomly-appearing target word was presented. Subjects were required to listen to the word list and raise their hands each time they heard the target word. Simultaneously, they were required to complete the Wisconsin Card Sorting Test. Accuracy scores for target word identification and card sorting responses were calculated.

In the procedure used by Blackwell and Bates (1995), subjects were presented a visual string of two, four, or six target digits that they were to memorize. The string was followed immediately by an individual sentence, presented auditorily, that was judged for its grammaticality. After the subjects made their grammaticality judgment, they saw another series of digits that either matched or did not match the digits in the target set and were asked to decide whether the string was the same or different from the sequence that preceded the sentence. The task therefore required that subjects keep unrelated and arbitrary material in memory while making a grammaticality judgment. An accuracy score was calculated for grammaticality judgments with and without digits. Reaction times were also collected.

Table 12-3   Linguistic Dual-Task Measures

LEVEL	TASK	REFERENCE
Lexical/Sublexical	Simultaneous semantic categorization and lexical decision under binaural listening	Arvedson & McNeil, 1987
	Target word identification among monosyllabic words (auditory vigilance) while completing card sorting task	LaPointe & Erickson, 1991
	Spoken digit monitoring for pattern of 3 consecutive odd numbers during recognition memory task for semantically related and unrelated word pairs	Fischler et al., 1994, as cited in Fischler 2000
	Picture naming in close sentences and tone discrimination or semantic categorization decision for words	Ferreira & Pashler, 2002; Hula et al., 2007
Sentence	Tone discrimination, semantic categorization, lexical decision, grammaticality judgment, and phrase completion in varying combinations under binaural listening	Murray, 2000; Murray et al., 1997
	Picture description and tone discrimination (2 or 3 tones)	Murray et al., 1998; Hula & McNeil, 2008
	Grammaticality judgment while holding increasing numbers of digits (2, 4, 6) in mind	Blackwell & Bates, 1995
	Visual-manual tracking during comprehension for sentences and stories of increasing complexity	Granier et al., 2000; McNeil et al., 2004
	Concurrent judgment of probe word relatedness and syllable counting following sentence presentation	Tompkins et al., 2002

Box 12-2

Why Dual Tasks?

Capacity theories originated when interference was observed between tasks that are executed simultaneously. This led to the assumption that psychological processes require processing structures as well as commitment of some amount of processing resources. Selectivity of attention is the result of limited availability of a processing resource.

Dual-task performance provides clues regarding how efficiently humans allocate resources (attention) to competing tasks. A resource can be viewed as any provision for processing. In a single resource model, attention is conceived as a general pool of energy that is limited but can be distributed over simultaneous demands. This model emphasizes the concept of effort (energy needed to meet demands of a task, i.e., concentration, motivation, arousal). The amount of capacity allocated is determined by the effort or attention that is needed for a task. Alternatively, a multiple resource approach has been proposed that argues for a variety of multiple, specific, and different resources that nonetheless retain a nonspecific general resource. This approach distinguishes among resources based on dimensions of processing modality (auditory vs. visual), stage (encoding vs. central processing vs. response), and code (spatial vs. verbal).

To the extent that two tasks or processes make demands on different sets of resources, they can be performed concurrently. Task difficulty places varying demands on resources at different stages of dual task execution. Task success depends on the complexity of the task components, familiarity with the components, some combination of the two, and the general level of arousal. Practice and task demands are strongly related (as tasks become highly practiced, demands on limited resources decrease to the point of automaticity).

Of course audiotapes for presenting the listening tasks included in the table can be developed using simple audio-editing software that is included on most computers or is available for downloading on the internet at no cost.

At least two dual-task methods are available commercially for clinical use and provide additional resources for implementing dual-task assessment with language-disordered patients. As described above, the Stroop task requires patients to read words and name colors simultaneously and is therefore a dual task. McNeil et al., (2011) suggest that this is a relatively easy task to include in language assessment procedures that extends beyond more traditional assessment. In the Telephone Switch subtest of the *Test of Everyday Attention* (Robertson, Ward, Ridgeway, & Nimmo-Smith, 1994), patients must search for targets among distractors in a simulated telephone directory while simultaneously counting strings of tones presented on an audiotape.

INTERVENTION FOR ACQUIRED LANGUAGE DISORDERS ASSOCIATED WITH ATTENTIONAL IMPAIRMENT

Treatment programs for attentional problems are either restorative or compensatory. Restorative treatments generally attempt to re-establish the cognitive function of attention through repetitive drills (e.g., Cicerone, 2002; Couillet et al., 2010; Gray, Robertson, Pentland, & Anderson, 1992; Niemann, Ruff, & Baser, 1990) while compensatory treatments (otherwise referred to as specific-skills training) attempt to improve the re-learning of functionally important activities requiring attention (e.g., self-care activities, driving, and reading). A meta-analysis suggests that compensatory training significantly improves performance on specific skills requiring attention while direct cognitive retraining methods do not affect outcomes significantly (Park & Ingles, 2001; Park & Barbuto, 2005; but see also Rohling et al., 2009, for evidence of significant improvements following direct attention process training).

Sohlberg (2005; Sohlberg et al., 2003) has organized attention treatments into six distinct approaches: (1) direct training of attention processes, (2) specific skills training, (3) training metacognitive strategies specific for managing attention deficits, (4) training the use of specific aids to compensate for attention deficits, (5) environmental modification/task accommodation, and (6) collaboration-focused approaches. Using the definitions provided above, direct attention process training is a restorative approach while the remaining five approaches are compensatory.

Park and Barbuto (2005) further suggest that restorative treatments may be more effective for improving specific cognitive deficits, whereas compensatory treatments appear to be more effective for the treatment of consciously accessible cognitive processes.

Restorative Approaches

A number of studies have been undertaken to investigate whether interventions aimed at direct attention retraining might result in improved language outcomes. Thomas-Stonell, Johnson, Schuller, and Jutai (1994) evaluated whether any gains resulting from intervention using a computer-based program designed to remediate cognitive-communication skills would generalize to a battery of standardized neuropsychological tests. The program (no longer available) focused on five skill areas: attention, memory/word retrieval, comprehension of abstract language, organization, and reasoning/problem solving. Most of the tasks required integration of skills from two or more areas. No description of the task themselves was provided. The battery of tests was selected to provide test scores in these five areas. Twelve participants between the ages of 12 and 21 with a history of TBI due primarily to motor vehicle accidents and of varying severity were randomly assigned to a remediation group and a control group to assess the effectiveness of the program. The remediation group received 8 weeks of intervention using the computer program; those in the control group received traditional therapy/community school programs during this period. Significant group differences emerged on a battery of standardized tests measuring composite language skills but not on any of the other cognitive tests including the *PASAT*.

Dotson et al. (2008) investigated whether increased engagement of intact attentional mechanisms found in the right hemispheres of fluent aphasic (left-brain damaged) patients might result in improved picture naming performance. The study was motivated by Coslett's (1999) spatial registration hypothesis, which suggests that individuals with disrupted spatial processing will perform less well on verbal tasks when they are linked to locations mediated by an impaired (i.e., contralesional) spatial system (see previous discussion under attentional and language impairments due to stroke). Attention was manipulated by presenting picture stimuli on a computer in the ipsilesional hemispace and gradually moving the location of presentation to the center of the computer screen. Two mechanisms of action for any improvements resulting from this treatment were proposed: (1) a change in the neural substrates for language characterized by transfer of language to perilesional cortex or the intact hemisphere or (2) improved word learning due to increased engagement of an intact attentional apparatus. Two of the three aphasic patients in the study demonstrated improved naming accuracy. Because generalization of improved naming was observed for untrained items, the authors concluded that either the neural mechanisms of attention that underlie word finding or the neural mechanism for word finding itself were changed as a result of treatment.

Crosson and colleagues (2007) also investigated the effects of this spatial attention manipulation on picture naming as well as a treatment focused on intention in a large group of patients with chronic nonfluent aphasia. Attention was defined as the ability to select one source of information for further processing from among multiple competing sources. Attention is closely associated with posterior sensory cortices; language performance is affected by attention deficits in patients with parietal lesions when the stimuli are presented on either the left or the right sides. Intention was defined as the ability to select among several competing actions for execution and initiation ("executive attention"). Intention mechanisms are associated with frontal action systems. More specifically, the left pre-supplementary motor cortex areas underlying intention for word generation as well as complex hand movements have been found to overlap. These areas are, in turn, connected to left lateral prefrontal cortex (LPFC), which is associated with word production.

Because the right hemisphere has been associated with word production in chronic aphasia, Crosson and colleagues hypothesized that it may be possible to facilitate recovery from aphasia through an intention treatment that exploits the right LPFC. Treatment consisted of picture naming trials presented on a computer monitor with alerting stimuli and correction procedures as necessary. These were accompanied by a complex left hand movement (lifting the lid on a box and pressing a button on a device within the box) to initiate picture presentation. Three phases were conducted using unique sets of 50 items; the complex movement was replaced with a non-meaningful circular hand gesture in the third trial to allow use outside of treatment. Comparison was made to attention treatment consisting of picture naming trials presented on computer monitor in left hemispace with alerting stimuli to left of center and correction procedures as necessary. After the alerting stimuli disappeared, the pictures would appear immediately in the upper, middle, or lower portion of the left side. Three phases were conducted using unique sets of 50 line drawings of objects with changes

in the number and duration of the alerting stimuli over each phase. The authors predicted that the intention treatment would enhance picture naming more than the attention treatment because it addressed action mechanisms that are typically impaired in nonfluent aphasia.

Improved naming performance was observed during both treatments for those patients with moderate to severe word-finding impairment. Significantly greater increments of gain were observed between phases for the intention treatment versus the attention treatment. Generalization to untrained stimuli was also observed for both treatments, but was greater for the intention treatment. No differential response to the two treatments was observed for those patients with profound word-finding impairment. Fewer of these patients demonstrated treatment gains or generalization to untrained items. While the results did not confirm the authors experimental hypotheses, Crosson and colleagues concluded that intention and attention treatment showed potential as treatments for nonfluent aphasia.

Helm-Estabrooks, Connor, and Albert (2000) examined the effects of an attention training program on auditory comprehension skills in two patients with chronic mixed nonfluent aphasia and marked auditory comprehension impairment. Training was hierarchically organized and began with nonlinguistic tasks of sustained attention and progressed to tasks requiring selective and alternating attention (symbol cancellation, trail making, repeated graphomotor patterns, auditory continuous performance, and sorting). Both cases demonstrated small improvements in auditory comprehension at the end of the training program.

Kohnert (2004) also administered a "cognitive" intervention consisting of non-linguistic tasks to a bilingual (Spanish-English) patient with severe nonfluent aphasia to assess the outcomes on both nonverbal skills and language performance. The tasks included card sorting to target perception and categorization skills, simple math computations (addition, subtraction), visual letter and number searches for sustained and alternating attention, and several tasks for high-level attention from a computer-based program. Interactions were carried out in Spanish during the first month of the program and in English during the second. Improvements were observed on all treated tasks while modest gains were observed on language measures in both languages. No attempt was made to compare the results of a second, language-oriented treatment to the outcomes achieved with the non-linguistic intervention.

Attention Process Training

Two commercially-available training programs, *Attention Process Training (APT)* (Sohlberg & Mateer, 1986) and *Attention Process Training-II (APT-II)* (Sohlberg et al., 2001) have received extensive evaluation with regard to treatment outcomes. *APT* is a theoretically-motivated program that uses a series of hierarchically-organized tasks (e.g., detection of auditorily presented number targets, auditorily presented strings of stimuli with response requirements of increasing difficulty or recorded in background noise, simultaneous sequencing exercises, multilevel card sorting) to remediate deficits of focused, sustained, selective, alternating, and divided attention. *APT-II* is also designed to address deficits in attentional processing but in individuals with mild brain dysfunction. The program is modeled after *ATP* (i.e., the activities are organized to address sustained, alternating, selective, and divided attention) and targets difficulties in coping with distraction, reduced mental control, and problems shifting attention between different activities.

Sohlberg and Mateer (1987) evaluated the effectiveness of *ATP* in four brain-injured subjects attending a day program with varying etiologies (aneurysm, gunshot wound, closed-head injury), severities (mild to severe), and times post onset (14–48 months). The treatment program was administered over 30 weeks; changes in performance on the Paced Auditory Serial Addition Test (*PASAT*) (Gronwall, 1977) in the absence of changes in general cognitive abilities were expected to provide evidence for the effectiveness of the attention training program.

Two subjects with mild to moderate attention deficits performed within normal limits on the *PASAT* and two subjects with severe attention deficits achieved scores within the mildly-impaired range on the *PASAT* after treatment. These improvements were not routinely associated with improvements on a measure of visual processing (Spatial Relations subtest, Woodcock-Johnson Psycho-Educational Battery [Woodcock & Johnson, 1977]) suggesting that the attentional improvements were due to the treatment. The authors interpreted these results as support for a process-specific approach to attentional remediation.

Others have suggested, however, that the observed improvements reported by Sohlberg and Mateer (1987) following *APT* may have been the result of specific skill learning rather than increased attentional functioning (Park, Proulx, and Towers, 1999). That is, *APT* may target the same specific skills that are required for performance on a given outcome measure (in this case, the *PASAT*). Any improvements following intervention then are simply a function of the amount of overlap between the skills targeted in process training and those required on the outcome measure and not a function of improved attention. Park et al. (1999) investigated this hypothesis in a group of 23 participants with traumatic brain injuries. Two outcome measures, the *PASAT* and the consonant trigrams task (a measure of memory under conditions of distraction), were used to evaluate the effects of *APT*. Performance on the *PASAT* was expected to improve following treatment because *APT* provides practice on attentional functions that underlie the *PASAT*. Performance on the consonant trigrams task was not expected to improve because *APT* does not target the cognitive functions underlying this task. Park et al. (1999) found that performance on the *PASAT* as well as on the consonant trigrams task improved following *APT*. Furthermore, improvement on the *PASAT* was not different from the improvement shown by control subjects following repetition of the test. The results suggested that some aspects of *APT* affected performance on the consonant trigrams task and that improvements following *APT* are due not necessarily to improved attentional functioning.

Sohlberg, McLaughlin, Pavese et al., (2000) compared *APT* to a program of therapeutic support to determine how well process training would influence patient performance in naturalistic settings. Using a crossover design, two groups of patients, each consisting of 7 randomly-assigned individuals with acquired brain injuries of varying etiologies, sites of lesion, and severity, received two blocks of treatment in different orders. In one treatment block, patients received 24 hours of *APT*; in the other, they received 10 hours of brain injury education and supportive listening. Both treatments were conducted over a 10-week period. Prior to beginning treatment and following completion of each treatment block, the participants were administered an extensive neuropsychological attention battery and questionnaires to assess any improvements in daily living. The results suggested that practice, whether from exposure to *APT* or from repeated testing, improved the patients' performance. Brain injury education also appeared to improve the patients' attitudes. Because the tasks used in *APT* were different from those used in the neuropsychological assessment, the authors concluded that improvement on standardized testing represented generalization of learning from process training. Similar to Park et al. (1999), the authors concluded that the improvements were not associated with general enhancements to attentional functioning but rather to executive skills that are associated with a subset of *APT* tasks.

Pero, Incoccia, Caracciolo, et al. (2006) also evaluated the effectiveness of *ATP* while attempting to overcome the problems associated with use of the *PASAT* as a single outcome measure. Two patients with chronic, severe TBI participated in the study; the first patient received 85 sessions of training while the second received 75 sessions. The *Test for Attentional Performance* (see Table 12-2) was administered to assess alertness, vigilance (sustained attention), selective attention, and divided attention. The *Test of Everyday Attention (TEA)* was also administered to assess whether *APT* generalizes to functional contexts. One patient demonstrated deficits in all areas except for reaction to warning. The second patient showed severe deficits in response time and selective attention but preserved alertness and vigilance.

Following training, both patients improved on some but not all tests of attention. *APT* was found to be ineffective in modifying response speed but more effective in producing improvements in selective and divided attention. Results obtained from the *TEA* paralleled those obtained on the *TAP*. The findings provide support for the selective effects of *APT*.

Barker-Collo, Feigin, Lawes, et al. (2009) undertook a randomized controlled trial to investigate the effectiveness of *APT* for attentional deficits arising from stroke. Seventy-eight participants with acute stroke (mean approximately 18 days time post onset) of all pathological types were randomized to either an *APT* group or a group receiving standard care (undefined). They were screened using standard tests of auditory and visual sustained, selective, divided, and alternating attention and also completed several tests to evaluate broader outcomes regarding quality of life. Assessments were repeated at 5 weeks and 6 months. Participants in the *APT* group received up to 30 hours of treatment (mean = 13.5 hours). The combined auditory and visual attention score from the *Integrated Visual Auditory Continuous Performance Test (IVA-CPT)* (Sandford & Turner, 2000) was used as the primary outcome measure. *APT* had a significant, positive effect on attention as measured by the *IVA-CPT* when compared to the group receiving standard care. Differences were not observed for any of the other attention or quality of life assessments. The authors concluded that *APT* had a positive effect on these patients and that early, post-stroke rehabilitation for attentional deficits may be warranted.

Similar results have been observed in patients with mild TBI following intervention with *APT-II* (Palmese & Raskin, 2000). After the administration of 10-week individualized programs based upon extensive neuropsychological assessment of three patients, one patient demonstrated significant improvement, one was improved on four of seven measures, and the last showed selective improvement on a few measures. In the latter patient, the improvement included increased performance on the consonant trigrams test, further suggesting that in some patients, *APT* influences select cognitive skills rather than general attentional capacity.

Direct Process Training for Acquired Language Disorders

Based on the observation that the language problems in some individuals with acquired language disorders (particularly those with mild impairments) may be associated with attentional deficits, several studies have been undertaken to evaluate the effectiveness of *APT-II* as a treatment for improving language performance following brain damage. Coelho (2005) administered *APT-II* to a 50-year-old woman with chronic aphasia (10 months after onset of stroke) to improve reading comprehension and reading rate. Reading comprehensions scores, based on responses to comprehension questions regarding magazine articles, improved from approximately 40% to 60% accuracy to 83% accuracy over the course of treatment. Reading rate, as indicated by words per minute, remained variable throughout treatment. Post-treatment gains on the *Reading Comprehension Battery for Aphasia—Second Edition* (LaPointe & Horner, 1998) and the *Gray Oral Reading Tests—Fourth Edition* (Wiederholt & Bryant, 2001) were interpreted as further support for improved reading outcomes secondary to *APT-II*. However, improvement on the *Western Aphasia Battery (WAB)* (Kertesz, 1982) for skills not targeted by the intervention was also observed and raised questions regarding the specificity of the outcomes.

Sinotte and Coelho (2007) replicated Coelho's study with a 60-year-old woman with mild anomic aphasia 6 months after onset of a left frontal hemorrhagic stroke. Following 16 sessions of *APT-II* over a 5-week period, less variability but otherwise few changes were observed in the patient's reading comprehension accuracy. Reading rate did not change appreciably. Clinical improvement was observed on a formal test of attention (*Test of Everyday Attention*) while small but insignificant improvements were observed on the GORT-4 and the *WAB*.

Murray, Keeton, and Karcher (2006) also used *APT-II* to treat a 57-year-old man with chronic, mild conduction aphasia. Following administration of an extensive neuropsychological battery, deficits in repetition, high-level auditory comprehension, and spoken language, working memory deficits, and mildly impaired attention for timed tasks were identified. After more than 50 hours of training, the patient demonstrated faster response latencies to a paragraph listening task but no other improvements on other measures of auditory comprehension. Nominal improvements were observed on attention and memory tests that were unrelated to the treatment tasks. Murray et al. concluded that structured attention programs such as *APT-II* may not provide "a viable or efficient approach to treating concomitant attention problems in patients with aphasia" (pp. 55–56).

Youse and Coelho (2009) investigated whether attention training would facilitate conversational discourse for two individuals with long-standing TBI. Two treatment protocols were administered in the same sequence: *APT-II* followed by *Interpersonal Process Recall,* a social skills–based procedure. Neither approach produced meaningful improvements in attention or conversation.

Language-Specific Approach

What do the outcomes reported from these restorative approaches suggest for the treatment of acquired language disorders associated with attentional impairments? The general conclusion appears to be that restorative training focused on improving attention results in improvements for the specific skills that underlie the training tasks themselves as well as any standardized tests that draw upon these same skills. Thus, restorative treatments that rely on cognitive training for improved attention are not likely to generalize to language processing (see Rohling et al., 2009).

These observations, as well as those of previous investigations of the effectiveness of attention rehabilitation (Sturm, Willmes, Orgass, & Hartje, 1997; Park & Ingles, 2001), argue that treatment for any specific attention deficits associated with language processing require specific training that is language-based. Therefore, of the two types of intervention described above (restorative versus compensatory), the compensatory approach using language-based treatment for such attentional deficits appears to be the more desirable choice because (a) the remediation has as its goal improved attention in service to a specific skill (i.e., listening comprehension, speaking) and (b) the attentional requirements for the skill are consciously available and indexed by a number of linguistic devices (e.g., grounding, windowing, topicalization, anaphora, and others).

For the remainder of this chapter, I present a framework for a specific skill-based approach to the remediation of acquired language disorders due to attentional impairment. Following from previous work, the intervention is targeted toward individuals with no more than moderate language and attentional deficits. The proposed framework is theoretically motivated and addresses many of the principles for successful language

intervention that have been identified in this review. Appendix 12-1 provides recommendations for an assessment battery related to individuals with acquired language disorders and attentional impairments. Appendix 12-2 provides a treatment protocol for such individuals based on a list of principles derived from the current literature. It is important to note that little can be said about the efficacy of this approach as no such intervention has been published (to my knowledge) nor investigated previously. Nonetheless, the approach is based on a synthesis of the available evidence to date and provides a potential next step for improving treatments for acquired language disorders of attentional origin.

Principles of Treatment

The principles underlying the language-based approach described here are also presented in Table 12-4. Fischler (2000) suggested that "training on attentional focus and resource management may prove helpful" but that such training "should be done within the **language domain** to the extent possible" (p. 367). Hula and McNeil (2008) hypothesize that "the relevant aspects of resources or working memory that change with intervention are those that are deployed and consumed only when they are being utilized in the service of the specific linguistic tasks that are challenging for the individual" (p. 184). The tasks in the current approach are language-based and emphasize recruitment of attentional resources in the service of language processing as well as management of resources during dual-task processing.

Fischler also notes that different patterns of interference in the allocation of attention occur as a result of tasks that impose **increasing attentional demands.** Murray et al. (1998) recognize a continuum of processing automaticity wherein production of incomplete or simple utterances has fewer costs to processing resources than more complete and complex syntactic forms. The complexity of these language-based tasks increases across the level of intervention (lexical versus sentence processing), the requirements of the tasks (e.g., picture naming versus discrimination of lexical targets; simple sentence construction versus anaphoric search in complex sentences), and the amount of competition for attentional resources (single versus dual-task requirements).

The goal of any treatment focusing on language and attention should be to **automatize attentional recruitment for language.** Carr and Hinckley (this volume) summarize this principle succinctly in stating that "most theories of skill acquisition are built around some version of the idea that attended processing gives

Table 12-4   Principles for Language-Specific Attentional Training

PRINCIPLE	REFERENCE
1. Train attentional focus and resource management for language	Fischler, 2000; Hula & McNeil, 2008
2. Increase attentional demands	Fishler, 2000; Murray et al., 1998
3. Automatize attentional recruitment for language	Murray, 1999; Carr &
a. Consistent practice	Hinckley, this volume
b. External versus internal focus	
c. Feedback concerns success or failure of performance on language task, not step by step attentional control	
4. Engage undamaged attentional mechanisms in non-dominant hemisphere	Coslett, 1999
5. Incorporate linguistic devices to focus attention	
a. Alternating subject selection for sentence production	Myachykov & Posner, 2005
b. Sentence focus structure	Cutler & Fodor, 1979
c. Anaphoric reference	Myachykov & Posner, 2005
d. Interpretation of grounding elements	Langacker, 2008
e. Event windowing	Talmy, 2003

way to automatic processing with practice." Performances that draw heavily on attention can be replaced by well-practiced habits, reducing or perhaps even eliminating the need for the guidance, temporary storage, and decision-making processes provided by what we now call working memory (James, 1890, as cited by Carr & Hinckley). Murray (1999) has suggested that extensive repetition of language tasks might make language processes more automatic, and thus less resource demanding, when the attentional impairment of the language-disordered individual is due to capacity limitations.

Language, of course, has as its goal successful communication of a speaker's or listener's intended message. The focus of automatic language processing then is not on how the message was achieved but rather whether the message was received. This has been referred to as internal versus external focus. According to Carr and Hinckley, the difference between internal and external focus is attending to what one is *doing* (internal focus) versus attending to input from the outside world about what one is *achieving* (external focus). Language users are externally focused and rely on listener feedback to determine whether the goals of their communication have been met.

This specific-skill approach establishes automatic language processing by engaging the patient in consistent and repetitive practice of language tasks. The focus is on whether or not the patient has achieved the desired response. Feedback concerns success or failure of performance on the language task and not step by step attentional control of language processing.

As indicated above, the approach is based on a hierarchy of increasingly more complex language tasks. For the simplest task, picture naming, procedures are included to **engage attentional mechanisms in the right cerebral hemisphere** by moving the locus of stimulus presentation into left hemispace. Based on the evidence to date, this modification is appropriate for language-impaired individuals with left hemisphere brain damage. Finally, the language tasks themselves **exploit linguistic devices that are known to focus attention** during language processing. These include alternating subject selection for sentence production, sentence focus structure, anaphoric reference, interpretation of grounding elements, and event windowing. Previous approaches (e.g., process training) have been guided by the assumption that attention operates independently of the tasks for which it's recruited, such as language. Thus, in the case of the language interventions described above, attention has been assigned responsibility for selecting verbal information, maintaining such information online, and providing adequate resources to support complex processing. What such approaches have not considered, however, is (a) the manner in which language influences attention and (b) the effects of language disruption on attentional processing. As the outcomes regarding attentional treatments for language disorders have shown, it is not enough to simply attend to language if the goal is to improve language processing. Rather, it appears that the language systems of individuals with acquired language disorders must be challenged to enlist attention in a meaningful way if improved outcomes are to be realized.

REFERENCES

Alberoni, M., Baddeley, A., Della Sala, S., Logie, R., & Spinnler, H. (1992). Keeping track of a conversation: Impairments in Alzheimer's disease. *International Journal of Geriatric Psychiatry, 7*, 39–646.

Alexander, M. P. (2002). Disorders of language after frontal lobe injury: Evidence for the neural mechanisms of assembling language. In D. T. Stuss, & R. T. Knight (Eds.), *Principles of frontal lobe function* (pp. 159–167). New York: Oxford University Press.

Alladi, S., Xuereb, J., Bak, T., Nestor, P., Knibb, J., Patterson, K., & Hodges, J. R. (2007). Focal cortical presentations of Alzheimer's disease. *Brain, 130*, 2636–2645.

Altmann, G. T. M. (1996). Accounting for parsing principles: From parsing preferences to language acquisition. In T. Inui, & J. L. McClelland (Eds.), *Attention and performance XVI: Information integration in perception and communication* (pp. 479–500). Cambridge, MA: The MIT Press.

Ansaldo, A. I., Arguin, M., & Lecours, A. R. (2004). Recovery from aphasia: A longitudinal study on language recovery, lateralization patterns, and attentional resources. *Journal of Clinical and Experimental Neuropsychology, 26*(5), 621–627.

Arvedson, J. C., & McNeil, M. R. (1987). Accuracy and response times for semantic judgments and lexical decisions with left- and right-hemisphere regions. *Clinical Aphasiology, 17*, 188–201.

Ayora, P., Janssen, N., Dell'Acqua, R., & Alario, F. X. (2009). Attentional requirements for the selection of words from different grammatical categories. *Journal of Experimental Psychology: Learning, Memory, and Cognition, 35*(5), 1344–1351.

Barker-Collo, S. L., Feigin, V. L., Lawes, C. M. M., Parag, V., Senior, H., & Rodgers, A. (2009). Reducing attentions deficits after stroke using attention process training: A randomized controlled trial. *Stroke, 40*(10), 3293–3298.

Belleville, S., Chertkow, H., & Gauthier, S. (2007). Working memory and control of attention in persons with Alzheimer's disease and mild cognitive impairment. *Neuropsychology, 21*(4), 458–469.

Blackwell, A., & Bates, E. (1995). Inducing agrammatic profiles in normals: Evidence for the selective vulnerability of morphology under cognitive resource limitation. *Journal of Cognitive Neuroscience, 7*(2), 1–49.

Blake, M. L., Duffy, J. R., Myers, P. S., & Tompkins, C. A. (2002). Prevalence and patterns of right hemisphere cognitive/communication deficits: Retrospective data from an inpatient rehabilitation unit. *Aphasiology, 16*(4), 537–547.

Blake, M. L. (2009). Inferencing processes after right hemisphere brain damage: Effects of contextual bias. *Journal of Speech, Language, and Hearing Research, 52*, 373–384.

Brickencamp, R., & Zillmer, E. (1998). *The d2 Test of Attention.* Seattle, WA: Hogrefe & Huber Publisher.

Brookshire, R. H., & Nicholas, L. E. (1997). *The Discourse Comprehension Test—Second Edition.* Albuquerque, NM: PICA Programs.

Broadbent, D. E., Cooper, P. F., FitzGerald, P., & Parkes, K. R. (1982). The Cognitive Failures Questionnaire (CFQ) and its correlates. *British Journal of Clinical Psychology, 21*, 1–16.

Callicott, J. H., Mattay, V. S., Bertolino, A., Finn, K., Coppola, R., Frank, J. A., . . .Weinberger, D. R. (1999). Physiological characteristics of capacity constraints in working memory as revealed by functional MRI. *Cerebral Cortex, 9*, 20–26.

Carr, T. H., & Hinckley, J. J. (2012). Attention: Architecture and process. In R. K. Peach & L. P. Shapiro (Eds.), *Cognition and acquired language disorders* (pp. 61–93). St. Louis, MO: Mosby.

Castel, A. D., Balota, D. A., & McCabe, D. P. (2009). Memory efficiency and the strategic control of attention at encoding: Impairments of value-directed remembering in Alzheimer's disease. *Neuropsychology, 23*(3), 297–306.

Caspari, I., Parkinson, S. R., LaPointe, L. L., & Katz, R. C. (1998). Working memory and aphasia. *Brain and Cognition, 37*, 205–223.

Cicerone, K. D. (1997). Clinical sensitivity of four measures of attention to mild traumatic brain injury. *The Clinical Neuropsychologist, 11*(3), 266–272.

Cicerone, K. D. (2002). Remediation of "working attention" in mild traumatic brain injury. *Brain Injury, 16*(3), 185–195.

Coelho, C. (2005). Direct attention training as a treatment for reading impairment in mild aphasia. *Aphasiology, 19*(3), 275–283.

Coelho, C. A. (2007). Cognitive-communication deficits following TBI. In N. D. Zasler, D. I. Katz & R. D. Zafonte (Eds.), *Brain injury medicine: Principles and practice* (pp. 895–910). New York: Demos.

Conners, C. K. (2004). *Conners' Continuous Performance Test II Version 5 (CPT-II Version 5).* San Antonio, TX: Pearson.

Couillet, J., Soury, S., Lebornec, G., Asloun, S., Joseph, P. A., Mazaux, J. M., & Azouvi, P. (2010). Rehabilitation of divided attention after severe traumatic brain injury: A randomised trial. *Neuropsychological Rehabilitation, 20*(3), 321–339.

Coventry, K. R., Lynott, D., Cangelosi, A., Monrouxe, L., Joyce, D., & Richardson, D. C. (2010). Spatial language, visual attention, and perceptual stimulation. *Brain and Language, 112*, 202–213. doi:10.1016/j.bandl.2009.06.001

Coslett, H. (1999). Spatial influences on motor and language function. *Neuropsychologia, 37*, 695–706.

Crosson, B. (2000). Systems that support language processes: Attention. In S. E. Nadeau, L. J. Gonzalez Rothi, & B. Crosson (Eds.), *Aphasia and language: Theory to practice* (pp. 372–398). New York: The Guilford Press.

Crosson, B. (2008). An intention manipulation to change lateralization of word production in nonfluent aphasia: Current status. *Seminars in Speech and Language, 29*(3), 188–199.

Crosson, B., Fabrizio, K. S., Singletary, F., Cato, M. A., Wierenga, C. E., Parkinson, R. B., Sherod, . . . Gonzalez Rothi, L. J. (2007). Treatment of naming in nonfluent aphasia through manipulation of intention and attention: A phase 1 comparison of two novel treatments. *Journal of the International Neuropsychological Society, 13*, 582–594.

Cutler, A., & Fodor, J. A. (1979). Semantic focus and sentence comprehension. *Cognition, 7*(1), 49–59.

Daneman, M., & Carpenter, P. A. (1980). Individual differences in working memory and reading. *Journal of Verbal Learning and Verbal Behavior, 19*, 450–466.

Davidson, J. E., Irizarry, M. C., Bray, B. C., Wetten, S., Galwey, N., Gibson, R., . . . Monsch, A. U. (2009). An exploration of cognitive subgroups in Alzheimer's disease. *Journal of the International Neuropsychological Society,* 1–11.

Deschaine, D., & Peach, R. K. (2008, November). The cognitive basis for microlinguistic changes in discourse after TBI. Poster presented to the annual convention of the American-Speech-Language Hearing Association, Chicago, IL.

Dotson, V. M., Singletary, F., Fuller, R., Koehler, S., Moore, A. B., Gonzalez Rothi, L. J., & Crosson, B. (2008). Treatment of word-finding deficits in fluent aphasia through the manipulation of spatial attention: Preliminary findings. *Aphasiology, 22*(1), 103–113.

Druks, J., & Masterson, J. (2000). *An object and action naming battery.* London: Psychology Press.

Ellis, C., & Peach, R. K. (2009). Sentence planning following traumatic brain injury. *NeuroRehabilitation, 24,* 255–266.

Erickson, R. J., Goldinger, S. D., & LaPointe, L. L. (1996). Auditory vigilance in aphasic individuals: Detecting nonlinguistic stimuli with full or divided attention. *Brain and Cognition, 30,* 244–253.

Ferreira, V. S., & Pashler, H. (2002). Central bottleneck influences on the processing stages of word production. *Journal of Experimental Psychology: Learning, Memory, and Cognition, 28*(6), 1187–1199. doi:10.1037//0278-7393.28.6.1187

Filley, C. M. (2002). The neuroanatomy of attention. *Seminars in Speech and Language, 23*(2), 89–98.

Fillingham, J. K., Sage, K., & Lambon Ralph, M. A. (2006). The treatment of anomia using errorless learning. *Neuropsychological Rehabilitation, 16*(2), 129–154.

Fischler, I. (2000). Attention, resource allocation, and language. In S. E. Nadeau, L. J. Gonzalez Rothi, & B. Crosson (Eds.), *Aphasia and language: Theory to practice* (pp. 348–370). New York: The Guilford Press.

Fodor, J. D., & Frazier, J. (1980). Is the human sentence parsing mechanism an ATN? *Cognition, 8,* 418–459.

Foldi, N. S., Lobosco, J. J., & Schaefer, L. A. (2002). The effect of attentional dysfunction in Alzheimer's disease: Theoretical and practical implications. *Seminars in Speech and Language, 23*(2), 139–150.

Frattali, C. M., Holland, A. L., Thompson, C. K., Wohl, C., & Ferketic, M. (2003). *Functional Assessment of Communication Skills for Adults (ASHA FACS).* American Speech-Language-Hearing Association: Rockville, MD.

Frazier, L., & Fodor, J. D. (1978). The sausage machine: A new two-stage parsing model. *Cognition 6,* 291–325.

German, D. J. (1989). *The Test of Adolescent and Adult Word-Finding.* Austin, TX: Pro-Ed.

Goodglass, H., Kaplan, E., & Barresi, B. (2000). *Boston Diagnostic Aphasia Examination—Third Edition (BDAE-3).* San Antonio, TX: The Psychological Corporation.

Granier, J. P., Robin, D. A., Shapiro, L. P., Peach, R. K., & Zimba, L. D. (2000). Measuring processing load during sentence comprehension: Visuomotor tracking. *Aphasiology, 14*(5), 501–513. doi:10.1080/026870300401270

Gray, J. M., Robertson, I., Pentland, B., & Anderson, S. (1992). Microcomputer-based attentional retraining after brain damage: A randomised group controlled trial. *Neuropsychological Rehabilitation: An International Journal, 2*(2), 97–115.

Green, S. M., Rich, J. B., & Parks, N. W. (2003). Moderators of verbal cueing effects on novel naturalistic actions in stroke. *Journal of the International Neuropsychological Society, 9,* 150.

Gronwall, D. (1977). Paced Auditory Serial Addition Task (PASAT): A measure of recovery from concussion. *Perceptual and Motor Skills, 44,* 367–373.

Hagen, C. (1984). Language disorders in head trauma. In A. Hollan (Ed.), *Language disorders in adults: Recent advances* (pp. 245–281). San Diego: College Hill Press.

Heaton, R. K., Chelune, G. J., Talley, J. L., Kay, G. G., & Curtis, G. (1993). *Wisconsin Card Sorting Test (WCST) manual, revised and expanded.* Odessa, FL: Psychological Assessment Resources.

Helm-Estabrooks, N., Connor, L. T., & Albert, M. L. (2000). Treating attention to improve auditory comprehension in aphasia. *Brain and Language, 74,* 445–501. doi:10.1006/brln.2000.2372

Helm-Estabrooks, N. (1992). *Aphasia Diagnostic Profiles (ADP).* Austin, TX: Pro-Ed.

Hinchliffe, F. J., Murdoch, B. E., Chenery, H. J., Baglioni, A. J., & Harding-Clark, J. (1998). Cognitive-linguistic subgroups in closed-head injury. *Brain Injury, 12*(5), 369–398.

Holland, A. L., Frattali, C. M., & Fromm, D. (1999). *Communication Activities of Daily Living—Second Edition (CADL-2).* Austin, TX: Pro-Ed.

Huisingh, R., Bowers, L., LoGiudice, C., & Orman, J. (2005). *The WORD Test 2—Adolescent.* East Moline, IL: LinguiSystems.

Hula, W. D., & McNeil, M. R. (2008). Models of attention and dual-task performance as explanatory constructs in aphasia. *Seminars in Speech and Language, 29*(3), 169–187.

Hula, W. D., McNeil, M. R., & Sung, J. E. (2007). Is there an impairment of language-specific attentional processing in aphasia? *Brain and Language, 103,* 240–241.

Hyndman, D., Pickering, R. M., & Ashburn, A. (2008). The influence of attention deficits on functional recovery post stroke during the first 12 months after discharge from the hospital. *Journal of Neurology, Neurosurgery, & Psychiatry, 79,* 656–663.

Jung-Beeman, M. (2005). Bilateral brain processes for comprehending natural languages. *Trends in Cognitive Sciences, 9*(11), 512–518.

Kempler, D., Andersen, E. S., & Henderson, V. W. (1995). Linguistic and attentional contributions to anomia in Alzheimer's disease. *Neuropsychiatry, Neuropsychology, & Behavioral Neurology, 8*(1), 33–37.

Kertesz, A. (1982). *Western Aphasia Battery.* New York: Grune & Stratton.

Kertesz, A. (2006). *Western Aphasia Battery—Revised Edition (WAB-R).* San Antonio, TX: Pearson.

Kohnert, K. (2004). Cognitive and cognate-based treatments for bilingual aphasia: A case study. *Brain and Language, 91*(3), 294–302. doi:10.1016/j.bandl.2004.04.001

Knopman, D. S., Roberts, R. O., Geda, Y. E., Boeve, B. F., Pankratz, V. S., Cha, R. H., . . . Petersen, R. C. (2009). Association of prior stroke with cognitive function and cognitive impairment: A population-based study. *Archives of Neurology, 66*(5), 614–619.

Knudsen, E. L. (2007). Fundamental components of attention. *Annual Review of Neuroscience, 30,* 57–78.

Langacker, R. L. (2008). *Cognitive grammar: A basic introduction.* New York: Oxford University Press.

LaPointe, L. L., & Erickson, R. J. (1991). Auditory vigilance during divided task attention in aphasic individuals. *Aphasiology, 5*(6), 511–520.

LaPointe, L. L., & Horner, J. (1998). *Reading Comprehension Battery for Aphasia—Second Edition (RCBA-2).* Austin, TX: Pro-Ed.

Levin, H. S. (1981). Aphasia in closed head injury. In M. T. Sarno (Ed.), *Acquired aphasia.* New York: Oxford University Press.

Levinoff, E. J., Saumier, D., & Chertkow, H. (2005). Focused attention deficits in patients with Alzheimer's disease and mild cognitive impairment. *Brain and Cognition, 57,* 127–130.

Lezak, M. D., Howieson, D. B., & Loring, D. W. (2004). *Neuropsychological assessment* (4th ed.). New York: Oxford University Press.

Lomas, J., Pickard, L., Bester, S., Elbard, H., Finlayson, A., & Zoghaib, C. (1989). The Communicative Effectiveness Index (CETI): Development and psychometric evaluation of a functional communication measure for adult aphasia. *Journal of Speech and Hearing Disorders, 54,* 113–124.

MacLeod, C. M. (1992). The Stroop task: The "gold standard" of attentional measures. *Journal of Experimental Psychology: General, 121,* 12–14.

Manly, T., & Robertson, I. H. (2005). The Sustained Attention to Response Test (SART). In L. Itti, G. Rees & J. K. Tsotsos (Eds.), *Neurobiology of attention* (pp. 337–339). Amsterdam: Elsevier.

Mapou, R. L., & Mateer, C. A. (1996). Understanding, evaluating and managing attention disorders following traumatic brain injury. *Journal of Head Trauma Rehabilitation, 11*(2), 1–16.

McNeil, M. R., Hula, W. D., & Sung, J. E. (2011). The role of memory and attention in aphasic language performance. In J. Guendouzi, F. Loncke & M. Williams (Eds.), *The handbook of psycholinguistic & cognitive processes: Perspectives in communication disorders.* LEA, Taylor & Francis.

McNeil, M. R., Kim, A., Lim, K., Pratt, S., Kendall, D., Pompon, R., . . . Dickey, M. (2010). *Automatic activation, interference and facilitation effects in persons with aphasia and normal adult controls on experimental CRTT-R-Stroop tasks.* Paper presented at the Clinical Aphasiology Conference, Isle of Palms, South Carolina.

McNeil, M. R., Doyle, P., Hula, W. D., Rubinsky, H., Fossett, T. R. D., & Matthews, C. T. (2004). Using resource allocation theory and duel-task methods to increase the sensitivity of assessment in aphasia. *Aphasiology, 18*(5), 521–542.

Mesulam, M. (1990). Large-scale neurocognitive networks and distributed processing for attention, language, and memory. *Annals of Neurology, 28,* 597–613.

Mesulam, M. (1998). From sensation to cognition. *Brain, 121,* 1013–1052.

Moosbrugger, H., Goldhammer, F., & Schweizer, K. (2006). Latent factors underlying individual differences in attention measures: Perceptual and executive attention. *European Journal of Psychological Assessment, 22*(3), 177–188.

Murray, L. L. (1999). Review attention and aphasia: Theory, research and clinical implications. *Aphasiology, 13*(2), 91–111.

Murray, L. L. (2000). The effects of varying attentional demands on the word retrieval skills of adults with aphasia, right hemisphere brain damage, or no brain damage. *Brain and Language, 72,* 40–72.

Murray, L. L. (2002). Attention deficits in aphasia: Presence, nature, assessment, and treatment. *Seminars in Speech and Language, 23*(2), 107–116.

Murray, L. L., Holland, A. L., & Beeson, P. M. (1997). Auditory processing in individuals with mild aphasia: A study of resource allocation. *Journal of Speech, Language, and Hearing Research, 40,* 792–808.

Murray, L. L., Holland, A. L., & Beeson, P. M. (1998). Spoken language of individuals with mild fluent aphasia under focused and divided-attention conditions. *Journal of Speech, Language, and Hearing Research, 41,* 213–227.

Murray, L. L., Keeton, R. J., & Karcher, L. (2006). Treating attention in mild aphasia: Evaluation of attention process training-II. *Journal of Communication Disorders, 39,* 37–61.

Myachykov, A., & Posner, M. I. (2005). Attention in language. In L. Itti, G. Rees & J. K. Tsotsos (Eds.), *Neurobiology of attention* (pp. 324–329). Boston: Elsevier.

Myers, P. S., & Blake, M. L. (2008). Communication disorders associated with right-hemisphere damage. In R. Chapey (Ed.), *Language intervention strategies in aphasia and related neurogenic communication disorders* (5th ed., pp. 963–987). Philadelphia: Lippincott Williams & Wilkins.

Neils, J., Roeltgen, D. P., & Greer, A. (1995). Spelling and attention in early Alzheimer's disease: Evidence for impairment of the graphemic buffer. *Brain and Language, 49,* 241–262.

Nicholas L. E., & Brookshire, R. H. (1993). A system for quantifying the informativeness and efficiency of the connected speech of adults with aphasia. *Journal of Speech and Hearing Research. 36,* 338–350.

Niemann, H., Ruff, R. M., & Baser, C. A. (1990). Computer-assisted attention retraining in head-injured individuals: A controlled efficacy study of an outpatient program. *Journal of Consulting and Clinical Psychology, 58*(6), 811–817.

Palmese, C. A., & Raskin, S. A. (2000). The rehabilitation of attention in individuals with mild traumatic brain injury, using the APT-II programme. *Brain Injury, 14*(6), 535–548.

Parasuraman, R., & Haxby, J. V. (1993). Attention and brain function in Alzheimer's disease: A review. *Neuropsychology, 7*(3), 242–272.

Park, N. W., & Barbuto, E. (2005). Treating attention impairments: Review with a particular focus on naturalistic action rehabilitation. In P. W. Halligan, & D. T. Wade (Eds.), *The effectiveness of rehabilitation for cognitive deficits* (pp. 81–90). New York: Oxford University Press.

Park, N. W., & Ingles, J. L. (2001). Effectiveness of attention rehabilitation after an acquired brain injury: A meta-analysis. *Neuropsychology, 15*(2), 199–210.

Park, N. W., Proulx, G., & Towers, W. M. (1999). Evaluation of the attention process training programme. *Neuropsychological Rehabilitation, 9*(2), 135–154.

Peach, R. K. (1992). Factors underlying neuropsychological test performance in chronic severe traumatic brain injury. *Journal of Speech and Hearing Research, 35,* 810–818.

Peach, R. K., Rubin, S. S., & Newhoff, M. (1994). A topographic event-related potential analysis of the attention deficit for auditory processing in aphasia. *Clinical Aphasiology, 22,* 81–96.

Peck, K. K., Moore, A. B., Crosson, B. A., Gaiefsky, M., Gopinath, K. S., White, K., & Briggs, R. W. (2004). Functional magnetic resonance imaging before and after aphasia therapy: Shifts in hemodynamic time to peak during an overt language task. *Stroke, 35,* 554–559.

Pero, S., Incoccia, C., Caracciolo, B., Zoccolotti, P., & Formisano, R. (2006). Rehabilitation of attention in two patients with traumatic brain injury by means of "attention process training." *Brain Injury, 20*(11), 1207–1219. doi:10.1080/02699050600983271

Ponsford, J., & Kinsella, G. (1991). The use of a rating scale of attentional behaviour. *Neuropsychological Rehabilitation, 1,* 241–257.

Ramscar, M., Matlock, T., & Boroditsky, L. (2009). Time, motion, and meaning: The experiential basis of abstract thought. In K. S. Mix, L. B. Smith, & M. G. (Eds.), *The spatial foundations of language and cognition* (pp. 67–82). Oxford: Oxford University Press.

Ramscar, M., Matlock, T., & Dye, M. (2009). Running down the clock: The role of expectation in our understanding of time and motion. *Language and Cognitive Processes.*

Robertson, I. H., Manly, T., Andrade, J., Baddeley, B. T., & Yiend, J. (1997). "Oops!": Performance correlates of everyday attentional failures in traumatic brain injured and normal subjects. *Neuropsychologia, 35*(6), 747–758.

Robertson, I. H., Ward, T., Ridgeway, V. & Nimmo-Smith, I. (1994). *The test of everyday attention.* Bury St. Edmunds: Thames Valley Test Company.

Rohling, M. L., Faust, M. E., Beverly, B., & Demakis, G. (2009). Effectiveness of cognitive rehabilitation following acquired brain injury: A meta-analytic re-examination of Cicerone et al.'s (2000, 2005) systematic reviews. *Neuropsychology, 23*(1), 20–39.

Sandford, J. A., & Turner, A. (2000). *Integrated Visual and Auditory Continuous Performance Test manual.* Richmond, VA: BrainTrain.

Sarno, M. T., Buonaguro, A., & Levita, E. (1986). Characteristics of verbal impairment in closed head injured patients. *Archives of Physical Medicine and Rehabilitation, 7,* 400–405.

Schretlen, D. (1997). *Brief Test of Attention professional manual.* Odessa, FL: Psychological Assessment Resources.

Shallice, T. (1982). Specific impairments of planning. *Philosophical Transactions of the Royal Society of London Series B, 298,* 199–209.

Sinotte, M. P., & Coelho, C. A. (2007). Attention training for reading impairment in mild aphasia: A follow-up study. *Neuropsychological Rehabilitation, 22,* 303–310.

Smith, A. (1991). *The Symbol Digit Modalities Test.* Los Angeles: Western Psychological Services.

Sohlberg, M. M. (2005). Can disabilities resulting from attentional impairments be treated effectively? In P. W. Halligan, & D. T. Wade (Eds.), *The effectiveness of rehabilitation for cognitive deficits* (pp. 91–102). New York: Oxford University Press.

Sohlberg, M. M., Avery, J., Kennedy, M., Ylvisaker, M., Coelho, C., Turkstra, L., & Yorkston, K. (2003). Practice guidelines for direct attention training. *Journal of Medical Speech-Language Pathology, 11*(3), xix–xxxix.

Sohlberg, M. M., Johnson, L., Paule, L., Raskin, S. A., & Mateer, C. A. (2001). *Attention process training-II: A program to address attentional deficits for persons with mild cognitive dysfunction* (2nd ed.). Wake Forest, NC: Lash & Associates.

Sohlberg, M. M., & Mateer, C. A. (1986). *Attention Process Training (APT).* Puyallup, WA: Association for Neuropsychological Research and Development.

Sohlberg, M. M., & Mateer, C. A. (1987). Effectiveness of an attention-training program. *Journal of Clinical and Experimental Neuropsychology, 9*(2), 117–130.

Sohlberg, M. M., McLaughlin, K. A., Pavese, A., Heidrich, A., & Posner, M. I. (2000). Evaluation of attention process training and brain injury education in persons with acquired brain injury. *Journal of Clinical and Experimental Neuropsychology, 22*(5), 656–676.

Spreen, O. & Benton, A. L. (1977). *Neurosensory Center Comprehensive Examination for Aphasia—Revised Edition (NCCEA).* Victoria, BC: University of Victoria, Neuropsychology Laboratory.

Stierwalt, J., & Murray, L. L. (2002). Attention impairment following traumatic brain injury. *Seminars in Speech and Language, 23*(2), 129–138.

Strauss, E., Sherman, E. M. S., & Spreen, O. (2006). *A compendium of neuropsychological tests: Administration, norms, and commentary—Third Edition.* New York: Oxford University Press.

Sturm, W., Longoni, F., Weis, S., Specht, K., Herzog, H., Vohn, R., . . . Willmes, K. (2004). Functional reorganization in patients with right hemisphere stroke after training of alertness: A longitudinal PET and fMRI study in eight cases. *Neuropsychologia, 42,* 434–450.

Sturm, W., Willmes, K., Orgass, B., & Hartje, W. (1997). Do specific attention deficits need specific training? *Neuropsychological Rehabilitation, 7*(2), 81–103.

Swinney, D. (1979). Lexical access during sentence comprehension: (Re)consideration of context effects. *Journal of Verbal Learning and Verbal Behavior, 18,* 645–659.

Talmy, L. (2003). The windowing of attention in language. *In Toward a cognitive semantics volume I: Concept structuring systems* (pp. 258–309). Cambridge, MA: The MIT Press.

Taube-Schiff, M., & Segalowitz, N. (2005). Linguistic attention control: Attention shifting governed by grammaticized elements of language. *Journal of Experimental Psychology: Learning, Memory, and Cognition, 31*(3), 508–519.

Thomas-Stonell, N., Johnson, P., Schuller, R., & Jutai, J. (1994). Evaluation of a computer-based program for remediation of cognitive-communication skills. *Journal of Head Trauma Rehabilitation, 9*(4), 25–37.

Tombaugh, T. N., & Rees, L. (2008). Computerized test of information processing. North Tonawanda, NY: MHS.

Tompkins, C. A., Baumgaertner, A., Lehman, M., & Fassbinder, W. (2000). Mechanisms of discourse comprehension impairment after right hemisphere brain damage: Suppression in lexical ambiguity resolution. *Journal of Speech, Language, and Hearing Research, 43,* 62–78.

Tompkins, C. A., Blake, M. L., Baumgaertner, A., & Fassbinder, W. (2002). Characterising comprehension difficulties after right brain damage: Attentional demands of suppression function. *Aphasiology, 16*(4/5/6), 559–572.

Tompkins, C. A., Bloise, C. G. R., Timko, M. L., & Baumgaertner, A. (1994). Working memory and inference revision in brain damaged and normally aging adults. *Journal of Speech, Language, and Hearing Research, 37*, 896–912

Tompkins, C. A., Fassbinder, W., Scharp, V. L., & Meigh, K. M. (2008). Activation and maintenance of peripheral semantic features of unambiguous words after right hemisphere brain damage in adults. *Aphasiology, 22*(2), 119–138.

Tompkins, C. A., Scharp, V. L., Meigh, K. M., & Fassbinder, W. (2008). Course coding and discourse comprehension in adults with right hemisphere brain damage. *Aphasiology, 22*(2), 204–223.

van Zomeren, A., & Brouwer, W. (1992). In J. Crawford, D. Parker, W., & McKinlay (Eds.), *A handbook of neuropsychological assessment* (pp. 241–266). Hillsdale, NJ, England: Lawrence Erlbaum Associates, Inc.

van Zomeren, A. H., & Spikman, J. M. (2005). Testing speed and control: The assessment of attentional impairments. In P. W. Halligan, & D. T. Wade (Eds.), *The effectiveness of rehabilitation for cognitive deficits* (pp. 71–80). New York: Oxford University Press.

Wechsler, D. (1997). *Wechsler Adult Intelligence Scale—Third Edition (WAIS-III)*. San Antonio, TX: Psychological Corporation.

Whelan, B., Murdoch, B., & Bellamy, N. (2007). Delineating communication impairments associated with mild traumatic brain injury: A case report. *Journal of Head Trauma Rehabilitation, 22*(3), 192–197.

Wiederholt, J. L., & Bryant, B. R. (2001). *The Gray Oral Reading Tests—Fourth Edition*. Austin, TX: Pro-Ed.

Wiig, E. H., & Secord, W. A. (1989). *Test of Work Knowledge—Expanded Edition (TLC-E)*. San Antonio, TX: The Psychological Corporation.

Willmott, C., Ponsford, J., Hocking, C., & Schonberger, M. (2009). Factors contributing to attentional impairments after traumatic brain injury. *Neuropsychology, 23*(4), 424–432. doi:10.1037/a0015058

Wilson, B. A., Alderman, N., Burgess, P. W., Emslie, H., & Evans, J. J. (1996). *Behavioural Assessment of the Dysexecutive Syndrome*. Bury St. Edmunds, England: Thames Valley Test Company.

Wilson, B. A., Cockburn, J., & Halligan, P. W. (1987). *Behavioral Inattention Test manual*. Fareham, UK: Thames Valley Test.

Woodcock, R., & Johnson, B. (1977). *Woodcock-Johnson Psycho-Educational Battery*. Boston, MA: Teaching Resources Corporation.

Ylvisaker, M., Hanks, R., & Johnson-Green, D. (2003). Rehabilitation of children and adults with cognitive-communication disorders after brain injury. *ASHA Supplement, 23*, 59–72.

Ylvisaker, M., Szekeres, S. F., & Feeney, T. (2008). Communication disorders associated with traumatic brain injury. In R. Chapey (Ed.), *Language intervention strategies in aphasia and related neurogenic communication disorders* (5th ed., pp. 879–962). Philadelphia: Lippincott Williams & Wilkins.

Youse, K. M., & Coelho, C. A. (2009). Treating underlying attention deficits as a means for improving conversational discourse in individuals with closed head injury: A preliminary study. *Neuropsychological Rehabilitation, 24*(4), 355–364.

Zimmermann, P., & Fimm, B. (1995). *The Test for Attentional Performance (TAP)*. English version 1.02. Herzogenrath: Psytest.

An Assessment Battery for Patients with Acquired Language Disorders due to Attentional Impairment

Area of Assessment	Recommended Test
General language	Aphasia Diagnostic Profiles (ADP) (Helm-Estabrooks, 1992)
	Boston Diagnostic Aphasia Examination—Third Edition (BDAE-3) (Goodglass, Kaplan, & Barresi, 2000)
	Neurosensory Center Comprehensive Examination for Aphasia (NCCEA) (Spreen & Benton, 1977)
	Western Aphasia Battery—Revised (WAB-R) (Kertesz, 2006)
Oral naming/word meaning	Object and Action Naming Battery (Druks & Masterson, 2000)
	Test of Adolescent and Adult Word Finding (German, 1989)
	The WORD Test 2—Adolescent (Huisingh, Bowers, LoGiudice, & Orman, 2005)
Higher-level language	Discourse Comprehension Test—Second Edition (Brookshire & Nicholas, 1997)
	Test of Language Competence—Expanded Edition (TLC-E) (Wiig & Secord, 1989)
Functional language	Communicative Effectiveness Inventory (CETI) (Lomas et al., 1989)
	Functional Assessment of Communication Skills for Adults (ASHA FACS) (Frattali, Holland, Thompson, Wohl, & Ferketic, 2003)
	Communication Activities of Daily Living—Second Edition (CADL-2) (Holland, Frattali, & Fromm, 1999)
Selective attention, sustained attention, attentional switching	Test of Everyday Attention (Robertson, Ward, Ridgeway, & Nimmo-Smith, 1994)
Attention allocation (dual-task performance)	Stroop Test (MacLeod, 1992)
Processing speed	Paced Auditory Serial Addition Test (PASAT) (Gronwall, 1977)
Ecological attention outcomes	Rating Scale of Attentional Behaviour (Ponsford & Kinsella, 1991
	Cognitive Failures Questionnaire (Broadbent, Cooper, FitzGerald, & Parkes, 1982)

A Language-Specific Approach to the Treatment of Acquired Language Disorders Associated with Attention Deficits

Attention Manipulation	Treatment
Lexical Processing	
Spatial attention	1. Picture stimuli are presented in ipsilesional hemispace for naming and gradually moved to the center of visual space. Accuracy of naming for trained and untrained items assessed to evaluate improvement.
Attention allocation	2. Patient listens to word lists and raises hand when target word heard while simultaneously completing card sorting task. Accuracy measured for target word identification and card sorting responses.
Sentence Processing	
Focused attention	1. Patient describes a dynamic event with semantically-reversible objects using external cues to determine the syntactic subject. Events are presented using pictures and/or object manipulations.
	Event: A brown bear kissing a black bear
	Cue: Brown bear
	Response: *The brown bear is kissing the black bear.*
	Cue: Black bear
	Response: *The black bear was kissed by the brown bear.*
	Event: A black bear giving a donkey to a brown bear
	Cue: Black bear
	Response: *The black bear is giving the donkey to the brown bear.*
	Cue: Brown bear
	Response: *The brown bear was given the donkey by the black bear.*
	2. Place embedded topics at the beginnings of sentences to improve attention to, and comprehension for, sentences; subsequently withdraw topicalization of target words.
	Topicalized sentence (Cutler & Fodor, 1979):
	Candid, the story was, that the reporter with the daily newspaper was responsible for.
	Which reporter was responsible for the story?
	Which story was the reporter responsible for?
	Sentence without topicalization:
	The opening of the concert was spoiled by the director's outburst.
	Which opening was spoiled by the director's outburst?
	Whose outburst spoiled the opening?

Attention Manipulation	Treatment
Sentence Processing	
Focused attention—cont'd	3. Present sentences with anaphoric pronouns that require a cognitive search for the antecedent Anaphoric sentences: *Kevin left after he found the envelope.* Who found the envelope? *Mary told John during the party about the woman he was going to meet.* Who was going to meet the woman? *The man who investigated Charley over the previous three years told the woman how much he hates him.* Who does the man hate? 4. Present sentences that use nominal grounding elements Articles (a, the): *The girl in the class likes a boy.* Do we know which girl likes the boy? Do we know which boy the girl likes? Demonstratives (this, that, these, those): *This evidence should satisfy those detectives.* Is the evidence close at hand? Are the detectives close at hand? Quantifiers (all, most, some, every, each, any): *All of the buildings were badly damaged but most of the animals escaped.* Did any of the buildings escape damage? Did any of the animals escape harm? 5. Present sentences that use clausal grounding elements Tense: *Jim says that he is injured.* *Jim says that he was injured.* *Jim said that he is injured.* *Jim said that he was injured.* Is Jim saying that he is injured now? Is Jim saying now that he is injured? Modals (may, can, will, shall, must): *You might help me shovel the snow for a change.* *You must help me shovel the snow for a change.* Is there a chance you won't help me with the snow? Are you required to help me shovel the snow?

Continued

Attention Manipulation	Treatment
Sentence Processing	
Focused attention—cont'd	6. Identify core elements of a sentence using windowing Path windowing*: *The ball that was hit by the pitcher sailed like a rocket on a line drive to the outfield wall.* Initial windowing: How was the ball hit? *The ball that was hit by the pitcher sailed like a rocket.* Medial windowing: What kind of a hit was it? *The ball that was hit by the pitcher sailed on a line drive.* Final windowing: Where did the hit go? *The ball that was hit by the pitcher sailed to the outfield wall.* *The example is for open path windowing. See text for examples of <u>closed</u> and <u>fictive</u> path windowing. Phase windowing: *The car battery continued to die and I kept recharging it.* Departure phase windowing: What did the car battery do? *The car battery continued to die.* Return phase windowing: What did I do? *I kept recharging the battery.* Factuality windowing: *I wasn't in the meeting last week.* Comparison frame: What would be the opposite of this event? *I was in the meeting last week.* *I went to the meeting last week because I was scheduled to speak.* Comparison frame: What would you have done if you were not scheduled to speak at the meeting last week? *I would not have gone to the meeting because I was not scheduled to speak.*
Attention allocation	7. Patients memorize a string of 2–6 digits presented visually, judge the grammaticality of a sentence presented auditorily, and then verify whether another string of digits matches the preceding string. Accuracy scores are calculated for the grammaticality judgments with and without the strings of digits. Sentence stimuli include errors of auxiliary and determiner omission, agreement, and transposition in early and late positions (see Blackwell & Bates, 1995, for list of sentences).

CHAPTER 13

Management of Communication Deficits Associated with Memory Disorders

CHAPTER OUTLINE

Nadine Martin

The memory subsystems described in Chapters 5 and 9 support language processing, verbal learning, and human communication in different ways. Impairment of each subsystem has consequences for the integrity of language processing and functional communication. Thus, assessment of language disorders should include an evaluation of short-term and long-term memory and other cognitive control processes (e.g., attention and executive functions). Additionally, the close association of memory and language processing indicates a need to develop treatment approaches that address both language and memory abilities. This need may seem obvious in the rehabilitation of communication disorders associated with traumatic brain injury and degenerative memory disorders (e.g., semantic dementia), as the memory disorders clearly instigates the communication disorder. Acquired aphasia, on the other hand, might seem to be primarily a language disorder and less obviously related to memory abilities. However, the memory disorder present in aphasia is not one of long-term memory or encoding new memories. Rather, it is a disturbance of short-term memory (STM) processes that are intrinsic to language processing. Recent approaches to treatment of adult-onset and developmental language disorders focus on improving short-term memory abilities to improve language function.

It is essential that students and practitioners of speech-language pathology and neuropsychology become aware of the ways in which different types of memory support language function and how impairment to these memory systems affect language processing and functional communication. This chapter reviews three types of memory impairments that have direct and/or indirect consequences for language processing and communication: memory encoding disorders (anterograde amnesia) associated with head injury, semantic memory deficits associated with progressive neurological disease, and short-term maintenance of verbal representations in aphasia. This is not an exhaustive list of memory disorders, but each illustrates a different type of memory support to language function progressing from least direct (encoding new memories) to semi-direct (semantic memory that is expressed via language) to most direct (short-term maintenance of language representations). The review of these three memory related communication impairments will include guidelines for assessment and a discussion of current approaches to rehabilitation. It is anticipated that the reader will become familiar with the indirect and direct ways in which impaired memory processes can impact language function and communication.

ENCODING NEW MEMORIES FOLLOWING TRAUMATIC BRAIN INJURY (TBI)

Nature of the Impact on Language and Communication

Specific language impairments following traumatic brain injury do occur, but are not common and are associated with more focal injuries. One language disorder that *is* quite common following a head injury is anomia (Heilman, Safran, & Geshwind, 1971), and the severity of this symptom is directly related to the severity of the injury (Levin, Grossman, & Kelly, 1976). Memory disorders following TBI are quite common and occur in conjunction with impairments to other cognitive processes such as attention and executive functioning. The nature of the memory disorder is a difficulty in encoding new information into long-term memory (Coelho, DeRuyter, & Stein, 1996; Ylvisaker, Szekeres, & Feeney, 2008). Curtiss, Vanderploeg, Spencer, and Salazar (2001) used cluster analyses to examine memory encoding and the involvement of short- and long-term memory processes in TBI. They identified impairments of three memory processes in this population: memory consolidation, retention of memories and retrieval of memories. Furthermore, they determined that those individuals with retrieval difficulties also demonstrated "memory control" problems (perseveration of responses). It has been hypothesized that the memory encoding difficulty may be related to impairments of the hippocampal system, which has been associated with consolidation of new memories (Nadel & Moscovitch, 1997).

An impaired ability to encode new memories does not affect language processing directly, but does disrupt verbal learning ability. It also can affect functional communication in several ways. The inability to learn new verbal information will make any effort to return to school or job training a challenge at best. It will also affect activities of daily living that require remembering specific sets of verbal information for a short period. For example, someone might be given directions somewhere or they might have new instructions for medicine regimen). The language in these instructions is not new, but the assembly of known words *is* new and must be encoded, understood, and retrieved in the short term. In addition to difficulties with specific tasks of daily living that involve language, memory retrieval impairment will make conversational interactions difficult. If there are breakdowns in functional communication, there is a risk that the person with TBI will become socially withdrawn (Ylvisaker et al., 2008), which in turn impact communication further. Rehabilitation approaches emphasize compensatory strategies to help the individual cope with these memory difficulties.

Assessment

Memory disorders are just one of several cognitive abilities that are impaired after head injury. Other disorders that may affect functional communication include disorders of attention and executive functions. Assessment of memory disorders and associated communication impairments should include standardized tests of memory (Butters & Delis, 1995), standardized assessments of language and communication (Turkstra, Coelho, & Ylvisaker, 2005), as well as non-standardized assessment of language and communication (Coelho, Ylvisaker, & Turkstra, 2005).

Standardized Memory Scales

Typically, standardized memory scales are included in a neuropsychological evaluation. Nonetheless, speech-language pathologists should be familiar with these tests and the interpretation of the test results. The most widely used memory scale is the Wechsler Memory Scale—Revised (WMS-R, Wechsler, 1987). It includes 13 subtests assessing many aspects of memory including short-term digit span, immediate recall of verbal and nonverbal material, delayed recall, visual memory, and verbal learning. Williams (1991) developed the Memory Assessment Scales, which are similar to the WMS-R, but include some additional tasks that measure cued recall, recognition, memory for proper names, and list-learning. This latter task allows for observation of learning strategies and error types that occur (Butters & Delis, 1995). This kind of information is directly relevant to the development of a rehabilitation protocol for the person with cognitive impairments following head injury. Fostering the development of efficient learning strategies is an important goal in cognitive rehabilitation. Thus, it is important to know what strategies, good or bad, the person with TBI is using to learn new information. Other tests of verbal learning include the Rey Auditory Verbal Learning Test (Rey, 1941, 1964) and the California Verbal Learning Test (CVLT; Delis, Kramer, Kaplan, & Ober, 1987). The typical procedure used in a verbal learning test is to first present a list of unrelated words five times and ask for immediate recall of the list after each presentation. These are the learning trials. They are followed by a second list of unrelated words presented one at a time. This is the interference task. Following this, the examinee is asked to recall the first list. Assessment of learning is gauged by number of items recalled after the interference task, but also the CVLT includes measures of strategies used by the examinee and errors that occurred during the list-learning task.

Standardized Tests of Cognitive-Based Communication Disorders

Assessment of language and memory function after traumatic brain injury can be challenging for the speech and language pathologist because standardized language and communication tests are not necessarily designed with this population in mind. Moreover, even those tests that assess functional communication do not address the functional language and communication needs outside the clinical setting. Nonetheless, standardized tests provide a starting point to evaluate the client's functional communication abilities relative to normative data or some standard of typical communication behavior (Turkstra et al., 2005). These measures can also serve to identify starting points in treatment.

In response to a growing need for guidelines to the assessment of language and communication abilities after TBI, the Academy of Neurological Communication Disorders and Sciences Practice Guidelines Group (ANCDS) developed a set of guidelines for speech-language pathologists (Turkstra et al., 2005). The committee evaluated 84 tests recommended by speech-language pathologists in a survey on assessment and an additional 40 tests recommended by publishers. After an initial screening, tests that did not include traumatic brain injury as a target population were eliminated, leaving 31 tests for the next stage of the evaluation, which considered the reliability and validity criteria of the tests. The criteria established by the Agency for Health Care Policy Research (www.ahrq.gov.clinic.epc; reported by Turkstra et al., 2005) were met by only 7 of the 31 tests. These included:

1. American Speech-Language-Hearing Association Functional Assessment of Communication Skills in Adults (ASHA-FACS)
2. Behavior Rating Inventory of Executive Function (BRIEF; Gioia, Isquith, Guy, & Kenworthy, 2000)
3. Communication Activities of Daily Living, Second Edition (CADL-2; Holland, Frattali, & Fromm, 1999)
4. Functional Independence Measure (FIM), Uniform Data Set for Medical Rehabilitation
5. Repeatable Battery for the Assessment of Neuropsychological Status (RBANS; Randolph, 2001)
6. Test of Language Competence—Expanded (Wiig & Secord, 1989)
7. Western Aphasia Battery (WAB; Kertesz, 1982)[1]

Turkstra et al. (2005) note some important themes that are shared by these measures. In the context of the International Classification of Functioning, Disability and Health (ICF) Model, some of these tests address impairment level and activity/participation levels of function. They also note that these measures are not designed specifically for cognitive communication impairments associated with traumatic brain injury. Although they can be adapted for use with this population, there is still a need for assessment measures designed specifically for this population.

Nonstandardized Assessment of Cognitive-Communication Impairment

As noted above, standardized assessments of language and communication disorders provide only a starting point of understanding the communication needs of someone with a traumatic brain injury. The eventual development of a comprehensive standardized battery to address the needs of this population will be a welcome advance in rehabilitation medicine. Until that is accomplished, nonstandardized assessment procedures can be used to fill in the assessment gaps not addressed by current standardized communication measures. It is important to note, however, that nonstandardized tests will always have a place in assessment of communication abilities associated with TBI. In particular, they are necessary to assess communication functions and abilities in real-world contexts, which vary across individuals. Thus, nonstandardized observations should be used to document (1) performance in real-world settings, (2) demands of those real-world settings, (3) competencies of the client's communication partners, and (4) changes in these circumstances (Coelho et al., 2005).

A nonstandardized assessment approach that is commonly used in rehabilitation of people with head injury is discourse analysis. This is a valuable means of gaining insight into a client's functional language abilities, as performance on single word and sentence processing measures may seem unimpaired. A survey by Coelho et al. (2005) indicated that speech-language pathologists working with individuals with TBI used two types of discourse analysis in their assessments of communication ability, monologic and conversational. Memory impairments potentially could affect either type of discourse, because maintaining a theme across sentences in a story or in the context of a conversation requires encoding information and maintaining it in working memory. Results of the survey indicated that typical measures obtained from monologic discourse samples included cohesion of meaning across sentences, grammatical complexity of sentences, thematic unity, accuracy of information content, productivity and efficiency of narrative, lexical selection, and propositional content. Some consistent observations reported by participants in the survey were that individuals with TBI are less verbal overall, and their narratives less efficient and coherent. In particular, the content of narratives was not always accurate or well organized. In the survey of conversational discourse studies in TBI a consistent finding was difficulty in initiation of and maintenance of conversation topics. Additionally, content errors and word finding episodes were reported. Memory disorders associated with TBI as well as some executive function impairments can account for these difficulties.

---

[1]Note that this test has been revised since publication of this report, WAB-R, Kertesz, 2006

Coelho et al. (2005; see also Ylvisaker, Szekeres, & Feeney, 2008) emphasize the need for dynamic, ongoing assessment to identify factors that will influence performance, including strategies used by the client, potential ways to modify a task, context effects, and environmental supports. The goal of a dynamic assessment is to determine how these factors can be modified to optimize a person's communication abilities and develop an effective intervention plan.

Consistent with the dynamic assessment approach, Ylvisaker and colleagues have developed a protocol that they term "contextualized hypothesis testing" (Ylvisaker & Feeney, 1998; Ylvisaker et al., 2008). This approach emphasizes the need for ongoing assessment of abilities and environmental factors in rehabilitation of communication impairments in TBI. There are a multitude of factors that can affect communication ability and success in functional communication environments. These ever-changing factors include those relating to a person's cognitive abilities and those relating to his/her real-life circumstances. A key motivation for using an ongoing hypothesis testing strategy is that there are multiple factors that may or may not be contributing to the communication success or failure of individuals with TBI. These include the memory disorder, speed of processing, language ability, knowledge base, and executive function abilities (e.g., attention, orientation, working memory self-monitoring). The combination of spared and impaired abilities in TBI will vary from person to person and will change over the course of recovery. It is critical to keep abreast of changes in a person's overall cognitive/language profile in order to adjust the rehabilitation program accordingly.

For the speech-language pathologist working in a setting that provides service for individuals with TBI, the benefits of using the contextual hypothesis testing approach will be enhanced by collaboration with other professionals who work with the client's cognitive/emotional abilities and/or the client's environment. Such collaboration provides more information to form and test hypotheses about approaches to rehabilitation that will be most beneficial to the client. It is also recommended that a portion of the hypotheses testing be carried out in contexts that at least simulate environmental settings that will be encountered by the client with TBI (Coelho et al., 2005; Ylvisaker & Feeney, 1998). For good reasons, clinical settings are different from the real-life environment in many ways. They control for distractions and variables that confound diagnoses of language disorders and, in so doing, enable optimal performance of someone with TBI (or other impairment) on diagnostic and treatment activities. This is an important approach to the overall assessment of

someone's language and cognitive abilities after brain injury, of course. However, the clinical environment does not reflect the real world in which the client will be faced with numerous and frequently changing variables that will challenge his/her functional communication every day. Therefore, it is important that clinicians find ways to assess a client's performance in his/her real life environment or in a setting that simulates the kinds of challenges the client will face outside the clinic.

Perhaps the most important recommendation of Ylvisaker and colleagues is that assessment needs to be ongoing and should continue for months or years depending on the circumstances of client and rehabilitation setting. Early assessments at the onset of TBI will need to be repeated to accommodate rapid changes that often occur in the first year post-trauma. The constellation of potential cognitive, emotional, and social impairments is complex and the true extent of a disability may not be apparent until there is time to observe interactions of the individual with his/her environment. Some difficulties noted early on may not be problematic to overall function until later stages of rehabilitation that involve, for example, vocational goals. Finally, they note that a person's emotional response to his/her disability is something that changes over time and depending on circumstances. This is an aspect of TBI rehabilitation that must be assessed periodically to ensure that support systems are responsive to the needs of the client.

Approaches to Rehabilitation

It should be apparent from the review of approaches to assessment of functional communication in TBI that there are a multitude of cognitive, social, and behavioral abilities and factors to be considered in this disorder. Given the idea that assessment and rehabilitation of TBI continuously yield information relevant to the evolving needs and circumstances of someone with TBI as he/she recovers, treatment strategies will need to be dynamic and consider all cognitive, executive, and social functions. For example, treatment does not involve just working on memory or just working on attention. Treatment must address these fundamental functions and in the context of real-life settings that the client will face. Thus, the first and most important consideration in fashioning a rehabilitation program for someone with TBI is that it will be very individualized. This is not to say that it will be totally unique, although parts of it may be. Rather, techniques and strategies to foster redevelopment or establishment of fundamental cognitive skills and functional/social communication abilities should be based on general approaches to cognitive rehabilitation and the unique needs, abilities, and disabilities of the client. This approach, which, by necessity, will involve the client's input, is reflected in a program of rehabilitation developed by Kennedy & Coelho (2005) that aims to develop self-monitoring and self-control of memory and learning in TBI. They emphasize the importance of a person with TBI learning to self-monitor the accuracy of his/her memory performance, be it retrieval of long- or short-term memories. This means that whatever specific memory retraining strategies are employed in a rehabilitation program, they need to be accompanied by additional training in monitoring the outcomes of memory "exercises." This will enable the client to be more aware of when he/she needs to review something to be remembered or to ask for additional information or repetition of information.

One means of promoting independent self-monitoring of memory functions is the use of a diary or memory notebook. A number of studies indicate the usefulness of this approach (Kreutzer, Wehman, Condor, & Morrison, 1989; Sohlberg & Mateer, 1989). Training to use a memory notebook is sometimes conducted in two stages (Sohlberg & Mateer, 1989; Squires, Hunkin, & Parkin, 1997). In the first stage, the client learns novel paired associates and uses the notebook to look up the responses. This helps to establish a habit of looking up information in the notebook. In the second stage, this new behavior is applied to looking up information in the notebook about everyday events (Squires et al., 1997).

Apart from the larger strategy of improving self-monitoring of memory abilities, there are the tasks and strategies used in the clinic to foster direct improvement in memory ability and/or to develop compensatory strategies that will compensate for memory limitations. Memory drills designed to stimulate immediate and short-term recall of information are somewhat effective, but effects of these exercises do not generalize to new environments or other tasks. Verbal elaboration is a technique used to promote improved encoding of information, and visual imagery is sometimes used to help this process. These approaches may be effective in the short-term, but it has been observed that spontaneous use of the strategies is rare and transfer to real-world situations is difficult (Mateer, Kerns, & Eso, 1996).

One approach that has been shown to effectively foster learning in the context of memory encoding difficulties is the use of errorless learning strategies. This approach minimizes or eliminates any opportunity for errors to occur during learning. Errorless learning is best understood as a set of task manipulations that can be incorporated into most treatments for memory impairments. Drawing from several sources in the literature

on errorless learning (Baddeley, Wilson, & Watts, 1995; Evans, Wilson, Schuri, et al., 2000; Wilson, Baddeley, Evans, & Shiel, 1994). Sohlberg, Ehlhardt, & Kennedy (2005) summarized the following practices that are effective in reducing or eliminating errors:

1. breaking down the targeted task into small, discrete steps or units;
2. providing sufficient models *before* the client is asked to perform the target task;
3. encouraging the client to avoid guessing;
4. immediately correcting errors;
5. carefully fading prompts. (p. 272)

The effects of errorless learning are believed to be mediated by implicit memory, knowledge that is learned without conscious recollection of what has been learned (Anderson & Craik, 2006; Baddeley & Wilson, 1994; Page, Wilson, Shiel, et al., 2006). The prevention of error in the learning process minimizes any priming of erroneous response by implicit memory, thus maximizing accurate encoding of the input. In contrast, explicit memory involves awareness and recollection of what is learned and the ability to adequately encode new memories. Errorful learning is exploited in tasks that involve overt evaluation of responses (e.g., trial and error learning; Sohlberg et al., 2005). This type of learning engages explicit memory processes, as correct and incorrect responses are integrated with long-term memories. Whereas explicit memory processes in TBI are impaired, implicit memory encoding remains viable (Baddeley & Wilson, 1994). This finding is supported by numerous studies of errorless learning for acquired memory disorders associated with various etiologies (e.g., TBI: Dou, Man, Ou, et al., 2006; Landis, Hanten, Levin, et al., 2006; amnesia: Baddeley & Wilson, 1994; Evans et al., 2000; Alzheimer's disease: Clare, Wilson, Breen, & Hodges, 1999; Clare, Wilson, Carter, et al., 2000; schizophrenia: O'Carroll, Russell, Lawrie, & Johnstone, 1999; herpes encephalitis: Parkin, Hunkin, & Squires, 1998; semantic dementia: Jokel, Cupit, Rochon, & Graham, 2007).

It is important for speech-language pathologists to be familiar with the principles of errorless and errorful learning and when to apply one or the other. In the case of memory disorders that impair the encoding of new memories, errorless techniques seem to be the most effective means of learning. The principles of errorless learning, repetitive, error-free experience with a particular task or stimulus, can be used to promote learning of all kinds of information or behaviors. Additionally, it is important to remember that treatment of memory disorders may require both direct and indirect strategies.

Approaches to assessment and rehabilitation of communication disorders associated with TBI include direct approaches to ameliorate memory encoding difficulties. However, there is a much greater focus on functional communication abilities. Addressing the communication needs of individuals with TBI necessarily involves consideration of their educational and social needs as well as their personal short- and long-term goals. Speech-language pathologists and neuropsychologists working with this population will be involved in collaborations with other professionals that have knowledge of the client's needs in these other domains of function that intersect with communication. For people who have had a traumatic brain injury, their disabilities are lifelong and will impact all aspects of their lives. However, these new circumstances are dynamic and ongoing change is to be expected. Thus, a key factor in a successful rehabilitation program for someone who has had a traumatic brain injury is the recognition that assessment of the client's personal and environmental conditions is ongoing and that intervention is adjusted accordingly.

SEMANTIC MEMORY DISORDERS

Nature of the Impact on Language and Communication

Semantic memory disorders associated with neurological degenerative disease affect long-term memory (LTM). LTM is also known as declarative memory and consists of semantic memory (knowledge of the world) and episodic memory (memory for personal experiences). LTM supports language processing indirectly as the conceptual knowledge base that is communicated and understood via language. Long-term declarative memory is contrasted with procedural memory, which supports skill learning and regulation of the execution of cognitive and motor skills. Whereas procedural memories are established via implicit learning, long-term declarative memories are formed via explicit learning. In the domain of language ability, Ullman, Corkin, Coppola, et al., (1997) proposed a model relating declarative memory to the mental lexicon, which stores word-specific knowledge, and procedural memory to the mental grammar, which supports rule-governed assembly of lexical representations into sentences. Impairment of procedural memory has been observed in Parkinson's disease and Huntington's chorea. This is most apparent in regulation of motor movements, but disturbances of grammatical abilities have also been observed (Ullman, et al., 1997).

Other degenerative neurological diseases such as frontal-temporal lobar disease (FTD) and Alzheimer's disease (AD) lead to degradation of the declarative memories (including semantic and episodic memories). The most prominent symptom of language disturbance in the *temporal* variant of FTD (also known as semantic dementia, SD) is anomia, which becomes more severe as the conceptual knowledge associated with words of a language deteriorates (Hodges, Patterson, Oxbury, & Funnel, 1992). Comprehension of words also becomes increasingly impaired as the disease progresses. Thus, in semantic dementia, the type of declarative memory that is vulnerable to the disease is factual memory about the world (semantic memory). Concepts that are expressed via language are degrading. In contrast, episodic memory, which is impaired in AD, is relatively preserved in SD. Semantic memories are also affected in AD, but differ in subtle ways from the impairment in SD. Evidence indicates that the nature of the semantic deficit in AD is a gradual degradation of distinguishing features among semantic concepts. This erosion makes it difficult to distinguish differences among related concepts (Garrard, Lambon Ralph, Patterson, et al., 2005; for review, Altmann & McClung, 2008). The difference in semantic impairment of SD and AD is evident in the types of errors that are made in picture naming. Errors produced by individuals with SD tend to be visual in nature (e.g., orange → ball, nail → pointed), indicating a loss of the concept itself. The picture naming errors of individuals with AD tend to be semantic coordinates (tiger → lion) or superordinates (tiger → apple) indicating a fuzziness about the features that distinguish members of a category (Altmann & McClung, 2008).

Despite the severe loss of conceptual meanings of words, other language abilities remain functional well into the course of the progressive dementia. Repetition is spared, as are abilities to distinguish words and non-words. Syntactic processing remains stable, even comprehension of thematic roles (Breedin & Saffran, 1999; Kempler, Curtis, & Jackson, 1987). Reading is characterized by progressive surface dyslexia (inability to read irregularly spelled words), and impaired comprehension as the lexical-semantic links break down. Reilly and Peele (2008) note that the relative preservation of nonsemantic domains of language makes it difficult to discern the presence of language impairment in casual conversation. However, a closer examination of the content of conversational speech and narratives typically reveals an overuse of closed class words, semantically "light" verbs (e.g., go vs. fly), and a paucity of nouns (e.g., Bird, Lambon Ralph, Patterson, & Hodges, 2000).

It is important to emphasize a distinction between the semantic impairment in stroke-related aphasia and that in semantic dementia. In aphasia, the difficulty is one of accessing semantics from words. Whereas in semantic dementia, semantic memories are degrading progressively, in aphasia, the difficulty lies in accessing semantics from lexical (word) representations (Antonucci & Reilly, 2008; Jefferies & Lambon Ralph, 2006; Martin, 2005). Thus, in aphasia, a word's meaning may be accessible on one task but not another, or accessibility might vary because of the memory load of the task (Martin, 2005, 2008). In semantic dementia, once the conceptual representations have degraded, there can be no connection with the words that were once used to express them. A study by Lambon Ralph, Graham, Patterson, and Hodges (1999) provides evidence of the conceptual nature of the anomia in semantic dementia. They found a strong positive correlation between the quality of conceptual definitions of objects and the ability to name the words.

Assessment

An early symptom that is a hallmark of Alzheimer's disease is episodic memory loss (Bayles, 1991), but there also can be difficulties in language processing (Kempler, Curtiss, & Jackson, 1987; Martin & Fedio, 1983) and working memory processes (Bayles, 2003). In contrast, the most prominent early symptom of semantic dementia is anomia and difficulty comprehending words (Reilly & Peele, 2008). Error types in naming are typically semantic paraphasias, often visually related to the target in some way. Another common symptom of semantic dementia is prosopagnosia (inability to recognize faces) and associative visual agnosia (impaired object recognition). These disturbances reflect the degrading conceptual representations that support the language system.

An important part of the assessment process in the case of semantic memory loss is the case history, including an interview with the primary caregiver (Bayles, 1991). Because of the progressive nature of this disorder, observations of changes in language and memory abilities observed by significant others are important to the diagnosis of semantic dementia. Hopper and Bayles (2008) provide a comprehensive list of formal tests that are appropriate for evaluating language and cognitive skills in dementia (Alzheimer's or semantic dementia). Effective screening measures include the story-retelling subtest on the Arizona Battery for Communication Disorders of Dementia (Bayles & Tomoeda, 1993) and the FAS Verbal Fluency Test (Borkowski, Benton, & Spreen, 1967). The story retelling test requires the person to listen to a story and retell it immediately after hearing it and then again 5 minutes after hearing it. Bayles and Tomoeda (1993) found that people with moderate Alzheimer's disease (and dementia typical of this disorder)

were unable to remember anything about the story after 5 minutes. Another screening test that is often used in this population is the Mini-mental State Examination (Folstein, Folstein, & McHugh, 1975). The test contains 11 items that focus on general cognitive abilities such as memory, orientation, and attention and more specific abilities such as language, calculation, and visual-spatial processing. Assessment of verbal fluency is another means of detecting word retrieval difficulties. Several language batteries have verbal fluency subtests, including the Arizona Battery for Communication Disorders of Dementia (Bayles & Tomoeda, 1993) and the Boston Diagnostic Aphasia Examination (Goodglass, Kaplan, & Barresi, 2000). The semantic verbal fluency task involves naming as many members of particular semantic category (e.g., animals) as one can in a specified period of time (e.g., 30 seconds or 1 minute). There are also letter fluency tasks that require naming words that begin with a particular letter. Word generation tasks tend to be difficult for people with dementia and consequently they are a sensitive measure of anomia at early stages of the illness. A more comprehensive evaluation of the language and memory abilities can be achieved with the full Arizona Battery for Communication Disorders of Dementia (Bayles & Tomoeda, 1993) and the Functional Linguistic Communication Inventory (Bayles & Tomoeda, 1994).

Part of a complete evaluation of language and cognitive abilities associated with degenerative neurological disease is an assessment of severity of the language and cognitive impairments. This information will help determine the level of functional care that a person with dementia needs and will help in determining goals for any kind of intervention to improve or maintain functional communication abilities. Hopper and Bayles (2008) recommend two scales that are used to document the progression of impairment to functional abilities: Global Deterioration Scale (Reisberg, Ferris, deLeon, & Crook, 1982) and a follow up to that test, the Functional Assessment Staging Scale (Reisberg, Ferris, & Franssen, 1985). Each of these use observation as the measure and include detailed descriptions of functional behaviors and impairments that are typically present at a particular stage of disease progression.

Approaches to Rehabilitation

When considering rehabilitation priorities for language impairment related to degenerative neurological disease, it may at first seem counterintuitive to provide language intervention that aims to improve language ability. Indeed, it is only in the last decade or so that clinicians and researchers have considered treatment approaches for people with semantic memory deficits that do more than compensate for the lost memories. Memory aids are still highly recommended to help the person with dementia to cope in his/her environment independently or with assistance from significant others for as long as is possible. Bourgeois and colleagues, for example, have demonstrated the usefulness of a memory aid (memory wallet) to enhance conversational skills of patients with AD (Bourgeois, 1990; Bourgeois & Mason, 1996). This kind of training, as might be expected, involves training of caregivers to work with the person with dementia (e.g., Hickey, Bourgeois, & Olswang, 2004). Although the goal is not to improve language and memory function per se, memory aids have an important impact on quality of life for the person with dementia and his/her significant others.

As our understanding of the exact nature of language impairment in semantic dementia improves, there has been an increasing focus on developing methods to improve language function in SD and AD by capitalizing on residual language abilities. Graham, Patterson, Pratt, and Hodges (2001) reported a seminal case study of DM, a 59-year-old male surgeon. Following a 2-year history of word-finding difficulties, the source of DM's anomia was determined to be semantic dementia. There were two central questions addressed in this study: (1) Would repeated practice on a set of vocabulary words provide short-term access to those words and (2) would it help to maintain access to that vocabulary from day to day. Several factors suggested this approach might be successful with DM. He had already made a list of words he could not reliably remember or produce. Also, he was highly motivated and expressed a willingness to practice every day.

Three sets of words were created. Words in Set 1 were practiced regularly for 2 weeks, and then words from Set 2 were practiced for 2 weeks. Performance improved with practice but dropped when practice was stopped. The third set of words was not practiced at all, but some improvement was noted in that set as well. It was concluded that relearning of names was possible in semantic dementia, but continued exposure and practice was needed. Graham et al. (2001) assessed DM's abilities after 2 years. DM continued to show improvement and maintenance of category fluency (naming members of categories). However, they also note that although he could name the objects, he could not provide semantic information about them. Also, his performance declined on The Pyramids and Palm Trees Test (Howard & Patterson, 1992), a nonverbal semantic tests of conceptual knowledge. They concluded that although the continued practice of object names supported retrieval of those names, it did not reverse the degradation of the semantic system.

Evidence that intensive practice can help to maintain access to words in semantic dementia comes from a treatment case study reported by Jokel, Rochon, and Leonard (2006) of a person with semantic dementia, AK, who was severely anomic. Their treatment protocol, like the approach used by Graham et al. (2001), involved intensive practice of objects that AK could once name. The training protocol included three groups of stimuli: words that AK understood but could not name, words that she could not understand or name, and words that she understood and could name. Immediately following treatment, there was improvement on words that AK could and could not understand before training. At a follow-up evaluation 1 month after therapy, these improvements remained only for those words that she could understand prior to therapy. Additionally, Jokel et al. (2006) provide evidence that the words AK understood and could name prior to treatment were less vulnerable to loss compared to untreated words that she knew and could name prior to treatment.

These two studies indicate the importance of residual comprehension of vocabulary to the success of a program to improve retrieval of word names. Although it is possible to stimulate short-term retrieval of vocabulary with intensive practice even for names whose meaning is not well retained, relearning in this context is short-lived compared to a context in which knowledge of the concept remains. Related findings by other researchers support this (e.g., Snowden, Griffiths, & Neary, 1999; Snowden & Neary, 2002). In an extensive review of treatments for word retrieval in semantic dementia, Henry, Beeson, and Rapcsak (2008) note that all evidence suggests that the ability to relearn vocabulary will be directly related to the residual semantic knowledge for those words. Consistent with this finding, it has been suggested that training vocabulary in SD should focus on a finite set of words that are relevant to the individual rather than focus on retraining lost vocabulary (Reilly, Martin, & Grossman, 2005). Henry et al. (2008) also suggest that drawing on relatively spared episodic memories in SD may enhance the effects of repeated practice of vocabulary.

Language rehabilitation in dementia aims to maximize functional language and slow progression of vocabulary loss over the course of a progressively dementing illness. There are two broad approaches to language rehabilitation with this population, the use of memory aids and repeated practice in the production of personally relevant words that the individual with SD is able to comprehend. Speech-language pathologists should be familiar with both approaches and be ready to use both in treating the language impairments in this population. Additionally, involvement of significant others and caregivers in the language maintenance program will maximize the beneficial effects of these approaches on functional communication.

VERBAL STM IMPAIRMENT IN APHASIA: IMPAIRED MAINTENANCE OF WORD REPRESENTATIONS IN STM

Nature of the Impact on Language and Communication

People with aphasia invariably demonstrate impairments of verbal STM and many have difficulty with language tasks that involve working memory and verbal learning. There is an extensive history of research on the cognitive organization of language processing and short-term memory systems. Language processing and verbal STM are often discussed as separate systems with the latter being a temporary store for phonological representations of utterances longer than a single word. Verbal span tasks exemplify this relationship; a sequence of verbal units is heard, held in STM, and repeated in the same serial order. Separation of STM and word processing seems intuitive, as we also store other types of cognitive and sensory information temporarily. Consistent with this model, the verbal STM impairment in aphasia also has been viewed as separate from the language impairment (Shallice & Warrington, 1970).

In contrast to the "separate systems" view, more recent proposals claim that the verbal STM impairment in aphasia is due to an impairment of a process that maintains activation of word representations over the course of language comprehension or production (Berndt & Mitchum, 1990; Martin, 2008; R. Martin, Shelton, & Yaffee, 1994; Martin & Gupta, 2004; Saffran, 1990; Saffran & Martin, 1990). There is much evidence supporting the view that verbal STM and word processing *are* related functionally and in terms of their cognitive organization. From the literature on verbal span abilities of normal speakers, we know that span capacity varies depending on the characteristics of the items to be recalled. Span is greater for digits than words (Brener, 1940) and greater for words than non-words (Hulme, Maughan, & Brown, 1991). Span capacity also is influenced by linguistic factors: phonological similarity (Conrad & Hull, 1964), word frequency (Hulme, Roodenrys, Schweickert, et al., 1997; Watkins & Watkins, 1977), and semantic similarity (Brooks & Watkins, 1990; Crowder, 1979; Poirier & Saint Aubin, 1995; Shulman, 1971). Additionally, studies of verbal STM impairments associated with aphasia have demonstrated quite dramatic effects of

lexical and semantic factors (e.g., frequency and imageability) on item recall in verbal span (Hanley & Kay, 1997; Martin & Saffran, 1997) and serial order (Martin & Bunta, 2007). The relationship of short-term activation maintenance processes and word processing can be understood in the context of an interactive activation (IA) model of word processing (Figure 13-1) that has been used to account for word processing impairment in aphasia (Dell, Schwartz, Martin, et al., 1997). Two parameters control the activation of phonological, lexical, and semantic representations of words in the lexical network: connection weight and decay rate. Dell et al. (1997) demonstrated that word processing impairments in aphasia could be accounted for as damage to these two processing parameters, leading to a reduction in strength of activation (connection weight impairment) and/or the ability to maintain activation of representations (decay rate impairment).

Figure 13-1 shows how repetition of even a single word requires maintenance of activated semantic and phonological representations over time. Martin & Saffran (1997) proposed that this temporal aspect of word processing is what links word processing and verbal STM and is an integral part of processing single or multiple word utterances. Martin & Gupta (2004) proposed further that the word processing and verbal STM impairments are related on a severity continuum: Less severe impairment of the "activation-maintenance" function results in a difficulty maintaining activation of multiple word utterances. On verbal span tasks this difficulty is manifested as a reduction in verbal STM capacity. More severe impairments of activation-maintenance result in difficulty maintaining activation of even single words, leading to a profile of aphasia as well as a reduction of verbal STM capacity. Empirical evidence supports this proposal. Verbal span is positively associated with word processing ability (Martin & Gupta, 2004) and with verbal learning ability (Freedman & Martin, 2001; Martin & Saffran, 1999). Martin, Saffran, and Dell's (1996) seminal case study of NC, a person with deep dysphasia, demonstrated that word processing abilities improve in tandem with recovery from aphasia. Additionally, the size of word span varies depending on the kind of task used to assess span, task demands and the degree of semantic or phonological impairment (Martin & Ayala, 2004).

Evidence of the intimate relationship between word processing and verbal STM has important clinical implications for approaches to diagnosis and treatment of language disorders in aphasia (Martin, 2000, 2008). In some sense, these recent findings reflect the views of the 19th century neurologist, Grashey (1885), who once postulated that short-term decay of linguistic

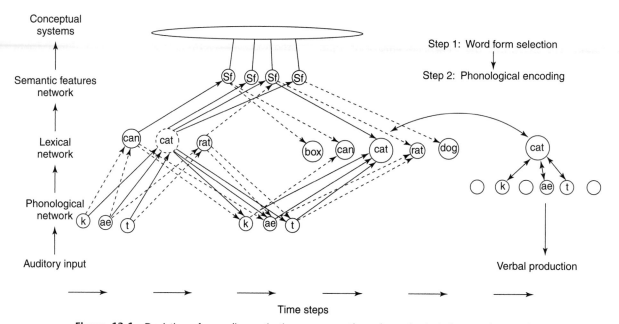

Figure 13-1   Depiction of spreading activation processes throughout the lexical network over the course of repeating a single word. Activation spreads from phoneme representations to lexical forms and semantic representations. Once activated, a representation begins to decay, but then is refreshed by feedback activation from subsequently activated representations. The feedforward-feedback cycles continue until a word is needed for production, at which time, the most highly activated lexical representation is selected and phonologically encoded.

representations was a possible cause of aphasia. Although this view was controversial in its day (Bartels & Wallesch, 1996), the data from recent studies are consistent with this view. Apart from this theoretical consideration, the STM impairment in aphasia can have consequences for functional communication that warrant consideration. As noted, verbal STM impairments are pervasive in aphasia. Individuals with mild aphasia or seemingly no residual aphasia may still have difficulty with short-term retention of language. It is not uncommon for individuals with mild aphasia to complain of functional language difficulty in day-to-day conversational situations. Short-term memory and other cognitive functions (e.g., attention and executive processing) that support language production and comprehension are most challenged in these contexts. Thus, there is a need for incorporation of measurements in aphasia evaluations that are sensitive to language processing under conditions of increased short-term working memory load. It should be noted that short-term memory considerations are just one of several other cognitive abilities that enable processing of language, attention (e.g., Hula & McNeil, 2008; Tseng, McNeil, & Milenkovic, 1993) and executive functions

(Miyake, Emerson, & Friedman, 2000). There is a need for better assessment of these abilities in aphasia as well. It is beyond the scope of this chapter to consider these, but the reader is referred to several of the chapters on memory, attention, and executive function in this text for further discussion.

In what follows, I discuss some of the recent advances in assessment and treatment of word processing disorders in aphasia that reflect the view of aphasia as a processing disorder affecting the ability to activate and/or maintain activation of language representations over the course of comprehension and production of language.

Assessment

Current assessment batteries for aphasia lack measures of verbal STM, although it is not uncommon for clinicians to include standard or informal measures of digit or word span as part of a language assessment. A simple measure of digit or word span, however, does not provide a subjective or objective measure of language function under conditions of increased short-term memory load or increased interference (invoking the need for executive functions). There are tests of functional language—for example, the Communicative

Activities of Daily Living—Second Edition (CADL-2; Holland, Frattali, & Fromm, 1999)—which measure language function in everyday communication situations. Certainly, these situations involve contexts in which STM load will be taxed. In that sense, such measures of functional language provide a useful global assessment of a person's ability to communicate in contexts that draw upon STM and executive processing resources to support language function. However, they do not provide a quantifiable measure of someone's sensitivity to short-term memory load effects on language function. This kind of assessment is needed if we are to develop treatments that focus on STM processing components of aphasia.

Assessments of the effects of STM load on language function would have another important use. For individuals with mild aphasia, there are few means to identify the nature of their language impairment. Typical language measures for aphasia involve single-word processing tasks. Such tasks are often successfully completed by someone with mild aphasia. There are no formal measures targeting mild aphasia in use today, and conventional assessment batteries of aphasia (e.g., Western Aphasia Battery—Revised, Kertesz, 2006) are not sensitive to mild language processing impairments (Ross & Wertz, 2004). It is only on measures of verbal STM (e.g., R. Martin et al., 1994; Ween, Verfaellie, & Alexander, 1996), attention (Murray, Holland, & Beeson, 1998; Murray, Keeton, & Karcher, 2006), or sentence processing (Martin & Freedman, 2001; R. Martin & He, 2004) that language difficulties become evident. Thus, there is a clinical need for assessment batteries that are sensitive to semantic and phonological impairments affecting both single *and* multiple word processing and which examine other cognitive processes that affect language processing. These assessments would provide a more complete diagnostic profile of the communication impairments associated with aphasia that would better inform the development of treatment strategies that focus on language content (semantic, phonological representations) and language processing (access to, maintenance and retrieval of language content).

Martin, Kohen, and Kalinyak-Fliszar (2008; in preparation) have developed a comprehensive test battery designed to assess language and verbal STM abilities in aphasia, the Temple Assessment of Language and Short-term Memory in Aphasia (TALSA). This test is described briefly here and also in Appendix 13-1. The TALSA battery includes some standard tests of language processing, but also has several unique features: Part 1 includes word processing tasks that probe semantic and phonological abilities. These tasks vary in difficulty and incorporate

variations affecting STM and/or executive processing load. Two variations involve inclusion of a 5-second interval between stimulus and response or between two stimuli to be compared. In one variation, the interval is unfilled (silent) allowing assessment of the ability to passively maintain activation of representations (passive STM). The other interval condition is "filled" (participant reads aloud numbers that appear on a computer screen). This variation assesses the ability to maintain activation of representations in the context of verbal interference (STM plus executive processing). Box 13-1 illustrates how these intervals are incorporated into two language tasks, phoneme discrimination judgments and word/non-word repetition.

Two other subtests vary STM and executive processing requirements in a different way, by increasing the number of items that need to be held in verbal STM (the working memory load) while making a judgment of similarity (synonymy and rhyming judgments). These are illustrated in Box 13-2.

Part 2 includes span tasks that vary phonological, lexical, and semantic characteristics of the stimuli. These include (1) digit and word span, (2) word span with words of high and low frequency and high and

---

Box 13-1

Examples of STM Variations on Typical Word Processing Tasks Used in Assessment of Aphasia: Incorporation of Intervals

EXAMPLE 1. INTERVALS BETWEEN TWO STIMULI TO BE JUDGED FOR SIMILARITY
Task: Judgments of Phonological Similarity
Are the two words you hear the same or different?
    Response: Yes or No.
1-sec Unfilled interval: apple.axle.Response
5-sec Unfilled interval: apple . . . *5 sec* . . . axle.
    Response
5-sec Filled interval: apple *sees and says:* "6 2 8 1 3."
    axle. Response.

EXAMPLE 2. INTERVAL BETWEEN STIMULUS AND RESPONSES
Task: Word and Non-word repetition.
Listen to the word (or non-word) and repeat it after
    the cue.
1-sec Unfilled interval: apple.cue: Response
5-sec Unfilled: apple . . . *5 sec* . . . cue: Response
5-sec Filled: apple *sees and says* "7 4 3 8 6." cue:
    Response

Box 13-2

Examples of STM Variations on Typical Word Processing Tasks Used in Assessment of Aphasia: Varying the Number of Items to Hold in Short-Term Working Memory

TASK 1. SYNONYMY TRIPLETS

3-choice condition: Which two words are most similar in meaning?

sorrow* grief* confusion
violin* clarinet fiddle*

2-choice condition: Which of these two words is most similar in meaning to the word in the middle?

*grief *sorrow confusion
clarinet *fiddle *violin

TASK 2. RHYMING TRIPLETS

Which two words rhyme?

grapes* drapes* ground
dice mouse* house*

Which word rhymes with the word in the middle?

grapes* drapes* ground
dice house* mouse*

---

low imageability, (3) word and non-word span, and (4) semantic and phonological probe memory span.

The memory load conditions in Part 1 and the span tasks in Part 2 enable assessment of the source of a language impairment (primarily semantic or phonological or both) and type of processing impairment (slowed activation or difficulty maintaining activation of word) at *all* levels of severity. The single word processing tasks vary from easy to hard and are useful for assessment of moderate and severe language impairments. Additionally, the interval conditions of the word processing tasks and the span tasks that vary semantic and phonological content are sensitive to spared and impaired semantic and phonological abilities in people with mild aphasia and can guide appropriate treatment approaches for this group.

Approaches to Rehabilitation

In conjunction with an increased interest in the contribution of STM to language processing and its impairment in aphasia, several attempts to treat the STM deficit in aphasia have been reported. Koenig-Bruhin and Studer-Eichenberger (2007) investigated the effectiveness of a treatment to improve temporary storage of verbal information by a person with reproduction

conduction aphasia. They based their study on the premise that repetition and STM impairments stem from premature decay of the activation of representations in STM (Martin & Saffran, 1992). Training involved repetition of sentences that were 4 to 7 words long and with increasing delays between the stimulus and response. Gains were observed in sentence repetition as well as span for digits and words.

A study by Majerus, Van der Kaa, Renard, and colleagues (2005) was designed to directly target the phonological short-term memory deficits of their participant, BJ, who presented with a word span of 3 and non-word span of 2. Evaluation of BJ's language and STM abilities revealed that although he could retain semantic information in STM, maintaining phonological information was impaired. Majerus et al. (2005) used delayed repetition tasks that required holding in STM meaningful and meaningless phonological information for increasingly longer periods. They trained repetition of over 250 pairs of bi-syllabic words or non-words that differed by a single consonant. The first step was to have BJ repeat the item pairs immediately after hearing the stimuli. Once phonological production was stabilized in this condition, item pairs were repeated after a 5-second-filled interval. Treatment was carried out for 16 months (2 times per week) and resulted in modest improvements of digit and non-word span, non-word repetition, rhyme judgments, and, by the participant's self-report, improvement in comprehension in conversational contexts involving more than two participants.

Francis, Clark, and Humphreys (2003) targeted the STM deficit of a person with aphasia by requiring the repetition of sentences that gradually increased in length and complexity. Their participant, BG, presented with impaired sentence repetition and impaired comprehension. Background testing led the investigators to conclude that BG's comprehension impairment was due mainly to her STM impairment. They predicted that improvement of her STM deficit (manifested as better repetition of longer and more complex sentences) would generalize to improved comprehension. Their prediction was confirmed in part. Improvement was observed on some measures of sentence comprehension (the Token Test), but BG's comprehension of sentences with reversible semantic roles was impaired as it had been prior to treatment. These studies as well as others that target short-term maintenance of representations (e.g., "spaced retrieval" therapy [Fridriksson, Holland, Beeson, & Morrow, 2005]) indicate the feasibility of a treatment approach for aphasic word and sentence processing disorders that focuses on improvement of the ability to maintain activation of the representations of words.

Recently, Martin and colleagues (in press, 2011) have developed a treatment protocol that addresses the processing deficits in aphasia, slowed activation and/or activation maintenance. The approach is summarized in Appendix 13-2. The protocol is flexible in that it can be applied to phonological and/or semantic processing of single word or multiple word utterances. The treatment task is repetition of words, non-words, word pairs, or word triplets that are varied in ways to stimulate semantic and/or phonological processing. An STM component is incorporated into the treatment by conducting it under three conditions that vary the interval between stimulus and response: 1-second Unfilled (1-sec UF), 5-second Unfilled (5-sec UF), and 5-second Filled (naming numbers that appear on a computer screen, 5-sec F). The third condition also introduces a dual task, thereby engaging executive processes. Stimulus variations at each level are presented hierarchically from easier to more difficult. Treatment is applied at the interval condition designated for the first treatment application followed by treatment to the *same stimuli* at the remaining interval conditions. Performance on the TALSA battery determines the starting point of treatment and is based on (1) type of language impairment (semantic or phonological), (2) severity (affecting processing of single or multiple words), and (3) STM component (interval at which performance falters).

The aim of this treatment approach is to improve language processing ability and functional communication by improving the ability to activate and maintain activation of word representations sufficiently over the course of comprehension and production of single and multiple words. A prediction of this treatment approach is that improvement of these fundamental abilities that support word processing should generalize to content and tasks beyond those used in treatment. Data from two treatment studies by Martin and colleagues illustrate the effectiveness of this treatment approach in this regard. The first is a case study of a person with conduction aphasia (Kalinyak-Fliszar, Kohen, Martin, et al., 2008; Kalinyak-Fliszar, Kohen, & Martin, in press, 2011). FS, a 55-year-old, right-handed female, was 29 months post-onset at the time she began treatment. Her performance on the TALSA battery (described above) indicated good semantic processing at the single word level, but moderately impaired phonological processing, especially in production tasks such as repetition and naming. She was enrolled in the phonological training protocol that began with repetition of three-syllable words, progressing to two- and three-syllable non-words. Each stimulus type was practiced at the three interval conditions so as to gradually increase the amount of time

she had to "hold" the word or non-word in STM before repeating it. Pre- and post-treatment data indicate that FS made gains in repetition of all four types of stimuli in this module with substantial effect sizes in the treatment and maintenance phases of the protocol. The most compelling data from this study are the gains made on language and STM measures following therapy. FS's performance on standardized tests either improved or was maintained on all measures. On the TALSA battery she improved on rhyming and synonymy triplet judgments, word pair repetition, and span tasks. These tasks increase memory load, but in different ways than the treatment task, indicating improvement of a fundamental ability that generalized to other tasks.

In a second study (Kohen, McCluskey, Kalinyak-Fliszar, & Martin, in preparation; Martin, Kohen, McCluskey, et al., 2009), this treatment approach was applied in a case of Wernicke aphasia. KX, a 69-year-old right-handed female, sustained two left cerebrovascular accidents (CVAs) within 1 year. Her most recent infarct was over 6 years before she was enrolled in this study. Results of her neuropsychological and language tests were consistent with a moderate-severe Wernicke-type aphasia. Because KX demonstrated impairments of both input phonological and semantic processing, she was enrolled in the treatment protocol to that targeted both abilities. The stimuli chosen for training were words varied for frequency and imageability and these were presented for repetition at the three interval conditions. These stimuli engage phonological representations as a repetition task, but also stimulate activation of lexical and semantic representations. The results indicated that repetition abilities improved for the treated words, especially for the 1-sec UF and 5-sec UF conditions. Criteria were reached for HI-HF words and HI-LF words in the 1-sec UF condition and for the HI-LF words in the 5-sec UF and 5-sec F interval conditions. Criteria were often reached within three treatment sessions and sometimes during baseline. Additionally, small but consistent improvement of untreated words was noted for all conditions. Anecdotal evidence of positive results of therapy includes observations of better self-monitoring and turn-taking skills in conversation and other functional communication activities.

These case studies of a treatment that aims to improve processing of language (activation and activation maintenance of language representations) are promising because they indicate generalization to untrained stimuli in the treatment protocol and to other tasks that engage STM in ways that differ from the treatment task. Synonymy judgments engage working memory processes and span tasks involve holding more items in memory, not holding a single item in memory for a longer time. The outcomes of the treatments for FS and KX suggest improvement of a fundamental ability to maintain activation of representations in the course of processing words. Additional case studies are needed to learn more about the potential usefulness of this approach to aphasia treatment. In principle, the processing approach should be applicable to all types of aphasia and the methods described here can be adapted to language tasks other than repetition.

Verbal STM impairments in aphasia reflect the most direct involvement of memory in language and language impairment. As such, assessment and treatment approaches will necessarily focus directly on language processing abilities. Although outcomes of treatment should result in improved functional communication, the treatments of this particular memory-related language disorder will involve direct, impairment-based approaches. Viewing aphasia as a form of STM impairment is a somewhat new perspective of the disorder. It is part of a recent paradigm shift in aphasia rehabilitation from a focus on treating content of language to treating processing of language. This is not to say that methods of aphasia rehabilitation have never focused on processing. Verbal cueing methods and priming treatments do just that. At this juncture, however, there is an increasing interest in understanding the dynamics of language processing and development of treatment strategies that build on that understanding.

ACKNOWLEDGMENTS

Preparation of this chapter was supported by grants from the National Institutes of Health (NIDCD), R01 DC 01924–14 and R21 DC008782–02 to Temple University (PI: N. Martin). The ideas put forth in this chapter were fostered by many helpful discussions with my colleagues and friends, Matti Laine, Gary Dell, Myrna Schwartz, Ruth Fink, Francine Kohen and Michelene Kalinyak-Fliszar, and my mentor and dear friend, the late Eleanor Saffran. I am grateful to them as well as the many people with aphasia and word production disorders whom I have had the privilege to know and work with over the years.

REFERENCES

Anderson, N. D., & Craik, F. I. M. (2006). The mnemonic mechanisms of errorless learning. *Neuropsychologia, 44,* 2806–2813.

Altmann, L., & McClung, J. S. (2008). Effects of semantic impairment on language use in Alzheimer's disease. *Seminars in Speech and Language, 29*(1),18–30.

Antonucci, S. M., & Reilly, J. (2008). Semantic memory and language processing: A primer. *Seminars in Speech and Language, 29*(1), 5–17.

Baddeley, A. D., & Wilson, B. A. (1994). When implicit learning fails: Amnesia and the problem of error elimination. *Neuropsychologia, 32,* 53–68.

Baddeley, A. D., Wilson, B. A., & Watts, F. (1995). *Handbook of memory disorders.* West Sussex, UK: John Wiley & Sons.

Bartels, C., & Wallesch, C. W. (1996). Nineteenth-century accounts of the nature of the lexicon and semantics: Riddles posed by the case of Johann Voit. In C. Code, C-W. Wallesch, Y. Joanette, & A. R. Lecourse (Eds.), *Classic cases in neuropsychology* (chap. 5, pp. 53–68). Hove, UK: Psychology Press.

Bayles, K. A. (1991). Alzheimer's disease symptoms: Prevalence and order of appearance. *Journal of Applied Gerontology, 10, 4,* 419–430.

Bayles, K. A. (2003). Effects of working memory deficits on the communicative function of Alzheimer's dementia patients. *Journal of Communication Disorders, 26,* 209–219.

Bayles, K. A., & Tomoeda, C. K. (1993). *Arizona Battery for Communication Disorders of Dementia.* Austin, TX: Pro-Ed.

Bayles, K. A., & Tomoeda, C. K. (1994). *The Functional Linguistic Communication Inventory.* Austin, TX: Pro-Ed.

Berndt, R. S., & Mitchum, C. C. (1990). Auditory and lexical information sources in immediate recall: Evidence from a patient with deficit to the phonological short-term store. In G. Vallar & T. Shallice (Eds.), *Neuropsychological impairments of short-term memory.* Cambridge, UK: Cambridge University Press.

Bird, H., Lambon Ralph, M. A., Patterson, K., & Hodges, J. R. (2000). The rise and fall of frequency and imageability: Noun and verb production in semantic dementia. *Brain and Language, 73,* 17–49.

Borkowski, J. G., Benton, A. L., & Spreen, O. (1967). Word fluency and brain damage. *Neuropsychologia 5,* 135–140.

Bourgeois, M. S. (1990). Enhancing conversation skills in Alzheimer's disease using a prosthetic memory aid. *Journal of Applied Behavior Analysis, 23,* 29–42.

Bourgeois, M. S., & Mason, L. A. (1996). Memory wallet intervention in an adult day care setting. *Behavioral interventions: Theory and practice in residential and community-based clinical programs. 11,* 3–18.

Breedin, S. D., & Saffran, E. M. (1999). Sentence processing in the face of semantic loss: A case study. *Journal of Experimental Psychology: General 1999, 128*(4), 547–562.

Brener, R. (1940). An experimental investigation of memory span. *Journal of Experimental Psychology, 26,* 467–482.

Brooks III, J. O., & Watkins, M. J. (1990). Further evidence of the intricacy of memory span. *Journal of Experimental Psychology: Learning, Memory, and Cognition, 16*(6), 1134–1141.

Butters, N., & Delis, D. C. (1995). Clinical assessments of memory disorders in amnesia and dementia. *Annual Review of Psychology, 46,* 493–523.

Clare, L., Wilson, B. A., Breen, K., & Hodges, J. R. (1999). Errorless learning of face-name associations in early Alzheimer's disease. *Neurocase, 5*(1), 37–46.

Clare, L., Wilson, B. A., Carter, G., Breen, K., Gosses, A., & Hodges, J. R. (2000). Intervening with everyday memory problems in dementia of Alzheimer type: An errorless learning approach. *Journal of Clinical & Experimental Neuropsychology, 22*(1), 132–146.

Coelho, C. A., DeRuyter, F., & Stein, M. (1996). Treatment efficacy: Cognitive-communicative disorders resulting from traumatic brain injury in adults. *Journal of Speech and Hearing Research, 39*, S5–S17.

Coelho, C., Ylvisaker, M., & Turkstra, L. S. (2005). Nonstandardized assessment approaches for individuals with traumatic brain injuries. *Seminars in Speech and Language, 26*(4), 223–241.

Conrad, R., & Hull, A. J. (1964). Information, acoustic confusion and memory span. *British Journal of Psychology, 55*, 429–432.

Crowder, R. G. (1979). Similarity and order in memory. In G. H. Bower (Ed.), *The psychology of learning and motivation: Advances in research and theory* (Vol. 13, pp. 319–353). New York: Academic Press.

Curtiss, G., Vanderploeg, R. D., Spencer, J., & Salazar, A. M. (2001). Patterns of verbal learning and memory in traumatic brain injury. *Journal of the International Neuropsychological Society, 7*, 574–585.

Delis, D. C., Kramer, J. H., Kaplan, E., & Ober, B. A. (1987). *California Verbal Learning Test Manual—Adult Version* (Res. ed.). New York: The Psychological Corporation.

Dell, G. S., Schwartz, M. F., Martin, N., Saffran, E. M., & Gagnon, D. A. (1997). Lexical access in aphasic and non-aphasic speakers. *Psychological Review, 104*(4), 801–838.

Dou, Z. L., Man, D. W. K., Ou, H. N., Zheng, J. L., & Tam, S. F. (2006). Computerized errorless learning-based memory rehabilitation for Chinese patients with brain injury: A preliminary quasi-experimental clinical design study. *Brain Injury, 20*(3), 219–225.

Evans, J. J., Wilson, B. A., Schuri, U., Andrade, J., Baddeley, A., Bruna, O., Canavan, T., . . . & Taussik, I. (2000). A comparison of "errorless" and "trial-and-error" learning methods for teaching individuals with acquired memory deficits. *Neuropsychological Rehabilitation, 10*(1), 67–101.

Folstein, M. F., Folstein, S. E., & McHugh, P. R. (1975). Minimental state. A practical method for grading the cognitive state of patients for the clinician. *Journal of Psychiatric Research 12*(3), 189–198.

Francis, D. R., Clark, N., & Humphreys, G. W. (2003). The treatment of an auditory working memory deficit and the implications for sentence comprehension abilities in mild "receptive" aphasia. *Aphasiology, 17*, 723–750.

Freedman, M. L., & Martin, R. C. (2001). Dissociable components of short-term memory and their relation to long-term learning. *Cognitive Neuropsychology, 18*, 193–226.

Fridriksson, J., Holland, A. L., Beeson, P., & Morrow, L. (2005). Spaced retrieval treatment of anomia. *Aphasiology, 19*, 99–109.

Garrard, P., Lambon Ralph, M. A., Patterson, K., Pratt, K. H., & Hodges, J. R. (2005). Semantic feature knowledge and picture naming in dementia of Alzheimer's type: A new approach. *Brain and Language, 93*, 79–94.

Gioia, G. A., Isquith, P. K., Guy, S. C., & Kenworthy, L. (2000). *Behavior Rating Inventory of Executive Function*. Odessa, FL: Psychological Assessment Resources.

Goodglass, H., Kaplan, E., & Barresi, B. (2000). *Boston Diagnostic Aphasia Examination—3*, Philadelphia: Taylor & Francis, Ltd.

Graham, K. S., Patterson, K., Pratt, K. H., & Hodges, J. R. (2001). Can repeated exposure to "forgotten" vocabulary help alleviate word-finding difficulties in semantic dementia? An illustrative case study. *Neuropsychological Rehabilitation, 11*, 429–454.

Grashey, H. (1885). Uber Aphasie und ihre BEziehung zur Wahrnehmung. *Archive fur Psychiatrie und Nervenkrankeiten, 16*, 654–688. De Bleser, R. (Trans.) (1989). [On aphasia and its relations to perception.] *Cognitive Neuropsychology, 6*, 515–546.

Hanley, J. R., & Kay, J. (1997). An effect of imageability on the production of phonological errors in auditory repetition. *Cognitive Neuropsychology, 14*(8), 1065–1084.

Heilman, K. M., Safran, A., & Geshwind, N. (1971). Closed head trauma and aphasia. *Journal of Neurology, Neurosurgery, and Psychiatry, 34*, 265–269.

Henry, M. L., Beeson, P. M., & Rapcsak, S. Z. (2008). Treatment for anomia in semantic dementia. *Seminars in Speech and Language, 29*(1), 60–70.

Hickey, E. M., Bourgeois, M. S., & Olswang, L. B. (2004). Effects of training to converse with nursing home residents with aphasia. *Aphasiology, 18*(5/6/7), 625–637.

Hodges, J., Patterson, K., Oxbury, S., & Funnel, E. (1992). Semantic dementia progressive aphasia with temporal lobe atrophy, *Brain, 115*, 1783–1806.

Holland, A., Frattali, C., & Fromm, D. (1999). *Communication activities of daily living* (2nd ed.). Austin, TX: Pro-Ed.

Hopper, T., & Bayles, K. A. (2008). Management of neurogenic communication disorders associated with dementia. In R. Chapey, *Language intervention strategies in adult aphasia* (5th ed., chap. 35, pp. 988–1008). Baltimore, MD: Lippincott, Williams, & Wilkins.

Howard, D., & Patterson, K. (1992). *The Pyramids and Palm Trees Test*. Bury St. Edmonds, UK: Thames Valley Test Company.

Hula, W. D., & McNeil, M. R. (2008). Models of attention and dual-task performance as explanatory constructs in aphasia. *Seminars in Speech and Language, 29*(3), 169–187.

Hulme, C., Maughan, S., & Brown, G. (1991). Memory for familiar and unfamiliar words: Evidence for a long-term memory contribution to short-term span. *Journal of Memory and Language, 30*, 685–701.

Hulme, C., Roodenrys, S., Schweickert, R., Brown, G. D., Martin, A., & Stuart, G. (1997). Word frequency effects on short-term memory tasks: Evidence for reintegration process in immediate serial recall. *Journal of Experimental Psychology: Learning, Memory and Cognition, 23*, 1217–1232.

Jefferies, E., & Lambon Ralph, M. A. (2006). Semantic impairment in stroke aphasia versus semantic dementia: A case-series comparison. *Brain (129)*, 2132–2147.

Jokel, R. J., Cupit, J., Rochon, E. A., & Graham, N. L. (2007). Errorless re-training in semantic dementia using MossTalk Words. *Brain and Language, 103*, 205–206.

Jokel, R., Rochon, E., & Leonard, C. (2006). Treating anomia in semantic dementia: Improvement, maintenance, or both? *Neuropsychological Rehabilitation, 16*, 241–256.

Kalinyak-Fliszar, M., Kohen, F. P., Martin, N., DeMarco, A., & Gruberg, N. (2008). Remediation of language and short-term memory deficits in aphasia. Presented at American Speech-Language-Hearing Association Convention, Chicago, November 20–22, 2008.

Kalinyak-Fliszar, M., Kohen, F. P., & Martin, N. (in press, 2011). Remediation of language processing in aphasia: Improving activation and maintenance of linguistic representations in (verbal) short-term memory. Aphasiology.

Kennedy, M. R. T., & Coelho, C. (2005). Self-regulation after traumatic brain injury: A framework for intervention of memory and problem solving. *Seminars in Speech and Language, 26*(4), 242–255.

Kempler, D., Curtis, S., & Jackson, C. (1987). Syntactic preservation in Alzheimer's disease. *Journal of Speech and Hearing Research, 30*, 343–350.

Kertesz, A. (1982). *Western Aphasia Battery*. San Antonio, TX: Psychological Corporation.

Kertesz, A. (2006). *Western Aphasia Battery—Revised*. San Antonio, TX: Pearson.

Koenig-Bruhin, M., & Studer-Eichenberger, F. (2007). Therapy of verbal short-term memory disorders in fluent aphasia: A single case study. *Aphasiology, 21*(5), 448–458.

Kohen, F. P., McCluskey, M., Kalinyak-Fliszar, M., & Martin, N. (in preparation). Treatment of word processing and verbal short-term memory impairments in a case of Wernicke's aphasia.

Kreutzer, J., Wehman, P., Conder, R., & Morrison, C. (1989). Compensatory strategies for enhancing living and vocational outcome following traumatic brain injury. *Cognitive Rehabilitation, 7*, 30–35.

Lambon Ralph, M. A., Graham, K., Patterson, K., & Hodges, J. (1999). Is a picture worth a thousand words? Evidence from concept definitions by patients with semantic dementia. *Brain and Language, 70*, 309–335.

Landis, J., Hanten, G., Levin, X., Li, L., Ewing-Cobbs, J., Duron, W., & High, W. Jr. (2006). Evaluation of the errorless learning technique in children with traumatic brain injury. *Archives of Physical Medicine and Rehabilitation, 87*(6), 799–805.

Levin, H. S., Grossman, R. G., & Kelly, P. J. (1976). Aphasic disorder in patients with closed head injury. *Journal of Neurology, Neurosurgery, and Psychiatry, 39*, 1062–1070.

Majerus, S., Van der Kaa, M. A., Renard, C., Van der Linden, M., & Poncelet, P. (2005). Treating verbal short-term memory deficits by increasing the duration of temporary phonological representations: A case study. *Brain and Language, 95*(1), 174–175.

Martin, A., & Fedio, P. (1983). Word production and comprehension in Alzheimer's disease: The breakdown of semantic knowledge. *Brain and Language, 19*, 124–141.

Martin, N. (2000). Word processing and verbal short-term memory: How are they connected and why do we want to know? *Brain and Language, 71*, 149–153.

Martin, N. (2005). Verbal and nonverbal semantic impairment in aphasia: An activation deficit hypothesis. *Brain and Language, 95*, 251–252.

Martin, N. (2008). The role of semantic processing in short-term memory and learning: Evidence from aphasia. In A. Thorn & M. Page (Eds.), *Interactions between short-term and long-term memory in the verbal domain* (chap. 11, pp. 220–243). Hove and New York: Psychology Press.

Martin, N., & Ayala, J. (2004). Measurements of auditory-verbal STM in aphasia: Effects of task, item and word processing impairment. *Brain and Language, 89*, 464–483.

Martin, N., & Bunta, F. (2007). Effects of lexical processing on primacy effects in repetition of words and nonwords: Evidence from aphasia. *Brain and Language, 103*, 183–184.

Martin, N., & Gupta, P. (2004). Exploring the relationship between word processing and verbal STM: Evidence from associations and dissociations. *Cognitive Neuropsychology, 21*, 213–228.

Martin, N., Kohen, F. P., & Kalinyak-Fliszar, M. (2008). *A diagnostic battery to assess language and short-term memory deficits in aphasia*. Presented at Clinical Aphasiology Conference, Jackson Hole, WY, June 24–28, 2008.

Martin, N., Kohen, F. P. & Kalinyak-Fliszar, M. (May 23–27, 2010). A processing approach to the assessment of language and verbal short-term memory abilities in aphasia. Presented at Clinical Aphasiology Conference, Charleston, SC May 23–27, 2010.

Martin, N., Kohen, F. P., Kalinyak-Fliszar, M. (in preparation). Assessment of language and verbal short-term memory abilities in aphasia.

Martin, N., Kohen, F. P., McCluskey, M., Kalinyak-Fliszar, M., & Gruberg, N. (2009). Treatment of a language activation maintenance deficit in Wernicke's aphasia. Presented at Clinical Aphasiology Conference, Keystone, CO, May 26–31, 2009.

Martin, N., & Saffran, E. M. (1992). A computational account of deep dysphasia: Evidence from a single case study. *Brain and Language, 43*, 240–274.

Martin, N., & Saffran, E. M. (1997). Language and auditory-verbal short-term memory impairments: Evidence for common underlying processes. *Cognitive Neuropsychology, 14*(5), 641–682.

Martin, N., & Saffran, E. M. (1999). Effects of word processing and short-term memory deficits on verbal learning: Evidence from aphasia. *International Journal of Psychology, 34*(5/6), 330–346.

Martin, N., Saffran, E. M., & Dell, G. S. (1996). Recovery in deep dysphasia: Evidence for a relation between auditory-verbal STM and lexical errors in repetition. *Brain and Language, 52*, 83–113.

Martin, R., & Freedman, M. (2001). Short-term retention of lexical-semantic representations: Implications for speech production. *Memory, 9*, 261–280.

Martin, R. C., Shelton, J., & Yaffee, L. (1994). Language processing and working memory: Neuropsychological evidence for separate phonological and semantic capacities, *Journal of Memory and Language, 33*, 83–111.

Martin, R. C., & He, T. (2004). Semantic short-term memory deficit and language processing: A replication. *Brain and Language, 89*, 76–82.

Mateer, C. A., Kerns, K. A., & Eso, K. L. (1996). Management of attention and memory disorders following traumatic brain injury. *Journal of Learning Disabilities, 29*(6), 618–632.

Miyake, A., Emerson, M. J., & Friedman, N. P. (2000). Assessment of executive functions in clinical settings: Problems and recommendations. *Seminars in Speech and Language, 21* (2), 169–185.

Murray, L., Holland, A. L., & Beeson, P. M. (1998). Spoken language of individuals with mild fluent aphasia under focused and divided-attention conditions. *Journal of Speech, Language, and Hearing Research, 41*, 213–227.

Murray, L. L., Keeton, R. J., & Karcher, L. (2006). Treating attention in mild aphasia: Evaluation of attention process training-II. *Journal of Communication Disorders, 39*, 37–61.

Nadel, L., & Moscovitch, M. (1997). Memory consolidation, retrograde amnesia and the hippocampal complex. *Current Opinion in Neurobiology, 7*, 217–227.

O'Carroll, R. E., Russell, H. H., Lawrie, S. M., & Johnstone, E. C. (1999). Errorless learning and the cognitive rehabilitation of memory-impaired schizophrenic patients. *Psychological Medicine, 29*(1), 105–112.

Page, M., Wilson, B. A., Shiel, A., Carter, G., & Norris, D. (2006). What is the locus of the errorless-learning advantage? *Neuropsychologia, 44*, 90–100.

Parkin, A. J., Hunkin, N. M., & Squires, E. J. (1998). Unlearning John Major: The use of errorless learning in the reacquisition of proper names following herpes simplex encephalitis. *Cognitive Neuropsychology, 15*(4), 361–375.

Poirier, M., & Saint Aubin, J. (1995). Memory for related and unrelated words: Further evidence on the influence of semantic factors immediate serial recall. *Quarterly Journal of Experimental Psychology, 48A*, 384–404.

Randolph, C. (2001). Repeatable battery for the assessment of neuropsychological status. San Antonio, TX: Psychological Corporation.

Reilly, J., Martin, N., & Grossman, M. (2005). Verbal learning in semantic dementia: Is repetition priming a useful strategy? *Aphasiology, 19*, 329–339.

Reilly, J., & Peele, J. E. (2008). Effects of semantic impairment on language processing in semantic dementia. *Seminars in Speech and Language, 29*(1), 32–43.

Reisberg, B., Ferris, S. H., & Franssen, E. (1985). An ordinal functional assessment tool for Alzheimer's-type dementia. *Hospital and Community Psychiatry, 36*, 593–595.

Reisberg, B., Ferris, S. H., deLeon, M. J., & Crook, T. (1982). The Global Deterioration Scale for assessment of primary degenerative dementia. *American Journal of Psychiatry, 139*, 1136–1139.

Rey, A. (1941). Psychological examination of traumatic encephalopathy. *Archives de Psychologie, 28*, 286–340.

Rey, A. (1964). *L'examen clinique en psychologie*. Paris: Presses Universitaires de France.

Roach, A., Schwartz, M. F., Martin, N., Grewal, R. S., & Brecher, A. (1996). The Philadelphia Naming Test: Scoring and rationale. In *Clinical Aphasiology* (Vol. 24, pp. 121–134). Austin, TX: Pro-Ed.

Ross, K. B., & Wertz, R. T. (2004). Accuracy of formal tests for diagnosing mild aphasia: An application of evidence-based medicine. *Aphasiology, 18*, 337–355.

Saffran, E. M., Schwartz, M. F., Linebarger, M. L., Martin, N., & Bochetto, P. (1988). *Philadelphia Comprehension Battery*. Unpublished.

Saffran, E. M. (1990). Short-term memory impairment and language processing. In A. Caramazza (Ed.), *Advances in cognitive neuropsychology and neurolinguistics*. Hillsdale, NJ: Erlbaum.

Saffran, E. M., & Martin, N. (1990). Neuropsychological evidence for lexical involvement in short-term memory. In G. Vallar & T. Shallice (Eds.), *Neuropsychological impairments of short-term memory*. Cambridge, UK: Cambridge University Press.

Shallice, T., & Warrington, E. K. (1970). Independent functioning of the verbal memory stores: A neuropsychological study. *Quarterly Journal of Experimental Psychology, 22*, 261–273.

Shelton, J., Martin, R. C., & Yaffee, L. (1992). Investigating a verbal short-term memory deficit and its consequences for language processing. In D. Margolin (Ed.), *Cognitive neuropsychology in clinical practice*. New York: Cambridge University Press.

Shulman, H. G. (1971). Similarity effects in short-term memory. *Psychological Bulletin, 75*, 399–415.

Snowden, J. S., Griffiths, H. L., & Neary, D. (1999). Semantic episodic memory interactions in semantic dementia: Implications for retrograde memory function. *Cognitive Neuropsychology, 13*, 1101–1137.

Snowden, J. S. & Neary, D. (2002). Relearning of verbal labels in semantic dementia. *Neuropsychologia, 40*, 1715–1728.

Sohlberg, M. M., & Mateer, C. A. (1989). Training use of compensatory memory books: A three stage behavioral approach. *Journal of Clinical and Experimental Neuropsychology, 11*, 871–891.

Sohlberg, M. M., Ehlhardt, L., & Kennedy, M. (2005). Instructional techniques in cognitive rehabilitation: A preliminary report. *Seminars in Speech Language Pathology, 26*, 268–279.

Squires, E. J., Hunkin, N. M., & Parkin, A. J. (1997). Errorless learning condition of novel associations in amnesia. *Neuropsychologia, 35*, 1103–1111.

Tseng, C.-H., McNeil, M., & Milenkovic, P. (1993). An investigation of attention allocation deficits in aphasia. *Brain and Language, 45*, 276–296.

Turkstra, L. S., Coelho, C., & Ylvisaker, M. (2005). The use of standardized tests for individuals with cognitive-communication disorders. *Seminars in Speech and Language, 26*(4), 215–222.

Ullman, M. T. (2004). Contributions of memory circuits to language: The declarative/procedural model. *Cognition, 92*, 231–270.

Ullman, M. T., Corkin, S., Coppola, M., Hickok, G., Growdon, J. H., Koroshetz, W. J., & Pinker, S. (1997). A neural dissociation within language: Evidence that the mental dictionary is part of declarative memory and that grammatical rules are processed by the procedural system. *Journal of Cognitive Neuroscience, 9*, 266–276.

Watkins, O. C., & Watkins, M. J. (1977). Serial recall and the modality effect. *Journal of Experimental Psychology: Human Learning and Memory, 3*, 712–718.

Wechsler, D. (1987). *Wechsler Memory Scale—Revised (WMS-R)*. New York: Psychological Corporation.

Ween, J. E., Verfaille, M., & Alexander, M. P. (1996). Verbal memory function in mild aphasia. *Neurology, 47*, 795–801.

Wiig, E., & Secord, W. (1989). *Test of language competence—expanded edition.* San Antonio, TX: Psychological Corporation.

Williams, J. M. (1991). *Memory assessment scales professional manual.* New York: Psychological Corporation.

Wilson, B. A., Baddeley, A., Evans, J., & Shiel, A. (1994). Errorless learning in the rehabilitation of memory impaired people. *Neuropsychological Rehabilitation, 4*, 307–326.

Ylvisaker, M., & Feeney, T. J. (1998). *Collaborative brain injury intervention: Positive everyday routines.* San Diego, CA: Singular Publishing Group.

Ylvisaker, M., Szekeres, S. F., & Feeney, T. J. (2008). Communication disorders associated with traumatic brain injury. In R. Chapey, *Language intervention strategies in adult aphasia* (5th ed., chap. 33, pp. 879–962). Baltimore, MD: Lippincott, Williams, & Wilkins.

13-1

A Diagnostic Battery for the Assessment of Language and Short-Term Memory Abilities in Aphasia

In this appendix, we describe briefly the purpose and contents of the Temple Assessment of Language and Short-Term Memory in Aphasia (TALSA). This test battery was designed to assess the effects of increased short-term memory load on language performance. The resulting profile from this test yields the following information:

(1) linguistic characteristics of language/STM impairment in aphasia at all levels of severity.
(2) processing nature of the language/STM impairment (weak activation or too-rapid decay of activated semantic and phonological representations),
(3) ability to activate and maintain activation of language representations in the contexts of increased memory load and verbal interference.

DESCRIPTION OF THE TALSA BATTERY

Part 1 includes word processing tasks that probe semantic and phonological abilities and vary in difficulty, allowing assessment of **all** levels of aphasia severity. Two variations of the tasks in Part 1 entail inclusion of a 5-second interval between stimulus and cue to respond (e.g., word-to-picture matching) or between two stimuli that need to be compared and judged on some dimension (e.g., phoneme discrimination). In one condition, the interval is unfilled (silent) allowing assessment of the ability to passively maintain activation of representations as time passes (the passive STM condition). The other 5-second interval condition is "filled" with the subject naming numbers on a computer screen. This condition assesses the ability to maintain activation of word representations in STM, but in the context of verbal interference. Part 1 also includes language tests that vary the memory load by increasing the number of words to be managed in two similarity judgment tasks (rhyming and synonymy triplet judgments).

Part 2 consists of verbal span measures that vary content of the words to be recalled in ways that make the span tasks sensitive to phonological or semantic levels of word representation.

The subtests of this first version of the *TALSA* battery are described briefly below. Normative data from 30 people with aphasia and 10 controls without aphasia or brain damage are available for this version (Martin, Kalinyak-Fliszar, & Kohen, 2010). A revised version is currently being developed in our laboratory. The battery is programmed for computer administration using E-Prime software. Readers are welcome to contact the author at nmartin@temple.edu for copies of the TALSA battery.

Part 1. Language Tests with Variations in Short-Term Memory Load

Input Phonological Processing Measures

Phoneme discrimination. Stimuli are word and non-word pairs that are identical or differ by one or two phonemes. Participants hear the stimulus pairs and determine whether they are the same or different.

Recognition of rhyming word and non-word pairs. Stimuli are word and non-word pairs that rhyme or do not rhyme. The participant listens to the stimulus pairs and decides whether they rhyme or not.

Input Lexical-Semantic Processing Measures

Lexical comprehension. A spoken word is matched to one of four pictures that are members of the same semantic category. The picture follows the spoken word after one of the three interval conditions.

Category judgments. This test measures the ability to access knowledge of category membership through spoken and written words presented simultaneously (verbal semantics) and through pictures (conceptual semantics). Two items (words or pictures) are presented in succession (at one of the three interval conditions). The task is to decide whether the two items are members of the same semantic category.

Measures that Involve Output Processing

Word and non-word repetition. Stimuli are words and non-words matched for length and CVC structure. The participant hears the stimulus and repeats it on cue after one of the three designated intervals.

Picture naming. (Adapted from the Philadelphia Naming Test, Roach, Schwartz, Martin, et al., 1996.) There are three sets of pictures, consisting of one-, two- and three-syllable names. Syllable length and word frequency are balanced across all three sets. A picture appears on the screen for 2000 milliseconds, followed by a cue to name (beep) after one of the three interval conditions.

Multiple-Word Utterances with STM Variations

Word string repetition. This test includes word pairs and word triplets that are phonologically related (initial phoneme overlap), categorically related or unrelated. Participants hear the word string and attempt to repeat it after one of the three interval conditions.

Sentence repetition task. There are two sets sentence stimuli: (1) simple declarative sentences with a noun phrase, verb phrase, and prepositional phrase (e.g., The boy walked the dog in the park) for repetition and (2) the same sentences padded with two modifiers (e.g., The *tall* boy walked the dog in the *public* park). Each sentence is presented auditorily and the participant is asked to repeat the sentence when a cue is provided after one of the three intervals.

Sentence comprehension. (Adapted from the Philadelphia Comprehension Battery, Saffran, Schwartz, Linebarger, et al., 1988.) This test examines comprehension of sentences that represent five syntactic structure types: Simple Active Declarative, Passive, Subject Relative Clause, Object Relative Clause, Locatives. All sentences have an agent and a patient, but half are semantically reversible. The participant hears the sentence, and after one of the three interval conditions, is presented with two pictures and points to the matching picture. There are two foil types. Lexical foils replace the agent or patient with another object or being (The policeman shoots the robber vs. the policeman shoots the dog). Reversible foils reverse the objects or beings in the agent and patient roles (The policeman shoots the robber vs. The robber shoots the policeman).

Measures of Lexical-Semantic and Phonological Processing that Vary Working Memory Load by Number of Items to Be Compared

Rhyming triplet judgments. The task is to decide which of two words rhyme with a target word or which two of three words rhyme when pictures are presented simultaneously with their spoken names. Stimuli are one-syllable, pictureable nouns with consonant-vowel structures: CVC, CCVC, CCVCC, CVCC. In one version, three pictures are presented diagonally on the page from top-left to bottom right. Their names are presented auditorily, in the same sequence as the picture display. Two of the picture names rhyme and the non-rhyming foil overlaps phonologically with one or two of the rhyming words in one of three ways: same initial phoneme (fan, pan, pail), same stressed vowel, (bag, rag, cat) or same final phoneme. This format requires holding three word pairs (e.g., *bag-rag, bag-cat, cat-rag*) in STM. In a second version, the same three pictures are presented diagonally as before, but the center picture is highlighted. Its name is presented first (e.g., *fan*) followed by the names of the other two pictures (e.g., *pan, pail*). The task is to determine which of these two words (*pan* or *pail*) rhymes with the target word (*fan*). In this task only two word pairs need to be held in short-term working memory (*fan-pan, fan-pail*). The dependent measure is proportion correct. Thirty pairs are tested in each of two formats: three-pair comparisons and (two-pair comparisons).

Synonymy triplet judgments. The task is to determine which of two words is most similar in meaning to a target word or which two of three words are most similar in meaning. The word triplets consist of concrete and abstract nouns and verbs). Two formats vary the memory load on performance and task requirements as described for the rhyming triplet judgment task.

Part 2. Span Measures with Language Variations

Span tasks are varied for the items (digits, words or non-words) and language characteristics of items to be recalled. Lexical-semantic and phonological variations include frequency, imageability, semantic category, and lexicality. Spans for "serial order" and "in any order" are calculated using a formulas developed by R. Martin and colleagues (e.g., Shelton, Martin, & Yaffee, 1992). These are described in the test instructions.

Digit and word spans. Verbal short-term memory span for digits and words is assessed by means of a pointing task and a repetition task. For the digit span task, number sequences (1–7 items) are generated from a finite set of nine digits (1–9), but with no repeats of digits within a string. Word sequences are generated from a finite set of nine imageable, high frequency words and matched for syllable length to the digits. In the repetition span, the participant repeats the sequence in order after hearing the entire list. In the pointing span, the participant points to the digits on a visual array (randomly changed on each trial), displayed after the digits are heard.

Repetition span for words varied for frequency and imageability. This test measures repetition for word strings (1–6 words in length) that consist of one and two-syllable words varied by frequency (F) and imageability (I) in four ways: HF-HI, LF-HI, HF-LI, LF-LI. Frequency and imageability variations are presented randomly within a string length condition. Participants hear the sequence of words and attempt to repeat it immediately in serial order.

Word–non-word span. The word span measure includes high imageability–high frequency words in each of four string-length conditions (2–5 words). All words are one to two syllables long. Non-word span stimuli (string lengths 1–5) are derived from the items in the word span test by changing two to three phonemes, sampling equally from initial, medial, and final positions of the word. Presentation of word and non-word conditions is blocked. Participants listen to each string and attempt to repeat it immediately in serial order.

Probe span tests of identity STM, semantic STM, and phonological STM. These tests were adapted from a paradigm developed by Martin, et al. (1994). Probe memory tasks are especially useful to assess language and STM deficits in people with milder aphasia who perform at ceiling on many tests in Part 1 of this battery. The participant hears a string of words followed by a spoken probe word. The task is to judge whether the probe is related to one of the words in the string. Half of the probes are unrelated to any word in the string. The other half of the probe words are related in some way to one of the words in the string, depending on the condition: semantic probe—one word in the string is from the same category as the probe word; phonologic probe—one word in the string rhymes with the probe word; identity probe—one word in the string is identical to the probe word. String lengths start at one and continue to seven for the semantic and phonologic probes. There are 12 string lengths for the identity probe.

13-2

A Treatment Protocol to Improve Activation and Maintenance of Activated Phonological and/or Semantic Representations of Words

Treatment Protocol

The protocol includes semantic and phonological modules, each with two parts: (1) single words and (2) word strings. Stimulus variations in all modules are presented hierarchically from easier to more difficult. There are three interval conditions for each module, a 1-sec UF, 5-sec UF, and 5-sec F.

Treatment Schedule

Treatment will be applied to a stimulus variation within a module beginning at one of the three intervals. Treatment can then be applied to the *same* stimuli at the next interval condition (Protocol 1 below, e.g., from 1 second unfilled to 5-second filled conditions) or to the next stimulus variation (Protocol 2 below, e.g., from three-syllable words to two-syllable non-words).

Treatment of Short-term Word Activation and Maintenance Impairments

Protocol 1 — Phonological Module

Variations	Interval condition		
	1-sec Unfilled	5-sec Unfilled	5-sec Filled
Level 1			
Lo image-Hi freq 2 syllable words	—————————→		
Non-words 2 syllables	—————————→		
Level 2			
Phonologically related word pairs	—————————→		
Lo image-Hi freq word pairs	—————————→		
Lo image-Lo freq word pairs	—————————→		

Protocol 1 — Phonological + Semantic Module

Variations	Interval condition		
	1-sec Unfilled	5-sec Unfilled	5-sec Filled
Level 1			
Hi image-Hi freq 2 syllable words	—————————→		
Lo image-Hi freq 2 syllable words	—————————→		
Level 2			
Categorically-related word pairs	—————————→		
Hi image-Hi freq word pairs	—————————→		
Lo image-Hi freq word pairs	—————————→		

Protocol 2 — Phonological Module

Variations	Interval condition		
	1-sec Unfilled	5-sec Unfilled	5-sec Filled
Level 1			
Lo image-Hi freq 2 syllable words	↓	↓	↓
Non-words 2 syllables			
Level 2			
Phonologically related word pairs			
Lo image-Hi freq word pairs	↓	↓	↓
Lo image-Lo freq word pairs			

Protocol 2 — Phonological + Semantic Module

Variations	Interval condition		
	1-sec Unfilled	5-sec Unfilled	5-sec Filled
Level 1			
Hi image-Hi freq 2 syllable words	↓	↓	↓
Lo image-Hi freq 2 syllable words			
Level 2			
Categorically-related word pairs			
Hi image-Hi freq word pairs	↓	↓	↓
Lo image-Hi freq word pairs			

Training Procedure

The training task in our studies has been repetition of a stimulus variation (words or non-words) in one of three interval conditions. It is important to note that the interval variations could be applied to other tasks. Feedback can be provided via a hierarchical cueing procedure if needed.

At What Level and Interval Condition Does Treatment Begin?

The module and interval condition to begin treatment depends upon factors related to performance on the Temple University Assessment of Language and Short-Term Memory in Aphasia (see Appendix 13-1). For example, assignment would depend on whether the word processing impairment affects semantic and/or phonological representations of words and at which interval condition activation maintenance of representations begins to falter. The treatment protocol has been designed to be **flexible** so that results of the TALSA Battery will determine the level, module and interval condition at which treatment will be applied, as well as the variation at which to initiate and progress through treatment.

CHAPTER 14

Treating Communication Problems in Individuals with Disordered Language

CHAPTER OUTLINE

Swathi Kiran and Chaleece Sandberg

The focus of this chapter will be on providing impairment-based therapy to persons with disordered language. The field of aphasiology has seen an evolution of classification of language disorders in adults. Most of the classification systems are based on etiology, symptoms, or a combination of etiology and symptoms; however, no one classification system has proven to be successful in classifying language disorders to the satisfaction of both clinicians and researchers. For example, Broca's aphasia is the term used for a collection of symptoms including word-finding difficulties, relatively preserved auditory comprehension, poor repetition, and non-fluent speech. This is a useful classification for clinicians because it immediately creates a picture of the patient. On the other hand, a researcher studying Broca's aphasia will soon discover that patients with Broca's aphasia can also exhibit agrammatism to varying degrees, which can interfere with comprehension; or apraxia, which can confound scores on word-finding measures. For this reason, the ideal scenario for clinicians and researchers is to determine each individual's specific language strengths and deficits and target each language deficit during therapy.

This chapter will first highlight the primary communication characteristics resulting from disturbances within the domain of language. Several sub-domains of language are elaborated, namely comprehension and production of phonological, orthographic, semantic, syntactic and discourse/pragmatic aspects of language

(Figure 14-1). Next, general guidelines for assessment and some specific examples of currently used assessments will be discussed. Finally, an evidence-based review of the treatment literature for the last 10 years will be presented. From this review, effective treatment techniques for each type of impairment will be selected and described for use in clinical practice. The current chapter utilizes a theoretical framework presented by Ellis and Young (Ellis & Young, 1988) that is pertinent to comprehension and production of spoken and written words. Disorders specific to the semantic system will be discussed within interactive activation models (Dell, 1986) and syntactic disorders will be discussed within theoretical frameworks proposed by Garrett (1980) and Caplan (1992).

Even though the chapter is organized into discrete levels of language processing, it is important to understand that language processing deficits in adults are not isolated modules of impairment but oftentimes are manifest as overlapping and analogous deficits that span across levels of language of processing. For instance, there is some overlap in the nature of deficits observed in orthographic aspects and phonological aspects of language processing. Likewise, there is some overlap between semantic aspects and phonological aspects of language processing. Therefore, when identifying a patient's specific language deficit and developing a treatment, one must acknowledge the possibility of overlapping behavioral markers across different levels of language.

LANGUAGE DISORDERS

Phonological Aspects of Language Disorders

Comprehension

Spoken language is comprehended from auditory input. Sound waves are decoded by the auditory system into small linguistic units we recognize as phonemes. This process is carried out by the auditory analysis system. Certain sequences of phonemes form units of meaning called morphemes. Morphemes that can stand alone are called words. Word forms are stored in the auditory input lexicon, which functions as a mechanism to verify the existence of a word in the individual's repertoire. Meanings of words are accessed from the semantic system. Although deficits in each of these systems will be described separately, keep in mind that these systems are intrinsically connected and, most often, more than one system is impaired.

Deficits in comprehension can occur at any level of phonological processing. Persons with impairment of only the auditory analysis system are said to have *pure word deafness*. These individuals have problems decoding speech, but are able to identify environmental sounds. This means that repetition and comprehension of speech are severely impaired, but other language functions are intact.

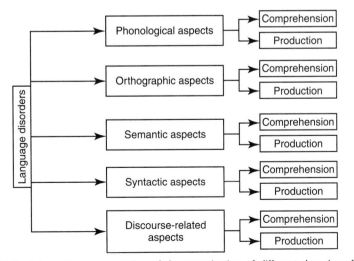

Figure 14-1 Schematic representation of the organization of different domains of language that defines the layout of the chapter.

Production

Spoken language production begins with a concept, which is then activated in the semantic system. This concept gains a phonological word form in the speech output lexicon. Once the word form is activated in the speech output lexicon, phoneme sequences are retrieved at the phoneme level, speech movements are planned by the motor cortex, and speech is produced.

Deficits in production can occur at any level of output processing or at the level of the semantic system itself. A disruption in the connection between the auditory analysis system and the phoneme level results in *auditory phonological agnosia*. Persons with this disorder exhibit poor repetition of nonwords, but intact lexical decision and repetition of real words with the use of the intact semantic system route. Deficits of the semantic system in particular will be discussed in another section. Deficits in the speech output lexicon and phoneme level result in mixed paraphasias. Mixed paraphasias are some combination of a semantic and a phonemic paraphasia. For example, if the target is *moustache* and the person says *whisper,* the error is in activating the word form *whisker* and assigning /p/ in the place of /k/. Deficits at the phoneme level result in phonemic paraphasias. Phonemic paraphasias can also occur as the result of verbal apraxia. Verbal apraxia is a deficit in the motor planning of phoneme sequences. Apraxia is distinguishable from dysarthria by the often preserved pronunciation of automatic phrases.

Orthographic Aspects of Language Disorders

Comprehension

Written language is comprehended from visual input. The visual analysis system decodes the written letters that form words. The words formed by certain combinations of letters are stored in the visual input lexicon, which accesses the meaning of the visual word form from the semantic system. The process of assigning a phoneme to a written letter is carried out via grapheme-to-phoneme conversion and can be independent from the lexicon and semantic system.

Persons with impairment of the visual analysis system and visual input lexicon have difficulty decoding and recognizing written language, but may be able to correctly assign phonemes to orthography, using the grapheme-to-phoneme conversion route. This is considered to be a peripheral dyslexia called *pure alexia* or letter-by-letter reading. Other types of peripheral dyslexia include *neglect dyslexia* and *attentional dyslexia*, which result from cognitive impairments described in

Chapter 8 of this book. *Phonological dyslexia* results from impairment of grapheme-to-phoneme conversion. These individuals are forced to rely on the whole-word semantic route and therefore read both regular and irregular real words with relatively high accuracy, but are unable to read nonwords and unfamiliar words. In contrast to phonological dyslexia, *surface dyslexia* results from impairment of the visual input lexicon and semantic system. These individuals exhibit impaired reading of irregular words, but preserved ability to read regular words and nonwords. Additionally, the person's ability to retrieve the meaning of the word relies on his/her pronunciation such that *stood* may be read as *stewed* activating the meaning relating to food rather than the meaning related to position. *Deep dyslexia* is a manifestation of an impairment comprising both the semantic system and the grapheme-to-phoneme conversion mechanism. Persons with deep dyslexia produce semantic paraphasias and/or morphological errors; show effects of imageability, concreteness, and word class; and exhibit impairment reading nonwords, often substituting real words (e.g., *bride* for *bripe*).

Production

The production of written language, like spoken language, begins with a concept, which is then activated in the semantic system. Once the concept activates a word form in the graphemic output lexicon, an abstract representation of the letters is activated in the graphemic buffer, which is thought to behave like working memory, storing the abstract letter forms until the specific letter forms can be activated. From here, a word can either be spelled orally or written. Specific letter forms (e.g., upper/lowercase, print/cursive style) are activated at the allograph level. Graphomotor patterns are then planned and executed by the motor system. The process of assigning a written letter to a phoneme is carried out via phoneme-to-grapheme conversion and can be independent from the lexicon and semantic system.

Persons with impairment at the allograph level present with letter substitutions of visually similar letters. Deficits at the graphemic buffer produce both oral and written spelling errors such as addition, deletion, substitution, and transposition of letters. These deficits in writing are referred to as peripheral dysgraphias. *Phonological dysgraphia* refers to a deficit in phoneme-to-grapheme conversion. Persons with phonological dysgraphia retain the ability to spell familiar words, both regular and irregular, but have difficulty spelling nonwords. In contrast to phonological dysgraphia, lexical agraphia or *surface dysgraphia* refers to a writing deficit that occurs at the level of the graphemic output lexicon. These individuals exhibit impairments in spelling irregular words or homophones, but relatively preserved spelling of regular words and nonwords. *Deep dysgraphia*, like deep dyslexia, involves the semantic system. Persons with deep dysgraphia produce semantic errors during free writing and writing to dictation, have difficulty writing nonwords, and the accuracy of their written output is affected by psycholinguistic factors such as imageability and word class.

Semantic Aspects of Language Disorders

This section will describe aspects of deficits in language function that involve the semantic system and the processing of the meanings of words for comprehension and production. The semantic system receives input from several modalities: auditory verbal/nonverbal input, visual verbal/nonverbal input, tactile input, olfactory input, and gustatory input. These semantic representations appear to be organized within the semantic system hierarchically, but also in somewhat overlapping categories (Rogers & McClelland, 2003). Deficits in semantic processing, affecting either comprehension or production of language, can be modulated by psycholinguistic factors and semantic category factors. Psycholinguistic factors that affect linguistic performance include imageability, concreteness, familiarity, frequency, age of acquisition, and word class (Luzzatti, Raggi, Zonca, et al., 2002; Nickels & Howard, 1995). Semantic category factors include the category itself, animacy, and typicality (Kiran & Thompson, 2003a; Shelton & Caramazza, 1999). Based on the several studies that have examined semantic processing deficits in persons with aphasia, it is clear that a selective fractionation of the semantic system can occur resulting in specific loss of a semantic category, a certain hierarchical level of a category, the inputs and output modalities into the semantic system or in the automatic processes involved (read Shelton & Caramazza, 1999; Tyler & Moss, 2001).

Access to the semantic system and activation within the semantic system can be explained via interactive activation models (Dell, 1986). Lexical access involves the following steps (Dell, 1986; Dell & O'Seaghdha, 1992; Dell, Schwartz, Martin, Saffran, & Gagnon, 1997). The semantic units receive external input (e.g., visual presentation of the picture *cat*). Activation spreads to all potential semantic nodes and down to the phonological units linked to those semantic nodes. The semantic and phonological units are connected bi-directionally, so semantic units receive input from activated phonological units. This positive feedback activates phonological neighbors of the target (e.g., *mat*, *sat*), semantic neighbors of the target (e.g., *dog*), and both semantically

and phonologically related words (e.g., *rat*). The most highly activated word node is selected. A phonological frame is then activated, which represents the syllabic structure of the word, and is involved in the retrieval of phonemes. Interactive activation models are appealing because of their flexibility in explaining both comprehension and production impairments. Comprehension and/or production errors could result from incomplete/incorrect activation of semantic nodes, incomplete/incorrect activation of phonological nodes, or failures in the bi-directional links between the semantic and phonological nodes.

Comprehension

Disruptions in the semantic system itself or in semantic access result in deficits in comprehension of language and can be manifest in several ways. As noted before, deep dyslexia is a reading disorder that results from damage to the semantic system, with errors reflecting deficits in processing the meanings of words. A deficit at the level of the auditory input lexicon results in *word meaning deafness*. These individuals exhibit difficulty understanding the meaning of spoken words but intact repetition, reading comprehension, spontaneous speech, and writing to dictation. A deficit at the level of the connection between the auditory input lexicon and the semantic system results in *semantic access dysphasia*. These individuals have intact semantic representations in the semantic system as evidenced by semantic judgment tasks as well as an intact auditory input lexicon as evidenced by a lexical decision task. However, impaired comprehension of the meanings of auditorily presented words indicates problems accessing the semantic representation.

Production

Disruptions of the semantic system also result in deficits in production of language. As mentioned previously, deep dysgraphia, like deep dyslexia, involves the semantic system. Persons with deep dysgraphia produce semantic errors during free writing and writing to dictation, have difficulty writing nonwords, and are affected by psycholinguistic factors such as imageability and word class. Deficits in verbal output, such as semantic paraphasias, neologisms, and mixed paraphasias in confrontation naming, word generation, and spontaneous speech can all be signs of damage to the semantic system.

Syntactic Aspects of Language Disorders

The rules that we use to generate sentences are collectively referred to as syntax or grammar and can produce an unlimited number of different novel sentences. We also use these rules to decode novel sentences for comprehension. Disruptions in this rule system can take the form of *agrammatism*, which refers to a general disuse of function words, omission or misuse of morphology, errors in sentence structure, and deficits in sentence comprehension. *Paragrammatism* refers to a general misuse of function words and morphology, but relative preservation of sentence structure. This section discusses the role that syntax plays in disorders of comprehension and production of sentences.

Comprehension

Comprehension of sentences requires not only an understanding of the meanings of the words in the sentence, but also an understanding of how the relationships between words in a sentence influence the overall meaning of the message. While reading or listening to a sentence, the average reader/listener parses the sentence, assigning syntactic structure to its parts (e.g., noun, verb, etc.) and mapping thematic roles onto the syntactic structures (e.g., agent, theme, etc.). Generally, the comprehension of a sentence is affected by the type of verb (e.g., transitive, intransitive, dative) and the number of arguments (e.g., one place verb, two place verbs, three place verbs) (Shapiro, 1997). Further, sentences that require movement of a clause (e.g., *It was the lady who the man kissed*) are considered to be more difficult than canonical sentences (e.g., *The man kissed the lady*). Persons with agrammatism either cannot reliably use their syntactic parser or cannot reliably map thematic roles onto syntactic structures, or both (Caplan, Baker, & Dehaut, 1985; Schwartz, Linebarger, Saffran, & Pate, 1987). Often, these individuals rely on a heuristic route for sentence comprehension, using real world knowledge and canonical word order to extract meaning. Therefore, non-reversible sentences (e.g., *The girl ate a cake*) are easier to comprehend than reversible sentences (e.g., *The girl pulled the boy*) and canonical sentences (e.g., *The boy kissed the girl*) are easier to comprehend than noncanonical sentences *(The boy was kissed by the girl)*.

Production

The production of a syntactically sound sentence as proposed by Garrett (1980) requires roughly six steps: (1) the formation of a message, (2) the assignment of thematic roles, (3) the selection of lexical items, (4) the assignment of syntactical and morphological items, (5) the selection of phonological forms, and (6) the planning of articulatory movements. Persons with agrammatism often omit function words and morphological endings during sentence production and may even have difficulty producing these forms

during reading or repeating of single words. Persons with paragrammatism often make substitution errors with function words and morphological endings during sentence production. Further, paragrammatism may reflect a disturbance in the ability to monitor the speech planning process (Butterworth & Howard, 1987). The omission or substitution of function words and morphological endings suggests impairment of the assignment of syntactical and morphological items during sentence planning.

Persons with agrammatism also exhibit reduced length and complexity in sentence production. Factors involved include reduced production of verbs, bias toward verbs that take fewer arguments (e.g., intransitive and transitive verbs, but rarely dative verbs), and reduced complexity of sentence structure (e.g., absence of embedded clauses) (Kim & Thompson, 2000; Thompson, Shapiro, Tait, Jacobs, & Schneider, 1996). Additionally, some agrammatic patients have difficulty generating logical relationships between lexical elements and may therefore produce sentences in which semantic aspects, such as animacy, influence word order rather than syntactic aspects, such as thematic roles (Saffran, Schwartz, & Marin, 1980). Recent studies have shown that patients typically classified as having Wernicke's aphasia also show problems with assigning accurate syntactic information (Faroqi-Shah & Thompson, 2003), reaffirming the notion that classical aphasia syndromes do not always result in unique and nonoverlapping language characteristics.

Discourse-Related Aspects of Language Disorders

Sometimes a person will score well on tests of specific language functions, such as naming, repetition, reading, and writing, but still present with abnormal language use in conversation or monologues. This suggests a deficit at the discourse level.

Comprehension

Discourse comprehension, or the ability to understand spoken or written text, requires a combination of language and cognitive skills for successful execution. In addition to the ability to understand the phonology, semantics, and syntax of the material, reasoning abilities such as drawing inferences and the ability to monitor information are needed to understand complex forms of discourse (Kamhi, 1997). In the process of reading or hearing a piece of discourse, the individual draws upon a range of skills including setting goals and expectations, problem solving, and shifting (van Dijk, 1987). An important aspect of conversational discourse is pragmatics. Conversation depends upon the ability for each conversational partner to understand the intended meaning of an utterance. This requires attention to the context in which the utterance is given, knowledge of each meaning that a word can have and assignment of the correct meaning to the correct context, and attention to visual (body language) and/or prosodic cues.

Production

Impairments in pragmatics not only decrease a person's ability to comprehend conversation, but also to produce natural conversation. Successful conversation also relies upon pragmatic factors of production such as initiation, topic maintenance, and turn-taking. Another important form of discourse is the monologue: retelling a story or personal event, generating a novel story, explaining a procedure, or describing a picture. Impairments in monologic discourse are evidenced as decreased cohesion, decreased grammatical complexity, decreased and/or inaccurate information content, and disorganized narrative structure. Such impairments also contribute to disruptions in effective and natural conversation.

ASSESSMENT

Overall Goals of Assessment

The World Health Organization (WHO) International Classification of Functioning, Disability, and Health (ICF, http://www.who.int/classifications/icf/en/) is the international standard framework for describing health and disability. This classification system describes diseases/injuries using body function and structure, activity and participation, and environmental factors. Therefore, the main goals of assessment are to differentially diagnose the language disorder and to describe its relationship with body function and structure, how it will affect the patient's activities and participation, and how environmental factors will affect recovery as well as activities of daily living.

It is important to obtain information from the neurologist regarding the etiology of the language disorder before the assessment begins to determine the factors that precipitated the problem, which areas of the brain are affected, and the progression of the disease. This information will help guide the clinician's choice of assessment materials and inform the patient's prognosis for recovery. For example, if the patient has primary progressive aphasia or semantic dementia, then assessment and treatment will focus more on molding the environment to increase participation in activities of daily living: preparing the patient and his/her caretaker(s) for the eventual language decline, monitoring

the language decline, preserving as much language function as possible through language training, and training the patient/caregiver to use augmentative means of communication. On the other hand, if the patient has aphasia due to cerebrovascular accident, then assessment and treatment will focus more on language training to increase participation in activities of daily living: identifying preserved language functions and using those to train and reorganize lost language functions.

General Considerations

When performing an assessment, the clinician should consider the patient's age; general health status; pre-morbid factors; current social, cultural, and emotional situation; and any previous treatment or concurrent treatment. It is important to know details regarding the patient's physical and mental health status so that accommodations can be made for physical limitations, such as paralysis/paresis, as well as for cognitive limitations, such as visual field cuts. Pre-morbid factors, such as education level, bilingualism, developmental language or learning disabilities, history of health problems (including vision and hearing), history of drug or alcohol abuse, history of psychiatric disorders, and so on, are important to document during the assessment because they can influence the extent to which a person can recover language function. It is important to determine the social support that is available for the patient, the cultural values of the patient and his/her family, the activities in which the patient is expected to or wishes to participate, and the patient's emotional stability and motivation to participate in therapy. Finally, it is important to determine the previous therapy or concurrent therapy in which the patient may be participating in order to optimize each type of therapy. Knowledge of previous therapy will help the clinician to build on the previous clinician's work. Concurrent participation in physical therapy, occupational therapy, and speech/language therapy can be maximally beneficial if the therapists work together to create an integrative therapy program.

General Guidelines of Testing

Whether using standardized or non-standardized measures of language function, it is important for the clinician to make general observations of the patient that may not be captured by the specific linguistic measures. The clinician's initial impression is of utmost importance during an evaluation because it is the most objective impression of the patient's strengths and limitations. The clinician should garner as much information as possible about the following: Is the patient responsive?

How appropriate are the responses? How well does she/he comprehend questions? Is the patient pragmatically appropriate? How does the patient communicate? If with gestures, can she/he be understood? If speaking, how intelligible is the speech? Is the patient oriented to time, place, and person and responding to the environmental situation? The answers to these questions will assist the clinician in creating a comprehensive report of the patient's language profile.

When choosing a test or battery of tests, it is good to begin with tests that give key information about all language modalities, such as the Western Aphasia Battery (WAB-R; Kertesz, 2006) or Boston Diagnostic Aphasia Examination (BDAE-3; Goodglass, Kaplan, & Barresi, 2000). The patient's functional level can be determined with information from an initial patient or family interview or information from the referring specialist. When administering standardized tests, it is important to: (a) follow the test protocol, (b) administer all subtests, and (c) pace the testing according to the patient's ability.

To maintain objectivity during an assessment, the clinician should refrain from "leading" the patient. The purpose of an assessment is to establish exactly what the patient's strengths and weaknesses are. If help in achieving the correct answer is given, even inadvertently, this should be noted and included in the assessment report. Maintaining a healthy balance between friendly encouragement and objectivity is a difficult, yet necessary part of performing a quality assessment. Regardless of the testing environment, it is always important to consider the patient's level of motivation, to treat the patient like an adult, and to speak more clearly to the patient rather than more loudly to facilitate comprehension.

Supplementary Assessments: Testing Selective and Specific Language Impairments

Supplementary tests should be given in conjunction with a broad standardized test battery in order to determine each specific language deficit that is contributing to the patient's overall language deficit.

Phonological Assessment
Comprehension

Assessment of the integrity of the auditory phonological analysis system can be accomplished through the use of subtests such as those found in the Psycholinguistic Assessment of Language (PAL; Caplan & Bub, unpublished) and Psycholinguistic Assessment of Language Processing in Aphasia (PALPA; Kay, Lesser, & Coltheart, 1992). These tests utilize auditorily presented nonword minimal pairs and/or rhyming judgment to examine the patient's ability to decode the word at the phoneme level. The use of nonwords ensures that the patient is not relying on the semantic system for decoding. Comparing performance on a nonword repetition task with performance on a real word repetition task can reveal problems with the link between the auditory analysis system and the phonological output buffer. A good test of the phonological input lexicon is an auditory lexical decision task compared to a visual lexical decision task. If the auditory lexical decision score is lower than the visual lexical decision score, but nonword repetition is intact, the deficit can be assumed to be at the level of the phonological input lexicon.

Production

Pinpointing deficits in phonological processing during production can be a bit tricky because deficits in language production can be due to a variety of factors. It is important, therefore, to first dismiss dysarthria and apraxia as possible culprits. Next, deficits in semantic processing must be ruled out. This can be accomplished by testing each input and output modality with the same set of items and performing additional tests to assess semantic system integrity. Again, subtests of the PAL and the PALPA require production of different types of words/nonwords. If all verbal output modalities (i.e., repetition, reading, and verbal naming) are affected, then it can be assumed that the deficit lies at the level of the speech output lexicon. Additionally, a pseudoword reading task can help identify phonological processing deficits.

Orthographic Assessment
Comprehension

Reading can be assessed with test batteries designed specifically for reading assessment, such as the Reading Comprehension Battery for Aphasia (RCBA-2; LaPointe & Horner, 1998) or the Gray Oral Reading Tests (although only standardized up to age 18) (GORT-4; Wiederholt & Bryant, 2001), or through subtests of other standardized measures, such as the PALPA. The goal of the reading assessment would be to identify the locus of the reading problem. Therefore, a compilation of tasks such as reading words that increase in letter length, reading regularly versus irregularly spelled words, reading pseudowords, and identifying pictures that match written words can help identify pure alexia, surface dyslexia, phonological dyslexia, and deep dyslexia.

Production

Specific test batteries for assessing written language in adults with acquired language disorders are not currently available; however, writing subtests from standardized test batteries such as the WAB, BDAE, and PALPA can sufficiently capture a patient's specific writing deficits. Again, the goal of the writing assessment would be to identify the locus of the problem. Tasks such as written picture naming, writing regular versus irregular words, writing pseudowords, and writing automatics (e.g., alphabet, numbers 1–20, name and address) can help identify peripheral agraphias, surface agraphia, phonological agraphia, and deep agraphia.

Semantic Assessment

One way to determine the integrity of the semantic system without the confounding effects of deficits in reading, writing, auditory processing, or speech is through semantic judgment tasks. In these tasks, individuals are asked to judge the similarity of concepts represented by pictures. One such test is included in the Pyramids and Palm Trees Test (PAPT; Howard & Patterson, 1992). Poor performance suggests that the features of each concept that overlap are not available for analysis, indicating a disruption in the semantic system.

Because anomia is a key feature of aphasia and language disorders in general, several tests are available to measure naming function. The Boston Naming Test (BNT; Goodglass, Kaplan, & Weintraub, 1983), the Test of Adolescent/Adult Word Finding (TAWF; German, 1990), and the Peabody Picture Vocabulary Test (PPVT-4; Dunn & Dunn, 2007)/Expressive Vocabulary Test (EVT-2; Williams, 2007) are a few of the tests specifically designed to measure naming. Many overall language batteries include subtests of naming objects, naming pictures, generating words in a category (e.g., animals, words that start with the letter _, etc.), and matching pictures to spoken or written words. It is important to include both spoken and written items to determine if the naming deficit is influenced by specific input or output modalities. Also, it is important to include animate and inanimate items, abstract and concrete items, items from different word classes, and items from several different semantic categories in order to determine whether or not the naming deficit is influenced by animacy, concreteness, imageability, word class, or semantic category. Other psycholinguistic factors to consider are word frequency, familiarity, and age of acquisition.

Syntactic Assessment

Comprehension

Sentence comprehension can be measured through tests designed specifically for the purpose, such as the Auditory Comprehension Test for Sentences (Shewan, 1979), the Philadelphia Comprehension Battery (Saffran, Schwartz, Linebarger, et al., unpublished), and the Northwestern Sentence Comprehension Test (Thompson, unpublished-b). Subtests of the WAB, BDAE, PALPA, and PAL also measure sentence comprehension, as does the Revised Token Test (RTT; McNeil & Prescott, 1978).

Production

Sentence production can be measured through subtests of the PAL, or using subtests from the Northwestern Assessment of Verbs and Sentences (NAVS; Thompson, unpublished-a) that elicit specific sentence structures. In general, it is relatively easy for clinicians to obtain a narrative sample of a simple picture description task using pictures from the WAB, BDAE, or other material. Once the patient's utterances are transcribed, the sentences/utterances can be subjected to a linguistic analysis of discourse (Saffran, Berndt, & Schwartz, 1989) in order to determine various aspects of syntactic structures.

Discourse Assessment

Conversational and monologic discourse can be assessed with nonstandardized techniques such as discourse analysis. In this technique, discourse is elicited through descriptive, narrative, procedural, or conversational tasks and analyzed using structured discourse analysis procedures. The Profile of Communicative Appropriateness (Penn, 1985) and Damico's Clinical Discourse Analysis (1985) analyze pragmatic aspects of discourse, Quantitative Production Analysis (QPA, Saffran, et al., 1989) analyzes syntactic aspects of discourse, Correct Information Unit (CIU) analysis (Nicholas & Brookshire, 1993) measures the informativeness of discourse, and Type Token Ratio (TTR) is a measure of lexical diversity (see Malvern & Richards, 2002, for a discussion of D, which is a variant of TTR that can be used with large and varying sample sizes). Recently, Wright and colleagues (2008; 2005) developed an analysis of main events that measures a patient's ability to provide the relationships and causation among elements in a story, above and beyond the informativeness and efficiency of the narrative. This analysis, in conjunction with a standard discourse analyses (e.g., TTR, CIU), shows promise as a sensitive tool for detecting treatment effects on narrative discourse in patients with aphasia. Comprehension of spoken and written discourse can be evaluated through the Discourse Comprehension Test (DCT; Brookshire & Nicholas, 1997). This test consists of spoken and written stories with corresponding questions that assess comprehension of directly stated and implied main ideas and details.

Finally, functional communication can be assessed with formal measures, such as the Communication Activities of Daily Living test (CADL-2; Holland, Frattali, & Fromm, 1999) and Porch Index of Communicative Ability (PICA-R; Porch, 2001), or rating scales, such as the American Speech-Language-Hearing Association Functional Assessment of Communication Skills for Adults (ASHA FACS; Ferketic, Frattali, Holland, et al., 2003).

TREATMENT

Overall Goals of Treatment

Once a patient's specific language impairments have been established, the overarching goal of treatment is to facilitate the general use of language for communication in order to increase the activities and participation of the patient. Treatment works toward reducing language impairment by increasing the efficacy of the residual language capacity and/or introduces compensatory strategies such as writing, drawing, or gesturing to aid the patient in conveying his/her message. Additionally, it may be helpful, especially for persons with progressive language disorders, to adapt the environment to facilitate better communication. For persons with non-progressive language disorders, the main goal of treatment should be to help him/her regain language function. Although compensatory strategies are important for the facilitation of communication, overreliance on them encourages learned nonuse of the impaired function (Taub et al., 1994).

General Considerations

The patient's physical and mental health status must be considered before beginning a therapy program. It is important to make sure that the patient is medically stable prior to beginning therapy in order to keep from doing harm to the patient by introducing too much stimulation (Holland & Fridriksson, 2001; Marshall, 1997). However, it is also important to take advantage of the spontaneous recovery that occurs within first few weeks after a brain injury to help maximize treatment effects (Hillis, 2005).

In addition to considering aspects of the patient, aspects of the therapy programs that are available for use must also be considered. Do any of the available programs target your patient's specific impairments? How effective is the therapy? Can it be modified to be more specific or more effective? Some programs will be perfect for your patient as is; others may need to be adapted for your patient's specific needs or to increase the effectiveness of the chosen therapy program. Some programs are readily adaptable; others are not meant to be used in conjunction with other techniques. Two ways of adapting therapy for increased effectiveness are constraint-induced language therapy (CILT; alternatively referred to as CIAT (constraint-induced aphasia therapy) or intensive language-action therapy (Pulvermuller, Neininger, Elbert, et al., 2001) and the complexity account of treatment efficacy (CATE; Thompson, Shapiro, Kiran, & Sobecks, 2003). These techniques are discussed in detail in Box 14-1. In addition, the duration of treatment and frequency of treatment (number of sessions per week) need to be considered prior to beginning a therapy program. Generally, increasing the intensity of treatment (Bhogal, Teasell, & Speechley, 2003) and/or the complexity of the material being trained (Thompson, 2007) results in increased effectiveness of therapy.

Treatment Research

In the past 10 years, research of treatments for language disorders has flourished. Efficacy of existing treatments has been examined as well as exploratory research into new methodologies. This section will review the research literature from the past 10 years and suggest promising treatment methodologies. Treatment studies were retrieved from the Academy of Neurologic Communication Disorders and Sciences (ANCDS) Aphasia Treatment Website (www.aphasiatx.arizona.edu) as well as from the PubMed and PsychINFO databases. The studies reviewed below were evaluated by Beeson and colleagues based on guidelines described in their website (noted above). For a reader to judge the effectiveness of a treatment outcome in a research study, however, there are no clear metrics that are standardized across different studies. One approach is to evaluate the effect size of either the direct effect or the generalization effect. The direct effect is the effect on the actual trained material. This is similar to a final exam in most courses in which the material being tested is exactly the material that was covered in the course. The effect size is calculated by subtracting the average performance on the material before training from the average performance on the material after training and dividing by the standard deviation of the performance before training. The larger the effect size the more robust the treatment effect (for benchmarks specific to a treatment domain, see Beeson & Robey, 2008). The generalization effect is the effect that the training had on related, but untrained material. This is akin to taking the GRE (Graduate Record Examination) in which the material being tested is related to what you learned in your undergraduate coursework but may not be exactly the material that

Box 14-1

Give Your Standard Therapy a New Twist

Standard aphasia therapy is standard because it has repeatedly been successful in improving language deficits in aphasia. However, just because something works doesn't mean that it can't be improved. Aphasia researchers are constantly looking for new ways to improve language therapy, making it more efficient and more effective.

One way to do that is to apply a technique from another field, such as physical therapy, to language therapy. Taub and colleagues (1993) developed a program to improve movement in chronic stroke patients in which the unaffected limb is placed in a constraining device such as an oven mitt, a sling, or a brace and the patient is forbidden to use that limb to carry out daily functions for a specified amount of time each day. This is called constraint-induced movement therapy (CIMT); it is intense and the improvements are monumental. The success of CIMT led aphasia researchers to apply the technique to language therapy.

Pulvermuller and colleagues (2001) were the first to successfully apply constraint-induced therapy to the domain of language for use in chronic aphasia, resulting in a program called CILT (constraint-induced language therapy), CIAT (constraint-induced aphasia therapy), and most recently, intensive language-action therapy. Often, patients can communicate very well using gestures and writing even though their verbal output is quite limited. In this study, the researchers discouraged the use of gestures and writing when they were not accompanied by verbal output and gradually constrained verbal output to a specific model of phrase production. The protocol used in the Pulvermuller study was a therapeutic game similar to "Go Fish," and was administered intensively at 3 hours a day for 10 days. Subsequent studies used similar methods and found similarly positive results (see Cherney, Patterson, Raymer, et al., 2008, for a review). Although there are several variations of this therapy approach that have been examined, the important principles that guide this therapy are massed practice, focusing on verbal communication and functional communication topics.

Another way to boost treatment effects is by starting with more complex material rather than working up slowly from simple to complex material. This may seem counterintuitive, but it's important to remember that persons with aphasia are not starting from scratch; the majority have simply lost some ability to express or comprehend what they already know.

Thompson and colleagues (2003) systematically tested the use of complex versus simple material in treatment for persons with aphasia while training sentence comprehension and production with TUF (treatment of underlying forms). They found that training more complex syntactic structures resulted not only in improvement of those structures, but also in generalization to less complex syntactic structures of the same type. On the other hand, training less complex structures did not result in generalization to more complex structures, only improvement in the trained structure. This effect is called the Complexity Account of Treatment Efficacy (CATE).

In the years since, Kiran and colleagues (Edmonds & Kiran, 2006; Kiran, 2007; Kiran, 2008; Kiran & Abbott, 2007; Kiran & Johnson, 2008; Kiran & Roberts, 2010; Kiran, Sandberg, & Abbott, 2009; Kiran & Thompson, 2003b) have performed a series of experiments testing the complexity hypothesis in the semantic domain in both monolingual and bilingual patient populations. Semantic complexity can come in several forms: Atypical members of a category are more complex than typical members of a category, abstract words are more complex than concrete words, and, in the case of bilingual aphasia, words in the weaker language are more complex than those in the stronger language. These studies have shown that training complex items results not only in improvement of the trained items, but also generalization to untrained less complex items; however, training less complex items results in improvement of the trained items, but not generalization to untrained complex items.

---

was covered in each of your courses. In patients with language disorders, generalization can be to standardized language tests or to a related, but different set of materials. The generalization effect size is calculated in the same manner as the direct effect size. It is helpful to keep this information in mind when reading treatment research articles.

Treatment for Phonological Impairments

Comprehension

Treatments for pure word deafness and auditory phonological agnosia have not been well researched. Tessier and colleagues (2007) utilized an errorless learning paradigm to successfully train phoneme discrimination and recognition in a patient with word deafness. Stefanatos and colleagues (2005; 2008) recently proposed a temporal processing deficit in word deafness and suggested altering the rate of speech in treatment to facilitate the perceptual discrimination of speech.

Production

Phonological cueing hierarchies are a common method of training word retrieval and usually start with the first phoneme, then the first syllable, then repetition of the whole word, although they can be expanded to include nonword rhymes (Wambaugh, Linebaugh, Doyle, et al., 2001). This cueing technique for increasing word retrieval has been shown to be effective in isolation (Herbert, Best, Hickin, et al., 2001; Hickin, Best, Herbert, et al., 2002; Wambaugh, 2003; Wambaugh, Cameron, Kalinyak-Fliszar, et al., 2004; Wambaugh, Doyle, Martinez, & Kalinyak-Fliszar, 2002; Wambaugh et al., 2001) or when combined with orthographic, tactile, and/or semantic cueing hierarchies (Abel, Schultz, Radermacher, et al., 2005; Abel, Willmes, & Huber, 2007; Cameron, Wambaugh, Wright, & Nessler, 2006; Conroy, Sage, & Lambon Ralph, 2009; DeDe, Parris, & Waters, 2003; Fink, Brecher, Schwartz, & Robey, 2002).

Another technique that can target phonological naming deficits is errorless learning (see Fillingham, Hodgson, Sage, & Ralph, 2003, for a review), which can simply be repetition of the target (Fillingham, Sage, & Lambon Ralph, 2005a, 2005b, 2006) or a reversed cueing hierarchy (Abel et al., 2005; Abel et al., 2007). Spaced retrieval is a form of errorless learning in which the repetition of a target is conducted over increasingly longer intervals and has recently been applied in patients with aphasia (Fridriksson, Holland, Beeson, & Morrow, 2005).

Training specific phonological processes using tasks such as rhyming judgment, identifying the first/last phoneme, minimal pair discrimination, and segmenting/blending have also shown positive results for increasing naming (Corsten, Mende, Cholewa, & Huber, 2007; Franklin, Buerk, & Howard, 2002; Fridriksson et al., 2005; Kendall, Rosenbek, Heilman, et al., 2008; Laganaro, Pietro, & Schnider, 2003; Raymer & Ellsworth, 2002). Additionally, these types of treatments have been combined with gesture or semantic training (Rodriguez, Raymer, & Rothi, 2006; Rose, Douglas, & Matyas, 2002; Spencer et al., 2000).

Phonological aspects of naming have also been trained through context, where pictures with phonologically similar names are presented simultaneously for confrontation naming (Fisher, Wilshire, & Ponsford, 2009). Similarly, contextual repetition priming is a treatment approach in which phonologically or semantically similar pictures are simultaneously and repeatedly presented for naming. Patients with phonological deficits generally appear to benefit more from this treatment than patients with semantic impairments (Martin, Fink, & Laine, 2004; Renvall, Laine, Laakso, & Martin, 2003). Some studies have shown better recovery of naming in persons with phonologically-based anomia after semantically focused training (Raymer, Kohen, & Saffell, 2006; Wambaugh et al., 2001).

To summarize, when evaluating and developing treatment options for phonological impairments, it is advantageous to identify the locus of impairment prior to selecting a treatment strategy that is most applicable for the corresponding impairment (see Table 14-1 for examples of behavioral markers of phonological impairments and corresponding treatment strategies).

Treatment for Orthographic Impairments

Treatment for Acquired Dyslexias

Two general reading treatment approaches, Multiple Oral Reading (MOR) and Oral Reading for Language in Aphasia (ORLA) (see Cherney, 2004, for a review), have been developed for improving reading skills in patients with language disorders. In MOR, the patient repeatedly reads sentences or paragraphs aloud. This treatment has had positive results for the remediation of letter-by-letter reading (Beeson, Magloire, & Robey, 2005) but may not be sufficient for mild reading deficits (Mayer & Murray, 2002). In ORLA, the clinician reads to the patient, then with the patient, and then patient reads on his/her own, all the while pointing to each read word. This treatment has also been shown to be a successful reading treatment (Orjada & Beeson, 2005). Other reading treatments are more specific to the level of deficit.

For phonological dyslexia, patients have been trained to blend CV and VC bigraphs to form CVC words, mirrored by a similar writing treatment (Bowes & Martin, 2007); to identify, discriminate, and blend phonemes, graphemes, and syllables (Kendall, Conway, Rosenbek, & Gonzalez-Rothi, 2003); to read function or less-imageable words by pairing them with high-imageable word homophones or near-homophones (Friedman, Sample, & Lott, 2002; Lott, Sample, Oliver, et al., 2008); and to build up to reading sentences one word at a time, repeating all previous words each time (Lott, Sperling, Watson, & Friedman, 2009). Also, irregular words have been targeted by training phoneme contrasts for letters (e.g., *c* pronounced either /k/ or /s/) (Peach, 2002).

Table 14-1 Behavioral Markers for Phonological Impairment and Corresponding Treatment Strategies

Behavioral Marker

Impaired phoneme discrimination
Pure word deafness—inability to identify spoken speech
Impaired segmenting/blending
Phonological paraphasias during naming, repeating, and reading
Impaired phonological processing abilities

Examples of Strategies for Use in Treatment of Phonological Impairments	Evidence
Rhyme judgment	Spencer et al. (2000), Franklin et al. (2002), Raymer et al. (2002), Doesborgh et al. (2004a)
Segmenting phonemes/syllables	Doesborgh et al. (2004a), Kendall et al. (2008)
Blending phonemes/syllables	Doesborgh et al. (2004a), Kendall et al. (2008)
Minimal pair discrimination	Corsten et al. (2007), Tessier et al. (2007)
Perceptual discrimination task	Stefanatos et al. (2005, 2008)
Monitor and correct phonetic speech errors	Franklin et al. (2002)
Phonological cueing hierarchy	Herbert et al. (2001), Wambaugh et al. (2001, 2003, 2004, 2007), Hickin et al. (2002), DeDe et al. (2003)
Phonological and orthographic cues	Fillingham et al. (2005a, 2005b, 2006)
Identify syllable structure/stress pattern	Rose et al. (2002)
Start with repetition and fade repetition cues (errorless learning and spaced retrieval)	Abel et al. (2005, 2007); Fridriksson (2005); Fillingham et al. (2005a, 2005b, 2006)
Phoneme identification	Franklin et al. (2002), Raymer et al. (2002), Corsten et al. (2007), Tessier et al. (2007), Kendall et al. (2008)
Provide pictures to name that are semantically or phonologically similar (contextual priming)	Martin et al. (2004); Renvall et al. (2003); Fisher et al. (2009)

For deep dyslexia, patients have been trained to recognize CV and VC bigraphs, then blend them to form CVC words (Friedman & Lott, 2002; Kim & Beaudoin-Parsons, 2007); identify phonemes, letters, and retrain their correspondences (Kiran, Thompson, & Hashimoto, 2001) (see Appendix 14-1 for detailed protocol); associate an image with each word (Ska, Garneau-Beaumont, Chesneau, & Damien, 2003); and associate letters with sounds and use tactile cues for blending (Yampolsky & Waters, 2002). Stadie and Rilling (2006) found similar improvements in reading for a lexical treatment, which used a semantic prime for content words and a phonological prime for function words, and a non-lexical treatment, which trained grapheme-to-word associations, grapheme-to-phoneme associations, and blending. Kiran and Viswanathan (2008) treated a case of severe alexia by training both grapheme-to-phoneme correspondences and semantic features of the target items with positive results in both reading and written naming.

For pure alexia (letter-by-letter reading), an errorless learning technique has been used with tactile input to reinforce learning of letters (Sage, Hesketh, & Ralph, 2005).

Treatment for Acquired Dysgraphias

Anagram and Copy Treatment (ACT), which consists of rearranging letters to form the target word, then copying the word, and Copy and Recall Treatment (CART; see Appendix 14-1 for complete description) are successful therapies for writing deficits (see Beeson, 2004, for a review). CART has been shown to be successful in isolation (Beeson, Rising, & Volk, 2003; Orjada & Beeson, 2005) as well as when combined with ACT (Beeson, Hirsch, & Rewega, 2002). Murray and Karcher (2000) trained verb retrieval with an ACT-type treatment and then simple sentence construction using the trained verbs. CART has also been used to increase naming either alone (Wright, Marshall, Wilson, & Page, 2008) or combined with repetition (Beeson & Egnor, 2006). Using a method similar to CART, Kumar and Humphreys (2008) found greater improvement for high imageability words in persons with deep dysgraphia. A modified version of CART using mnemonic devices, such as a picture of glasses taking the place of the "oo" in the word *look,* increased irregular spelling more than the unmodified version (Schmalzl & Nickels, 2006).

Another interesting writing therapy utilizes spared sound/letter correspondences in persons with acquired dysgraphias by having patients rely on sound/letter correspondences to guess at the spelling of a word, then check their guess against a spell-checker (Beeson, Rewega, Vail, & Rapcsak, 2000; Beeson, Rising, Kim, & Rapcsak, 2008) (for a review see Beeson, 2004). Similarly, Rapp and Kane (2002) and Rapp (2005) implemented a "spell, study, spell" treatment wherein the patient attempts to spell a dictated word, sees and hears it spelled correctly, then attempts to spell again. This treatment appeared to be more successful for patients with deficits in the graphemic buffer. In an errorless learning paradigm, Sage and Ellis (2006) found that training orthographic neighbors of a target (i.e., words that overlap in spelling) increased target spelling as much as training the target in a person with a graphemic buffer disorder.

Additionally, phoneme-to-grapheme conversion and grapheme-to-phoneme conversion can be specifically and simultaneously targeted to improve both writing and reading (Kiran, 2005; Luzzatti, Colombo, Frustaci, & Vitolo, 2000). To summarize, there are several treatment strategies supported by empirical evidence that can be applied for patients with orthographic input and/or output impairments (Table 14-2). Again, identifying the locus of impairment facilitates the selection of the appropriate treatment strategy on a case-by-case basis.

Treatment for Semantic Impairments/ Lexical Retrieval Deficits

Anomia is a deficit in retrieving words from the semantic system and is the most pervasive language impairment in language disorders. Therefore, several methods have been proposed for treating deficits in word retrieval, including repetition, cueing, and semantic training techniques.

Repetition has been shown to improve lexical retrieval even without feedback regarding accuracy (Nickels, 2002). Raymer and Ellsworth (2002) showed no significant difference among rehearsal, phonologic, and semantic treatments for verb retrieval. As mentioned previously, errorless learning is a repetition method of treatment wherein the patient is given the target to repeat, and then cues are slowly faded until she/he can spontaneously produce the target. Spaced retrieval is a type of errorless learning wherein the time between correct repetitions is slowly increased. Fillingham and colleagues (2005a, 2005b) found that simple repetition errorless learning with no fading cues and no feedback regarding accuracy is similar in effectiveness to errorful learning wherein the patient is given the first phoneme and grapheme as cues for naming with no feedback.

Semantic cueing hierarchies start with the least semantic information and increase the amount of semantic information or context until the patient correctly names the target. Wambaugh and colleagues (2001; 2002; 2004; Wambaugh, 2003) have shown semantic cueing hierarchies to be successful in patients with semantically based word finding deficits. Additionally, performance seems to improve when the orthographic form is added to the treatment (Wambaugh & Wright, 2007). Studies that have combined phonological and semantic information into cueing hierarchies have also resulted in improved word finding (Abel et al., 2005, 2007; Cameron et al., 2006; Conroy et al., 2009; Fink et al., 2002). Interestingly, increasing cues (errorful learning) and vanishing cues (errorless learning) have been shown to be equally effective methods of cue presentation (Abel et al., 2005, 2007; Conroy et al., 2009). Personalized cueing, wherein patients choose salient features or mnemonics as cues, can also be considered semantic cueing and has been shown to be successful in treating naming deficits (Freed, Celery, & Marshall, 2004; Marshall, Freed, & Karow, 2001; Marshall, Karow, Freed, & Babcock, 2002). Doesborgh, van de Sandt-Koenderman, Dippel, and colleagues (2004b) successfully implemented a computer program called Multicue that allowed patients to choose their own cues from four possible choices.

Contextual repetition priming is a treatment approach in which semantically or phonologically similar pictures are simultaneously and repeatedly presented for naming (Laine & Martin, 1996). Although some patients have shown interference during the semantic context condition, this treatment has shown short-term positive effects for patients with semantic deficits (Cornelissen, Laine, Tarkiainen, et al., 2003; Martin et al., 2004; Martin, Fink, Renvall, & Laine, 2006; Martin & Laine, 2000; Renvall, Laine, & Martin, 2005, 2007) and more sustained effects with additional semantic and phonologic tasks (Renvall et al., 2007).

Semantic training specifically targets semantic representations and their connections to each other. Semantic Feature Analysis (SFA) is a type of semantic training in which the patient is asked to provide different features for each word being trained (see Appendix 14-1 for detailed protocol) (Haarbaurer-Krupa, Moser, Smith, et al., 1985). This treatment is based on spreading activation models of the semantic system and has been shown to be successful in both individual treatment (Coelho, McHugh, & Boyle, 2000; Gordon, 2007) and group treatment (Antonucci, 2009). It has also been combined with Response Elaboration Training (RET) (Kearns, 1985) with positive outcomes (Conley & Coelho, 2003). A modified version of SFA has been used

Table **14-2**   Behavioral Markers for Orthographic Impairment and Corresponding Treatment Strategies

Behavioral Marker

No response in reading and/or writing
Semantic paraphasias in reading and/or writing
Phonemic paraphasias in reading and/or writing
Mixed paraphasias in reading and/or writing
Neologisms in reading and/or writing
Spelling errors and/or letter substitutions
Can read and/or write familiar words, but not unfamiliar words or pseudowords
Can read and/or write regular words and pseudowords, but not irregular words
Cannot write long words (i.e., orthographic buffer impairment)
Written naming more impaired than verbal naming

Examples of Strategies for Use in Treatment of Reading Impairments	**Evidence**
Retrain grapheme-to-phoneme correspondences	Kiran et al. (2001); Yamposkly & Waters (2002); Kendall (2003); Kiran & Viswanathan (2008)
Train phoneme contrasts for letters that map on to more than one sound	Peach (2002)
CV and VC bigraph training, then blending	Friedman & Lott (2002); Kendall (2003); Kim & Beaudoin-Parsons (2007); Bowes & Martin (2007)
Use tactile cues for blending (tap finger—single sound; drag finger—blend sounds)	Yampolsky & Waters (2002)
Repeat letter/word after clinician while reading and receiving tactile input (letter tracing) on the palm of the hand	Sage et al. (2005)
Pair function words or less imageable words with semantically salient homophones	Friedman et al. (2002); Lott et al. (2008)
Prime content words with semantically related words and function words with phonologically related words	Stadie & Rilling (2006)
Associate an image with each word	Ska et al. (2003)
Build up sentences one word at a time, repeating all previous words during each reading	Lott et al. (2009)
MOR (Multiple Oral Reading): passages are read aloud repeatedly	Mayer & Murray (2002); Cherney (2004); Beeson et al. (2005)
ORLA (Oral Reading for Language in Aphasia): clinician reads to the patient, then choral reading, then the patient reads alone	Cherney (2004); Orjada & Beeson (2005)

Examples of Strategies for Use in Treatment of Writing Impairments	**Evidence**
Retrain both phoneme-to-grapheme and grapheme-to-phoneme conversion skills	Luzzatti et al. (2000); Kiran (2005)
CART (Copy and Recall Treatment): patient copies the target word repeatedly, then tries to write word without a model	Beeson et al. (2002); Beeson et al. (2003); Orjada & Beeson (2005); Kumar & Humphreys (2008)
Modified CART using picture mnemonics on word cards	Schmalzl & Nickels (2006)
ACT (Anagram and Copy Treatment): patient rearranges letters to form the target word, then copies the word	Murray & Karcher (2000); Beeson et al. (2002);
Use preserved letter-to-sound correspondences to attempt word spelling, then use spell-checker	Beeson et al. (2000, 2008)
Patient attempts to spell the word, then studies the correct spelling visually and auditorily, then makes another attempt	Rapp & Kane (2002); Rapp (2005)
Train orthographic neighbors (words that overlap in spelling)	Sage & Ellis (2006)

to train more complex exemplars in a category in order to increase generalization to untrained items (Kiran, 2007, 2008; Kiran & Abbott, 2007; Kiran & Johnson, 2008; Kiran, Sandberg, & Abbott, 2009; Kiran & Thompson, 2003b). Wambaugh and Ferguson (2007) also modified SFA for verb retrieval with positive results.

Other treatments focusing on the semantic system have included tasks such as asking yes/no questions about features of the target (Raymer & Ellsworth, 2002); performing tasks that require semantic knowledge of the target (Davis & Harrington, 2006); semantic decision tasks, such as part-whole relationships, definitions, and categories (Doesborgh, van de Sandt-Koenderman, Dippel, et al., 2004a); using circumlocution to arrive at the target word (Francis, Clark, & Humphreys, 2002); and spoken/written word to picture matching (Raymer et al., 2006). Rose and Douglas (2008) compared a semantic treatment that involved describing the use and shape of the target object with an iconic gesture treatment and a combined semantic/gesture treatment and found that although all three treatments improved naming, there were larger effect sizes for the semantic and combined semantic/gesture treatments. Table 14-3 provides examples of various behavioral markers that can be observed with patients who have semantic impairments and corresponding treatment strategies that have garnered empirical support.

Treatment of Syntactic Impairments

Comprehension

Treatment of Underlying Forms (TUF) is a syntactic treatment that trains thematic roles (i.e., agent and theme) as well as the movement that occurs to form noncanonical sentences and uses complex sentences for maximal generalization (see Thompson & Shapiro, 2005, for a review; see also Shapiro & Thompson, 2006; see Appendix 14-1 for detailed protocol). TUF has been shown to be successful in treating syntactic comprehension deficits (Jacobs & Thompson, 2000). In another vein, Hoen, Golembiowski, Guyot, and colleagues (2003) showed that training non-linguistic cognitive sequences (e.g., training the sequence 123–231 so that when given the first three letters GBT, the patient knows the next three letters are BTG) improves comprehension of relative sentences (e.g., *It was the man who the woman hugged*).

Production

One syntactic treatment to improve the grammaticality of patient utterances is mapping therapy (Byng, 1988), during which patients are systematically trained to associate grammatical elements with their thematic roles (i.e., agent and theme) and asked to produce sentences based on the trained thematic roles (Rochon, Laird,

Bose, & Scofield, 2005). This type of treatment has been delivered in an errorless learning paradigm with similar results to the traditional approach (Wierenga, Maher, Moore, et al., 2006). TUF has also been successfully used to improve syntactic production (Dickey & Thompson, 2007; Jacobs & Thompson, 2000; Murray, Ballard, & Karcher, 2004; Thompson et al., 2003).

Another focus of grammatical production is the retrieval and proper inflection of verbs and retrieval of the correct argument structure for each verb. Webster, Morris, and Franklin (2005) successfully trained verb retrieval with semantic tasks, verb/argument association with plausibility tasks, and sentence generation with an argument generation task. Bastiaanse, Hurkmans, and Links (2006) treated verb production at the word and sentence level by using sentence completion for both infinitive and inflected verb retrieval, and then trained sentence construction with anagrams. Schneider and Thompson (2003) compared a semantic treatment for verb naming with a treatment focusing on the argument structure of the verb and found that both treatments improved verb naming. In another study, a semantic-based treatment to improve lexical retrieval of content words in a sentence context by promoting systematic retrieval of verbs and their thematic roles resulted in generalization to sentence production for sentences containing trained verbs and to untrained semantically related verbs (Edmonds, Nadeau, & Kiran, 2009). Faroqi-Shah (2008) compared a morphophonological treatment that included auditory discrimination of differently inflected verbs, morphology generation, and oral/written transformation from one inflection to another to a morphosemantic treatment that included anomaly judgment, sentence completion with the correct inflection, and sentence construction. Both improved verb morphology, but morphosemantic treatment generalized to narratives.

Finally, AAC devices have been used to train the construction of certain sentences. Patients have been taught to assign a special symbol to the agent of a sentence and move pictures around to form the correct construction (Weinrich, Boser, McCall, & Bishop, 2001). Table 14-4 provides examples of aspects of sentence comprehension and production that can be impaired in individuals with language disorders and examples of treatment strategies that can be employed with such individuals.

Treatment of Discourse Impairments

In addition to treating specific language impairments, the clinician should work on overall discourse impairments and/or pragmatic impairments in higher functioning patients. This type of treatment utilizes more realistic situations and sentences and can include conversing with familiar partners and incorporate activities of daily living.

Table **14-3** Behavioral Markers for Semantic Impairment and Corresponding Treatment Strategies

Behavioral Marker

Semantic paraphasias during naming
Circumlocutions
Word generation as impaired as confrontation naming
Naming impairment across all modalities
Unable to match spoken and/or written words with pictures and/or objects
Unable to match semantically related words and/or pictures
Category specific impairments (e.g., only impaired in naming animals)

Examples of Strategies for Use in Treatment of Semantic Impairments	**Evidence**
Phonological cueing hierarchy	Wambaugh et al. (2001, 2002, 2003, 2004)
Semantic cueing hierarchy	Wambaugh et al. (2001, 2002, 2003, 2004)
Combined semantic and phonological cueing hierarchy	Fink et al. (2002); Abel et al. (2005, 2007); Cameron et al. (2006); Conroy et al. (2009)
Personalized cues	Marshall et al. (2001, 2002); Freed et al. (2004)
Train iconic gestural cues	Rose et al. (2002); Rose & Douglas (2008)
Multicue: a computer program that allows the user to choose his/her cues	Doesborgh et al. (2004b)
Provide tactile cues for first grapheme/phoneme	DeDe et al. (2003)
Have the patient categorize items	Kiran & Thompson (2003); Kiran (2007, 2008); Kiran & Abbott (2007); Kiran et al. (2009)
Ask the patient yes/no questions about semantic features	Raymer & Ellsworth (2002); Kiran & Thompson (2003); Kiran (2007, 2008); Kiran & Abbott (2007); Kiran et al. (2009);
Have the patient name to definition	Kiran & Abbott (2007); Kiran et al. (2009)
Create a semantic map for each item, listing a variety of semantic features for each item	Coelho et al. (2000); Conley & Coelho (2003); Kiran & Thompson (2003); Boyle (1995, 2004); Gordon (2007); Wambaugh & Ferguson (2007); Kiran (2007, 2008); Kiran & Abbott (2007); Kiran et al. (2009); Antonucci (2009)
RET (Response Elaboration Training): repeat and expand patient's responses in treatment	Conley & Coelho (2003)
Repeatedly present items with no feedback regarding accuracy	Nickels (2002); Fillingham et al. (2005a, 2005b, 2006)
Use increasing cues for deficits in semantic memory and vanishing cues for deficits in semantic access	Abel et al. (2005, 2007)
Encourage circumlocution until the target is reached	Francis et al. (2002)
Spoken/written word to picture matching	Raymer et al. (2006)
Provide pictures to name that are semantically or phonologically similar (contextual priming)	Cornelissen et al. (2003); Martin et al. (2000, 2004, 2006); Renvall et al. (2005, 2007)
Have the patient perform tasks that require semantic knowledge	Davis & Harrington (2006)

Some discourse treatments have focused on training both the patient and the conversational partner of the patient to use strategies to prevent or repair communication breakdowns during conversation (Cunningham & Ward, 2003; Fox, Armstrong, & Boles, 2009; Hopper, Holland, & Rewega, 2002) (see Appendix 14-1 for detailed protocol from Hopper et al., 2002). Promoting Aphasics Communicative Effectiveness (PACE) (see Davis, 2005, for a review) is a conversational training program for the patient that promotes the exchange of new information, equal participation of clinician and patient, the ability to use any communicative modality, and functional feedback from the clinician. Manheim, Halper, and Cherney (2009) trained a patient to use a computer program with recorded narrative scripts as models for improving conversation. A device called Sentence Shaper has been developed that relieves the patient of the processing load of creating sentences by

Table **14-4**   Behavioral Markers for Syntactic Impairment and Corresponding Treatment Strategies

Behavioral Marker

Lack of function words, limited morpheme use
Abnormal word order
Overuse of simple sentence structures (i.e., active sentences only)
Overuse of simple verbs (i.e., no verbs that require more than two arguments)
Decreased sentence comprehension with increased sentence complexity
Canonical word order interpretation of non-canonical sentences
Overreliance on world knowledge for sentence interpretation

Strategies for Use in Treatment of Syntactic Impairments	**Evidence**
Thematic role assignment (match agents/themes with noun phrases in the sentence) for sentence comprehension	Jacobs & Thompson (2000)
Map thematic roles to noun phrases in the sentence during sentence comprehension	Jacobs & Thompson (2000); Thompson et al. (2003); Murray et al. (2004); Rochon et al. (2005), Wierenga et al. (2006); Dickey & Thompson (2007)
Train movement of noun phrases to construct non-canonical sentences	Jacobs & Thompson (2000); Thompson et al. (2003); Murray et al. (2004); Dickey & Thompson (2007)
Work on morphological elements of verbs for sentence production	Faroqi-Shah (2008)
Verb/argument structure tasks	Schneider & Thompson (2003); Webster (2005)
Sentence completion tasks	Bastiaanse et al. (2006)
Train non-linguistics sequences to facilitate access to grammar	Hoen et al. (2003)
Use AAC to construct active and passive sentences	Weinrich et al. (2001)

providing a workspace for constructing sentences before producing them and after training and use has been shown to improve narratives both with and without the device (Linebarger, McCall, & Berndt, 2004; see Linebarger & Schwartz, 2005 for a review; McCall, Virata, Linebarger, & Berndt, 2009).

Other researchers have attempted to improve discourse by using it as a context for treatment. Peach and Wong (2004) focused a syntactic treatment at the discourse level by using story retelling as a way to elicit sentences and provide feedback as to the grammaticality of the sentences. The patient's syntactic errors decreased and information units increased. Murray, Timberlake, and Eberle (2007) introduced a discourse training module into a TUF treatment protocol by having the patient use one of the trained sentences in a five-sentence written narrative during each session. Robson (2001) incorporated a written treatment with a PACE-like treatment where the patient was able to practice using writing to convey information when the verbal form was not available. Herbert and colleagues (2003) trained patients who had finished a treatment for word retrieval on tasks that increasingly resembled conversation. Rider and colleagues (2008) found that simply training word retrieval using SFA increased the use of those trained items during subsequent narrative performance that required those items. Table 14-5 provides

examples of various behavioral markers in discourse comprehension and production and examples of treatment strategies that can be applied to improve discourse abilities in patients with language disorders.

Biological Treatment Approaches

Recently, some researchers have been exploring different avenues for treatment, such as pharmacology and electrical stimulation techniques (e.g., rTMS, tDCS), that directly influence the neural processes associated with language use (see Small & Llano, 2009, for a review). For example, memantine, a drug which is normally used to treat Alzheimer's disease, was combined with CIAT to produce more favorable outcomes than either treatment alone (Berthier et al., 2009). Similarly, repetitive transcranial magnetic stimulation (rTMS) and transcranial direct current stimulation (tDCS) have been used in conjunction with behavioral therapy with positive outcomes (Baker, Rorden, & Fridriksson, 2010; Naeser, Martin, Treglia, et al., 2010). For a more thorough explanation of these techniques, see Box 14-2.

Summary of Treatment Studies

Research focused on developing effective therapies for patients with language disorders has generated a remarkable body of research providing clinicians with a wide range of treatment options to choose from.

Table **14-5** Behavioral Markers for Pragmatic/Discourse Impairment and Corresponding Treatment Strategies

Behavioral Marker

Word finding difficulties during conversation
Problems with initiation, topic maintenance, and turn-taking
Decreased cohesion, grammatical complexity, information content
Inability to process pragmatic cues
Inability to draw inferences from stories

Strategies for Use in Treatment	**Evidence**
Train the conversational partner	Hopper et al. (2002); Cunningham & Ward (2003); Fox et al. (2009)
PACE (Promoting Aphasics Communicative Effectiveness): focus on exchanging new information, equal participation of patient and clinician, use any modality to communicate, receive functional feedback	Robson (2001); Davis (2005)
Train sentence production and word retrieval to improve discourse	Herbert et al. (2003); Peach & Wong (2004); Murray et al. (2007); Rider et al. (2008)
Sentence Shaper: computer program that acts as a workspace for constructing sentences prior to production to alleviate processing demands of conversation	Linebarger et al. (2004); McCall et al. (2009)

Almost all of these studies, however, are pre-efficacy studies, evaluating the success of a specific treatment with a small number of participants. In order to prescribe a certain form of therapy relative to a current gold standard, efficacy treatment studies need to be conducted, of which there are very few. Until then, clinicians need to sift through the available empirical research to decide which therapy approach has sufficient evidence to merit its application to specific types of patients. In the process of choosing a specific therapy approach for a patient one must consider several factors, including the theoretical basis for the work, the robustness of the experimental design, the number of participants, the reliability and validity of outcome measures, statistical power, and issues with confounding variables. For a more detailed approach to evaluating the evidence from empirical studies examining the effectiveness of specific therapies, the Academy of Neurologic Communication Disorders and Sciences (ANCDS) Aphasia Treatment website (http://aphasiatx.arizona.edu) provides descriptions about the criteria used to classify the research evidence based on research quality.

Treatment for Language Impairments in Degenerative Diseases

Most of the focus of this chapter has been on reviewing the evidence available for treating individuals with nonprogressive language impairments (i.e., language impairments subsequent to cerebrovascular disease or trauma). In individuals with progressive language impairments such as primary progressive aphasia and dementia, research has focused on the combined pharmacological and behavioral management of these syndromes. Additionally, behavioral therapies reflect an integration of language, cognitive stimulation, and caregiver education. With regard to therapies for individuals with dementia, there have been several published systematic reviews of studies aiming to improve cognitive, functional, and caregiver education (Bayles, Kim, Chapman, et al., 2006; Hopper, Mahendra, Kim, et al., 2005; E. S. Kim, Cleary, Hopper, et al., 2006; Mahendra, Kim, Bayles, et al., 2005; Zientz, Rackley, Chapman, et al., 2007a; Zientz, Rackley, Chapman, et al., 2007b).

RECOVERY PATTERNS OBSERVED WITH FUNCTIONAL IMAGING TECHNIQUES

The recovery of language function in persons with language disorders is normally assessed with behavioral measures. This is the simplest and most cost-effective way to see if your therapy program is actually working for your patient. It has also been the most practical way to ascertain the effectiveness of new treatment protocols in the research literature until recently. The improved functionality and increased availability of functional imaging techniques, such as functional magnetic resonance imaging (fMRI) and magnetoencephalography (MEG), have made it possible to observe neurophysiological changes associated with language recovery. The results from tools such as these, coupled with behavioral data, greatly enhance our understanding of the neural mechanisms

Box 14-2

Electrify Your Therapy

Two new techniques are rapidly gaining popularity in aphasia treatment research: transcranial magnetic stimulation (TMS) and transcranial direct current stimulation (tDCS).

TMS uses strong magnetic fields placed over the scalp to create an electrical field which induces an electrical current in the neural tissue, changing the way neurons communicate with each other. Normally, rTMS (repetitive transcranial magnetic stimulation) is used for aphasia therapy. In conventional rTMS, the pulse (i.e., change in magnetic field from 0 to 3 tesla) is repeated at a certain frequency. If the rate is at or below 1 Hz (1 pulse per second), then the effect will be inhibitory, if the rate is above 1 Hz, then the effect will be excitatory.

Naeser and colleagues (2005) used slow wave rTMS to induce inhibitory effects in the right hemisphere homologue of Broca's area in four patients with chronic nonfluent aphasia. They found that just 20 minutes of rTMS per day, five days a week for two weeks improved picture naming significantly in this group.

tDCS uses electrical current delivered through the scalp via electrodes to either increase or decrease neuronal excitability. The polarity of the current flow determines the amount of excitability; anodal stimulation (A-tDCS) increases excitability and cathodal stimulation (C-tDCS) decreases excitability (Wagner et al., 2007).

In a recent study, Baker and colleagues (2010) used A-tDCS to excite left-hemisphere language areas in 10 patients with chronic aphasia during language therapy. An fMRI scan was used to place electrodes at the point of highest cortical activity during correct picture naming for each patient. For five consecutive days, patients were given 1 mA (milli-ampere) of current for 20 minutes while performing a computerized word-to-picture matching task. At post-test, items that were trained during A-tDCS improved significantly more than those that were trained during the sham condition.

---

underlying behavioral changes and the conclusions that can be made regarding the natural recovery process, the effectiveness of treatment, and the way the two interact.

For example, Saur, Lange, Baumgartner, and colleagues (2006) mapped the progress of recovery of language function in 14 patients with aphasia from the acute stage to the chronic stage using repeated fMRI scans and behavioral tests. They found that during the acute stage (1–2 days post-stroke), there was very little activity in the spared tissue of the language areas of the left hemisphere; during the subacute stage (about 12 days post-stroke), there was activation in both the left-hemisphere language areas and their right-hemisphere homologues, with the peak activation in the right hemisphere; and during the chronic stage (about 10 months post-stroke), the peak activation shifted back to the left hemisphere in the spared tissue of the language areas, which was associated with improvements on behavioral measures of language function.

Another example is a recent study in which 26 patients with aphasia were scanned with fMRI before and after 30 hours of treatment for word retrieval. The patients who showed gains in treatment also showed increased activation in spared left-hemisphere language areas post-treatment when compared with pretreatment (Fridriksson, 2010). These results challenge previously held beliefs, suggesting that transfer of language function to the right hemisphere may be maladaptive

rather than supportive for persons with some sparing of language areas in the left hemisphere.

CONCLUSIONS

The field of rehabilitation of language disorders in adults has expanded considerably over the last twenty years. Additionally, our understanding of the mechanisms underlying behavioral changes subsequent to treatment has benefited from recent advances in neuro-imaging techniques such as fMRI and MEG. Clearly, improvements in language processing abilities induced by treatment can be mapped onto the brain. It is also clear now that the nature of treatment provided may influence the recruitment of regions to support recovery. Consequently, clinicians need to be very judicious about selecting appropriate treatments for their patients as the neurobehavioral outcomes of the rehabilitation can be beneficial or detrimental depending upon the treatment employed. Understanding the basis for language processing in normal individuals and the different ways in which language can be impaired goes a long way to ensure appropriate treatment choices for this population. Ultimately, the goal of this field is to have "treatment prescriptions" for specific types of language disorders based on empirical behavioral evidence and supported by neuroscience data indicating functional changes in the brain.

REFERENCES

Abel, S., Schultz, A., Radermacher, I., Willmes, K., & Huber, W. (2005). Decreasing and increasing cues in naming therapy for aphasia. *Aphasiology, 19*(9), 831–848.

Abel, S., Willmes, K., & Huber, W. (2007). Model-oriented naming therapy: Testing predictions of a connectionist model. *Aphasiology, 21*(5), 411–447.

Antonucci, S. M. (2009). Use of semantic feature analysis in group aphasia treatment. *Aphasiology, 23*(7), 854–866.

Baker, J. M., Rorden, C., & Fridriksson, J. (2010). Using transcranial direct-current stimulation to treat stroke patients with aphasia. *Stroke, 41*(6), 1229–1236. doi: STROKEAHA.109.576785 [pii] 10.1161/STROKEAHA.109.576785

Bastiaanse, R., Hurkmans, J., & Links, P. (2006). The training of verb production in Broca's aphasia: A multiple-baseline across-behaviours study. *Aphasiology, 20*(2), 298–311.

Bayles, K. A., Kim, E. S., Chapman, S. B., Zientz, J., Rackley, A., Mahendra, N., . . . Cleary, S. J. (2006). Evidence-based practice recommendations for working with individuals with dementia: Simulated presence therapy. (Academy of Neurologic Communication Disorders and Sciences Bulletin Board)(Clinical report). *Journal of Medical Speech—Language Pathology, 14*(3), xiii(9).

Beeson, P. M. (2004). Remediation of written language. *Topics in Stroke Rehabilitation, 11*(1), 37–48.

Beeson, P. M., & Egnor, H. (2006). Combining treatment for written and spoken naming. *Journal of the International Neuropsychological Society, 12*(6), 816–827. doi: S1355617706061005 [pii] 10.1017/S1355617706061005

Beeson, P. M., Hirsch, F. M., & Rewega, M. A. (2002). Successful single-word writing treatment: Experimental analyses of four cases. *Aphasiology, 16*(4), 473–491.

Beeson, P. M., Magloire, J. G., & Robey, R. R. (2005). Letter-by-letter reading: natural recovery and response to treatment. *Behavioral Neuroscience, 16*(4), 191–202.

Beeson, P. M., Rewega, M. A., Vail, S., & Rapcsak, S. Z. (2000). Problem-solving approach to agraphia treatment: Interactive use of lexical and sublexical spelling routes. *Aphasiology, 14*(5), 551–565.

Beeson, P. M., Rising, K., Kim, E. S., & Rapcsak, S. Z. (2008). A novel method for examining response to spelling treatment. *Aphasiology, 22*(7–8), 707–717. doi: 10.1080/02687030701800826

Beeson, P. M., Rising, K., & Volk, J. (2003). Writing treatment for severe aphasia: Who benefits? *Journal of Speech Language and Hearing Research, 46*(5), 1038–1060.

Beeson, P. M., & Robey, R. R. (2008). *Meta-analysis of aphasia treatment outcomes: Examining the evidence*. Paper presented at the Clinical Aphasiology Conference, Jackson Hole, WY.

Berthier, M. L., Green, C., Lara, J. P., Higueras, C., Barbancho, M. A., Davila, G., & Pulvermuller, F. (2009). Memantine and Constraint-Induced Aphasia Therapy in Chronic Poststroke Aphasia. *Annals of Neurology, 65*(5), 577–585. doi: 10.1002/ana.21597

Bhogal, S. K., Teasell, R., & Speechley, M. (2003). Intensity of aphasia therapy, impact on recovery. *Stroke, 34*(4), 987–992. doi: 10.1161/01.str.0000062343.64383.d0

Bowes, K., & Martin, N. (2007). Longitudinal study of reading and writing rehabilitation using a bigraph-biphone correspondence approach. *Aphasiology, 21*(6), 687–701.

Boyle, M. (2004). Semantic feature analysis treatment for anomia in two fluent aphasia syndromes. *American Journal of Speech-Language Pathology, 13*(3), 236–49.

Boyle, M., & Coelho, C. A. (1995). Application of semantic feature analysis as a treatment for aphasic dysnomia. *American Journal of Speech Language Pathology, 4*(4), 94–98.

Brookshire, R. H., & Nicholas, L. E. (1997). *Discourse Comprehension Test* (2nd ed.). Albuquerque: PICA Programs.

Butterworth, B., & Howard, D. (1987). Paragrammatisms. *Cognition, 26*(1), 1–37.

Byng, S. (1988). Sentence processing deficits: Theory and therapy. *Cognitive Neuropsychology, 5*(6), 629–676. doi: http://dx.doi.org/10.1080/02643298808253277

Cameron, R. M., Wambaugh, J. L., Wright, S. M., & Nessler, C. L. (2006). Effects of a combined semantic/phonologic cueing treatment on word retrieval in discourse. *Aphasiology, 20*(2), 269–285.

Capilouto, G. J., Wright, H. H., & Wagovich, S. A. (2006). Reliability of main event measurement in the discourse of individuals with aphasia. *Aphasiology, 20*(2–4), 205–216.

Caplan, D. (1992). *Language: Structure, processing, and disorders*. Cambridge: The MIT Press.

Caplan, D., Baker, C., & Dehaut, F. (1985). Syntactic determinants of sentence comprehension in aphasia. *Cognition, 21*(2), 117–175. doi: 0010–0277(85)90048–4 [pii]

Caplan, D., & Bub, D. (unpublished). *Psycholinguistic Assessment of Language (PAL)*.

Cherney, L. R. (2004). Aphasia, alexia, and oral reading. *Topics in Stroke Rehabilitation, 11*(1), 22–36.

Cherney, L. R., Patterson, J. P., Raymer, A., Frymark, T., & Schooling, T. (2008). Evidence-based systematic review: Effects of intensity of treatment and constraint-induced language therapy for individuals with stroke-induced aphasia. *Journal of Speech Language and Hearing Research, 51*(5), 1282–1299. doi: 10.1044/1092–4388(2008/07–0206)

Coelho, C. A., McHugh, R. E., & Boyle, M. (2000). Semantic feature analysis as a treatment for aphasic dysnomia: A replication. *Aphasiology, 14*, 133–142.

Conley, A., & Coelho, C. A. (2003). Treatment of word retrieval impairment in chronic Broca's aphasia. *Aphasiology, 17*(3), 203–211.

Conroy, P., Sage, K., & Lambon Ralph, M. (2009). The effects of decreasing and increasing cue therapy on improving naming speed and accuracy for verbs and nouns in aphasia. *Aphasiology, 23*(6), 707–730.

Cornelissen, K., Laine, M., Tarkiainen, A., Jarvensivu, T., Martin, N., & Salmelin, R. (2003). Adult brain plasticity elicited by anomia treatment. *Journal of Cognitive Neuroscience, 15*(3), 444–461.

Corsten, S., Mende, M., Cholewa, J. R., & Huber, W. (2007). Treatment of input and output phonology in aphasia: A single case study. *Aphasiology, 21*(6), 587–603.

Cunningham, R., & Ward, C. (2003). Evaluation of a training programme to facilitate conversation between people with aphasia and their partners. *Aphasiology, 17*(8), 687–707.

Damico, J. S. (1985). Clinical discourse analysis: A functional approach to language assessment. In C. S. Simon (Ed.), *Communication skills and classroom success: Assessment of language-learning disabled students* (pp. 165–204). San Diego: College-Hill Press.

Davis, A. G. (2005). PACE revisited. *Aphasiology, 19*(1), 21–38.

Davis, C., & Harrington, G. (2006). Intensive semantic intervention in fluent aphasia: A pilot study with fMRI. *Aphasiology, 20*(1), 59–83.

DeDe, G., Parris, D., & Waters, G. (2003). Teaching self-cues: A treatment approach for verbal naming. *Aphasiology, 17*(5), 465–480.

Dell, G. S. (1986). A spreading-activation theory of retrieval in sentence production. *Psychological Review, 93*(3), 283–321.

Dell, G. S., & O'Seaghdha, P. G. (1992). Stages of lexical access in language production. *Cognition, 42*(1–3), 287–314.

Dell, G. S., Schwartz, M. F., Martin, N., Saffran, E. M., & Gagnon, D. A. (1997). Lexical access in aphasic and non-aphasic speakers. *Psychological Review, 104*(4), 801–838.

Dickey, M. W., & Thompson, C. K. (2007). The relation between syntactic and morphological recovery in agrammatic aphasia: A case study. *Aphasiology, 21*(6), 604–616.

Doesborgh, S. J. C., van de Sandt-Koenderman, M. W. E., Dippel, D. W. J., van Harskamp, F., Koudstaal, P. J., & Visch-Brink, E. G. (2004a). Effects of semantic treatment on verbal communication and linguistic processing in aphasia after stroke: A randomized controlled trial. *Stroke, 35*(1), 141–146. doi: 10.1161/01.str.0000105460.52928.a6

Doesborgh, S. J. C., van de Sandt-Koenderman, M. W. M. E., Dippel, D. W. J., van Harskamp, F., Koudstaal, P. J., & Visch-Brink, E. G. (2004b). Cues on request: The efficacy of Multicue, a computer program for wordfinding therapy. *Aphasiology, 18*(3), 213–222.

Dunn, L. M., & Dunn, D. M. (2007). *Peabody Picture Vocabulary Test—Fourth Edition (PPVT-4)*. San Antonio: AGS Publishing/Pearson Assessments.

Edmonds, L. A., & Kiran, S. (2006). Effect of semantic naming treatment on crosslinguistic generalization in bilingual aphasia. *Journal of Speech Language and Hearing Research, 49*(4), 729–748. doi: 49/4/729 [pii] 10.1044/1092-4388(2006/053)

Edmonds, L. A., Nadeau, S. E., & Kiran, S. (2009). Effect of Verb Network Strengthening Treatment (VNeST) on Lexical Retrieval of Content Words in Sentences in Persons with Aphasia. *Aphasiology, 23*(3), 402–424. doi: 10.1080/02687030802291339

Ellis, A. W., & Young, A. W. (1988). *Human Cognitive Neuropsychology* (Augmented ed.). Hove, UK: Erlbaum.

Faroqi-Shah, Y. (2008). A comparison of two theoretically driven treatments for verb inflection deficits in aphasia. *Neuropsychologia, 46*(13), 3088–3100.

Faroqi-Shah, Y., & Thompson, C. K. (2003). Effect of lexical cues on the production of active and passive sentences in Broca's and Wernicke's aphasia. *Brain and Language, 85*(3), 409–426.

Ferketic, M., Frattali, C., Holland, A., Thompson, C., & Wohl, C. (2003). *Functional Assessment of Communication Skills for Adults (ASHA FACS)*: American Speech-Language-Hearing Association.

Fillingham, J., Hodgson, C., Sage, K., & Ralph, M. A. L. (2003). The application of errorless learning to aphasic disorders: A review

of theory and practice. *Neuropsychological Rehabilitation: An International Journal, 13*(3), 337–363.

Fillingham, J., Sage, K., & Lambon Ralph, M. (2005a). Further explorations and an overview of errorless and errorful therapy for aphasic word-finding difficulties: The number of naming attempts during therapy affects outcome. *Aphasiology, 19*(7), 597–614.

Fillingham, J., Sage, K., & Lambon Ralph, M. (2005b). Treatment of anomia using errorless versus errorful learning: Are frontal executive skills and feedback important? *International Journal of Language & Communication Disorders, 40*(4), 505–523.

Fillingham, J., Sage, K., & Lambon Ralph, M. (2006). The treatment of anomia using errorless learning. *Neuropsychological Rehabilitation, 16*(2), 129–154.

Fink, R., Brecher, A., Schwartz, M. F., & Robey, R. R. (2002). A computer-implemented protocol for treatment of naming disorders: Evaluation of clinician-guided and partially self-guided instruction. *Aphasiology, 16*(10), 1061–1086.

Fisher, C. A., Wilshire, C. E., & Ponsford, J. L. (2009). Word discrimination therapy: A new technique for the treatment of a phonologically based word-finding impairment. *Aphasiology, 23*(6), 676–693.

Fox, S., Armstrong, E., & Boles, L. (2009). Conversational treatment in mild aphasia: A case study. *Aphasiology, 23*(7), 951–964.

Francis, D. R., Clark, N., & Humphreys, G. W. (2002). Circumlocution-induced naming (CIN): A treatment for effecting generalization in anomia? *Aphasiology, 16*(3), 243–259.

Franklin, S., Buerk, F., & Howard, D. (2002). Generalized improvement in speech production for a subject with reproduction conduction aphasia. *Aphasiology, 16*(10), 1087–1114.

Freed, D., Celery, K., & Marshall, R. C. (2004). CASE STUDY—Effectiveness of personalised and phonological cueing on long-term naming performance by aphasic subjects: A clinical investigation. *Aphasiology, 18*(8), 743–757.

Fridriksson, J. (2010). Preservation and modulation of specific left hemisphere regions is vital for treated recovery from anomia in stroke. [Article]. *Journal of Neuroscience, 30*(35), 11558–11564. doi: 10.1523/jneurosci.2227–10.2010

Fridriksson, J., Holland, A. L., Beeson, P., & Morrow, L. (2005). Spaced retrieval treatment of anomia. *Aphasiology, 19*(2), 99–109. doi: 10.1080/02687030444000660

Friedman, R. B., & Lott, S. N. (2002). Successful blending in a phonological reading treatment for deep alexia. *Aphasiology, 16*(3), 355–372.

Friedman, R. B., Sample, D. M., & Lott, S. N. (2002). The role of level of representation in the use of paired associate learning for rehabilitation of alexia. *Neuropsychologia, 40*(2), 223–234.

Garrett, M. F. (Ed.). (1980). *Levels of processing in sentence production* (Vol. 1). London: Academic Press.

German, D. J. (1990). *Test of Adolescent Adult Word Finding (TAWF)*. Austin, TX: Pro-Ed.

Goodglass, H., Kaplan, E., & Barresi, B. (2000). *Boston Diagnostic Aphasia Examination—Third Edition (BDAE-3)*. Austin, TX: Pro-Ed.

Goodglass, H., Kaplan, E., & Weintraub, S. (1983). *Boston Naming Test*. Philadelphia: Lea & Febiger.

Gordon, J. K. (2007). A contextual approach to facilitating word retrieval in agrammatic aphasia. *Aphasiology, 21*(6), 643–657.

Haarbaurer-Krupa, J., Moser, L., Smith, G., Sullivan, D., & Szekeres, S. F. (1985). Cognitive rehabilitation therapy: Middle stages of recovery. In M. Yvilsaker (Ed.), *Head injury rehabilitation: Children and adolescents*. San Diego: College Hill Press.

Herbert, R., Best, W., Hickin, J., Howard, D., & Osborne, F. (2001). Phonological and orthographic approaches to the treatment of word retrieval in aphasia. *International Journal of Language & Communication Disorders, 36* Suppl, 7–12.

Herbert, R., Best, W., Hickin, J., Howard, D., & Osborne, F. (2003). Combining lexical and interactional approaches to therapy for word finding deficits in aphasia. *Aphasiology, 17*(12), 1163–1186.

Hickin, J., Best, W., Herbert, R., Howard, D., & Osborne, F. (2002). Phonological therapy for word-finding difficulties: A re-evaluation. *Aphasiology, 16*(10–11), 981–999.

Hillis, A. (2005). Stages and mechanisms of recovery from aphasia. *Japanese Journal of Neuropsychology, 21*(1), 35–43.

Hoen, M., Golembiowski, M., Guyot, E., Deprez, V., Caplan, D., & Dominey, P. F. (2003). Training with cognitive sequences improves syntactic comprehension in agrammatic aphasics. *Neuroreport, 14*(3), 495–499.

Holland, A. L., Frattali, C., & Fromm, D. S. (1999). *CADL-2 Communication Activities of Daily Living* (2nd ed.). Austin: Pro-Ed.

Holland, A. L., & Fridriksson, J. (2001). Aphasia management during the early phases of recovery following stroke. *American Journal of Speech Language Pathology, 10*(1), 19–28. doi: 10.1044/1058–0360(2001/004)

Hopper, T., Holland, A., & Rewega, M. (2002). Conversational coaching: Treatment outcomes and future directions. *Aphasiology, 16*(7), 745–761.

Hopper, T., Mahendra, N., Kim, E. S., Azuma, T., Bayles, K. A., Cleary, S. J., & Tomoeda, C. K. (2005). Evidence-based practice recommendations for working with individuals with dementia: spaced-retrieval training. *Journal of Medical Speech–Language Pathology, 13*(4), xxvii(8).

Howard, D., & Patterson, K. (1992). *The Pyramids and Palm Trees Test*. Bury St. Edmunds: Thames Valley Test Company.

Jacobs, B. J., & Thompson, C. K. (2000). Cross-modal generalization effects of training noncanonical sentence comprehension and production in agrammatic aphasia. *Journal of Speech Language and Hearing Research, 43*(1), 5–20.

Kamhi, A. G. (1997). Three perspectives on comprehension: Implications for assessing and treating comprehension problems. *Topics in Language Disorders, 17*(3), 62–74.

Kay, J., Lesser, R. P., & Coltheart, M. (1992). *The Psycholinguistic Assessment of Language Processing in Aphasia (PALPA)*. Hove, UK: Erlbaum.

Kearns, K. (1985). Response elaboration training for patient initiated utterances. *Clinical Aphasiology, 15*, 196–204.

Kendall, D. L., Conway, T., Rosenbek, J., & Gonzalez-Rothi, L. (2003). Case study—Phonological rehabilitation of acquired phonologic alexia. *Aphasiology, 17*(11), 1073–1095.

Kendall, D. L., Rosenbek, J. C., Heilman, K. M., Conway, T., Klenberg, K., Gonzalez Rothi, L. J., & Nadeau, S. E. (2008).

Phoneme-based rehabilitation of anomia in aphasia. *Brain and Language, 105*(1), 1–17.

Kertesz, A. (2006). *Western Aphasia Battery—Revised (WAB-R)*: Harcourt Assessment, Inc.

Kim, E. S., Cleary, S. J., Hopper, T., Bayles, K. A., Mahendra, N., Azuma, T., & Rackley, A. (2006). Evidence-based practice recommendations for working with individuals with dementia: Group reminiscence therapy (care and treatment of dementia). *Journal of Medical Speech–Language Pathology, 14*(3), xxiii(12).

Kim, M., & Beaudoin-Parsons, D. (2007). Training phonological reading in deep alexia: Does it improve reading words with low imageability? *Clinical Linguistics and Phonetics, 21*(5), 321–351. doi: 777792763 [pii] 10.1080/02699200701245415

Kim, M., & Thompson, C. K. (2000). Patterns of comprehension and production of nouns and verbs in agrammatism: Implications for lexical organization. *Brain and Language, 74*(1), 1–25.

Kiran, S. (2005). Training phoneme to grapheme conversion for patients with written and oral production deficits: A model-based approach. *Aphasiology, 19*(1), 53–76.

Kiran, S. (2007). Complexity in the treatment of naming deficits. *American Journal of Speech Language Pathology, 16*(1), 18–29. doi: 16/1/18 [pii] 10.1044/1058–0360(2007/004)

Kiran, S. (2008). Typicality of inanimate category exemplars in aphasia treatment: Further evidence for semantic complexity. *Journal of Speech Language and Hearing Research, 51*(6), 1550–1568. doi: 10.1044/1092–4388(2008/07–0038)

Kiran, S., & Abbott, K. P. (2007). Effect of abstractness on treatment for generative naming deficits in aphasia. *Brain and Language, 103*(1–2), 92–94. doi: DOI 10.1016/j.bandl.2007.07.060

Kiran, S., & Johnson, L. (2008). Semantic complexity in treatment of naming deficits in aphasia: Evidence from well-defined categories. *American Journal of Speech Language Pathology, 17*(4), 389–400. doi: 10.1044/1058–0360(2008/06–0085)

Kiran, S., & Roberts, P. M. (2010). Semantic feature analysis treatment in Spanish-English and French-English bilingual aphasia. *Aphasiology, 24*(2), 231–261.

Kiran, S., Sandberg, C., & Abbott, K. (2009). Treatment for lexical retrieval using abstract and concrete words in persons with aphasia: Effect of complexity. *Aphasiology, 23*, 835–853.

Kiran, S., & Thompson, C. K. (2003a). Effect of typicality on online category verification of animate category exemplars in aphasia. *Brain and Language, 85*(3), 441–450.

Kiran, S., & Thompson, C. K. (2003b). The role of semantic complexity in treatment of naming deficits: Training semantic categories in fluent aphasia by controlling exemplar typicality. *Journal of Speech Language and Hearing Research, 46*(3), 608–622.

Kiran, S., Thompson, C. K., & Hashimoto, N. (2001). Training grapheme to phoneme conversion in patients with oral reading and naming deficits: A model-based approach. *Aphasiology, 15*, 855–876.

Kiran, S., & Viswanathan, M. (2008). Effect of model-based treatment on oral reading abilities in severe alexia: A case study. *Journal of Medical Speech–Language Pathology, 16*(1), 43(17).

Kumar, V. P., & Humphreys, G. W. (2008). The role of semantic knowledge in relearning spellings: Evidence from deep dysgraphia. *Aphasiology, 22*(5), 489–504.

Laganaro, M., Pietro, M. D., & Schnider, A. (2003). Computerised treatment of anomia in chronic and acute aphasia: An exploratory study. *Aphasiology, 17*(8), 709–721.

Laine, M., & Martin, N. (1996). Lexical retrieval deficit in picture naming: implications for word production models. *Brain and Language, 53*(3), 283–314. doi: S0093–934X(96) 90050–4 [pii] 10.1006/brln.1996.0050

LaPointe, L. L., & Horner, J. (1998). *Reading Comprehension Battery for Aphasia (RCBA-2).* Austin, TX: Pro-Ed.

Lindamood, P. C., & Lindamood, P. D. (1998). *The Lindamood phoneme sequencing program for reading, spelling, and speech.* Austin, TX: Pro-Ed.

Linebarger, M., McCall, D., & Berndt, R. S. (2004). The role of processing support in the remediation of aphasic language production disorders. *Cognitive Neuropsychology, 21*(2–4), 267–282.

Linebarger, M., & Schwartz, M. (2005). AAC for hypothesis testing and treatment of aphasic language production: Lessons from a "processing prosthesis." *Aphasiology, 19*(10), 930–942.

Lott, S. N., Sample, D. M., Oliver, R. T., Lacey, E. H., & Friedman, R. B. (2008). A patient with phonologic alexia can learn to read "much" from "mud pies." *Neuropsychologia, 46*(10), 2515–2523.

Lott, S. N., Sperling, A. J., Watson, N. L., & Friedman, R. B. (2009). Repetition priming in oral text reading: A therapeutic strategy for phonologic text alexia. *Aphasiology, 23*(6), 659–675.

Luzzatti, C., Colombo, C., Frustaci, M., & Vitolo, F. (2000). Rehabilitation of spelling along the sub-word-level routine. *Neuropsychological Rehabilitation: An International Journal, 10*(3), 249—278.

Luzzatti, C., Raggi, R., Zonca, G., Pistarini, C., Contardi, A., & Pinna, G. D. (2002). Verb-noun double dissociation in aphasic lexical impairments: The role of word frequency and imageability. *Brain and Language, 81*(1–3), 432–444. doi: S0093934X01925362 [pii]

Mahendra, N., Kim, E. S., Bayles, K. A., Hopper, T., Cleary, S. J., & Azuma, T. (2005). Evidence-based practice recommendations for working with individuals with dementia: Computerassisted cognitive interventions (CACIs). *Journal of Medical Speech–Language Pathology, 13*(4), xxxv(10).

Malvern, D., & Richards, B. (2002). Investigating accommodation in language proficiency interviews using a new measure of lexical diversity. *Language Testing, 19*(1), 85–104. doi: 10.1191/0265532202lt221oa

Manheim, L. M., Halper, A. S., & Cherney, L. (2009). Patientreported changes in communication after computer-based script training for aphasia. *Archives of Physical Medicine and Rehabilitation, 90*(4), 623–627.

Marshall, R. C. (1997). Aphasia treatment in the early postonset period: Managing our resources effectively. *American Journal of Speech Language Pathology, 6*(1), 5–11.

Marshall, R. C., Freed, D. B., & Karow, C. M. (2001). Learning of subordinate category names by aphasic subjects: A comparison of deep and surface-level training methods. *Aphasiology, 15*(6), 585–598.

Marshall, R. C., Karow, C. M., Freed, D. B., & Babcock, P. (2002). Effects of personalized cue form on the learning of subordinate category names by aphasic and non-brain-damaged subjects. *Aphasiology, 16*(7), 763–771.

Martin, N., Fink, R., & Laine, M. (2004). Treatment of word retrieval deficits with contextual priming. *Aphasiology, 18*(5), 457–471.

Martin, N., Fink, R. B., Renvall, K., & Laine, M. (2006). Effectiveness of contextual repetition priming treatments for anomia depends on intact access to semantics. *Journal of the International Neuropsychological Society, 12*(6), 853–866. doi: S1355617706061030 [pii] 10.1017/S1355617706061030

Martin, N., & Laine, M. (2000). Effects of contextual priming on impaired word retrieval. *Aphasiology, 14*(1), 53–70.

Mayer, J. F., & Murray, L. L. (2002). Approaches to the treatment of alexia in chronic aphasia. *Aphasiology, 16*(7), 727–743.

McCall, D., Virata, T., Linebarger, M. C., & Berndt, R. S. (2009). Integrating technology and targeted treatment to improve narrative production in aphasia: A case study. *Aphasiology, 23*(4), 438–461.

McNeil, M. R., & Prescott, T. E. (1978). *Revised Token Test*: University Park Press.

Murray, L. L., Ballard, K., & Karcher, L. (2004). Linguistic specific treatment: Just for Broca's aphasia? *Aphasiology, 18*(9), 785–809.

Murray, L. L., & Karcher, L. (2000). A treatment for written verb retrieval and sentence construction skills. *Aphasiology, 14*(5), 585–602.

Murray, L. L., Timberlake, A., & Eberle, R. (2007). Treatment of underlying forms in a discourse context. *Aphasiology, 21*(2), 139–163.

Naeser, M. A., Martin, P. I., Nicholas, M., Baker, E. H., Seekins, H., Kobayashi, M., et al. (2005). Improved picture naming in chronic aphasia after TMS to part of right Broca's area: An open-protocol study. *Brain and Language, 93*(1), 95–105. doi: S0093–934X(04)00227–5 [pii] 10.1016/j.bandl.2004.08.004

Naeser, M. A., Martin, P. I., Treglia, E., Ho, M., Kaplan, E., Bashir, S., et al. (2010). Research with rTMS in the treatment of aphasia. *Restorative Neurology and Neuroscience, 28*(4), 511–529. doi: 10.3233/rnn-2010–0559

Nicholas, L. E., & Brookshire, R. H. (1993). A system for quantifying the informativeness and efficiency of the connected speech of adults. *Journal of Speech & Hearing Research, 36*(2), 338.

Nickels, L. (2002). Improving word finding: Practice makes (closer to) perfect? *Aphasiology, 16*(10–11), 1047–1060.

Nickels, L., & Howard, D. (1995). Aphasic naming: What matters? *Neuropsychologia, 33*(10), 1281–1303. doi: 0028–3932(95) 00102–9 [pii]

Orjada, S., & Beeson, P. l. (2005). Concurrent treatment for reading and spelling in aphasia. *Aphasiology, 19*(3), 341–351.

Peach, R. (2002). Treatment for phonological dyslexia targeting regularity effects. *Aphasiology, 16*(8), 779–789.

Peach, R., & Wong, P. (2004). Integrating the message level into treatment for agrammatism using story retelling. *Aphasiology, 18*(5), 429–441.

Penn, C. (1985). The profile of communicative appropriateness: A clinical tool for the assessment of pragmatics. *South African Journal of Communication Disorders, 32*, 18–23.

Porch, B. A. (2001). *Porch Index of Communicative Ability—Revised (PICA-R).* Albuquerque: PICA Programs.

Pulvermuller, F., Neininger, B., Elbert, T., Mohr, B., Rockstroh, B., Koebbel, P., & Taub, E. (2001). Constraint-induced therapy of chronic aphasia after stroke. *Stroke, 32*(7), 1621–1626.

Rapp, B. (2005). The relationship between treatment outcomes and the underlying cognitive deficit: Evidence from the remediation of acquired dysgraphia. *Aphasiology, 19*(10), 994–1008.

Rapp, B., & Kane, A. (2002). Remediation of deficits affecting different components of the spelling process. *Aphasiology, 16*(4), 439–454.

Raymer, A. M., & Ellsworth, T. A. (2002). Response to contrasting verb retrieval treatments: A case study. *Aphasiology, 16*(10), 1031–1045.

Raymer, A. M., Kohen, F. P., & Saffell, D. (2006). Computerized training for impairments of word comprehension and retrieval in aphasia. *Aphasiology, 20*(2–4), 257–268.

Renvall, K., Laine, M., Laakso, M., & Martin, N. (2003). Anomia treatment with contextual priming: A case study. *Aphasiology, 17*(3), 305–328.

Renvall, K., Laine, M., & Martin, N. (2005). Contextual priming in semantic anomia: A case study. *Brain and Language, 95*(2), 327–341. doi: S0093–934X(05)00039–8 [pii] 10.1016/j.bandl.2005.02.003

Renvall, K., Laine, M., & Martin, N. (2007). Treatment of anomia with contextual priming: Exploration of a modified procedure with additional semantic and phonological tasks. *Aphasiology, 21*(5), 499–527.

Rider, J. D., Wright, H. H., Marshall, R. C., & Page, J. L. (2008). Using semantic feature analysis to improve contextual discourse in adults with aphasia. *American Journal of Speech Language Pathology, 17*(2), 161–172. doi: 10.1044/1058–0360 (2008/016)

Robson, J., Marshall, J., Chiat, S., & Pring, T. (2001). Enhancing communication in jargon aphasia: A small group study of writing therapy. *International Journal of Language & Communication Disorders, 36*(4), 471–488.

Rochon, E., Laird, L., Bose, A., & Scofield, J. (2005). Mapping therapy for sentence production impairments in nonfluent aphasia. *Neuropsychological Rehabilitation: An International Journal, 15*(1), 1–36.

Rodriguez, A. D., Raymer, A. M., & Rothi, L. J. G. (2006). Effects of gesture+verbal and semantic-phonologic treatments for verb retrieval in aphasia. *Aphasiology, 20*(2), 286–297.

Rogers, T. T., & McClelland, J. L. (2003). *Semantic cognition: A parallel distributed processing approach.* Cambridge, MA: MIT Press.

Rose, M., & Douglas, J. (2008). Treating a semantic word production deficit in aphasia with verbal and gesture methods. *Aphasiology, 22*(1), 20–41.

Rose, M., Douglas, J., & Matyas, T. (2002). The comparative effectiveness of gesture and verbal treatments for a specific phonologic naming impairment. *Aphasiology, 16*(10), 1001–1030.

Saffran, E. M., Berndt, R. S., & Schwartz, M. F. (1989). The quantitative analysis of agrammatic production: Procedure and data. *Brain and Language, 37*(3), 440–479.

Saffran, E. M., Schwartz, M. F., Linebarger, M. C., Martin, N., & Bochetto, P. (unpublished). *Philadelphia Comprehension Battery.*

Saffran, E. M., Schwartz, M. F., & Marin, O. S. (1980). The word order problem in agrammatism. II. Production. *Brain and Language, 10*(2), 263–280.

Sage, K., & Ellis, A. W. (2006). Using orthographic neighbours to treat a case of graphemic buffer disorder. *Aphasiology, 20*(9), 851–870.

Sage, K., Hesketh, A., & Ralph, M. A. L. (2005). Using errorless learning to treat letter-by-letter reading: Contrasting word versus letter-based therapy. *Neuropsychological Rehabilitation: An International Journal, 15*(5), 619–642.

Saur, D., Lange, R., Baumgartner, A., Schraknepper, V., Willmes, K., Rijntjes, M., & Weiller, C. (2006). Dynamics of language reorganization after stroke. *Brain, 129,* 1371–1384.

Schmalzl, L., & Nickels, L. (2006). Treatment of irregular word spelling in acquired dysgraphia: Selective benefit from visual mnemonics. *Neuropsychological Rehabilitation: An International Journal, 16*(1), 1–37.

Schneider, S., & Thompson, C. (2003). Verb production in agrammatic aphasia: The influence of semantic class and argument structure properties on generalisation. *Aphasiology, 17*(3), 213–241.

Schwartz, M. F., Linebarger, M. C., Saffran, E. M., & Pate, D. S. (1987). Syntactic transparency and sentence interpretation in aphasia. *Language and Cognitive Processes, 2*(2), 85–113.

Shapiro, L. P. (1997). Tutorial: an introduction to syntax. *Journal of Speech Language and Hearing Research, 40*(2), 254–272.

Shapiro, L. P. & Thompson, C. K. (2006). Training language deficits in Broca's aphasia. In Y. Grodzinsky and K. Amunts (Eds.), *Broca's Region.* Oxford University Press, 119–134.

Shelton, J. R., & Caramazza, A. (1999). Deficits in lexical and semantic processing: implications for models of normal language. *Psychonomic Bulletin Review, 6*(1), 5–27.

Shewan, C. M. (1979). *The Auditory Comprehension Test for Sentences.* Chicago: Biolinguistics Clinical Education Center Press.

Ska, B., Garneau-Beaumont, D., Chesneau, S., & Damien, B. (2003). Diagnosis and rehabilitation attempt of a patient with acquired deep dyslexia. *Brain and Cognition, 53*(2), 359–363.

Small, S. L., & Llano, D. A. (2009). Biological approaches to aphasia treatment. *Current Neurology and Neuroscience Reports, 9*(6), 443–450.

Spencer, K. A., Doyle, P. J., McNeil, M. R., Wambaugh, J. L., Park, G., & Carroll, B. (2000). Examining the facilitative effects of rhyme in a patient with output lexicon damage. *Aphasiology, 14*(5), 567–584.

Stadie, N., & Rilling, E. (2006). Evaluation of lexically and non-lexically based reading treatment in a deep dyslexic. *Cognitive Neuropsychology, 23*(4), 643–672.

Stefanatos, G., Gershkoff, A., & Madigan, S. (2005). Computer-mediated tools for the investigation and rehabilitation of auditory and phonological processing in aphasia. *Aphasiology, 19*(10), 955–964.

Stefanatos, G. A. (2008). Speech perceived through a damaged temporal window: Lessons from word deafness and aphasia. *Seminars in Speech and Language, 29*(3), 239–252. doi: 10.1055/s-0028-1082887

Taub, E., Crago, J. E., Burgio, L. D., Groomes, T. E., Cook, E. W., 3rd, DeLuca, S. C., & Miller, N. E. (1994). An operant approach to rehabilitation medicine: Overcoming learned nonuse by shaping. *Journal of Experimental Analysis of Behavior, 61*(2), 281–293. doi: 10.1901/jeab.1994.61-281

Taub, E., Miller, N. E., Novack, T. A., Cook, E. W., 3rd, Fleming, W. C., Nepomuceno, C. S., . . . Crago, J. E. (1993). Technique to improve chronic motor deficit after stroke. *Archives of Physical Medical Rehabilitation, 74*(4), 347–354.

Tessier, C., Weill-Chounlamountry, A., Michelot, N., & Pradat-Diehl, P. (2007). Rehabilitation of word deafness due to auditory analysis disorder. *Brain Injury, 21*(11), 1165–1174. doi: 781945296 [pii] 10.1080/02699050701559186

Thompson, C. (2007). Complexity in language learning and treatment. *American Journal of Speech–Language Pathology, 16*(1), 3–5. doi: 16/1/3 [pii] 10.1044/1058-0360(2007/002)

Thompson, C. (unpublished-a). *Northwestern Assessment of Verbs and Sentences—Revised.*

Thompson, C. (unpublished-b). *Northwestern Sentence Comprehension Test.*

Thompson, C., & Shapiro, L. (2005). Treating agrammatic aphasia within a linguistic framework: Treatment of underlying forms. *Aphasiology, 19*(10–11), 1021–1036. doi: 10.1080/02687030544000227

Thompson, C., Shapiro, L., Kiran, S., & Sobecks, J. (2003). The role of syntactic complexity in treatment of sentence deficits in agrammatic aphasia: The complexity account of treatment efficacy (CATE). *Journal of Speech, Language, and Hearing Research, 46*(3), 591–607.

Thompson, C., Shapiro, L. P., Tait, M. E., Jacobs, B. J., & Schneider, S. L. (1996). Training wh-question production in agrammatic aphasia: Analysis of argument and adjunct movement. *Brain and Language, 52*(1), 175–228. doi: S0093-934X(96)90009-7 [pii] 10.1006/brln.1996.0009

Tyler, L. K., & Moss, H. E. (2001). Towards a distributed account of conceptual knowledge. *Trends in Cognitive Science, 5*(6), 244–252.

van Dijk, T. A. (1987). Episodic models in discourse processing. In R. Horowitz & S. J. Samuels (Eds.), *Comprehending oral and written language* (pp. 161–196). San Diego, CA: Academic Press, Inc.

Wagner, T., Fregni, F., Fecteau, S., Grodzinsky, A., Zahn, M., & Pascual-Leone, A. (2007). Transcranial direct current stimulation: A computer-based human model study. *NeuroImage, 35*(3), 1113–1124. doi: 10.1016/j.neuroimage.2007.01.027

Wambaugh, J. (2003). A comparison of the relative effects of phonologic and semantic cueing treatments. *Aphasiology, 17*(5), 433–441.

Wambaugh, J., Cameron, R., Kalinyak-Fliszar, M., Nessler, C., & Wright, S. (2004). Retrieval of action names in aphasia: Effects of two cueing treatments. *Aphasiology, 18*(11), 979–1004.

Wambaugh, J., Doyle, P. J., Martinez, A. L., & Kalinyak-Fliszar, M. (2002). Effects of two lexical retrieval cueing treatments on action naming in aphasia. *Journal of Rehabilitation Research and Development, 39*(4), 455–466.

Wambaugh, J., & Ferguson, M. (2007). Application of semantic feature analysis to retrieval of action names in aphasia. *Journal of Rehabilitation Research and Development, 44*(3), 381–394.

Wambaugh, J., Linebaugh, C. W., Doyle, P. J., Martinez, A. L., Kalinyak-Fliszar, M., & Spencer, K. A. (2001). Effects of two cueing treatments on lexical retrieval in aphasic speakers with different levels of deficit. *Aphasiology, 15*(10), 933–950.

Wambaugh, J., & Wright, S. (2007). Improved effects of word-retrieval treatments subsequent to addition of the orthographic form. *Aphasiology, 21*(6), 632–642.

Webster, J., Morris, J., & Franklin, S. (2005). Effects of therapy targeted at verb retrieval and the realization of the predicate argument structure: A case study. *Aphasiology, 19*(8), 748–764.

Weinrich, M., Boser, K. I., McCall, D., & Bishop, V. (2001). Training agrammatic subjects on passive sentences: Implications for syntactic deficit theories. *Brain and Language, 76*(1), 45–61.

WHO. (2001). International Classification of Functioning, Disability, and Health (Vol. WHA54.21). Geneva: World Health Organization.

Wiederholt, J. L., & Bryant, B. R. (2001). *Gray Oral Reading Tests—Fourth Edition (GORT-4)*. Austin, TX: Pro-Ed.

Wierenga, C. E., Maher, L. M., Moore, A. B., White, K. D., McGregor, K., Soltysik, D. A., . . . Crosson, B. (2006). Neural substrates of syntactic mapping treatment: An fMRI study of two cases. *Journal of the International Neuropsychological Society, 12*(01), 132–146. doi: doi:10.1017/S13556 1770606019X

Williams, K. T. (2007). *Expressive Vocabulary Test—Second Edition (EVT-2)*: AGS Publishing/Pearson Assessments.

Wright, H. H., Capilouto, G. J., Wagovich, S. A., Cranfill, T. B., & Davis, J. E. (2005). Development and reliability of a quantitative measure of adults' narratives. *Aphasiology, 19*(3–5), 263–273.

Wright, H. H., Marshall, R. C., Wilson, K. B., & Page, J. L. (2008). Using a written cueing hierarchy to improve verbal naming in aphasia. *Aphasiology, 22*(5), 522–536.

Yampolsky, S., & Waters, G. (2002). Treatment of single word oral reading in an individual with deep dyslexia. *Aphasiology, 16*(4), 455–471.

Zientz, J., Rackley, A., Chapman, S. B., Hopper, T., Mahendra, N., & Cleary, S. (2007a). Evidence-based practice recommendations: caregiver-administered active cognitive stimulation for individuals with Alzheimer's disease. (ANCDS Bulletin Board). *Journal of Medical Speech–Language Pathology, 15*(3), xxvii(8).

Zientz, J., Rackley, A., Chapman, S. B., Hopper, T., Mahendra, N., Kim, E. S., & Cleary, S. J. (2007b). Evidence-based practice recommendations for dementia: educating caregivers on Alzheimer's disease and training communication strategies. (Clinical report). *Journal of Medical Speech–Language Pathology, 15*(1), liii(12).

14-1

Sample Treatment Protocols

PHONOLOGICAL TREATMENT

The phonological treatment used by Kendall and colleagues (2008) will be outlined. This approach was adapted from the Lindamood Phoneme Sequencing Program (LiPS; Lindamood & Lindamood, 1998), which is a well-known and successful program for children with phonological processing disorders.

The steps are as follows:

Stage 1: Consonants and vowels in isolation

1. *Exploration of sounds.* The clinician presents a picture of a mouth making the sound and asks the patient to look in the mirror and repeat the sound after the clinician. Feedback is given regarding accuracy and the patient is asked to describe what he/she saw and felt during sound production.
2. *Motor description.* The clinician describes how each articulator contributes to production of the sound. The patient is asked to make the sound, and then describe how it is made. The clinician provides feedback and probes for more information, if necessary.
3. *Perception task.* The clinician makes the sound and asks the patient to choose the sound from an array of mouth pictures. The clinician provides feedback and probes incorrect responses until correct.
4. *Production task.* The clinician elicits sound production via repetition, mouth picture cue, or motor description. Feedback is provided and incorrect responses are probed until correct.
5. *Graphemes.* The clinician places grapheme tiles on the table with the mouth pictures and trains the patient to match each tile with its corresponding sound. This is accomplished using mouth pictures and motor descriptions. Once the patient can reliably match sound to grapheme, the grapheme tiles are then used in steps 3 and 4 above. The patient must achieve 80% accuracy for three consecutive treatment sessions to move on to stage 2.

Stage 2: Syllables

1. *Perception task.* The clinician produces a sound combination and asks the patient to combine either the mouth pictures or the grapheme tiles to match the target. The clinician provides feedback.
2. *Production task.* The clinician uses combinations of either the mouth pictures or the grapheme tiles representing syllables to elicit first each sound in isolation, then the blended syllable. The clinician then asks the patient to judge whether or not his/her production was correct. Next, one sound is changed and the patient is asked to say the old syllable, identify what has changed, and then say the new syllable. The patient must achieve 80% accuracy across three sessions to progress from one- to two- to three-sound syllables and from one- to two-syllable combinations.

ORTHOGRAPHIC TREATMENTS

Reading. Grapheme-to-phoneme treatment has been successful in remediating both phonological and deep dyslexia.

The steps are as follows (Kiran et al., 2001):

1. The clinician selects a word from the training set and asks the patient to read it. Feedback regarding accuracy is provided and then the clinician provides the word and asks the patient to repeat it.
2. The clinician asks the patient to spell the target aloud and then provides accuracy feedback. If the patient is unable to spell the word, the clinician spells the word aloud and asks the patient to repeat it.
3. The clinician presents the letters of the target word as well as an equal number of letters that are not in the target word in a random sequence and asks the patient to select the letters of the target word. If the patient does not select the correct letters, the clinician provides feedback and

helps the patient to select the correct letters, requiring the patient to say the letters aloud as she/he selects them.

4. The clinician presents each letter of the target word to the patient in a random order and asks the patient to identify the presented letter. Accuracy feedback is given and incorrect responses are corrected by the clinician, who then asks the patient to repeat the correct letter name.

5. The clinician forms the target word with the letters and then asks the patient to say each letter aloud while pointing to it. The clinician asks the patient to read the word aloud. This step is practiced until the patient can perform the task twice unaided.

The clinician repeats steps 3 through 5 and then presents the target word card for the participant to read aloud. Accuracy feedback is given and the clinician proceeds to the next word.

Writing. Copy and Recall Treatment (CART) is a well-researched and effective treatment for writing deficits. CART is carried out in a few simple steps (Beeson et al., 2003).

The steps are as follows:

1. The clinician selects a picture of the word to be written, names the item, and asks the patient to write the name of the item. Feedback is given regarding accuracy. If the patient correctly writes the word, the next word is chosen. If the patient incorrectly writes the word, the clinician moves on to step 2.

2. The clinician writes the word or shows the patient a previous correctly written example and asks the patient to write the word three times, giving accuracy feedback each time.

3. The clinician removes all written examples of the word and once again provides just the picture of the item. The clinician prompts the patient to write the word, gives feedback, covers the word, and asks the patient to write it again. This process is repeated three times and then the next item is presented.

4. For homework, the patient is given daily worksheets. Each worksheet has the target pictures with the written name and 20 lines for copying each word. Also, the patient is given a daily recall test page with pictures, but no written form.

SEMANTIC TREATMENT

Semantic Feature Analysis (SFA) is an effective, straightforward treatment for word retrieval deficits. One reason SFA is an appealing semantic treatment is in its flexibility. It has successfully been applied in a variety of ways, including with atypical items for greater generalization (Kiran & Johnson, 2008).

SFA is carried out in a few simple steps (Boyle & Coelho, 1995):

1. The patient attempts to name a pictured object. Regardless of whether or not the patient is successful, the clinician moves on to step 2.

2. The clinician places the picture in the middle of the table or a board with six semantic feature types listed around the perimeter: category, use, action, physical attribute, location, and association. For each item, the clinician asks the patient to provide the semantic features and can prompt the patient by asking: "What category does it belong to?" "What is it used for?" "What does it do?" "What does it look like?" "Where can you find it?" and "What does it remind you of?" The clinician writes down each semantic feature generated by the patient under the corresponding labels. If the patient cannot provide a feature, the clinician provides the feature.

3. If the patient is still unable to name the picture, the clinician provides the correct response and has the patient repeat it along with all of the semantic features. Success in naming each item correctly is reinforced, regardless of when it occurs. However, feature analysis is always carried out in its entirety before moving on to the next item.

SYNTACTIC TREATMENT

Treatment of Underlying Forms (TUF) is an effective treatment for sentence comprehension and production that generalizes to untrained items that share similar linguistic properties. It is recommended that Wh-movement (e.g., *The aunt saw the girl whom the boy kissed.*) and NP-movement (e.g., *The boy was kissed by the girl.*) sentences be used in TUF.

The steps for carrying out TUF are as follows (Dickey & Thompson, 2007):

1. A picture depicting the target sentence is placed in front of the patient (e.g., *The aunt saw the girl who the boy kissed.*).

2. Cards with each constituent part of each clause in the sentence (i.e., agent, theme, verb) are placed in front of the patient, arranged in two active sentences (e.g., THE AUNT SAW THE GIRL and THE BOY KISSED THE GIRL) with the WHO card set aside.

3. The clinician explains the steps required to make the target sentence, showing the patient how to identify thematic roles and demonstrating Wh-movement or NP-movement.

4. The patient uses the cards to reassemble the sentence and then reads the sentence aloud. The clinician will assist with this step, if necessary.

DISCOURSE TREATMENT

Conversational coaching is a formalized approach to teaching strategies to patients and their conversational partners. In this treatment, both the patient and the conversational partner participate in therapy.

The steps for conversational coaching are as follows (Hopper et al., 2002):

1. The clinician conducts a baseline observation to determine the strategies that both conversational partners use, which strategies are effective, which strategies are ineffective, and which strategies are missing, but may be useful.
2. The clinician then writes each strategy to be taught in large font on white paper and explains each strategy to both partners. Each strategy is reviewed before each session.
3. Short videotaped monologues are shown only to the patient, who is then responsible for relaying the story to his or her conversational partner. During this exercise, the clinician coaches both partners to use their respective strategies.

CHAPTER 15

Clinical Approaches to Communication Impairments Due to Executive Dysfunction

This book describes the impact of cognitive impairments on the communication functioning of individuals following acquired brain injury. Cognition can be broadly described as mental activities or operations involved in taking in, interpreting, encoding, storing, retrieving, and making use of knowledge or information and generating a response (Ylvisaker & Szekeres, 1994). Examples of cognitive processes attributed to the frontal lobes include the ability to focus attention to stimuli, remembering and learning, organizing information, reasoning, and problem solving. In addition to specific cognitive processes, the frontal lobes mediate executive control of thought and behavior. Such executive functions include goal setting, behavior planning and sequencing, goal oriented behavior, and initiation and evaluation of behavior (Lezak, 1993). Baddeley (1986) coined the term "dysexecutive syndrome" to characterize the range of impairments that commonly follow frontal lobe injury (Baddeley, 1986). Executive functions impact on all aspects of our daily behavior, including our ability to communicate.

This chapter will focus on approaches to taking executive functioning explicitly into account when treating communication difficulties after acquired brain injury. Executive functions are typically mediated by the frontal and prefrontal cortices (Stuss & Benson, 1984), and so the assessment and treatment approaches described in this chapter will be most relevant to populations who have damage in these regions. This is with recognition of the fact that executive functioning probably involves multiple component processes involving several brain regions working in concert (Keil & Kaszniak, 2002). Frontal injury can be focal, such as would occur with a stroke, or it can be diffuse, which is more typical of traumatic brain injury (TBI). Executive functioning can be compromised by disorders such as multiple sclerosis (O'Brien, Chiaravalloti, Goverover, & DeLuca, 2008), Alzheimer's disease (Marshall, Capilouto, & McBride, 2007) and even from cerebellar damage due to the links to the frontal cortex via cortico-ponto-cerebellar networks (Schweizer, Levine, Rewilak, et al., 2008). Many of the strategies discussed in this chapter are drawn from the TBI research literature, given the preponderance of executive functioning deficits that may follow this type of injury. Nonetheless, the ideas presented here will be useful to managing communication problems that arise from other acquired frontal injuries.

HOW DOES IMPAIRED EXECUTIVE FUNCTIONING AFFECT COMMUNICATION?

Executive impairment has been described as representing either a loss of drive or a loss of control that may translate into deficiencies (e.g., inertia, rigidity, poor conceptualization and planning) or excesses (such as disinhibition) of cognition and behavior (R. Tate, 1999; R. L. Tate, Lulham, Broe, et al., 1989). Inertia and rigidity can lead to a flat presentation, seeming disinterest in the conversation, and inability to generate and maintain topics. Alternatively, excesses can interfere due to frequent interruptions, disinhibited responses, swearing, and perseveration on topics. These inappropriate and disturbing communicative behaviors are difficult to manage, particularly when in a community setting such as a shopping center.

The relationship between executive functioning and communication difficulties after TBI was first enunciated three decades ago. A. L. Holland (1982) was perhaps the first to ask the classic question "When is aphasia aphasia?" raising the idea that if people with TBI were labeled as aphasic they would, in turn, receive inappropriate treatment that would fail to take their cognitive impairments into account. At about the same time, other researchers recognized this interplay between cognition and language, leading to the introduction of the term *cognitive-language disorder* (Hagen, 1984; Kennedy & DeRuyter, 1991). The first work in this area examined the relationship between cognitive disturbances following TBI and psycholinguistic aspects of language (Hagen, 1984). The impairments of attention, memory, sequencing, categorization, and associative abilities were seen to result in an impaired capacity to organize and structure incoming information, emotional reactions, and the flow of thought. Such impairments, Hagen argued, caused a disorganization of language processes. Cognitive disorganization is reflected through language use that is characterized by irrelevant utterances that may not make sense, difficulty inhibiting inappropriate utterances, word-finding difficulties, and problems ordering words and propositions. Prigatano, Roueche, and Fordyce (1985) described nonaphasic language disturbances following TBI including the problems of talkativeness, tangentiality, and fragmented thought processes. In the 1990s, the term *cognitive-communication disorder* emerged (Hartley, 1995) in recognition of the relationship

between impaired cognition and its wider ramifications for everyday communication skills.

The debate regarding the definition of "cognitive-linguistic" disorders continues with the proposition that the term lacks terminological clarity, which undermines the assessment of complex communication functioning (Body & Perkins, 2006). Nonetheless, it is now widely accepted that the communication difficulties following TBI are mostly the result of a combination of cognitive and linguistic impairments. In addition, it is also recognized that executive functioning impairments in the domains of attention, memory, organization, planning, flexible problem solving, and self awareness are consistently seen in people after TBI (Anderson, Bigler, & Blatter, 1995; Levin, Goldstein, Williams, & Eisenberg, 1991). These types of difficulties can have a significant deleterious impact on a person's day-to-day interactions leading to social communication impairments. Elements of discourse pragmatics, such as turn-taking and social judgment, and theory of mind elements (e.g., appreciation of another's perspective) may also be impaired due to executive dysfunction (McDonald & Pearce, 1998).

Many studies have shown that individuals with TBI experience difficulties during conversation. Poor conversational competence in individuals with TBI is the result of verbosity, inappropriate responses to social communication, poor topic maintenance, and reliance on additional conversational prompting provided by their communication partners (C. A. Coelho, Youse, & Le, 2002; Godfrey & Shum, 2000; Togher, Hand, & Code, 1997). It is thus not surprising that conversations with individuals with TBI have been described as less enjoyable, less interesting, and less rewarding (Bond & Godfrey, 1997; C. A. Coelho et al., 2002). This is problematic for individuals with TBI as conversation is fundamental for socializing and strengthening interpersonal relationships (C. A. Coelho et al., 2002). The assessment of executive functioning as it pertains to communication will be described in further detail in the next section.

ASSESSMENTS OF EXECUTIVE FUNCTIONING

A common aspect of all tests of executive function is that the patient is placed in a situation that requires them to respond to novel or non-routine demands with increasing levels of task complexity (Shallice, 1988). Assessments of executive functioning that includes an emphasis on communication functioning frequently rely on decontextualized tasks that use pen and paper, visual tasks, and objects. Unfortunately, the inherent structure of these assessments can enhance the performance of a person with frontal lobe impairment leading to failed diagnosis of executive functioning difficulties (Eslinger & Damasio, 1985). For example, usually testing is conducted in a quiet office, without distractions and with a clinician who coordinates the test administration, provides direction regarding rules, sets goals, and prompts the person when to start and when to stop the task. The core deficits inherent in executive functioning, namely establishing a functional framework to complete the operation, starting, stopping, tracking and switching, may be circumvented by the controlled nature of the assessment task (Manchester, Priestley, & Jackson, 2004).

STANDARDIZED TESTS OF EXECUTIVE FUNCTIONING THAT INCORPORATE COMMUNICATION

To guide practitioners regarding the best executive functioning tests to use in clinical practice, members of the Academy of Neurologic Communication Disorders and Sciences (ANCDS) Practice Guidelines Group (Turkstra, Coehlo, & Ylvisaker, 2005) published a list of the standardized norm-referenced tests that met established validity and reliability criteria for the TBI population. There were seven tests suggested (Box 15-1).

Box 15-1

Tests Recommended by the ANCDS Practice Guidelines Group

- American Speech-Language-Hearing Association Functional Assessment of Communication Skills in Adults (ASHA-FACS) (Frattali, Thompson, Holland, et al., 1995)
- Behavior Rating Inventory of Executive Function (BRIEF) (Gioia, Isquith, Guy, & Kenworthy, 2000)
- Communicative Activities of Daily Living (CADL-2) (A. Holland, Frattali, & Fromm, 1999)
- Functional Independence Measure (FIM, 1996)
- Repeatable Battery for the Assessment of Neuropsychological Status (RBANS) (Randolph, 2001)
- Test of Language Competence—Extended (TLC-E) (Wiig & Secord, 1989)
- Western Aphasia Battery—R (Kertesz, 2006)

Data from Turkstra, L. S., Coelho, C., & Ylvisaker, M. (2005). The use of standardized tests for individuals with cognitive-communication disorders. *Seminars in Speech & Language, 26*(4): 215–222.

As there is currently limited evidence with regard to standardized instruments for individuals for cognitive-communication disorders, the committee limited its recommendations to practice options. The recommendations were to use caution when evaluating people with brain injury using existing standardized tests; to consider standardized testing within a broader framework that incorporated factors such as the person's pre-injury characteristics, stage of recovery, and everyday communication demands; and to collaborate with other health professionals, particularly when considering the use of impairment-level cognitive tests (L. Turkstra, Ylvisaker, Coelho, et al., 2005).

Additionally, there are a plethora of executive functioning tests that do not specifically invoke language processing and therefore will not be discussed in this chapter (e.g., Rey-Osterrieth Complex Figure, Tower of London, Raven's Colored Progressive Matrices, and Wisconsin Card Sort Test). For a review of these assessments, the reader is referred to Keil & Kaszniak (2002).

Tests of Executive Functioning and Communication in Everyday Contexts: Standardized Tests

Rather, the focus of the assessments described here will be the evaluation of executive functioning that is associated with communication skills in everyday contexts, including standardized and non-standardized approaches, which are discussed in the next section. Executive functioning affects all aspects of our everyday activity (Ylvisaker & Feeney, 1998) and so evaluation tools have begun to emerge to capture these difficulties (Kilov, Togher, & Grant, 2009). The question of when to complete these assessments remains unanswered, although it was recently reported that executive functioning tests were more predictive of recovery if administered 5 months post-injury than at 8 weeks post-injury (Green, Colella, Hebert, et al., 2008). However, there is also evidence that executive functioning can be screened in the acute setting (Bennett, Ong, & Ponsford, 2005) using the Dysexecutive Questionnaire (DEX), which is a subtest of the Behavioral Assessment of the Dysexecutive Syndrome (BADS) (Wilson, Alderman, Burgess, et al., 1996). This battery includes a 20-item Dysexecutive Questionnaire (DEX) that samples the range of problems in four broad areas of likely change: emotional or personality changes, motivational changes, behavioral changes, and cognitive changes. The questionnaire has two versions, one of which is completed by the client (the DEX) and one of which is completed by a significant other who has close, preferably daily contact with the client (DEX-R). Bennett et al. (2005) found that while neuropsychologists and occupational therapists' ratings on the DEX were strongly associated with measures of executive functioning, the ratings of family members and people with TBI were not. This finding suggested that clinicians need to be judicious regarding when the DEX is administered and who completes it.

In general, the assessments described in this chapter are best administered in the sub-acute and chronic phases of recovery after an acquired brain injury. One reason for this is that difficulties often do not become evident until the person returns to his/her everyday situations, such as shopping, working, and conversing in group situations. It is also true that the severity and degree to which executive impairment manifests from one individual to the next varies enormously, influenced not only by the severity of the injury but also pre-morbid intelligence, motivation, and the nature of the task (Shallice & Burgess, 1991). In less severe cases, routine behavior previously learned may be carried out normally and basic skills retained. However, there may be a disruption of the capacity to focus attention voluntarily and to deal with novel situations adaptively. When deficits are more pervasive all behavior may be disrupted.

As the relationship between communication and executive functioning is clearly multifaceted, a variety of theoretical approaches have been taken to their evaluation. The complex nature of the area has also led to the development of multidisciplinary approaches to evaluation with considerable overlap between speech language pathology and neuropsychology. The resulting assessments developed over the past decade are innovative, reflective of everyday contexts, and encompass the latest technological advances, including: (1) the use of virtual reality (e.g., the Virtual Multiple Errands Test or VMET) (Rand, Rukan, Weiss, & Katz, 2009), (2) a focus on the intricacies of social interactions (the Awareness of Social Inference Test) (McDonald, Flanagan, & Rollins, 2002), and (3) an examination of the subtle cognitive-communication deficits arising from acquired brain injury called the Functional Assessment of Verbal Reasoning and Executive Strategies (FAVRES) (MacDonald, 1998).

The Virtual Multiple Errands Test

This test is based on the Multiple Errands Test (MET) (Alderman, Burgess, Knight, & Henman, 2003; Burgess, Alderman, Forbes, et al., 2006; Knight, Alderman, & Burgess, 2002), which is performed at a real shopping mall or in a hospital environment and involves the completion of various tasks, rules to adhere to, and a

specified time frame. For example, in the MET the individual is asked to buy six items, such as:

- Buy a bottle of mineral water
- Get a napkin from the coffee shop
- Buy a Kit-Kat chocolate bar
- Pick up an envelope that is waiting for you at the FOX shop and do what is necessary
- Get a visiting card from one of the shops
- Buy a bottle of orange juice

The individual is then given a set of rules to abide by, including, for example, "You are not allowed to go into the same shop more than once, and you are not allowed to buy more than two items at any shop." Finally, the individual is asked to meet the tester at a certain time at a preset location. The tester follows the participant around the shopping mall recording mistakes, with scoring relating to behaviors such as non-efficiency, rule breaking, and use of partial and complete mistakes in completing a task. The MET was moderately correlated with most of the items in the DEX (Alderman et al., 2003) demonstrating ecological validity. Two problems with the MET are the time consuming nature of completing this assessment and the requirement that the individual is independently ambulant.

Rand and colleagues (Rand, Katz, & Weiss, 2007) therefore used virtual reality technology to create a virtual mall. The Virtual Mall (VMall) is a functional virtual environment consisting of a large supermarket where individuals with acquired brain injury can engage in the complex task of shopping (Rand et al., 2007). The VMET is a virtual reality evaluation of the person engaged in an adapted version of the MET. While the VMET had moderate to high correlations with the MET in post-stroke participants and older healthy controls (Rand et al., 2009), further psychometric evaluation is needed. The types of mistakes made by the post-stroke participants were similar in both the real mall and the VMall, including problems with planning, difficulty with multitasking, and a lack of awareness of mistakes. This assessment offers a promising window into the future of evaluating executive functioning deficits. As virtual reality technology continues to improve, it may be possible to expand the communicative contexts the individual with acquired brain injury is asked to participate within while remaining in the clinic room. A limitation, however, is that in the current VMall there are no communicative interactions that mirror real-life interaction—the virtual reality platform merely offers the clinician an insight into the organization and planning of shopping, and the individual's response to distracters such as background music and announcements.

The Awareness of Social Inference Test (TASIT)

Executive functioning impairments have implications for the assessment of social communication skills. Social communication encompasses a complex array of components including, for example, the ability to make inferences, and to understand and make requests (McDonald, 1992, 1993; McDonald & Pearce, 1996, 1998; Pearce, McDonald, & Coltheart, 1998; L. S. Turkstra, McDonald, & Kaufman, 1995). This research has shown that a proportion of adults with TBI misinterpret conversational inferences generated by discrete speech acts. Given that linguistic performance is relatively normal in these people, it is thought that they have difficulty utilizing the contextual information necessary to generate these inferences. However, the nature of the contextual cues involved and whether any particular sources of contextual cues are more poorly processed is not well understood (McDonald, 2000).

Executive abilities related to concept formation and inhibition have been implicated in the capacity to interpret non-literal language (Martin & McDonald, 2006). Studying the effect of how indirect contextual information is detected by conversational speakers has led to advances in the study of sarcasm (McDonald, 2007; McDonald & Pearce, 1996), use of hints (McDonald & Sommers, 1993), and, more recently, theory of mind investigations with people with TBI (Bibby & McDonald, 2005; Martin & McDonald, 2005). It is thought that the ability to detect sarcasm is impaired in those with frontal injury because the frontal lobes control the executive processes that enable us to respond adaptively to novel stimuli by overriding routine, habit-driven responses. It is thought that damage to these processes may lead to more automatic responses, which are either stimulus-bound or habit driven. This leads to a reduced appreciation of inferential meanings in language because they are stimulus-bound to the most concrete aspects of the information given and are not able to suppress their tendency to respond in a routine way to such attributes. They are therefore unable to appreciate alternative meanings or associations (McDonald & Pearce, 1996). In McDonald and Pearce's (1996) study of 10 people with TBI it was determined that this group could interpret consistent verbal exchanges but had difficulty with literally contradictory (sarcastic) verbal exchanges. They found that the literal meaning of a sarcastic comment needed to be rejected in order for the inference to be detected.

Theory of mind concerns the ability to make judgments about the mental states of others. It is thought that this skill underpins the ability to interpret and predict how others will behave. The traditional approach to evaluating this skill is through the use of "false belief" and complex story tasks that examine how participants use conceptual or pictorial information about the beliefs of those depicted in the story. While this has been a tantalizing line of inquiry in the study of the unique frontal deficits that are associated with TBI, it seems that theory of mind is not a singular ability, and that the judgments made in these traditional story tasks could involve non–theory of mind inferential reasoning (Bibby & McDonald, 2005) and cognitive flexibility (Henry, Phillips, Crawford, et al., 2006). Nonetheless, people with severe TBI demonstrate specific impairments on tasks requiring them to make inferences about others' mental states when compared to control participants (Bibby & McDonald, 2005).

In response to these findings, McDonald and colleagues developed the Awareness of Social Inference Test (TASIT) (McDonald et al., 2002) which is an audiovisual clinical tool for the assessment of social perception. There are 3 parts: Part 1 assesses emotion recognition, Parts 2 and 3 assess the ability to interpret conversational remarks meant literally (i.e., sincere remarks and lies) or non-literally (i.e., sarcasm) as well as the ability to make judgments about the thoughts, intentions, and feelings of speakers. The subtests relating to executive functioning, namely Parts 2 and 3, comprise video vignettes where the participants watch brief dialogues between two actors. In Part 2 (Social Inference—Minimal), there are 15 vignettes; 5 where the exchange is sincerely meant, 5 where similar scripts were enacted sarcastically, and 5 where the scripts are literally paradoxical (i.e., they could only make sense if it was understood that one person was being sarcastic). After viewing each vignette, participants are required to answer questions regarding the speaker's (1) feelings, (2) beliefs, (3) intentions, and (4) meaning. In Part 3 of the TASIT (Social Inference—Enriched), there are 16 vignettes that provide additional information before or after the dialogue of interest to "set the scene." For example, two co-workers confide to each other that a party over the weekend was truly dreadful. This is followed by a scene with the host of the party in which he/she claims the party was a great success. In half the vignettes the scripts are enacted as a diplomatic lie, trying to make the best of a bad situation. In the remainder they are enacted sarcastically. As with Part 2, the ability to interpret vignettes is assessed via a set of 4 questions for each vignette.

The TASIT is an important advance in the assessment of social communication functioning. It is sensitive to disorders such as TBI (McDonald, Tate, Togher, et al., 2008), schizophrenia (Rankin, Salazar, Gorno-Tempini, et al., 2009), and the behavioral form of frontotemporal dementia (bvFTD) and Alzheimer's disease (Kipps, Nestor, Acosta-Cabronero, et al., 2009). The TASIT has adequate psychometric properties with demonstrated reliability and validity (McDonald, Bornhofer, Shum, et al., 2006) and is available in alternate forms.

The Functional Assessment of Verbal Reasoning and Executive Strategies (FAVRES)

The Functional Assessment of Verbal Reasoning and Executive Strategies (FAVRES) is an assessment tool designed specifically for the acquired brain injury population (MacDonald & Johnson, 2005). It is a reliable and discriminating measure for differentiating performances of those with and without ABI (MacDonald & Johnson, 2005). Importantly, it provides an evaluation of executive functions within everyday communication contexts. There are four functional tasks that simulate everyday life including: planning an event, scheduling a workday, making a decision, and building a case to solve a problem. While not designed specifically to comprehensively assess executive functions, the tasks in this assessment elicit aspects of executive functioning in simulated real-life contexts. For example, the Planning an Event subtest involves choosing a social event given certain restrictions, while the Scheduling subtest involves sequencing, organizing, and prioritizing important daily events with time constraints. The latter of these tasks was found to be the most powerful discriminator of whether participants with TBI returned to work (Isaki & Turkstra, 2000).

Non-standardized Approaches to Assessing Communication and Executive Functioning

All the tests described in this chapter have been standardized evaluations of some aspect of executive functioning and communication performance. We use executive functions every day in our interactions with others, however, and so ideally it would be beneficial to evaluate the effects of executive functioning deficits in these contexts. While there is a paucity of research in this area, there have been some attempts to provide frameworks for clinicians to examine executive functioning in real-life communication contexts. Two of these are to be discussed here. These include the concept of "collaborative contextualized hypothesis testing" proposed by Ylvisaker and colleagues (Ylvisaker & Feeney, 1998), and the General Behavioral Observation Form (Hartley, 1995).

Collaborative Contextualized Hypothesis Testing

This rather daunting title merely reflects the process of working out reasons for a person's difficulty in everyday social contexts. So, for example, if a person is having difficulty reading a chapter and answering questions about the content, there are a number of possible reasons this could be occurring, including problems with executive functioning (Table 15-1).

These are only some of the possible reasons a person may be having difficulty. Others include problems with visual acuity, memory, speed of information processing, language difficulties, and behavioral problems. Ylvisaker & Feeney (1998) suggest that the process of hypothesis testing is a dynamic one that should be conducted in collaboration with all members of the professional team, including family members. They suggest that this process is best conducted in real contexts in the individual's life. As people with TBI often perform well on standardized, structured tests, but fail in their everyday activities, Ylvisaker suggests they be evaluated in the situations where they are having difficulty. It is also suggested that this process is ongoing as consequences of a brain injury may not emerge for months or even years after the injury.

Table **15-1**	Some Hypotheses About Why a Person Has Difficulty with a Reading Comprehension Task
Executive Function	**Description of Underlying Problem**
Attention	Inadequate sustained attention, distractibility/weak filtering, inability to divide attention, difficulty shifting from the previous task
Orientation	Unclear orientation to the task
Working memory	Insufficient space in working memory to hold the task instructions, reading strategies, and information from the paragraph
Self-monitoring	Failure to recognize that the task is difficult and requires special strategic effort
Organization/ integration	Difficulty organizing information to comprehend the text, to understand how details relate to each other, to understand how the questions relate to the text, or to formulate an organized answer

From Coelho, C., Ylvisaker, M., & Turkstra, L. S. (2005). Nonstandardized assessment approaches for individuals with traumatic brain injuries. *Seminars in Speech & Language* (4), 223–241.

General Behavioral Observation Form

Examining communication in daily contexts is a challenge. One solution to simplify observing specific behaviors is the use of checklists. One such tool, called the General Behavioral Observation Form, was developed by Hartley (1995) as a way for raters to characterize an individual's cognitive functions, including attention, executive functions/meta-cognition, processing and response speed, emotional control, drive, motivation, and memory. The rater judges where the function is "within normal limits," "not able to judge," or is an "area of need." Under the heading "Executive Functioning" the following areas can be rated on this form:

- Awareness of deficits/errors
- Ability to identify goals
- Spontaneous use of strategies
- Awareness of strategies used
- Ability to accept/use feedback
- Self-correction of errors
- Flexibility in shifting tasks
- Level of effort/cooperation. (Hartley, 1995)

In Coelho et al.'s (2005) review of evidence on the use of non-standardized procedures for the assessment of people with TBI, it is recommended that collaborative contextualized hypothesis testing should be used for planning behavioral interventions and to provide supports for the person with TBI. The use of checklists is suggested to have face and content validity but requires ongoing investigation (Table 15-2).

Table 15-2	Summary of Executive Functioning Assessments
Standardized and recommended by ANCDS	• American Speech-Language-Hearing Association Functional Assessment of Communication Skills in Adults (ASHA-FACS) • Behavior Rating Inventory of Executive Function (BRIEF) • Communicative Activities of Daily Living (CADL-2) • Functional Independence Measure (FIM) • Repeatable Battery for the Assessment of Neuropsychological Status (RBANS) • Test of Language Competence—Extended (TLC-E) • Western Aphasia Battery—R
Assessments that evaluate executive functioning and communication in everyday contexts	• Virtual Multiple Errands Test (VMET) • The Awareness of Social Inference Test (TASIT) • Functional Assessment of Verbal Reasoning and Executive Strategies (FAVRES)
Non-standardized approaches to assessing communication and executive functioning	• Contextualized hypothesis testing • General Behavioral Observation form

TREATMENT OF EXECUTIVE FUNCTIONING TO IMPROVE COMMUNICATION OUTCOMES

The effect of damaged executive functioning on communication behavior and the clinical populations in whom this occurs have been described in detail by Cannizzaro and Coelho in Chapter 11. This section will provide an overview of the treatments that have been trialed in the management of executive functioning difficulties with a description of empirical research studies that have focused on executive functioning impairments and that have an impact on an aspect of communicative functioning or on some relevant aspect of everyday behavior where communication is a component.

Treating executive functioning with the view to improving communication outcomes is a relatively new field. As can be seen in the previous section, as assessments are developed and theoretical advances are made in a field, treatments typically follow. Recently, Kennedy and colleagues (2008) conducted an extensive review of intervention for the executive functions of problem solving, planning, organizing, and multitasking by adults with traumatic brain injury. They evaluated 15 studies that met stringent inclusion criteria, including 5 randomized controlled trial treatment studies. The precise executive function that was targeted varied across these studies, with some studies aiming for participants to make realistic predictions or self-monitor their performance during problem solving tasks (e.g., Cicerone & Giacino, 1992) while others emphasized setting and managing goals (e.g., Levine, Robertson, Clare, et al., 2000), managing time (Fasotti, Kovacs, Eling, & Brouwer, 2000), or initiating and sustaining steps in an organized sequence to carry out a functionally complex activity (e.g., Turkstra & Flora, 2002). Additional targets for intervention included improving participants' ability to self-regulate their emotions during problem based activities that also required strategic thinking and finally training strategic problem solving through verbal reasoning abilities (Marshall et al., 2004).

In this section, the treatment approaches for executive functioning deficits have been divided broadly into two sections. The first section describes the treatment approaches that have focused on the person with TBI learning to regulate their own behavior using a range of meta-cognitive strategies.

Meta-cognitive approaches include:

- Problem solving and problem awareness training
- Goal attainment scaling
- Time pressure management
- Verbal self-instruction
- Strategic thinking training

The second, less researched approach is the use of pharmacological interventions.

Where possible, the evidence base has been evaluated for treatments, which have been empirically validated in randomized controlled trials or well designed single case experimental design studies. These summaries are drawn from a downloadable file from PsycBITE (www.psycbite.com) that provides a summary of the paper, description of the method and results, and an overview of the rehabilitation program (Tate, Perdices, McDonald, et al., 2007). Each entry also displays a rating of methodological quality, the PEDro score (Maher, Sherrington, Herbert, et al., 2003) if the paper is a group comparison study and a SCED score (R. Tate, McDonald, Perdices, et al., 2008) if the paper is a single case experimental design. These ratings indicate the degree to which risks of bias were accounted for in the study design. They do not indicate the value of the treatment, but rather offer an indication of the robustness of the findings. Papers are only listed here if they score 5/10 or greater on the PEDro score, and 5/10 or greater on the SCED scale.

Meta-Cognitive Strategy Instruction Approaches

Treatments of executive functioning have been described as meta-cognitive strategy instruction (MSI) approaches, which train participants to solve problems, plan, or be better organized by training step-by-step procedures. Direct instruction is used to teach individuals to regulate their own behavior by breaking complex tasks into steps while thinking strategically (Ehlhardt, Sohlberg, Glang, & Albin, 2005). To be able to self-regulate, persons need to identify an appropriate goal and predict their performance in advance of the activity, identify possible solutions based on their general predictions, and self-monitor their performance and then change their behavior if they determine through self-assessment that the goal has not been met (Kennedy, Coelho, Turkstra, et al., 2008). Early studies commenced work on the obvious problem people with brain injury had in solving problems, and these are discussed in the next section.

Problem Solving Treatments

One of the earliest studies was undertaken by von Cramon and colleagues in 1991 (von Cramon, Matthes-von Cramon, & Mai, 1991). In this study 37 "poor" problem solvers were "randomly" assigned to either a 60-week, 25-session problem solving training (PST) ($n = 20$) or to a memory training (MT; $n = 17$) of comparable intensity and duration. In PST, participants identified problems and solutions, weighed the pros and cons of solutions, and monitored their performance after solutions were implemented. Those who received PST improved on a planning task and on standardized tests more than those who received memory training. Kendall and colleagues extended the work of von Cramon using the D'Zurilla & Goldfried (1971) model of social problem solving (Kendall, Shum, Halson, et al., 1997). In this model, social problem solving is conceptualized as consisting of four specific problem solving skills:

1. Problem definition and formulation of goals
2. Generation of alternative solutions
3. Selection of an appropriate solution, and
4. Implementation and verification of the solution

Kendall and colleagues developed a video assessment task to evaluate social problem solving skills with 15 participants with TBI and a matched control group. In addition, they administered the Social Problem Solving Inventory (Bellack, Sayers, Mueser, & Bennett, 1994) to both groups. Results indicated that individuals with TBI were impaired relative to the control group in their ability to recognize and define social problems and to generate a range of solutions. These differences only emerged during the video task. This led to the conclusion that treatment of social problem solving may be better directed at the early stages of the problem solving process (i.e., identifying and interpreting social problems and generating a range of possible solutions).

Training problem awareness, monitoring, and evaluation was further developed by Miotto and colleagues, with the aim of increasing insight and awareness of how difficulties impact on everyday tasks. In a cross-over study with two control groups, participants were trained to improve their attention and problem solving in an Attention and Problem Solving Rehabilitation Group (APS) (Miotto, Evans, Souza de Lucia, & Scaff, 2009). Thirty participants were allocated to one of three groups: (1) the APS group, (2) an information and education group who received an education booklet about brain injury and suggestions for cognitive exercises, and (3) a traditional treatment group who continued with their regular rehabilitation program. Prior to, immediately following the 10-week, once weekly group, and at 6 months' follow-up, participants were evaluated on the DEX, a modified Multiple Errands Task, and a comprehensive series of neuro-psychological assessments. In the APS group, the first 4 weeks focused on attention skills with the remaining 6 weeks of the training directed toward problem solving skills using the Attention and Problem Solving Framework (see diagram of the framework). This was a systematic approach to identifying ways of solving problems (reducing impulsivity) and managing/monitoring goal achievement through the development of a mental checking/goal management routine. Participants used self-monitoring sheets to record problems as they occurred in everyday life, and to develop an effective plan using a "STOP: THINK!" strategy, as a form of self-instruction to interrupt impulsive action (Figure 15-1). Practice was provided with hypothetical and real-life problems, and in the final stages of the program they were asked to plan and perform a day activity away from the treatment center using the problem solving framework. Results showed some improvement in the APS group on measures of executive functioning and there was some generalization to real-life activities.

Goal Attainment Scaling (GAS) (Table 15-3)

The Goal Attainment Scaling (GAS) technique is another example of meta-cognitive strategy training (Kiresuk & Sherman, 1968). Even though this procedure is now more than 40 years old, it is still in current use in rehabilitation settings (Schlosser, 2004). GAS involves the following steps (Kiresuk & Sherman, 1968): (a) specify a set of goals; (b) assign a weight for each goal according to priority; (c) specify a continuum of possible outcomes (worst expected outcome (−2), less than expected outcome (−1), expected outcome (0), more than expected outcome (+1), and best expected outcome (+2); (c) specify the criteria for scoring at each level; (d) determine current or initial performance; (e) intervene for a specified period; (f) determine performance attained on each objective; and (g) evaluate the degree of attainment. This approach was used to train 8 participants with TBI in a program that focused on "high" involvement with goal setting compared to a control group (the "low" involvement condition) of another 8 people with TBI who monitored progress towards goals (Webb & Glueckauf, 1994). Participants in the "high involvement" group learned the GAS procedure using a series of worksheets: an "Examples of Goal Definitions" worksheet and two other worksheets that focused on perceived goal progress and rating goal attainment levels from their own perspective. While both groups improved in their ability to set goals following the intervention, those in the "high" group were better than the

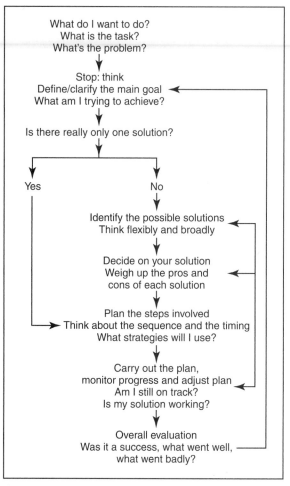

Figure 15-1 Attention and Problem Solving Framework. [From Miotto, E. C., Evans, J. J., Souza de Lucia, M. C., & Scaff, M. (2009). Rehabilitation of executive dysfunction: A controlled trial of an attention and problem solving treatment group. *Neuropsychological Rehabilitation: An International Journal, 19*(4), 517–540.]

"low" group 2 months following the end of treatment. The authors suggested that maintenance was facilitated by the active self-monitoring and the promotion of self-control needed to complete the GAS process. While the nature of the goals was not articulated in this paper, the principles of intervention could easily be applied to people with acquired communication disorders following brain injury.

Time Pressure Management (Table 15-4)

Time pressure management (TPM) is another executive functioning treatment that is of relevance to people with communication disorders in everyday contexts.

Table 15-3   Goal Attainment Scaling Treatment Studies

WEBB & GLUECKAUF (1994)
REHABILITATION
PSYCHOLOGY 39(3), 179–188

PEDro SCORE – 5/10
CLASS I EVIDENCE

Method/Results	Rehabilitation Program

Design
• Study type: RCT
• Population: n = 16 adults with a diagnosis of TBI (GOAT ≥ 80), 88% male, M = 27.4 years (1.9)
• Groups: Two groups based on participant's level of involvement in goal setting:
  1. High Involvement (HI)
  2. Low Involvement (LI)
Setting
Inpatient rehabilitation/community setting
Primary outcome measure/s
• Goal Attainment Scaling.
Secondary outcome measure/s
• None.
Result
Both groups improved from pre- to post-testing, but there was no statistical difference between HI and LI groups at post-treatment. However, at follow-up the HI group had maintained more goals while the LI group had returned to pre-treatment levels (between group statistics performed).
	Aim
	To examine whether the level of participant involvement in goal preparation affects specific rehabilitation outcomes
	Materials
	Goal blocks, specific goal worksheets
	Treatment plan:
	• Duration: 8 weeks (8 hours total)
	• Procedure: 1 session (1 hour) per week
	• Content: There were the three parts to the therapy:
	  1. *Orientation:* Both groups were given a detailed explanation of the goal setting process but more input expected from the HI than the LI group.
	  2. *Goal Setting:* Participants in both groups prioritized their goals (HI on wooden blocks and LI on paper), goals were behaviorally operationalized and goal attainment scaling performed.
	  3. *Goal Monitoring:* HI group taught the Goal Assessment technique, which includes reviewing goals, monitoring and rating own goal progress, and completing a goal follow-up diary. LI group monitored goals but did not use the technique.

Fasotti and colleagues (2000) tested the effectiveness of this approach by comparing it with "concentration therapy" (CT). In TPM treatment, the person with ABI learns to give themselves enough time to deal with the task at hand and therefore prevent or manage time pressure during everyday tasks such as having a conversation. The task was to listen to a videotaped story with the instruction to remember as much as possible. Fasotti and colleagues randomly assigned 22 participants with TBI to either the TPM or CT groups. In the TPM treatment, participants underwent three main stages: (1) participants were made aware of their disability and slowed information processing, (2) participants were trained in the "Let me give myself enough time" cognitive strategy, which involved four steps of self-instruction, including:

1. Recognizing the time pressure at hand,
2. Preventing as much time pressure as possible,
3. Dealing with the time pressure as quickly as possible and encouraging the patient to monitor themselves, and
4. Strategy application and maintenance, where TPM was practiced in increasingly complex conditions with increased distractions.

The concentration group was asked to watch and remember videos using four steps of self-instruction including:

1. Try to focus on and remember the main themes in the story.
2. Do not get distracted by irrelevant sounds from the surrounding environment.
3. Do not get distracted by your own irrelevant thoughts.
4. Try to imagine the things that are said.

While both groups improved following the training programs, the TPM group used more steps to identify solutions to problems and improved more on standardized tests, the benefits of which were maintained at 6 months post-treatment.

These two studies describe the use of problem solving training using similar elements of self-monitoring, self-recording of performance, making strategy decisions based on goals, and adjusting or modifying their performance based on this self-assessment or external feedback. Based on this evidence, Kennedy et al. (2008) suggested a Practice Standard for young to middle aged adults with TBI whereby meta-cognitive strategy instruction (MSI) should be used to improve

Table 15-4 Time Pressure Management Treatment Studies

FASOTTI, KOVACS, ELING, & BROUWER (2000) *NEUROPSYCHOLOGICAL REHABILITATION* 10(1), 47–65	PEDRO SCORE – 5/10 CLASS I EVIDENCE
Method/Results	**Rehabilitation Program**

Method/Results	Rehabilitation Program

Design
• Study type: RCT.
• Population: $n = 22$ (68% male, severe to very severe TBI with slowed processing speed, age 18–45 years).
 	
Groups
1. Experimental Group—TPM ($n = 12$, M = 26.1 years; SD= 8.1)
2. Control Group—concentration training ($n = 10$; M = 30.1 years, SD = 5.5)
 	
Setting
Not stated.
 	
Primary Outcome Measure/s
• Observation checklist to assess the use of the strategies when performing a new story task
• Neuropsychological tests of memory, attention and reaction time including:
• Rey 15 word test
• Rivermead Behavioural Memory Test
• PASAT
• Auditory Concentration Test
• Visual reaction time measures
 	
Secondary Outcome Measure/s
• Psychosocial well-being questionnaires and measures of general activity (number of social contacts and leisure activities).
 	
Result
Treatment was effective compared to the concentration training, with both an increased number of steps taken to reduce time pressure and a greater level of managing performance after training for the Experimental Group vs. Control Group. Some significant increases in attention and memory scores over time were found for the TPM group, but not for the control group. No significant group differences were found for psychosocial measures.
	Aim
	To improve information processing by teaching skills in Time Pressure Management (TPM) to compensate for mental slowness
	
	Materials
	9 videotaped short stories of 1–4 mins, video player, TV, cassette recorder, audio tape with recorded radio broadcasts (e.g., music and news), and telephone
	
	Treatment Plan
	• Duration: 2–3 weeks (mean length of training 7.4 hrs)
	• Procedure: Up to 3 sessions/wk, 1 hr/session
	
	Content
	Experimental Group:
	Based on models of Ylvisaker et al. (1987) and Meichenbaum (1977, 1980), 9 short stories are administered to enable teaching TPM strategies (e.g., a scenario is given: "Imagine you are outside a railway station in a strange town and you ask a passerby the way to the tourist office." The videotape shows a man giving directions. The patient is asked to repeat as much as possible).
	    Strategies are taught using self-instructional methods in 3 stages:
	1. Awareness of errors and deficits (given feedback)
	2. Acceptance and acquisition of the 4-step TPM strategy
	3. Application and maintenance in more challenging circumstances (e.g., more distracting environments)
	The training focuses on time pressure and its negative effects on task performance.
	    Control Group:
	    The same 9 short stories are administered, with 4 generic suggestions given to recall information.

problem solving, planning, and organizational skills deficits. They reported that the available evidence exceeded the minimum requirements set forth by the American Academy of Neurology for this level of recommendation. Kennedy et al. (2008) also suggested that there was less available evidence to support the maintenance of activity outcomes following the withdrawal of MSI treatment; however, there was sufficient positive evidence from three RCTs (Fasotti et al., 2000; Rath, Simon, Langenbahn, et al., 2003; Webb & Glueckauf, 1994) for it to be considered likely.

Verbal Self-Instruction (Table 15-5)

Verbal self-instruction is another strategy that has been employed to improve planning and organization (Cicerone & Wood, 1987; Turkstra & Flora, 2002). Turkstra & Flora (2002) used step-by-step organizational strategies and role play activities with a person with TBI whose aim was to return to work as a counselor. His difficulties arose when he attempted to take notes and write reports during interviews with clients. Through the use of over-learned carrier phrases and the structure of S.O.A.P.—that is, (S) subjective comments by the person interviewed; (O), objective data; (A), a

Table 15-5 Verbal Self-Instruction Treatment Studies

TURKSTRA & FLORA (2002) *JOURNAL OF COMMUNICATION DISORDERS 35,* 467–482	SCED SCORE – 5/10 CLASS III EVIDENCE
Method/Results	**Rehabilitation Program**
Design	***Aim***
• Study type: SSD; pre-post (A-B) single case design	To improve note taking and report writing accuracy.
• Participant: *n* = 1 called A.P. with a diagnosis of multiple TBIs with a severe TBI at age 26 yrs; coma duration = 1 week; severity = severe memory and executive impairment; years post-trauma = 23. A.P. was male, aged 49, having difficulty with work as a counselor due to executive functioning organization deficits.	***Materials*** Pen, paper, laptop, role play materials for cases
Setting	***Treatment Plan***
Community setting	• *Duration:* 21 sessions of 1 hour each over 10 weeks
Target Behavior Measure/s	• *Procedure:* Therapy sessions included 5 minutes conversation, 5 minutes writing to dictation, and 50 minutes on report writing
• Report writing accuracy	
• Self-reported level of ease with report-writing	• *Content:* Participant was trained to use the S.O.A.P. format used by health professionals to listen to, write notes about, and report on a case: (S) subjective comments by the person interviewed, (O), objective data, (A), a statement of the assessment, and (P) plans for the next session (see Appendix 15-1).
• Success in obtaining competitive employment	
Control Outcome Measure/s	
• Spelling accuracy	
• Discourse cohesion	
Result	
Training enabled A.P. to learn a procedure for reporting facts more accurately, eliminating extraneous information and increasing efficiency. Templates were adapted for inclusion in the work setting, and after multiple attempts A.P. found employment as a counselor.	

statement of the assessment; and (P), plans for the next session—which were used to help him listen to, write notes, and report on a case, the participant was able to improve his note taking and report writing performance and efficiency and ultimately he obtained employment as a counselor.

Treatment of Strategic Thinking (Table 15-6)

Strategic thinking is an automatic and unconscious process that we undertake when we need to solve a problem. In those cases where frontal damage has occurred, some authors have approached the difficulty of teaching problem solving strategies by instructional techniques focusing on explicit verbal reasoning (Fox, Martella, & Marchand-Martella, 1989; Marshall et al., 2004) or in one study the use of an instructional package called TEACH-M (Ehlhardt, Sohlberg, Glang & Albin, 2005). TEACH-M was based on evidence from special education and neuropsychological rehabilitation research. Four individuals with severe memory and executive functioning impairments were taught a multi-step procedure to facilitate learning and retention of an e-mail task.

In the Ehlhardt et al. (2005) study, three participants retained the email procedure after a 30-day break and all participants generalized their skills to an untrained interface. All participants reported enthusiasm for the teaching program, stating they would recommend it to a friend. Instructional components reported to be most helpful included instructor modeling of the steps and having four or five treatment sessions each week.

PHARMACOLOGICAL INTERVENTION

With increasingly sophisticated pharmacological advances, there have been a small number of studies examining the effectiveness of medication to manage cognitive behaviors following acquired brain injury. The use of bromocriptine was compared with a placebo with significant improvements for the drug treatment group on measures of executive function and in dual-task performance (McDowell, Whyte, & D'Esposito, 1998). However, other studies have shown no significant differences between treatment and placebo groups following the administration of methylphenidate (Speech, Rao, Osmon, & Sperry, 1993) or amantadine (Schneider, Drew-Cates, Wong, & Dombovy, 1999). In contrast, positive improvements in attention, memory, and naming skills were reported

Table 15-6   Strategic Thinking Treatment Studies

EHLHARDT, SOHLBERG, GLANG,
& ALBIN (2005) *BRAIN INJURY 19*(8), 569–583

SCED SCORE—8/10
CLASS III EVIDENCE

Method/Results

Design

- Study type: Single subject design. Multiple baselines across partici-pants, with follow-up 1 month post-treatment
- Participants: $n = 4$, etiology—TBI, coma duration > 1 month, severity-severe memory and executive impairment, years post-trauma $= 23.3$ (SD $= 6.9$)
  1. Participant 1: Male, aged 48
  2. Participant 2: Male, aged 47
  3. Participant 3: Female, aged 58
  4. Participant 4: Female, aged 36

Setting

Community setting: Local transitional living programs and support groups

Target Behavior Measure/s

- Number of correct steps completed in sequence on an e-mail task
- Number of correct steps completed, regardless of sequence, on an e-mail task
- Number of training sessions needed to reach mastery criterion (100% correct for 7/7 steps)

Primary Outcome Measure/s

- None

Result

Training enabled participants to learn a procedure for using an e-mail interface with 100% accuracy within 7–15 days. Treatment effect generalized to a novel e-mail interface and/or an unrelated computer game. Skills were maintained at 1 month post-training. Data were graph-ically presented but not statistically analyzed.

Rehabilitation Program

Aim

To improve procedural memory in participants with memory and executive impairment

Materials

Computer software to simulate an e-mail interface

Treatment Plan

- Duration: 7–15 days, number of total contact hours not specified.
- Procedure: Daily training sessions of unspecified duration.
- Content: Participants are trained to use a simulated e-mail interface to read and reply to e-mails from four hypothetical persons (doctor, counselor, dentist, and friend). There were four categories of e-mail messages: billing, appointments, direction to appointments, invitation to go out. The training method (TEACH-M) emphasizes task analysis, errorless learning, ongoing assessment of task performance, cumulative review of acquired skills, and frequent practice of skills.

---

for nine patients in a study of 20 people with TBI who received for Cerebrolysin (Alvarez, Sampedro, Perez, et al., 2003).

Improvements have also been reported in two people with severe chronic traumatic brain injury who were administered methylphenidate to reduce perseveration during conversation (Frankel & Penn, 2007). Both participants were noted to improve during the active drug phase with amelioration of perseverative manifestations, evidence of improved topic shift and contribution to conversation, and a greater capacity for reconstitution and working memory tasks.

CONCLUSIONS

Executive functioning deficits following acquired brain injury impact on all aspects of everyday functioning, including communication skills. While there is a paucity

of assessments to directly evaluate the interplay between executive functioning and communication, it is gratify-ing to see progress being made in this area with the publication of assessments such as the TASIT and the FAVRES. In addition to these new assessments, clini-cians need to be aware of the impact impaired execu-tive functioning can have on communication in daily life and to ensure that they are assessing these situa-tions routinely. Reliance on standardized communica-tion assessments that can ameliorate the effects of poor executive function can lead to misdiagnosis and there-fore inappropriate treatment recommendations. It is therefore critical to evaluate communication in condi-tions that resemble everyday situations.

In reviewing the treatment studies that have either directly or indirectly focused on communication out-comes, Kennedy et al. (2008) concluded that there was sufficient evidence to recommend meta-cognitive strat-egy instruction as a practice standard for young to middle aged adults for difficulty with planning, problem solving, and organization. There was also evidence for strategic thinking interventions for verbal reasoning in middle-aged adults with chronic disability. Treatment in everyday tasks and contexts is recommended, with a focus on self-regulation, self-monitoring, and use of activity and participation outcome measures. Treatments have been effective in both individual and group formats, and the "active ingredients" in successful executive functioning treatments have been described as having individualized goal setting, use of meta-cognitive strategies that encourage self-regulation, internalization or self-instruction, structure and practice in a variety of real-life environment, and explicit feedback or training in self-evaluation systems, such as the use of video-taped feedback (Kennedy et al., 2008; MacDonald & Wiseman-Hakes, 2010). Effective executive functioning treatments rely on clear step-by-step instructional techniques that build skills within everyday interactional tasks and that are meaningful for the individuals with brain injury and their families. It is expected that communication treatments will become increasingly sophisticated as our appreciation of the components of successful intervention advances. There is still some way to go with regard to identifying which components of the practice regime are most effective, or the duration and intensity of treatment that is needed to effect change. Incorporating experience dependent neuroplasticity principles (Kleim & Jones, 2008) into future treatment studies will assist this process of continued development of treatments. In the meantime, being aware of the essential ingredients identified to date will assist clinicians in designing treatments that are both clinically meaningful and maximally effective in the management of communication difficulties following acquired brain injury.

REFERENCES

Alderman, N., Burgess, P. W., Knight, C., & Henman, C. (2003). Ecological validity of a simplified version of the Multiple Errands Shopping Test. *Journal of the International Neuropsychological Society, 9*(1), 31–44.

Alvarez, X. A., Sampedro, C., Perez, P., Laredo, M., Couceiro, V., Hernandez, A., et al. (2003). Positive effects of Cerebrolysin on electroencephalogram slowing, cognition and clinical outcome in patients with postacute traumatic brain injury: an exploratory study. *International Clinical Psychopharmacology, 18*(5), 271–278.

Anderson, C., Bigler, E., & Blatter, D. D. (1995). Frontal lobe lesions, diffuse damage, and neuropsychological functioning in traumatic brain-injured patients. *Journal of Clinical and Experimental Neuropsychology, 17*, 900–908.

Baddeley, A. (1986). *Working memory*. Oxford, UK: Oxford University Press.

Bellack, A., Sayers, M., Mueser, K., & Bennett, M. (1994). Evaluation of social problem-solving in schizophrenia. *Journal of Abnormal Psychology, 103*, 371–378.

Bennett, P., Ong, B., & Ponsford, J. (2005). Measuring executive dysfunction in an acute rehabilitation setting: Using the dysexecutive questionnaire (DEX). *Journal of the International Neuropsychological Society, 11*(04), 376–385.

Bibby, H., & McDonald, S. (2005). Theory of mind after traumatic brain injury. *Neuropsychologia, 43*(1), 99–114.

Body, R., & Perkins, M. (2006). Terminology and methodology in the assessment of cognitive-linguistic disorders. *Brain Impairment, 7*(3), 212–222.

Bond, F., & Godfrey, H. P. D. (1997). Conversation with traumatically brain-injured individuals: a controlled study of behavioural changes and their impact. *Brain Injury, 11*(5), 319–329.

Burgess, P. W., Alderman, N., Forbes, C., Costello, A., Coates, L. M., Dawson, D. R., et al. (2006). The case for the development and use of "ecologically valid" measures of executive function in experimental and clinical neuropsychology. *Journal of the International Neuropsychological Society, 12*(2), 194–209.

Cicerone, K., & Giacino, J. (1992). Remediation of executive function deficits after traumatic brain injury. *NeuroRehabilitation, 2*, 12–22.

Cicerone, K., & Wood, J. (1987). Planning disorder after closed head injury: A case study. *Archives of Physical Medicine and Rehabilitation, 68*, 111–115.

Coelho, C., Ylvisaker, M., & Turkstra, L. S. (2005). Nonstandardized assessment approaches for individuals with traumatic brain injuries. *Seminars in Speech & Language, 4*, 223–241.

Coelho, C. A., Youse, K. M., & Le, K. N. (2002). Conversational discourse in closed-head-injured and non-brain-injured adults. *Aphasiology, 16*(4–6), 659–672.

D'Zurilla, T., & Goldfried, M. (1971). Problem solving and behavior modification. *Journal of Abnormal Psychology, 78*, 107–126.

Ehlhardt, L. A., Sohlberg, M., Glang, A., & Albin, R. (2005). TEACH-M: A pilot study evaluating an instructional sequence for persons with impaired memory and executive functions. *Brain Injury, 19*(8), 569–583.

Eslinger, P., & Damasio, A. (1985). Severe disturbance of higher cognition following bilateral frontal lobe oblation: Patient EVR. *Neurology, 35*, 1731–1741.

Fasotti, L., Kovacs, F., Eling, P. A. T. M., & Brouwer, W. H. (2000). Time pressure management as a compensatory strategy training after closed head injury. *Neuropsychological Rehabilitation: An International Journal, 10*(1), 47–65.

F. I. M. (1996). *Uniform data set for medical rehabilitation*. Buffalo, NY: University at Buffalo.

Fox, R. M., Martella, R. C., & Marchand-Martella, N. E. (1989). The acquisition, maintenance, and generalization of problem-solving skills by closed head-injured adults. *Behavior Therapy, 20*(1), 61–76.

Frankel, T., & Penn, C. (2007). Perseveration and conversation in TBI: Response to pharmacological intervention. *Aphasiology, 21*(10–11), 1039–1078.

Frattali, C. M., Thompson, C. M., Holland, A. L., Wohl, C. B., & Ferketic, M. M. (1995). ASHA FACS—A functional outcome measure for adults. *ASHA, April,* 40–46.

Gioia, G., Isquith, P., Guy, S., & Kenworthy, L. (2000). *Behavior Rating Inventory of Executive Function.* Odessa, FL: Psychological Assessment Resources.

Godfrey, H., & Shum, D. (2000). Executive functioning and the application of social skills following traumatic brain injury. *Aphasiology, 14*(4), 433–444.

Green, R. E., Colella, B., Hebert, D. A., Bayley, M., Kang, H. S., Till, C., et al. (2008). Prediction of return to productivity after severe traumatic brain injury: Investigations of optimal neuropsychological tests and timing of assessment. [Comparative Study Research Support, Non-U.S. Gov't]. *Archives of Physical Medicine & Rehabilitation, 89*(12 Suppl), S51–60.

Hagen, C. (1984). Language disorders in head trauma. In A. Holland (Ed.), *Language disorders in adults* (pp. 245–281). San Diego, CA: College Hill Press.

Hartley, L. L. (1995). *Cognitive-communicative abilities following brain injury: A functional approach.* San Diego, CA: Singular.

Henry, J. D., Phillips, L. H., Crawford, J. R., Ietswaart, M., & Summers, F. (2006). Theory of mind following traumatic brain injury: The role of emotion recognition and executive dysfunction. *Neuropsychologia, 44*(10), 1623–1628.

Holland, A., Frattali, C., & Fromm, D. (1999). *Communication activities of daily living: Second Edition—CADL-2.* Austin, TX: Pro-Ed.

Holland, A. L. (1982). When is aphasia aphasia? The problem of closed head injury. In R. H. Brookshire (Ed.), *Clinical Aphasiology Conference proceedings* (pp. 345–349). Minneapolis, MN: BRK Publishers.

Isaki, E., & Turkstra, L. (2000). Communication abilities and work re-entry following traumatic brain injury. *Brain Injury, 14*(5), 441–453.

Keil, K., & Kaszniak, A. W. (2002). Examining executive function in individuals with brain injury: A review. *Aphasiology, 16*(3), 305–335.

Kendall, E., Shum, D., Halson, D., Bunning, S., & Teh, M. (1997). The assessment of social problem-solving ability following traumatic brain injury. *Journal of Head Trauma Rehabilitation, 12* (3), 68–78.

Kennedy, M. R. T., Coelho, C., Turkstra, L., Ylvisaker, M., Moore Sohlberg, M., Yorkston, K., et al. (2008). Intervention for executive functions after traumatic brain injury: A systematic review, meta-analysis and clinical recommendations. *Neuropsychological Rehabilitation: An International Journal, 18*(3), 257–299.

Kennedy, M. R. T., & DeRuyter, F. (1991). Cognitive and language bases for communication disorders. In D. R. Beukelman & K. M. Yorkston (Eds.), *Communication disorders following traumatic brain injury: Management of cognitive, language and motor impairments* (pp. 123–190). Austin, TX: Pro-Ed.

Kertesz, A. (2006). *Western Aphasia Battery—Revised (WAB-R).* Oxford, UK: Pearson PsychCorp.

Kilov, A. M., Togher, L., & Grant, S. (2009). Problem solving with friends: Discourse participation and performance of individuals with and without traumatic brain injury. *Aphasiology, 23*(5), 584–605.

Kipps, C., Nestor, P., Acosta-Cabronero, J., Arnold, R., & Hodges, J. (2009). Understanding social dysfunction in the behavioral variant of frontotemporal dementia: The role of emotion and sarcasm processing. *Brain: A Journal of Neurology, 132*(3), 592–603.

Kiresuk, T., & Sherman, R. (1968). Goal attainment scaling: A general method for evaluating comprehensive community mental health programs. *Community Mental Health Journal, 4,* 443–453.

Kleim, J. A., & Jones, T. A. (2008). Principles of experience-dependent neural plasticity: Implications for rehabilitation after brain damage. *Journal of Speech, Language, and Hearing Research, 51*(1), S225–S239.

Knight, C., Alderman, N., & Burgess, P. W. (2002). Development of a simplified version of the multiple errands test for use in hospital settings. *Neuropsychological Rehabilitation, 12*(3), 231–256.

Levin, H., Goldstein, F., Williams, D., & Eisenberg, H. (1991). The contribution of frontal lobe lesions to the neurobehavioral outcome of closed head injury. In H. Levin, H. Eisenberg, & A. Benton (Eds.), *Frontal lobe function and dysfunction* (pp. 318–338). New York: Oxford University Press.

Levine, B., Robertson, I. H., Clare, L., Carter, G., Hong, J., Wilson, B. A., et al. (2000). Rehabilitation of executive functioning: An experimental-clinical validation of Goal Management Training. *Journal of the International Neuropsychological Society, 6*(3), 299–312.

Lezak, M. D. (1993). Newer contributions to the neuropsychological assessment of executive functions. *Journal of Head Trauma Rehabilitation, 8* (1), 24–31.

MacDonald, S. (1998). *Functional assessment of verbal reasoning and executive strategies.* Guelph, Canada: Clinical Publishing.

MacDonald, S., & Johnson, C. (2005). Assessment of subtle cognitive-communication deficits following acquired brain injury: A normative study of the functional assessment of verbal reasoning and executive strategies (FAVRES). *Brain Injury, 19*(11), 895–902.

MacDonald, S., & Wiseman-Hakes, C. (2010). Knowledge translation in ABI rehabilitation: A model for consolidating and applying the evidence for cognitive-communication interventions. *Brain Injury, 24*(3), 486–508.

Maher, C., Sherrington, C., Herbert, R., Moseley, A., & Elkins, M. (2003). Reliability of the PEDro scale for rating quality of randomized controlled trials. *Physical Therapy, 83,* 713–721.

Manchester, D., Priestley, N., & Jackson, H. (2004). The assessment of executive functions: Coming out of the office. *Brain Injury, 18*(11), 1067–1081.

Marshall, R. C., Capilouto, G. J., & McBride, J. M. (2007). Treatment of problem solving in Alzheimer's disease: a short report. *Aphasiology, 21*(2), 235–247.

Marshall, R. C., Karow, C. M., Morelli, C. A., Iden, K. K., Dixon, J., & Cranfill, T. B. (2004). Effects of interactive strategy modelling training on problem-solving by persons with traumatic brain injury. *Aphasiology, 18*(8), 659–673.

Martin, I., & McDonald, S. (2005). Evaluating the causes of impaired irony comprehension following traumatic brain injury. *Aphasiology 19*(8), 712–730.

Martin, I., & McDonald, S. (2006). That can't be right! What causes pragmatic language impairment following right hemisphere damage? *Brain Impairment 7*(3), 202–211.

McDonald, S. (1992). Communication disorders following closed head injury: New approaches to assessment and rehabilitation. *Brain Injury, 6*, 283–292.

McDonald, S. (1993). Pragmatic skills after closed head injury: Ability to meet the informational needs of the listener. *Brain and Language, 44*(1), 28–46.

McDonald, S. (2000). Neuropsychological studies of sarcasm. *Metaphor and Symbol, 15*(1–2), 85–98.

McDonald, S. (2007). The social and neuropsychological underpinnings of communication disorders after severe traumatic brain injury. In M. Ball & J. Damico (Eds.), *Clinical aphasiology: Future directions—a festschrift for Chris Code.* (pp. 42–71). New York: Psychology Press.

McDonald, S., Bornhofen, C., Shum, D., Long, E., Saunders, C., & Neulinger, K. (2006). Reliability and validity of the Awareness of Social Inference Test (TASIT): A clinical test of social perception. *Disability and Rehabilitation: An International, Multidisciplinary Journal, 28*(24), 1529–1542.

McDonald, S., Flanagan, S., & Rollins, J. (2002). *The Awareness of Social Inference Test.* Edmonds, UK: Thames Valley Test Company.

McDonald, S., & Pearce, S. (1996). Clinical insights into pragmatic theory: Frontal lobe deficits and sarcasm. *Brain and Language, 53*(1), 81–104.

McDonald, S., & Pearce, S. (1998). Requests that overcome listener reluctance: Impairment associated with executive dysfunction in brain injury. *Brain and Language, 61*, 88–104.

McDonald, S., & Sommers, P. v. (1993). Differential pragmatic language loss following closed head injury: Ability to negotiate requests. *Cognitive Neuropsychology, 10*, 297–315.

McDonald, S., Tate, R., Togher, L., Bornhofen, C., Long, E., Gertler, P., et al. (2008). Social skills treatment for people with severe, chronic acquired brain injuries: A multicenter trial. *Archives of Physical Medicine & Rehabilitation, 89*, 1648–1659.

McDowell, S., Whyte, J., & D'Esposito, M. (1998). Differential effect of a dopaminergic agonist on prefrontal function in traumatic brain injury patients. *Brain 121*(Pt 6), 1155–1164.

Miotto, E. C., Evans, J. J., Souza de Lucia, M. C., & Scaff, M. (2009). Rehabilitation of executive dysfunction: A controlled trial of an attention and problem solving treatment group. *Neuropsychological Rehabilitation: An International Journal, 19*(4), 517–540.

Meichenbaum, D. (1977). *Cognitive behaviour modification. An integrative approach.* New York: Plenum Press.

Meichenbaum, D. (1980). Self instructional methods. In F. H. Kaufer & A. Goldstein (Eds.), *Helping people change.* New York: Pergamon Press.

O'Brien, A. R., Chiaravalloti, N., Goverover, Y., & DeLuca, J. (Writer). (2008). Evidenced-based cognitive rehabilitation for persons with multiple sclerosis: A review of the literature. doi: DOI: 10.1016/j.apmr.2007.10.019

Pearce, S., McDonald, S., & Coltheart, M. (1998). Interpreting ambiguous advertisements: The effect of frontal lobe damage. *Brain and Cognition 38*(2), 150–164.

Prigatano, G. P., Roueche, J. R., & Fordyce, D. J. (1985). Non-aphasic language disturbances after closed head injury. *Language Sciences, 7*, 217–229.

Rand, D., Katz, N., & Weiss, P. L. (2007). Evaluation of virtual shopping in the VMall: Comparison of post-stroke participants to healthy control groups. *Disability and Rehabilitation: An International, Multidisciplinary Journal, 29*(22), 1710–1719.

Rand, D., Rukan, S. B.-A., Weiss, P. L., & Katz, N. (2009). Validation of the Virtual MET as an assessment tool for executive functions. *Neuropsychological Rehabilitation: An International Journal, 19*(4), 583–602.

Randolph, C. (2001). *Repeatable battery for the assessment of neuropsychological status.* San Antonio, TX: Psychological Corporation.

Rankin, K. P., Salazar, A., Gorno-Tempini, M. L., Sollberger, M., Wilson, S. M., Pavlic, D., et al. (2009). Detecting sarcasm from paralinguistic cues: Anatomic and cognitive correlates in neurodegenerative disease. *NeuroImage, 47*(4), 2005–2015.

Rath, J. F., Simon, D., Langenbahn, D. M., Sherr, R. L., & Diller, L. (2003). Group treatment of problem-solving deficits in outpatients with traumatic brain injury: A randomised outcome study. *Neuropsychological Rehabilitation, 13*(4), 461–488.

Schlosser, R. W. (2004). Goal attainment scaling as a clinical measurement technique in communication disorders: A critical review. *Journal of Communication Disorders, 37*(3), 217–239.

Schneider, W. N., Drew-Cates, J., Wong, T. M., & Dombovy, M. L. (1999). Cognitive and behavioral efficacy of amantadine in acute traumatic brain injury: An initial double-blind placebo-controlled study. *Brain Injury, 13*(11), 863–872.

Schweizer, T. A., Levine, B., Rewilak, D., O'Connor, C., Turner, G., Alexander, M. P., et al. (2008). Rehabilitation of executive functioning after focal damage to the cerebellum. *Neurorehabilitation & Neural Repair, 22*(1), 72–77.

Shallice, T. (1988). *From neuropsychology to mental structure.* Cambridge, UK: Cambridge University Press.

Shallice, T., & Burgess, P. (1991). Deficits in strategy application following frontal lobe damage in man. *Brain 114*, 727–741.

Speech, T. J., Rao, S. M., Osmon, D. C., & Sperry, L. T. (1993). A double-blind controlled study of methylphenidate treatment in closed head injury. *Brain Injury, 7*(4), 333–338.

Stuss, D. T., & Benson, D. F. (1984). Neuropsychological studies of the frontal lobes. *Psychological Bulletin, 95*(1), 3–28.

Tate, R. (1999). Executive dysfunction and characterological changes after traumatic brain injury: Two sides of the same coin? *Cortex, 35*(1), 39–55.

Tate, R., McDonald, S., Perdices, M., Togher, L., Schultz, R., & Savage, S. (2008). Rating the methodological quality of single-subject designs and n-of-1 trials: Introducing the Single-Case Experimental Design (SCED) Scale. *Neuropsychological rehabilitation, 18*(4), 385–401.

Tate, R., Perdices, M., McDonald, S., Togher, L., Schultz, R., & Savage, S. (2007). *PsycBITE rehabilitation summaries.* Sydney, AU: Psychologist's Registration Board of NSW.

Tate, R. L., Lulham, J. M., Broe, G. A., Strettles, B., & Pfaff, A. (1989). Psychosocial outcome for the survivors of severe blunt head injury: The results from a consecutive series of 100 patients. *Journal of Neurology, Neurosurgery, and Psychiatry, 52,* 1128–1134.

Togher, L., Hand, L., & Code, C. (1997). Analyzing discourse in the traumatic brain injury population:telephone interactions with different communication partners. *Brain Injury, 11*(3), 169–189.

Turkstra, L., Ylvisaker, M., Coelho, C., Kennedy, M., Sohlberg, M. M., Avery, J., et al. (2005). Practice guidelines for standardized assessment for persons with traumatic brain injury. *Journal of Medical Speech-Language Pathology, 13*(2), ix–xxxviii.

Turkstra, L. S., Coelho, C., & Ylvisaker, M. (2005). The use of standardized tests for individuals with cognitive-communication disorders. *Seminars in Speech & Language, 26*(4), 215–222.

Turkstra, L. S., & Flora, T. L. (2002). Compensating for executive function impairments after TBI: A single case study of functional intervention. *Journal of Communication Disorders, 35*(6), 467–482.

Turkstra, L. S., McDonald, S., & Kaufman, P. M. (1995). Assessment of pragmatic skills in adolescents after traumatic brain injury. *Brain Injury, 10*(5), 329–345.

von Cramon, D. Y., Matthes-von Cramon, G., & Mai, N. (1991). Problem-solving deficits in brain-injured patients: A therapeutic approach. *Neuropsychological Rehabilitation, 1*(1), 45–64.

Webb, P. M., & Glueckauf, R. L. (1994). The effects of direct involvement in goal setting on rehabilitation outcome for persons with traumatic brain injuries. *Rehabilitation Psychology Fall, 39*(3), 179–188.

Wiig, E., & Secord, W. (1989). *Test of Language Competence—Expanded Edition.* San Antonio, TX: Psychological Corporation.

Wilson, B., Alderman, N., Burgess, P., Emslie, H., & Evans, J. (1996). *Behavioural assessment of the dysexecutive syndrome: Test manual.* Cambridge, England: Thames Valley Test Company.

Ylvisaker, M., & Feeney, T. (1998). *Collaborative brain injury intervention: Positive everyday routines.* San Diego: Singular Publishing Group.

Ylvisaker, M., & Szekeres, S. F. (1994). Communication Disorders Associated with Closed Head Injury. In R. Chapey (Ed.), *Language Intervention Strategies in Adult Aphasia* (3rd ed., pp. 546–568). Baltimore, Maryland: Williams & Wilkins.

15-1

Suggested Treatment Protocols for Executive Functioning and Communication After Traumatic Brain Injury

Treatment Approach	Description
Social problem solving training (von Cramon et al., 1991; D'Zurilla & Goldfried, 1971; Kendall et al., 1997)	Ask the person to engage in the following aspects of problem solving in response to video stimuli. 1. Problem identification and formulation of goals 2. Generate alternative solutions 3. Weigh the pros and cons of solutions and select one 4. Implement the solution Kendall and colleagues used 12 videos of situations from 4 categories of problems: a. Refusing unreasonable requests b. Dealing with criticism c. Dealing with objectionable behavior from others d. Understanding nonverbal behavior Each 30-second video encapsulated the problem but did not resolve the conflict. Patients were asked to attempt each of the steps of problem solving separately. 1. To assess problem definition and formulation, participants were asked simply whether a problem existed in the video and if so, what it was. 2. The person was asked to generate as many possible solutions as they could. 3. They were then asked to choose the best possible solution and describe the possible consequences of the solutions. 4. Finally, the participants were asked to watch the video, and were given the problem and a selected solution. They were then asked to describe how they would implement that strategy (i.e., what would they say or do) and what they thought would happen as a result of their choice.
Attention and problem solving training (Miotto et al., 2009)	1. Problem awareness, monitoring and evaluation This step uses self-monitoring sheets to record problems as they occur in day-to-day life, receive education about brain injury and consequences of behavior, and complete exercises with different attentional demands (e.g., sustained, divided, selective). Tasks are provided that make demands on planning and goal management. Strategies taught include: using goal management training concepts of checking the mental blackboard, time management strategies, environment modification, cue cards, and watch alarms. 2. Developing a plan The goal is to teach clients to replace impulsive or inappropriate responses, based on the steps in Figure 15-1. Strategy: STOP:THINK! which is a form of self-instruction to interrupt impulsive action when faced with a problem. Practice is given in hypothetical and real-life situations. Clients are encouraged to generate a range of possible solutions to problems, using divergent thinking, and to create strategies to implement plans of action including attention strategies and memory aids. In the final stage, clients plan and perform an activity away from the center. 3. Initiating and implementing a plan Miotto and colleagues acknowledge that some people with TBI have difficulty translating attention into action. They recommend the use of compensatory mechanisms such as electronic reminder systems (e.g., alarms) in conjunction with external reminders (such as diaries, checklists).

Continued

Treatment Approach	Description
Goal setting treatment (Webb & Glueckauf, 1994)	This protocol describes the intervention given to a group of people with TBI who received treatment designed to facilitate high involvement (HI) in their goal setting over 8 individual sessions.
	1. Orientation
	A detailed description of the goal-setting process is provided and participants are encouraged to ask questions and discuss the importance of setting personal rehabilitation goals.
	2. Goal setting
	Each goal is written on small wooden blocks, which are then arranged in rank order from their most important to least important area. Examples of goal areas include: "socialization" and "community integration." Once they are prioritized, create a specific, behavioral goal based on the first goal priority.
	3. Goal monitoring
	Review each chosen goal with the person using worksheets designed so that he/she can describe perceived goal progress and rate goal attainment processes using the Goal Attainment Scale. The participants are asked to monitor their goals in a diary format as well as being verbally reviewed each week.
Time pressure management (TPM) (Fasotti et al., 2000)	The person learns to give himself/herself enough time to deal with a task (such as having a conversation) by preventing or managing time pressure.
	Three main stages to TPM:
	1. Participants are made aware of their disability and slowed information processing. They are asked to watch videos and recall as many details as they can. The amount they recall is given to them (a "reproduction score").
	2. Participants are trained to "Let me give myself enough time" strategy, which has 4 steps:
	a. Recognize the time pressure (Ask the question "Are there two or more things to done at the same time for which there is not enough time?" If yes, go to step 2, or else just do the task)
	b. Prevent as much time pressure as possible (Make a short plan of which things can be done before the actual task begins)
	c. Deal with the time pressure as quickly as possible (Make an emergency plan describing what to do in case of overwhelming time pressure)
	d. Encourage self-monitoring (Plan and emergency plan ready? Then use it regularly)
	3. In strategy application and maintenance, TPM is practiced in increasingly complex conditions with increased distractions (e.g., during the presentation of videotaped stories a radio was playing in the background, or the phone rang).
	A behavioral observation list was developed to assess the use of strategies during the treatment and were scored with 1 point each for each task:
	1. Asking for information about the content in the video in a concise and plain way
	2. Asking questions about the instructions
	3. Asking if the radio could be turned off or down
	4. Making a written plan on how to perform the task
	5. Reiterating the most important instructions
	6. Interrupting the video
	7. Asking the clinician for clarification
	8. Asking for a short pause

Treatment Approach	Description
Verbal self instruction (Turkstra & Flora, 2002)	21 therapy sessions of 1 hour each over 10 weeks to train a person with brain injury wanting to return to work as a counselor. The goal was to improve his note-taking and report writing. Each session included 5 minutes of writing to dictation (control task), and 50 minutes work on report writing.
	The S.O.A.P. format was used: (S), subjective comments by the person interviewed, (O) objective data from the session, (A), a statement of assessment, and (P) plans for the next session. The format was modified with the use of carrier phrases:
	Example:
	Client says _____
	O—Objective
	I see _____
	The client talked about _____
	I said to the client _____
	I explained _____
	A—Assessment
	My impression of this client is _____
	Her prognosis is _____
	P—Plan
	My recommended plan is _____.
	These carrier phrases were used both in the interview and in the report. The patient practices using the format in role-play sessions based on client scenarios, with at least one new case each session to facilitate generalization.
TEACH-M (Ehlhardt et al., 2005)	This is an instructional package that facilitates learning and retention of procedures for using a simple email interface.
	The TEACH-M components include:
	1. *Task analysis:* Know the instructional content. Break it into small steps. Chain steps together.
	2. *Errorless Learning:* Keep errors to a minimum during the acquisition phase. Model target steps before the client attempts a new step. Carefully fade support. If an error occurs, demonstrate the correct/skill right away and ask the client to do it again.
	3. *Assess performance* (initial): Assess skills before treatment; (ongoing)—probe performance at the beginning of each teaching session and/or before introducing a new step.
	4. *Cumulative review:* Review regularly previously learned skills.
	5. *High rates of correct practice trials:* Practice the skill several times. Spaced retrieval is helpful. This is one form of errorless learning that builds in review and practice with opportunities to recall the email steps over increasing intervals of time.
	6. *Meta-cognitive strategy training:* The prediction technique can be used to encourage active processing of the material. The reflection-prediction technique asks participants to reflect on their performance during the task analysis and practice phase and then predict which email steps would be easy and which would be difficult during the subsequent phase. Laminated screenshots of each of the email steps were used to facilitate this process.

Page numbers followed by *f* indicate figures; *t*, tables; *b*, boxes.